THE EYE AND SYSTEMIC DISEASE

THE EYE
and
SYSTEMIC
DISEASE

EDITED BY

Frederick A. Mausolf, M.D., M.Sc.

Assistant Professor of Ophthalmology, Department
of Ophthalmology, University of Chicago School
of Medicine, Chicago, Illinois;
formerly Instructor in Ophthalmology, Department
of Ophthalmology, University of Iowa
College of Medicine, Iowa City, Iowa

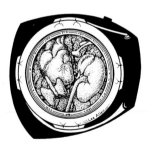

WITH 230 ILLUSTRATIONS

The C. V. Mosby Company
SAINT LOUIS 1975

Library of Congress Cataloging in Publication Data

Main entry under title:

The eye and systemic disease.

   Transactions of the biennial international symposium organized by the Dept. of Ophthalmology, University of Iowa College of Medicine.
   Bibliography: p.
   Includes index.
   1.   Ocular manifestations of general diseases—Congresses.
I.   Mausolf, Frederick A.   II.   Iowa.   University.
Dept. of Ophthalmology.   [DNLM: 1.   Eye
manifestations—Congresses.   WW475 I61e 1973]
RE65.D93   616.07'54   75-4851
ISBN 0-8016-3142-4

CB/CB/B   9   8   7   6   5   4   3   2

TO

Hermann M. Burian, M.D.

(1906—1974)

CONTRIBUTORS

William B. Bean, M.D.
Kempner Professor and Director, Institute for the Medical Humanities, University of Texas Medical Branch, Galveston, Texas.

Giambattista Bietti, M.D.
Head of the Department of Ophthalmology, Clinica Oculistica, University of Rome, Rome, Italy.

Giles G. Bole, Jr., M.D.
Professor of Internal Medicine, Physician-in-charge, Rackham Arthritis Research Unit, The University of Michigan Medical School, Ann Arbor, Michigan.

Michael C. Brain, D.M., F.R.C.P., F.R.C.P.(C)
Professor of Medicine, McMaster University, Hamilton, Ontario, Canada.

David G. Cogan, M.D.
Henry Willard Williams Professor of Ophthalmology, Emeritus, Harvard Medical School, Boston, Massachusetts.

M. Ulrich Dardenne, M.D.
Professor of Ophthalmology and Head of the Department for Microsurgery of the Eye, Bonn University Hospitals, Bonn, West Germany.

Jørn Ditzel, M.D., Ph.D.
Chief, Section of Endocrinology and Metabolism, Department of Medicine, Aalborg Regional Hospital, Aalborg, Denmark.

Donald S. Fredrickson, M.D.
Director of Intramural Research and Chief, Molecular Disease Branch, National Heart and Lung Institute, National Institutes of Health, Bethesda, Maryland.

Adnan H. Halasa, M.D.
Associate Professor of Ophthalmology, Department of Ophthalmology, American University Medical Center, Beirut, Lebanon.

Paul Henkind, M.D., Ph.D.
Professor and Chairman, Department of Ophthalmology, Albert Einstein College of Medicine, Montefiore Hospital and Medical Center, Bronx, New York.

Thomas P. Kearns, M.D.
Consultant in Ophthalmology, Mayo Clinic and Mayo Foundation; Professor of Ophthalmology, Mayo Medical School, Rochester, Minnesota.

Walter M. Kirkendall, M.D.
Professor and Director, Program in Internal Medicine, The University of Texas Medical School at Houston, Houston, Texas.

David L. Knox, M.D.
Associate Professor of Ophthalmology, Johns Hopkins University School of Medicine, Wilmer Ophthalmological Institute, Johns Hopkins Hospital, Baltimore, Maryland.

Malcolm N. Luxenberg, M.D.
Professor and Chairman, Department of Ophthalmology, Medical College of Georgia, Augusta, Georgia.

Donald S. McLaren, M.D., Ph.D.
Professor of Clinical Nutrition and Director of the Nutrition Research Program, School of Medicine, American University of Beirut, Beirut, Lebanon.

Frank W. Newell, M.D.
The Raymond Professor and Chairman, Department of Ophthalmology, The University of Chicago, Chicago, Illinois.

Harold O. Perry, M.D.
Consultant in Dermatology, Mayo Clinic and Mayo Foundation; Professor of Dermatology, Mayo Graduate School of Medicine, University of Minnesota, Rochester, Minnesota.

Steven M. Podos, M.D.
Professor of Ophthalmology, Washington University School of Medicine, St. Louis, Missouri.

David H. Solomon, M.D.
Professor and Chairman, Department of Medicine, UCLA School of Medicine, Los Angeles, California.

GUEST CONTRIBUTORS

Paul S. Ramalho, M.D., Ph.D.
Professor of Ophthalmology, St. Mary's Hospital, University of Lisbon, Lisbon, Portugal.

Michael D. Sanders, F.R.C.S., M.R.C.P.
Consultant in Ophthalmology, National Hospital and St. Thomas' Hospital, London, England.

FOREWORD

The biennial international symposiums organized by the Department of Ophthalmology in Iowa City have had important topics as their themes. I believe, however, that nothing could be more important than the role of the eye in systemic diseases.

The ocular manifestations of systemic affections have always played an important role in general medicine. In numerous cases these ocular findings and symptoms lead to the correct diagnosis of the generalized condition. In this symposium we wanted to stress this aspect of ophthalmology, and we believe that this collection of papers and discussions will renew the interest and emphasize the importance of the eye signs in systemic diseases.

In addition, this book underlines the fact that ophthalmology is not a surgical specialty, a medical specialty, a pediatric specialty, or any other kind of affiliated specialty. Ophthalmology is fortunate enough to be organ centered and therefore covers all aspects of diseases of the eye and its adnexa. Although in other areas of medicine only now do specialists of various disciplines get together to form a team such as the cardiologists and the cardiac surgeons, or the nephrologists and the kidney surgeons, we in ophthalmology are fortunate enough to have been organ oriented ever since ophthalmology was established as an independent specialty. With all the striking and phenomenal advances in ocular surgery, it is a worthwhile endeavor to underline the importance of medical ophthalmology.

All the credit for organizing and initiating this symposium goes to Dr. Frederick Mausolf, who was still a resident in our department. He has shown a tremendous amount of initiative, imagination, and perseverance, for which we are grateful. I sincerely hope that this book, which he has so elegantly masterminded, will have the deserved success.

Frederick C. Blodi, M.D.
Professor and Head,
Department of Ophthalmology,
Iowa City, Iowa
November 1974

PREFACE

During recent years there has been an increasing interest among ophthalmologists in the relationship of eye disease to general disease. This has been most evident in the evolution of neuro-ophthalmology into a recognized subspecialty among ophthalmologists. However, a look at the table of contents of the leading ophthalmic journals reveals that there is interest in a very wide range of systemic diseases—systemic ophthalmology. At the same time general physicians have advanced greatly in the understanding of the pathophysiology of many systemic diseases. The purpose of this symposium is to review and discuss recent advances in systemic ophthalmology. To achieve this goal, several of the world's leading ophthalmologists, internists, and dermatologists were included in the symposium faculty. The general format adhered to throughout most of this symposium was that a general review of the systemic diseases, emphasizing pathophysiology, was presented by either an internist or a dermatologist and the ophthalmic aspects were presented by an ophthalmologist. After each pair of presentations a panel discussion was conducted to integrate and expand the presented material.

The major subjects presented during the symposium included metabolic disease, collagen and rheumatic disease, nutritional disease, endocrine disease, diabetes mellitus, vascular disease, hematologic disease, gastrointestinal disease, and skin disease. Infectious disease and neurologic disease were specifically omitted because the former was the topic of the previous international symposium held in Iowa City and the latter will be the topic of a future symposium. Each individual symposium faculty member decided what diseases to present, and to what extent, in his lecture based upon his interest and the limited time available. Other topics of interest to the audience, composed of ophthalmologists, internists, family physicians, and dermatologists, were introduced during the panel discussions. The results were that most of the important areas of systemic ophthalmology were presented to some extent during this symposium.

A symposium of this magnitude requires the cooperation and effort of many individuals. First of all, appreciation must be expressed to Dr. F. C. Blodi, whose inspiration, cooperation, and guidance helped to make the symposium a success. All of the speakers must be congratulated for having delivered such excellent papers and for their act of participation in the panel discussions. After the meeting each speaker generously submitted a manuscript with illustrations for this transaction of the symposium. Credit must be also given to the staff of the University of Iowa Department of Ophthalmology both for suggestions in planning the symposium and for conducting the excellent panel discussions. Lee Allen prepared the necessary art work and Ogden Frazier the photography. Dr. Ron Zahoruk, of McMaster University, while a fellow at the University of Iowa, gave many useful suggestions toward the planning of the symposium. The Conference Center of the University of Iowa helped provide not only for the physical arrangements for the symposium, but also for the excellent meals and entertainment presented during the symposium. Mrs. Marlys Bartling had the difficult task of providing all the secretarial help for both the symposium and its transactions. Special credit must be given to Mr. Mel Chiles for applying his administrative skills to the planning and running of the symposium. The financial contributions of many companies were appreciated. Most of all, thanks must be expressed to those physicians who took the time out from their practices to attend the meeting on systemic ophthalmology. Their presence and active participation during the panel discussions clearly demonstrated that indeed there was a need for a symposium on systemic ophthalmology.

Frederick A. Mausolf

CONTENTS

1

The eye: gateway to medical wisdom

William B. Bean

The topic of my comments has been part of my occupation and preoccupation for many years. My theme concerns the unity of medicine. I think a disservice occurs to patients and to medicine when those taking care of the sick, and in particular, those who are ultraspecialists in medicine, forget the common theme and broad background of getting sick and getting well. I appear before you as a physician, and I know that most people here are ophthalmologists. Still I am not here to upset you. I feel at home with ophthalmologists. I hope you will feel at home with me.

There are two viewpoints I wish to present from the sayings of Peter Mayer Latham, an English clinician who was active about a 150 years ago. First of all, what he said about the eye is still germane to our problems today. As he addressed his clinical clerks, the undergraduate medical students of the time, he said, "If you desire to make pathological knowledge the groundwork of your credit and use-fulness through life, let me advise you not to allow the period of your pupilage to pass by without making a special study of diseases of the eye. Here you see almost all disease in miniature; and from the peculiar structure of the eye, you see them as though through a glass; and you learn many of the little wonderful details in the nature of the morbid processes, which, but for the observation of them in the eye, would not have been known at all. Let every one of you who has a few months to spare give them to the Eye Infirmary." Somewhere else he said, "The eye might have been intended to furnish us a little model for studying processes of disease and processes of reparation as they go on in all parts of the body so admirably does it answer this purpose." He has these things to say about specialization. "The study of our times has been chiefly to specialize and to localize disease, and it has had very useful results. But it has a tendency to narrow our views, and cripple our practice by setting up as many several pathologies within the body as there are several organs." And then again, "The very habit of dwelling long and minutely (as we needs must do if we would understand them) upon the facts which concern the pathology of one organ has brought us consciously to regard it as a single center of disease much more than it really is." And finally, "In proportion as we are more intent upon investigating the local processes of diseases in a particular organ,

1

scrutinizing them pathologically, and nicely weighing their diagnostic signs, there is a danger that our minds may be withdrawn from those larger views which regard their constitutional origin, and their consequent liability to fall upon any or all organs of the body."

Yesterday, some of us were privileged to hear several brilliant historical discourses. Dr. Snyder's remarkable recapitulation of Dr. Gould's life and doings may have sounded silly to those who are unfamiliar with history, and yet this is merely one of the vast concourse of errors from which some truth arose. Gould listed an awful lot of evil and many problems. He then formed the opinion that eye strain, the seventh of the deadly sins of civilization, was the ruination of almost everybody he saw or dealt with. This is simply one of the measures of overspecialization. Everything is seen through the narrow observer viewpoint of a man trained to think eye, ear, kidney, brain, or sex organs. But Gould, who was passionately concerned about correcting refractive errors absolutely, also believed that by doing a complete examination of his patients, getting a long and really remarkably lucid history, he would know much more about the patient as a person than he had ever learned from the physics of his eyeballs. What is not clear, is just the way he was able to adjust the mathematics of his compulsively correct refraction to the information he got in listening to and examining his patient. The history of medicine suggests that the doctors that have done the most good have been those who understood people. Indeed, Dr. Gould added a dimension of perception and skill that probably made up for his being a fanatic. A fanatic, defined in ironic terms by Santayana, is somebody who redoubles his effort when he loses sight of his objectives.

Now if I may talk of the importance of the whole person to each individual in this room in a holistic approach, let me, as the only Osler Professor in the world, give you a few comments about William Osler. Osler's family designated him for the ministry. As time went on, and in fact very early, he took no stock in this. Nonetheless, Osler had an early ambition to be an ophthalmologist and if he had received an appointment for a residency or internship, which he strove for valiantly, he would undoubtedly have been heard from in the field of ophthalmology. Osler is remembered by many people for many things. He wrote and crystallized into diamond-like sparkles many ideas and many wise thoughts. My reason for bringing up Osler is the fact that Osler's first professional bill, recorded in his own handwriting, was "Speck in the cornea, 50¢." Every bill he ever charged is recorded in splendid bound volumes now at the University of McGill in Montreal. It is interesting that several days later, the same problem occurred. We have, with another patient, another entry: "Removal of speck from the cornea, $1.00." A doubling of the fee may have meant a richer patient.

I now come to the main portion of my theme, that is, the crossroads where ophthalmology and general medicine deal with the same people, the same problems, the same material, and the same diseases. For the most part in recent years, they do not seem to be talking to each other. In a number of instances, whole disease complexes grew up side by side within one hospital or medical school community —with the ophthalmologists taking care of the eyeball part of it and internists, surgeons, and others taking care of the bodily part of it.

Nobody has ever really worked out the geography of the great Republic of Medicine. If one did, it could be shown that often two streams of thought, knowledge, and ideas flowed side by side with no confluence. Getting together would have made medicine move to its proper objectives much more rapidly and much more gracefully. When there is not intercommunication in any terrain where ideas should be common, progress is held back. In medicine, sick people cannot have the advantage of the understanding and care they should have. It becomes, in effect, the sterile narcissistic attitude of a miser or somebody who hoards learning and never arrives at the point of wisdom. When information is treated as trade secrets and something that patent rights and profit should be derived from, medicine deteriorates. Thus the care of the patient, which is the real concern of everyone in medicine, also suffers or perhaps is almost eliminated.

From very ancient records of medical history, the Egyptian papyruses with their lovely hieroglyphs tell us of specialization in Egypt. Some doctors treated wounds, some treated the vapors, and some treated small portions of the body. The doctor and the deity dealing with the eye probably were not more superspecialized than the medical physician priest who presided over the south end of the alimentary canal. These early proctologists went about in the land under magnificent term "shepherd of the anus." As far as one can make out from the really very obscure and very tiny fractions of pictures, hieroglyphs, and whatnot, ophthalmia was recognized. Since they did not understand light and vision, they could not understand refraction or vision.

One of the more encouraging things about medicine, though, is that as it developed over the next several thousand years, ophthalmology became recognized as a part of general biology, the wellness and illness of people, and became recognized as having its proper place in medicine. It was no monopoly, nor was it just a delightful experience for the dilettante. We need not go through the story of cataract operation and many others that developed perhaps independently but certainly along the way in India and in the Middle East, before the coming of Newton and his expounding of the physics of light. After physics invaded the sickroom, people stopped thinking of vision as a natural wonder or a miracle, and it was possible for ophthalmologists to make their first unique contribution.

I suppose if one wanted to bracket the modern change that brought ophthalmology out of the ancient Egyptian, Greek, and Latin sequence it might be pinpointed when Donders, studying all sorts of visual difficulty, was able to separate out those related to troubles with the lens and those related to irregularities in the cornea. When physics had reached this stage, correction for what could not be prevented became a reality.

Many people born with visual difficulties had been looked upon as stupid or idiotic or simply tossed into the river. It suddenly occurred to people who studied children born blind, and therefore without vision, or born deaf, and therefore mute, that such unfortunates were not necessarily stupid. Humane ways of dealing with them might change a black, bleak life in the dungeon into one with meaning and even pleasure.

Those of you who have been attending the various lectures have heard a most enchanting discourse on the story of eyeglasses or spectacles. Whether the surgery of minor changes in shape and structure of the eyeball will do away with eyeglasses is something beyond my competence and understanding.

With your permission, I will tell you about a few diseases in which the eye as well as other tissues of the body are likely to be involved. For a season they were the property of ophthalmologists. A miserly attitude or mere laziness kept them from sharing the information they had with other people.

Today we recognize sarcoidosis as a complicated disease characterized by abnormalities in immune mechanisms and remarkable kinds of granulomas. The dermatologists, Besnier and Boeck, had described cutaneous lesions and granulomatous lymph nodes. Then for a time sarcoidosis was recognized as Heerfordt's uveoparotid fever, but even earlier than that, the great Jonathan Hutchinson had described the trouble in the remarkable series of journals he edited entitled *Archives of Surgery*. For 11 years, through the 1890s, the Hutchinson of "Hutchinson's teeth" and "Hutchinson's eyes" (congenital syphilitic keratosis) edited this journal. It was quarterly, and there are two things about it that are quite remarkable. First of all, in the entire 11 years, there was never a single paper on surgery; so *Archives of Surgery* seems a rather strange title. The other thing is that every paper contributed to it was contributed by Jonathan Hutchinson, probably because editor Hutchinson was the sole reviewing body. Whether he ever turned any of his papers down is not for us to say, but nobody else got in. As an editor, I have been accused of having the monopoly on publishing my own papers, but I never went quite this far. If you think you have invented a rare disease, you should heed the advice of Osler by reading through Jonathan Hutchinson's *Archives of Surgery* and see if he did not describe it, and, indeed, sarcoidosis was described as Mortimer's malady after the Mrs. Mortimer who was the patient Jonathan Hutchinson described in detail and got his faithful, but really not very good, artist to draw a picture. Also, Hutchinson was the first to describe temporal arteritis, which is a disorder of extraordinary importance to ophthalmologists and perhaps of more importance to general physicians, for if they do not recognize it, they will not have their patient seen and treated promptly. And thus another blind person will be added to the list. Jonathan Hutchinson described sarcoidosis as follows: "I feel the less scruple in thus placing in juxtaposition cases which are possibly not identical in nature because I hold it to be important not to attempt to constitute species in nosology. The truth is probably that the various pathologic influences are capable of the most various combinations and that we have on all sides connecting links between maladies which have gained distinctive names. We do not, for instance, know enough to ask the cause of what we call lichen planus to be sure that it may not have a lupoid form when occurring in a tuberculous patient. Patient investigation and great care and observations of phenomena are needed before we can hope to arrive at the truth on these matters. I therefore thought it well at the present time to place those cases on record hoping that the future may furnish material for better elucidation."

It was my pleasure as an intern at Johns Hopkins on Longcope's service to find that he was working on sarcoidosis, though at the time I had not the vaguest idea what was really wrong with one of my favorite patients who had jaundice and nothing wrong with his skin. Longcope did a lot to clarify the matter of a disease that was protean in manifestations and did not belong just to ophthalmologists.

Marfan's syndrome is another disease of considerable interest. Marfan was a French doctor who took care of children, and he described what he called dolicho-stenomelia, that is, long, narrow, gracile fingers. Five or six years later, Achard called it arachnodactyly, or 'spider fingers,' and it has been only relatively recently that it has become known as Marfan's syndrome. For a long time the ophthalmologists knew all about the dislocation of the lens, the shimmering of the iris, and different color of the iris on the two sides and wrote learned papers on it. Williams, an ophthalmologist in Cincinnati, described it in 1876. But even the opthalmologists did not pay any attention to it for decades. I cannot explain that to a group of ophthalmologists. By the 1920s the ophthalmologists of the United States had written many papers and, indeed, monographs on it. But ophthalmologists did not seem to be much interested in the fact that it was a disease of the whole body.

It was not until the 1940s that the fact became recognized that it was a disorder of connective tissue throughout the whole body. The danger of tearing or shredding the aorta, bursting an aortic valve, and developing a disastrous and often, fatal dissecting hematoma of the aorta were much more important than the difficulty with dislocated lenses.

Now, instead of continuing on with the melancholy story of the separation of ophthalmology from general medicine, I am happy to report that it has been our good fortune to have a close and effective collaboration of ophthalmology and medicine. One of the very pleasant recollections of the early weeks when I came to Iowa City 25 years ago was talking to Dr. O'Brien and making arrangements for teaching ophthalmology to clinical clerks while they were on the medical service. Dr. Leinfelder and many others have continued this system. In this way, our staff, the students, the residents, and many others have learned a great deal in ophthalmology, and I am sure it has been good for the interns and residents in ophthalmology to see something of general medicine.

The woman with Marfan's syndrome, the second patient I ever saw with this disorder, was admitted on the obstetrical service at the Cincinnati General Hospital, and since I was interested in pellagra, they asked me to see her feet. She was trying to have a baby, but some radiologically invisible obstruction was preventing a normal exit. She had external strabismus because her lenses were detached from their moorings. The iris on both sides shimmered. She had pigeon breast, kyphoscoliosis, high arched palate, long gracile fingers, and systolic murmur.

Pseudoxanthoma elasticum, a badly named disease for the skin, looks more like pig skin and for a long time was the figurative stuffed trophy of two Scandinavian ophthalmologists, Grönblad and Strandberg, even though an occasional dermatologist or country doctor had described the disease. The term "angioid streaks" referred to disruptions in Bruch's membrane caused by its fragility and the tug of the extraocular muscles. This produces small eyeball quaking, when some of the internal stabilizing tissues of the globe are pried apart. If the ophthalmologists look a bit above the globe itself, they will see the peculiar "cigarette-paper scarring" characteristic of the disease in the eyelids. Skin that looks like and almost feels like shimmering, wet blotting paper.

Fabry's syndrome, another rare disease on which I will not need to go into detail, is caused by a completely specified, waxy material that either loves to get into smooth muscle or smooth muscle loves to get hold of it. In this syndrome the enzyme that usually degrades the material down to the next stage of its metabolism is ineffectual and accumulates. The disease was first recognized as a skin disorder. Little black spots in the bathing trunk area of men look as if a grinder set to grind pepper rather coarse had gone over the midportion of the body. Men with Fabry's syndrome often die of renal failure in the middle years though the exact relationship of the metabolic disorder to what happens in the kidneys is not completely worked out. Women may be identified as carriers if the doctor uses the slit lamp to see little hazy, wavy lines in the cornea. This does not interfere with vision. In the urine and in the slit-lamp view one may find little crystals, which under polarized light produce characteristic Maltese crosses. A large array of changes occur in the conjunctival and scleral vessels.

Another area of importance is the axilla. Even if any of you has ever been a student of freckles, I doubt if even those of you who had many when you were small have ever seen or paid attention to a minor phenomenon of capital importance. Freckles in the armpit indicate neurofibromatosis or pheochromocytoma. This is quite in distinction to Addison's disease where the armpit of a blond may become dark and ugly looking. Once Al Braley called to my attention the fact that strange things may occur in the cornea in a person with von Recklinghausen's disease, or neurofibromatosis, and pheochromocytoma. The lesion he showed me with the slit lamp is that of a large number of medullated nerves coursing down over the cornea where such nerves have no squatter's rights in adult life. Like the corneal lesions of Fabry's syndrome, they do not appear to the naked eye or with the ophthalmoscope but must be detected with the slit lamp. Although I realize that ophthalmologists are not noted for getting clinical clues from the axilla, I hope they sometimes look at the skin and other parts of the body that can be viewed without having the patient undress.

Another lesion is ochronosis, sometimes described as "Alcap, the obscure," basically alkaptonuria. The deposits of alkapton bodies give a strange look to cartilage and to the ear as well as the eyeball and should be familiar to all ophthalmologists.

Panchondritis, or polychondritis, often begins as a mild conjunctivitis or episcleritis, or perhaps a mild panophthalmia. It is a peculiar disease in which the cartilage looses its form, volume, and strength and becomes floppy and useless. The eyes rarely suffer very much, but the ears fall over and joints may become so insecure and unpredictable that they act like universal joints. Most persons who have died with this have had their tracheobronchial tree converted into a structure with about as much intrinsic character as the esophagus. Branches of the windpipe become flutter valves. Atelectasis leads to pneumonia and chronic or promptly fatal infection.

The congenital dysplastic angiopathy, which I prefer to call it, rather than the Sturge-Weber-Kalischer syndrome, is the combination of a birthmark, port-wine nevus of the face, and underlying chaos in the vascular arrangement and support of various structures including the brain. There are many related vascular anomalies such as the Lindau syndrome.

Masque biliaire is a periocular pigmentation of no clinical significance despite its French name. Traumatic asphyxia, which may produce quite spectacular bleeding in the conjunctiva and even in the sclera, as well as petechiae over the whole upper portion of the trunk, results from crushing injuries that suddenly put a vast thrust of pressure on the venous system in the terrain of the superior vena cava.

Nutrition disorders, including Wernicke syndrome, may in man be associated with total ophthalmoplegia, or paralysis of varying extraocular muscles, singly or in combination.

I have seen a retinal arteriovenous fistula in a patient who had hereditary hemorrhagic telangiectasia, or Osler's disease. I had no way of knowing whether this was truly a congenital lesion or whether a sudden hemorrhage near a retinal artery and vein during healing and restoration allowed an arteriovenous shunt to occur.

I will now present a poem* about medical specialists.

What makes a budding doctor see
Which is his special, specialty?
Does just the wise one do his dernest
To pass the Boards as an internist?
Does surgery recruit great thinkers
Or manic, money grabbing tinkers?
Do those with fears and wire twists
Find solace as psychiatrists?
Is it because their nostrils close
That some physicians pick the nose?
Are they frustrated engineers
Our orthopedic gadgeteers?
Do they reject frivolity
And people in pathology?
Do those who're blind or cannot hear
Confine themselves to eye or ear?
Do those who did not work in classes
Seek a career in fitting glasses?
Are skin disease's devotees
Lured by short hours but longish fees?
With technics of some famed fan dancers
While veiling, I'll suggest the answers.

I really think the message of my sermon is clear enough and I do not have to elaborate further. I am very much concerned in medicine of the future that we are being led into all kinds of devious paths. It certainly behooves us to see that our own house, the profession of medicine, is in order. To this end it seems to me to be enormously important that we work together as a single unified body. We think of people as whole people. Little would I like to denigrate the eye. We all know of its vast importance. But there are other parts of the body too. I wish to leave you with a brief lesson: the fact that the eyes have a head, and the head has a body, and the body has a head, and the head has eyes, and these are all part of a greater unity. I trust that the theme and what we will learn in this magnificient program, which has been arranged for you, will continue to illustrate what I think is a tremendously important aspect of medicine.

*Bean, W. B.: Careers in medicine, A.M.A. Arch. Intern. Med. **99:**847-858, June 1957.

REFERENCE

Bean, W. B., editor: Aphorisms from Latham, Iowa City, 1962, Prairie Press.

2

Hereditary systemic diseases of metabolism that affect the eye

Donald S. Fredrickson

In one of the most recent authoritative tabulations[58] there were nearly 2000 known mutations at different loci in human genes transmitted as mendelian traits. Many are harmless and do not qualify as diseases. Others are developmental defects that range from minor annoyance to lethality. A relatively small number, a few hundred at most, are recognized as hereditary disorders of metabolism whose manifestations are systemic and often quite pleomorphic. The outer limits of the "inborn errors of metabolism" are uncertain. There are members of unqualified standing, like sickle-cell anemia, in which the defective gene product and its resultants have been sufficiently well characterized to earn the name "molecular disease." Others, like pseudoxanthoma elasticum, to take one example, are provisional members, since the character of the responsible defect is quite obscure. Additional members are constantly being admitted by disclosure of new metabolic defects. The rate of such discovery has greatly accelerated over the past two decades and has formed one of the most absorbing chapters in modern medical history.

OCULAR INVOLVEMENT IN GENERAL

A survey of a number of recent and older compendiums[12, 22, 23, 57, 81, 90] suggests that about half of the inherited (systemic) metabolic diseases usually or always involve the eye, if we include the extraocular muscles and lids. This rough proportion is felicitously in line with an earlier ratio of little statistical, but some historical, significance, that obtaining in the Croonian Lectures of 1908, the fountainhead of the concept of "inborn errors" of metabolism. You may recall that Sir Archibald Garrod chose as his examples four disorders, two of which—alkaptonuria and albinism—have ocular manifestations.[32]

I have listed in Table 2-1 about 50 distinct forms of inherited metabolic disorders associated with ocular signs. Admittedly, I have taken a few liberties in including some outrageously nonspecific signs, like the jaundiced scleras expected in hereditary hemolytic anemias or hyperbilirubinemic states. Only major pheno-

8

Table 2-1. Ocular signs associated with hereditary metabolic disorders

Location	Disease	Abnormality	Proximate cause
Eyelids or oculomotor	Abetalipoproteinemia	Ptosis, ophthalmoplegia	
	Familial hyperlipoproteinemia (usually types II and III)	Xanthelasma	Cholesterol deposition
	Facioscapulohumeral progressive muscular dystrophy	Weakness of orbicularis oris muscle	?
	Gaucher's disease, type 2 (acute neuropathic)	Characteristic strabismus with hyperextension of neck	Destruction of cranial nerve ganglia
	Hyperkalemic periodic paralysis	Ophthalmoplegia	?
	Tangier disease	Ptosis, ophthalmoplegia	?
Sclera and conjunctiva	Alkaptonuria	Discoloration	Homogentisic acid deposition
	Cystinosis		Cystine deposition
	Ehlers-Danlos syndrome	Blue color	?
	Osteogenesis imperfecta	Blue color	?
	Fabry's disease	Vascular deformity	Glycolipid deposition in vessel walls
	Farber's disease	Granulomas	Ceramide accumulation
	Hemoglobinopathies Sickle-cell anemia (SS) Sickle cell–hemoglobin C disease (SC)	Vascular deformity	Sludging
	Hereditary hemolytic anemias	Jaundice	Hyperbilirubinemia
	Hereditary hyperbilirubinemia	Jaundice	Hyperbilirubinemia
Iris	Albinism	Depigmentation	Melanophore dysfunction
	Phenylketonuria	Depigmentation	Melanophore dysfunction
Cornea	Alkaptonuria	Pigmentation	Homogenistic acid deposition
	Cystinosis	? Clouding	Cystine? crystal deposits
	Fabry's disease	Clouding	Ceramide trihexoside? deposition
	Ehlers-Danlos syndrome	Deformities	
	Familial hyperlipoproteinemia (usually types II or III)	Arcus senilis	Cholesterol? deposition
	GM_1 gangliosidosis	? Clouding	Mucopolysaccharide deposition
	Hereditary amyloidosis	Dystrophy	Immunoglobulin? deposition
	Lecithin : cholesterol acyl transferase deficiency	Arcus senilis–like ring	Lipid? deposition
	Mannosidosis	Clouding	?
	Osteogenesis imperfecta	Arcus senilis Deformities	?
	Mucopolysaccharidoses (MPS)	Clouding	Mucopolysaccharide deposition
	Hurler	Clouding	
	Hunter	Deposition, no clouding	
	Scheie	Clouding	
	β-glucuronidase deficiency	Clouding	
	Maroteaux-Lamy	Clouding	
	Morquio	Clouding	

Continued.

Table 2-1. Ocular signs associated with hereditary metabolic disorders—cont'd

Location	Disease	Abnormality	Proximate cause
Cornea— cont'd	Mucolipidoses	Clouding	
	I-cell disease	Clouding	
	Pseudo-Hurler poly- dystrophy	Clouding	
	Mannosidosis		
	Tangier disease	Stromal deposits	Cholesteryl ester? storage
	Wilson's disease	Kayser-Fleischer ring	Cu++ deposition
Lens	Cerebrotendinous xanthoma- tosis	Cataracts	Cholestanol/cholesterol? deposition
	Ehlers-Danlos syndrome	Subluxation	
	Galactosemia	Cataracts	Dulcitol? accumulation
	Homocystinuria	Subluxation Cataracts	? Cystine deficiency
	Lowe's syndrome	Cataracts	?
	Marfan's syndrome	Subluxation	
	Myotonic dystrophy	Cataracts	?
	Pseudohypoparathyroidism	Cataracts	Secondary calcification
	Sulfite oxidase deficiency	Subluxation	?
	Weill-Marchesani syndrome	Cataracts Subluxation	?
	Wilson's disease	Cataracts	?
Vitreous	Hereditary amyloidosis with upper limb neuropathy	Opacities	?
Retina	Ehlers-Danlos syndrome	Detachment	Faulty collagen or elastic tissue
	Homocystinuria	Detachment, degen- eration	Faulty collagen or elastic tissue
	Marfan's syndrome	Detachment	Faulty collagen or elastic tissue
	Pseudoxanthoma elasticum	Degeneration (angi- oid streaks)	Faulty collagen or elastic tissue
	Farber's disease	Macular degenera- tion	Neuronal storage of lipids
	GM₁ gangliosidosis	Macular degenera- tion (cherry-red spot)	Neuronal storage of ganglioside
	GM₂ gangliosidosis (especially type I, Tay-Sachs disease)	Macular degenera- tion (cherry-red spot)	Neuronal storage of ganglioside
	Metachromatic leukodystrophy (late infantile with multiple sulfatase deficiencies)	Macular degenera- tion	Neuronal storage of sulfatide
	Niemann-Pick diseases (types A and C)	Macular degenera- tion (cherry-red spot)	Neuronal storage of sphingomyelin
	Homocystinuria	Optic atrophy	Glaucoma or thrombosis
	Krabbe's disease	Optic atrophy	Neuronal excess of galactosyl ceramide?
	Metachromatic leukodystrophy (late infantile and juvenile)	Optic atrophy	Neuronal accumulation of sulfatide
	Abetalipoproteinemia	Retinitis pigmentosa	?
	Albinism	Depigmentation	Melanophore dysfunction
	Cystinosis with nephropathy	Patchy depigmenta- tion	?

Table 2-1. Ocular signs associated with hereditary metabolic disorders—cont'd

Location	Disease	Abnormality	Proximate cause
Retina— cont'd	Mucopolysaccharidosis (Hunter's)	Retinitis pigmentosa	
	Refsum's syndrome	Retinitis pigmentosa	Phytanic acid deposi- tion??
	Diabetes mellitus	Vascular abnormality	?
	Fabry's disease	Vascular abnormality	Glycolipid deposition
	Familial hyperlipoproteinemia (types I or V)	Vascular abnormality (lipemia retinalis)	Reflectance from excess triglyceride-rich lipo- proteins in plasma
	Hemoglobinopathies Sickle-cell anemia (SS) Sickle cell–hemoglobin C disease (SC)	Vascular abnormality	Sludging
	Familial hypercholesterolemia (form of type II hyperlipo- proteinemia)	Xanthomatous de- posits	Deposition of cholesterol

typic variation is included, however; many of these disorders have been further degraded to subtypes illustrating important genetic heterogeneity. More for my instruction than for ophthalmologists, I have chosen to list conditions repetitively if they involve macroscopically different parts of the eye. About half of the conditions appear to affect more than one part. The cornea and retina suffer the most involvement; the lens, sclera, and conjunctiva are the next.

Despite the regularity of ocular involvement in these disorders, it is interesting that in only two or three, perhaps albinism, Fabry's disease, and Wilson's disease, are the eye lesions themselves sufficiently distinctive to afford a specific diagnosis. I refer you to the accompanying paper by Dr. Podos for more accurate description of the ocular lesions attending metabolic disease and confirmation of an amateur's impressions of their relative nonspecificity.

Proximate bases for eye lesions

As with many other manifestations of metabolic diseases, the exact basis of many of the lesions in the eye are poorly understood. I have attempted to summarize some of the mechanisms in Table 2-1. Often one can only presume that substances stored elsewhere in the body are accumulating in the cornea or that identical "connective-tissue disturbances" in joints are also operating to alter the shape of the globe or supports of the lens. Careful analysis of affected eyes is beginning to yield more specific information. One excellent example is the determination that it is not galactose or galactose-1-phosphate, but a product of their reduction in the lens, dulcitol (galactitol), which damages this tissue in galactosemia.[38] In cystinosis, cystine crystals have been positively identified in the conjunctiva, but there is still uncertainty as to whether it is this amino acid that collects in the cornea.[25] In the sphingolipidoses, it seems fairly certain that it is the immediate substrates of specific missing enzymes that cause ganglion cells to swell and produce macular degeneration. On the other hand, the mechanisms of retinal pigment changes in many of the lipidoses are quite obscure. In general, the biochemistry of the eye is less well charted than that of the liver or skin fibroblast.

KINDS OF DISEASES THAT AFFECT THE EYE
Further sorting

The disorders in Table 2-1 can be rearranged in several ways. One way is to arrange them according to the biochemical system involved. See outline below. It then appears that far and away the two major groups of disorders producing ocular involvement relate primarily to the metabolism of lipids and lipoproteins and the metabolism of collagen, elastins, and other elements of connective tissue.

The general nature of metabolic disorders producing ocular lesions is as follows:

Disordered metabolism of lipids or lipoproteins
  Abetalipoproteinemia
  Cerebrotendinous xanthomatosis
  Familial hyperlipoproteinemias
  Lecithin : cholesterol acyl transferase
    deficiency
  Refsum's disease
  Sphingolipidoses
    Fabry's disease
    Farber's disease
    GM₁ gangliosidoses
    GM₂ gangliosidoses
    Krabbe's disease
    Sphingomyelin lipidoses
    Sulfatide lipidoses
  Tangier disease
Disordered metabolism of connective tissues
  Collagen-elastic tissue
    Ehlers-Danlos syndrome
    Marfan's syndrome
    Osteogenesis imperfecta
    Pseudoxanthoma elasticum
  Homocystinuria
  Mannosidosis
  Mucolipidoses
    I-cell disease
    Pseudo-Hurler syndrome

Disordered metabolism of connective tissues—cont'd
  Mucopolysaccharidoses
    β-Glucosidase deficiency
    Hunter's syndrome
    Hurler's syndrome
    Maroteaux-Lamy syndrome
    Morquio's syndrome
    Sanfilippo syndromes A and B
    Scheie syndrome
Disordered amino acid metabolism
  Albinism
  Alkaptonuria
  Cystinosis?
  (Homocystinuria)
  Phenylketonuria
  Sulfite oxidase deficiency
Defective carbohydrate metabolism
  Diabetes mellitus
  Galactosemia
Defective or deficient transport proteins
  Sickle-cell diseases
  Wilson's disease?
Diseases of muscle
  Muscular dystrophies
  Periodic paralyses

Lipidoses

Nearly all the lipidoses so far identified affect the eye. Perhaps the only exceptions are *Wolman's disease* and *cholesteryl ester storage* disease and non-neuropathic Gaucher's disease. The nonneuropathic or adult form of Gaucher's disease is cited as producing a cherry-red spot in one reliable atlas,[91] but I am sure this was a mistaken diagnosis. The pingueculas described in very early patients with this disease seem no longer to be a significant or reliable feature. I have taken the liberty of placing the rarer, neuropathic form (type 2) of Gaucher's disease in Table 2-1 only to remind readers of the contribution of strabismus to the diagnostic facial appearance of affected infants.[28] As we shall presently discuss, all the other sphingolipidoses tend to cause serious damage to the optic nerve or neurons immediately behind the retina.

The eye lesions associated with the *familial hyperlipidemias* or hyperlipoproteinemias[27, 31] include xanthomas of the eyelids, arcus senilis, or lipemia retinalis; all are trivial and not threatening to sight. They gain their significance because of the frequency with which they are seen relative to most of the other metabolic diseases. Arcus senilis and xanthelasma also occur in the rare diseases *cerebrotendinous xanthomatosis*[71] and β-sitosterolemia.[7] In the former an undetermined metabolic defect leads to storage of cholestanol and cholesterol in skin, tendons, and central nervous system. In β-sitosterolemia, 10% to 20% of the circulating sterols include plant sterols like β-sitosterol and campesterol that normally are little absorbed. The inherited biochemical defects are unknown.

Corneal arcus and xanthelasma also frequently occur in the absence of hyperlipidemia. I do not believe the ophthalmologists need to order triglyceride or cholesterol measurements to determine the presence of hyperlipidemia[26] in their patients with such lesions. It is appropriate to ask the patient whether such tests have been performed at some time within the past 5 years; if not, the patient should be referred to a generalist or specialist who deals often with such common disorders.

We shall take up the lipoprotein deficiencies below. This leaves *Refsum's disease,* originally designated "heredopathia atactica polyneuritiformis."[70, 82] It is easier to remember it as *phytanic acid storage disease,* for defective oxidation of this compound leads to its accumulation in plasma. There is a deficient activity of phytanic acid oxidase,[82] a mitochondrial enzyme that catalyzes the α-hydroxylation of phytanic acid as a first step in its degradation. Phytanic acid and phytol are trace components of the diet, derived from plants. Although there is some evidence for lipid infiltration in nervous tissues, the fact has yet to be proved whether this lipid is phytanic acid and how its presence causes the ichthyotic skin lesions, the peculiarly changing peripheral polyneuropathy and cerebellar ataxia, or the retinitis pigmentosa, that usually occur in all patients with this disease.

Connective tissue disease

Most of the different phenotypes in the category of connective tissue disorders affect the eye, usually by altering the lens or its supports, the shape of the globe or quality of tissue immediately subjacent to the retina, or by deposition of material in the cornea.[17, 57] The molecular or enzymatic defects underlying the collagen and elastic tissue syndromes have still eluded pursuit; they are hidden in constituent macromolecules of very limited solubility and exasperating monotony of structure. The mucopolysaccharidoses and mucolipidoses are caused by deficient activity of lysosomal enzymes and will receive more attention below.

Homocystinuria is listed in the outline above as one of the connective tissue disorders, although nosologically it must also be considered as an abnormality in amino acid metabolism. An effect on connective tissue metabolism is evident only in the form attributable to deficiency of the enzyme cystathionine synthase in the liver. This enzyme lies in the pathway of methionine metabolism and catalyzes conversion of homocysteine and serine to cystathione.[33, 62] The enzyme block prevents the normal formation of cysteine and cystine and also probably affects the elaboration of connective tissue elements which are highly dependent on sulfation for normal structure. Cystathionine synthase deficiency leads to widespread loss of integrity of supporting tissues, most seriously apparent in blood vessels. In the eye, the lens is frequently displaced and there are cataracts. Optic atrophy may occur, secondary to glaucoma or thrombosis. There are other mutant genotypes that lead to homocystine or homocysteine accumulation in blood or urine. They are caused by interference with the N^5-methyl tetrahydrofolate–dependent conversion of homocysteine to methionine[62] and are not known to have any effect on the eye.

Defects in metabolism of other amino acids

Only a minority of the disorders involving metabolism or transport of amino acids cause any damage to the eye. An important exception is *albinism,* in which the conversion of tyrosine to melanin by melanophores is impaired by mutations at several genetic loci.[21] The decrease in pigmentation cited in Table 2-1 is the most common ocular change in albinism, but is only one among many more serious ones occurring in some forms. The most common of the aminoacidurias, *phenyl-ketonuria,* is marked in the eye only by depigmentation of the iris.[48] The single recorded instance of *sulfite oxidase deficiency*[43, 52] included subluxation of the lens among other more lethal abnormalities. The pigmentation of the sclera, conjunctiva, and cornea in *alkaptonuria* is a local expression of more dramatic deposition of polymerized homogentisic acid in cartilage and other tissues.[51] The latter results from widespread deficiency of the enzyme homogentisic acid oxidase. *Cystinosis* occurs in several forms. The phenotype associated with nephropathy is notable for crystalline deposits in the cornea and sometimes peripheral retinopathy.[74, 92] Probably some forms of cystinosis will eventually turn out to be lysosomal enzyme deficiencies.

Carbohydrate disorders

Although there are a number of inborn errors of carbohydrate metabolism, *diabetes mellitus* and *galactosemia* are the only ones that damage the eye. Diabetes, nevertheless, is undoubtedly the most common metabolic disease affecting the eye, a distinction derived from its high frequency in nearly all populations. It is ironic that the effect of diabetes on the vasculature of the eye and the many secondary changes in vision that may occur are well known, while the metabolic defect or defects underlying the disease have yet to be established.

Transport defects

The several *hemoglobinopathies* that are associated with sickling cause distortions of retinal vasculature that come close to being distinctive or pathognomonic. The sickle-cell (SS) or sickle cell–hemoglobin C (SC) hemoglobinopathies are examples of mutation-induced defects in a transport protein. A cascade of morbid events arises from single amino acid substitution in a lengthy protein chain. The first order resultant affects the shape of the erythrocyte; blood flow in small vessels is altered, followed by thrombosis, which can lead to further damage of the retina or other parts of the eye.[37] *Wilson's disease* may not belong properly in the category of a defective transport mechanism. A deficiency of ceruloplasmin has been shown usually to attend the tissue deposition of copper, but not necessarily to cause it.[4] The disease associated with one of the most classic of eye signs, the Kayser-Fleischer ring, still awaits clarification of its primary biochemical lesion.

Defective lipoprotein metabolism

Three inherited diseases listed under lipids and lipoproteins in the outline above may also be considered as transport defects. They are the severe lipoprotein deficiency states *abetalipoproteinemia* and *Tangier disease* and *lecithin : cholesterol acyl transferase (LCAT) deficiency*. Their features are summarized in Table 2-2. The first two of these diseases[30] are both indicated by hypocholesterolemia, which sometimes is the presenting sign. Beyond that they are quite different. Abetalipoproteinemia, sometimes called the Bassen-Kornzweig syndrome, represents a total failure of the normal mechanisms for transport of triglycerides in plasma. The lipoprotein species mainly involved in this process—chylomicrons, very low density lipoproteins (VLDL), and low-density lipoproteins (LDL)—are missing from plasma. Hence plasma glyceride concentrations, like that of cholesterol, are extremely low. The inherited defect is believed to involve availability of one of the major apoliproteins (apoB) that normally assists in movement of glycerides from hepatic and intestinal cells and in solubilization of these lipids in the extracellular fluids. The results include malabsorption of fat, thorny erythrocytes (acanthocytes), severe posterior column and cerebellar dysfunction, and retinitis pigmentosa. Cause of the nervous system lesions is unknown and is possibly related to availability of fat-soluble vitamins.

Tangier disease is rare, with 16 known examples. It is more compatible with a reasonably normal life than is abetalipoproteinemia. The lipoprotein pattern is characterized by a near absence of high-density lipoproteins (HDL), while some lower density lipoproteins are present in abnormally increased concentrations. Hence, plasma cholesterol is low, but the triglyceride concentration is normal or modestly elevated. The single most dramatic clinical findings are enlargement and a peculiar orange tint to the pharyngeal tonsils. This is a manifestation of widespread storage of cholesteryl esters in reticuloendothelial cells. Two aspects of Tangier disease are especially commended to the attention of ophthal-

Table 2-2. Dyslipoproteinemias associated with ocular lesions

Disease	C	TG	CE/C	Red blood cells	Neurologic signs	Malabsorption	Abnormal tonsils	Renal disease	Lipoprotein abnormality
Abetalipoproteinemia	Low	Low	Normal	Acanthocytes	+	+	0	0	Absent chylomicrons, LDL, and VLDL
Tangier disease	Low	High or normal	Normal	Normal	+	0	+	0	HDY low or absent, LDL low
LCAT deficiency	Normal or high	Normal or high	Low	Target cells	0	0	0	+	Abnormal VLDL and HDL composition

For eye changes, see Table 2-1.

C, Plasma cholesterol concentration; *TG,* plasma triglyceride concentrations; *CE/C,* percentage of plasma cholesterol esterified; *LDL,* low-density lipoproteins; *VLDL,* very low density lipoproteins; *HDL,* high-density lipoproteins.

mologists. One is lipid deposition in the cornea in adults with this disease. Vision is not affected, and the lens and retina are normal. The second is relapsing neuropathy, which may lead to either ptosis or inability to close the eye. We have seen one young patient with strabismus that could not be satisfactorily corrected by repeated operations. It is therefore possible that the neuropathy of Tangier disease may lead to abnormal motion of the eyeball. The basic lesion in Tangier disease is believed to lie in the synthesis or structure of apolipoproteins A-I or A-II.

Lecithin : cholesterol acyl transferase (LCAT) is the enzyme in plasma that accounts for most of the esterification of plasma cholesterol. LCAT deficiency thus far has been observed in three distantly related Norwegian families.[64] The chemical hallmark of the disorder is a reduction, in the absence of jaundice and other signs of hepatic parenchymal disease, of the proportion of cholesterol in plasma that is esterified (normally above 70%) to about 10% or less. Lipoproteins of abnormal structure are present in plasma and their presence seems to lead to lipid deposition in tissues, particularly the kidney. Renal failure may result. An accompanying sign is lipid deposition in the outer regions of the cornea.[34] The resulting arcus senilis is unusual in that it begins at the limbus, without the usual clear zone seen in the arcus accompanying more usual forms of hyperlipidemia. LCAT activity is considered necessary for normal lipoprotein formation and metabolism, hence the consideration of this disease as a "transport" disorder.

There is no specific treatment for abetalipoproteinemia, Tangier disease, or LCAT deficiency. Large amounts of vitamin A improve the night blindness of abetalipoproteinemia. In this disease there is also evidence of lipid peroxidation in tissues, including the heart. Supplements of vitamin A and E are therefore usually given to patients with abetalipoproteinemia.

Although the syndrome of *"familial hypolipidemia"* described by Hooft and collaborators[40] has been included among inherited diseases affecting the eye,[24] I have omitted it from Table 2-1. In the family described by Hooft et al., two siblings had hyperlipidemia, retarded development, a rash on the face and extremities, and nail changes. One of the two had tapetoretinal degeneration with no electroretinographic response. This peculiar disorder seems so similar to *acrodermatitis enteropathica,*[11] in which eye lesions are not characteristic, that one wonders if they are not the same condition. Since acrodermatitis entropathica does sometimes lead to very low levels (absence?) of β-lipoproteins,[93] conceivably it could lead to eye lesions similar to those in abetalipoproteinemia. The basic defect in this fascinating disorder, which empirically is corrected by diiodoquinone, is not known.

For completeness, I should note that I have also omitted mention of familial dysautonomia, which is also associated with corneal dystrophy,[35] but the metabolic nature of the disorder is not well enough known to permit ready classification.

Other disorders

Finally, the outline includes the *muscular dystrophies* and *periodic paralyses,* which may bring part of their puzzle to the attention of the ophthalmologist, particularly through nonspecific ophthalmoplegias and cataracts,[86] in the instance of *myotonic dystrophy.* The inherited disorders of muscle and bone, like the connective tissue diseases, will doubtless soon have their day. For the present it is the "lysosomal diseases" that are at the crest of attention.

LYSOSOMAL HYDROLASE DEFICIENCIES

I will devote the remainder of my discussion to the first group of diseases found in Table 2-3, where I have assembled those metabolic diseases whose defective gene product has either been identified or can be reasonably suspected. I have already mentioned most of the "nonlysosomal enzyme" deficiencies as well as the transport disorders and will turn now to defects in the function of the scavenger system represented by the lysosomes.

In 1965 Hers coined the term "inborn lysosomal diseases" to call attention to these cellular elements and the consequences of their dysfunction.[39] The lysosomes are intracellular vesicles in which are sequestered substances produced or taken up by the cell, the latter acquisition being mainly by the process of pinocytosis. The purpose is sequestration of materials from the rest of the intracellular environment so that they may be degraded by powerful enzymes that are

Table 2-3. Some hereditary metabolic diseases affecting the eye grouped according to known biochemical defects

Lysosomal hydrolase deficencies	
Sphingolipidoses	
GM$_1$ gangliosidoses	GM$_1$ ganglioside β-galactosidase(s)
GM$_2$ gangliosidoses	GM$_2$ ganglioside hexosaminidase A (and B)
Fabry's disease	α-Galactosidase
Krabbe's disease	Galactocerebroside β-galactosidase
Sulfatide lipidoses	Cerebroside sulfatase(s)
Sphingomyelin lipidoses	Sphingomyelinase
Farber's disease	Ceramidase
Mucopolysaccharidoses	
Hurler	α-L-Iduronidase
Hunter	Sulfiduronate sulfatase
Scheie	α-L-Iduronidase
β-Glucuronidase deficiency	
Mucolipidoses	
I-cell disease	Multiple enzyme deficiencies
Pseudo-Hurler polydystrophy	Multiple enzyme deficiencies
Mannosidosis	α-Mannosidase
Nonlysosomal enzyme deficiencies	
Albinism	Tyrosinase (in some forms)
Alkaptonuria	Homogentisic acid oxidase
Galactosemia	Galactose-1-phosphate uridyl transferase
	galactokinase
Homocystinuria	Cystathionine synthase
Phenylketonuria	Phenylalanine hydroxylase
Refsum's disease	Phytanic acid oxidase
Sulfite oxidase deficency	Sulfite oxidase
Defective transport proteins or lipoproteins	
Abetalipoproteinemia	? Apolipoprotein B
Hemoglobinopathies	Hemoglobin
Lecithin : cholesterol acyl transferase (LCAT) deficiency	Lecithin : cholesterol acyl transferase
Tangier disease	? Apolipoprotein A-I
Wilson's disease?	? Ceruloplasmin

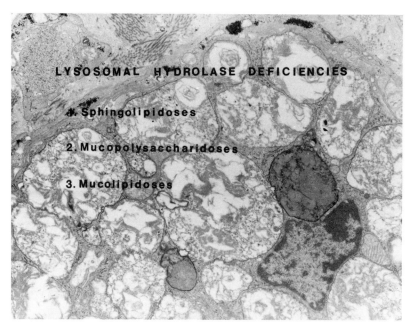

Fig. 2-1. Electron micrograph of bone marrow macrophage from patient with Niemann-Pick disease. The larger inclusion bodies, each delimited by a membrane and filled with amorphous "debris," are lysosomes. Three major groups of lysosomal hydrolase deficiency states that affect the eye are listed. (Courtesy Dr. Victor Ferrans, Bethesda, Md.; × 15,000.)

active at an acid pH. These include "acid hydrolases," which break ester bonds; glycosidases, which act at glycosidic linkages; phosphatases; sulfatases; and proteases or cathepsins. In the past decade genetically determined specific deficiencies among these enzymes have been elucidated in a host of diseases in which the electron microscope has revealed swollen lysosomes in multiple cell types (Fig. 2-1). Deficient protease activity has never been documented as the cause of disease, but a myriad of severe deficiencies in the activity of one or more acid hydrolases or glycosidases have been detected. Indeed, it may be said that had mutations not altered their effectiveness or activity, the existence of many of these enzymes would still be unproved.

General features

The lysosomal enzyme deficiency states that affect the eye fall into three main classes: sphingolipidoses, mucopolysaccharidoses, and mucolipidoses.

The sphingolipidoses and mucopolysaccharidoses basically involve defects in compounds having quite different basic structure but share a number of common features. Indeed, among them are certain "transition diseases" in which the metabolism of both sphingolipid and mucopolysaccharide is interfered with by primary deficiency of apparently only a single enzyme activity. For example, among the sphingolipidoses listed in Table 2-3, Farber's disease, GM_1 gangliosidosis, and certain variants of the sulfatide lipidoses are associated with bone or joint abnormalities and sometimes excess urinary secretion of mucopolysaccharide. On the other hand, the mental retardation in some of the mucopolysaccharidoses may prove to be from secondary interference with sphingolipid metabolism in the central nervous system. The "transition disorders" are sometimes classified as mucolipidoses,[79] but I have listed that group here especially to call attention to I-cell disease and the pseudo-Hurler syndrome, which are of special interest because it is believed they represent inadequate entry of lysosomal enzymes into the cell rather than true enzyme deficiency.[63]

Inheritance

A common feature of the lysosomal enzyme disorders is the requirement that the patient be homozygous for the abnormal allele in order for the disease to be apparent. In the normal genotype a considerable excess of enzyme activity is present, and although it is usually reduced detectably in the tissues of the heterozygote, catabolism of the substrate in question is usually not sufficiently limited to cause storage or disability. Thus, most of these disorders are inherited as autosomal recessives. The exceptions are those diseases in which the affected genetic locus lies on the X chromosome. In these instances, the male hemizygote has no normal allele to offset his inherited deficiency and expression of the disorder is complete. Because of normal, random suppression of one of the X chromosomes (Lyon hypothesis), female heterozygotes too may show disease although usually expression is milder. Only two known lysosomal disorders affecting the eye are X linked. One is Fabry's disease. The condition described in the ophthalmologic literature as Fleischer's dystrophy (cornea verticillata) appears to be a manifestation of Fabry's disease in the female heterozygote.[24] The other is the Hunter form of mucopolysaccharidoses, in which nearly all affected patients are males and the female heterozygote rarely shows involvement.[57]

The metabolic diseases in general, and the lysosomal storage diseases in particular, also provide some vivid examples of how different mutations affecting the chemical activity of the same protein lead to very different phenotypic expression. A different base substitution at the same codon might induce a different amino acid substitution in a protein chain, or mutations at slightly different loci on the same gene or cistron can produce changes in enzyme activity that are quantitatively not distinguishable by assay, but are easily visible clinically. "Allelism" is a term referring to the phenotypes produced by mutations of this sort. Reference is made below to Hurler and Scheie syndromes of the mucopolysaccharidoses as examples.[57] Another is found in the sphingomyelin disorders in which types A and B both involve severe sphingomyelinase deficiency, yet are dramatically different phenotypes. It is important to realize that such phenotypic variation is thus not capricious, but programmed; phenotype in affected sibs will be concordant, not type A in one and type B in another. "Genetic compounds" consisting of one allele for type A and one for type B may also be expected to occur and have been recognized tentatively in the mucopolysaccharidoses.[57]

Diagnosis

Nearly all of the lysosomal enzymes are present in circulating leukocytes or fibroblasts cultured from bone marrow, skin, or amniotic fluid. The skin fibroblast has been particularly helpful in both determining the biochemical defects in these mutants and permitting relatively simple diagnosis. Two workers, Dr. Roscoe Brady[8] and Dr. Elizabeth Neufeld[63] and their co-workers at the National Institutes of Health have had exceptional success in determining a number of the enzyme defects in the sphingolipidoses and mucopolysaccharidoses, respectively.

In these enzyme deficiencies, the fibroblasts tend to store the substrates of the defective enzyme. Lysosomes enlarge, the cells may become vacuolated, and differential staining may make the storage process more obvious. Such morphologic changes are rarely specific, however, and only measurement of specific enzyme activities, ideally using the natural substrate, permits definitive diagnosis. In the majority of these conditions, diagnosis of the homozygous abnormal genotype has also been accomplished by use of fetal fibroblasts cultured from amniotic fluid obtained between the sixteenth and twentieth weeks of pregnancy. It is now accepted medical practice to perform abortion, if the parents so request, when it has been determined that the fetus is homozygous abnormal for one of those defects associated with severe disability and shortened life-span.

Diagnosis of the heterozygote in the autosomal recessive disorders can be effectively achieved in only some of the lysosomal disorders, because the overlap of enzyme activities in normal cells and in those from heterozygotes often is too great. The most effective campaign to identify heterozygotes has been carried out in Tay-Sachs disease.[15] The high gene frequency among Ashkenazi Jews and a concerted effort to refine detection of subnormal enzyme activity have made this particularly possibile. In nearly all the other diseases, suspicion and subsequent detection of genetic hazard in the unborn offspring still depend on the prior birth of an affected sib.

Treatment

Means to replace missing lysosomal enzymes are presently on the frontier of research today. Attempts thus far to replace missing hydrolase activity with heterologous enzymes have not provided means of sustained therapy.[41, 53] Homologous enzyme replacement by infusions of normal plasma have met with some evidence of initial success in Fabry's disease[10, 54] and in the mucopolysaccharidoses.[18] Eventually, other means of instilling purified enzyme preparations under conditions that promote their entry into appropriate cells will have to be devised. A unique success has been observed in the transplantation of a normal kidney to patients with Fabry's disease[17]; the α-galactoside that is deficient in the patients is produced by the normal kidney. This protects the implanted kidney from destructive lipid deposition, but it is uncertain to what degree the normal enzyme is available to other tissues of the recipient.

Sphingolipidoses

The sphingolipids are a class of complex lipids that derive their name from the common constituent sphingosine (1,3-dihydroxy-2-amino-4-transoctadecene) or one of its congeners (Fig. 2-2). In sphingolipids, the single amino group is joined in peptide linkage to a long-chain fatty acid to form ceramide (labeled CER in Figs. 2-3 and 2-4). The distinguishing feature of the sphingolipids is the moiety joined in ester or glycosidic linkage to the C-1 hydroxyl of the sphingosine base (Figs. 2-2 to 2-4).

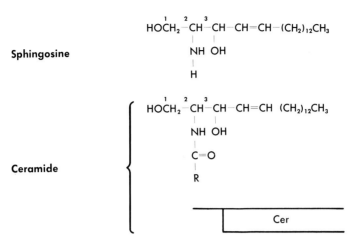

Sphingosine

Ceramide

Fig. 2-2. Structures of sphingosine and its acylated derivative, ceramide. The long-chain fatty acid moiety varies in its chain length, degree of unsaturation, or state of hydroxylation in different classes of sphingolipids. One of the ultimate steps in degradation of all sphingolipids is a splitting of the peptide bond between the amino group of carbon-2 of sphingosine and the fatty acid. In Farber's disease, the responsible enzyme, ceramidase, is believed to be deficient.

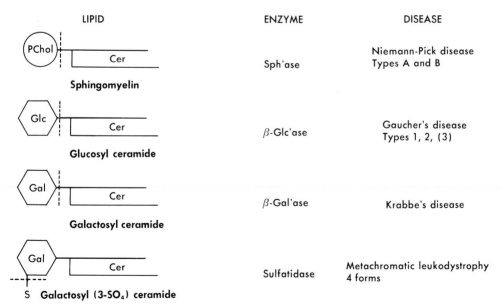

Fig. 2-3. The principal sphingolipid class (class I) stored in certain of the sphingolipidoses and enzyme deficiency involved. Note that only one of the sphingolipids, sphingomyelin, is a phospholipid; the others are glycolipids of varying complexity. *Cer,* Ceramide; *Gal,* galactose; *Glc,* glucose; *PChol,* phosphatidyl choline; *Sph,* sphingomyelin.

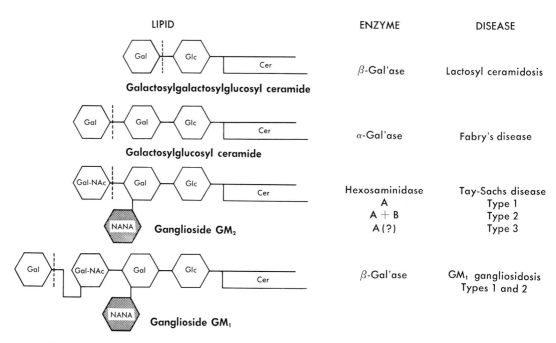

Fig. 2-4. Others among the sphingolipidoses (class II). The presence of *N*-acetylneuraminic acid, or sialic acid (NANA), is the hallmark of the gangliosides. *Gal-NAc, N*-acetylgalactos-amine; for other abbreviations see Fig. 2-3.

GM₁ gangliosidoses. Gangliosides are glycosphingolipids that contain at least one molecule of sialic acid (Fig. 2-4). They are found nearly exclusively in neural tissues and located mainly in ganglion cells, but small amounts of gangliosides are also found in many other tissues, notably including the liver, spleen, kidney, and retina. The structure of ganglioside GM₁ is shown in Fig. 2-4. This lipid accumulates in at least two phenotypes called, respectively, (1) *generalized gangliosidosis*[66] (the infantile form) and (2) *juvenile gangliosidosis.*[65] In addition to massive cerebral storage of ganglioside GM₁ and its asialo derivative, in both forms there also occurs visceral storage of both mucopolysaccharides (keratan sulfate–like polymers), and gangliosides. Concomitant interference with the catabolism of mucopolysaccharide thus adds Hurler syndrome–like skeletal changes and hepatosplenomegaly to the severe psychomotor damage, which quickly leads to death in the infantile form. About half the patients with generalized gangliosidosis develop a cherry-red spot on the macula. Clouding of the cornea is most unusual. The juvenile or "late infantile" form makes its appearance at 6 to 12 months and progresses more slowly. Its manifestations are primarily neurologic; bony deformities are mild or absent, and ocular lesions have not been observed.

The biochemical defect in GM₁ gangliosidosis was discovered by O'Brien and collaborators.[65] It is profound deficiency of the β-galactosidase required for splitting the terminal galactose residue from the ganglioside (Fig. 2-4), thus preventing its further catabolism. The same enzyme possibly may catalyze the breakdown of keratan sulfate. Alternatively the stored ganglioside products may interfere with the action of other enzymes involved in degradation of mucopolysaccharide.

GM₂ gangliosidoses. The product of the terminal cleavage of ganglioside GM_1 is ganglioside GM_2 (Fig. 2-4). Its terminal residue is *N*-acetylgalactosamine and a deficiency of the galactosaminidase catalyzing its removal would be expected to cause accumulation of ganglioside GM_2. This expectation is realized with disastrous consequences in at least three different phenotypic forms. The best known of these is *Tay-Sachs disease,* or GM_2 gangliosidosis type 1.[8, 77] The older term *amaurotic idiocy,* accompanied by eponyms or indication of the age onset, has fallen into disuse as biochemical markers have become available as a basis for classification.

Tay-Sachs disease becomes clinically expressed in infancy and its primary manifestations are entirely neurologic. A cherry-red spot is evident in nearly every instance and most of the infants become blind within the first 12 to 18 months of life. Affected children are usually dead by 3 years of age. Occasionally, a child whose sib has followed the expected course will itself develop cherry-red spots but then follow a more protracted course of central nervous system disability.

The hexosaminidase involved can be separated into several components, possibly monomer-dimer forms. The A component is grossly deficient in tissues in Tay-Sachs disease. A total deficiency of hexosaminidase activity occurs in the *"Sandhoff variant"* of GM_2 *gangliosidosis.*[72] The visceral storage of ganglioside GM_2, its asialo derivative, and very similar glycolipids that occurs in Tay-Sachs disease is much exaggerated in this form. A milder variant, in which hexosaminidase deficiency is less than either of the above types, has also been reported by several workers. The course is protracted; a cherry-red spot has not been reported, but optic atrophy and retinitis pigmentosa have been noted.[6, 88]

Fabry's disease. The breakdown of circulating leukocytes and erythrocytes releases large quantities of a membrane glycolipid called globoside. The first step in its degradation by lysosomal enzymes yields the compound galactosylgalactosylglucosyl ceramide (Fig. 2-4). This is further broken down by release of its terminal galactose through splitting of an α-glycosidic bond. A deficiency in activity of the responsible α-galactosidase causes widespread deposition of the ceramide trihexoside substrate in endothelial and smooth muscle cells of blood vessels, in ganglion cells and perineural cells of the autonomic nervous system, and in many other cells of the body, including the skin and cornea. The result is *Fabry's disease,*[20, 85] earlier known by its characteristic skin lesion *angiokeratoma corporis diffusum universale.*[68] The principal manifestations are recurrent crises of fever and burning pain in the extremities, edema, and renal dysfunction. The patients usually die prematurely from complications of vascular disease or hypertension. The changes in the eyes are characteristic. They include corneal dystrophy, presumably from ceramide trihexoside storage, and star-shaped opacities in the posterior part of the lens. In addition, the mural storage of glycolipids in the blood vessels of the retina and conjunctiva causes a revealing tortuosity. Reference has already been made to the X-linked nature of inheritance, causing the most severe form of the disease to appear in males. The heterozygous females, who often have an attenuated form of the disease, may have corneal dystrophy (Fleischer's dystrophy). Some success in treatment of this disorder by enzyme replacement has been mentioned above.

Galactosyl ceramide. The brain and the kidney normally contain appreciable amounts of the relatively simple glycolipids, galactosyl ceramide and its sulfuric acid ester (Fig. 2-3). In the brain they are primarily localized to the myelin sheath and are therefore present in very small quantities prior to myelination. Galactosyl ceramide must be distinguished from the other major cerebroside (hexosyl ceramide) in tissues that contain a single glucose residue. Glucosyl ceramide is one of the products on the degradative pathways of both gangliosides and the globoside mentioned above under Fabry's disease. Glucosyl ceramide is found in most tissues of the body other than brain, where it appears only early in development. It accumulates in Gaucher's disease, a β-glucoside deficiency state.[25]

Krabbe's disease. A similar β-galactoside deficiency has only recently been detected in *Krabbe's disease, or globoid cell leukodystrophy*[19, 54] (Fig. 2-3). This is a disease that appears at 3 to 6 months of age as progressive retardation with prominent long-tract signs, pseudobulbar palsy, cortical blindness, and optic atrophy. Reports of pathologic lesions have thus far been confined to the nervous tissue; there is severe demyelination, gliosis, and infiltration with unique globoid cells that are rich in galactosyl ceramide. For many years only a brain biopsy provided an antemortem diagnosis of Krabbe's disease. This can now be swiftly accomplished by measurement of galactosyl ceramide-β-galactosidase activity in peripheral leukocytes, serum, or cultured fibroblasts.

Sulfatide lipidoses. A portion of the galactosyl ceramides in the nervous system and in the kidney are sulfated at the carbon-3 of galactose (Fig. 2-3). The amounts of galactosyl ($3\text{-}SO_4$) ceramide increase rapidly during myelination and continue to accumulate in man until middle age. That an appreciable turnover of such sulfatides occurs normally becomes dramatically evident when the activity of one or more sulfatases is affected by mutation. This is attended by demyelination and accumulation of cerebroside sulfate in brain, peripheral nerves, liver, and kidney. These sulfatide lipidoses include several forms of *metachromatic leukodystrophy* (MLD).[60] Metachromasia refers to the ability of sulfated compounds like sulfatides, heparin, or chondroitin sulfate—among other anionic substances— to shift the absorption of certain cationic dyes to a shorter wavelength. Thus light of a longer wavelength is transmitted and dyes like cresyl violet, toluidine blue, or methylene blue appear pink or red. Increased urinary secretion of sulfatides in MLD can be detected as by tests for metachromasia, a nonspecific feature helpful in diagnosis when combined with other clinical signs.

The most common type of MLD appears at 12 to 18 months, hence the frequent name *late infantile form*. The course is progressive and is usually fatal in 5 to 15 years. The eye signs, as described by Cogan[13] include a grayish macula with a red spot in the center. Macular discoloration may be one of the earliest signs. The disease may also appear later in youth or adulthood. The characterization of tissue sulfatase activity is extensive, but still only partially complete. For years they have been most conveniently measured by use of nonphysiological substrates (arylsulfates). Arylsulfatase A activity has been shown to bear a close resemblance to tissue cerebroside sulfatase and to be different from arylsulfatase B. Arylsulfatase A and cerebroside sulfatase activities are greatly depressed in late, infantile MLD[44] and less so in adult MLD. A variant with multiple sulfatase deficiencies also occurs. Apparently the deficient enzymes include one or more that also act on mucopolysaccharides, for quantities of the latter also accumulate. Not unexpectedly these patients have bony deformities. They also have changes in the macular region of the retina.

Sphingomyelin lipidoses. Among the important structural lipids in nearly all cells, myelin, and circulating lipoproteins is sphingomyelin, a ceramide derivative in which phosphorylcholine, rather than a glycoside residue is esterified to the C-1 hydroxyl group of sphingosine (Fig. 2-3). There are a number of lipid storage diseases in which the tissue content of sphingomyelin is increased, nearly always concomitant with storage of unesterified cholesterol.[29] In two particular forms, such lipid storage is accompanied by severe tissue deficiency of the enzyme sphingomyelinase, which cleaves phosphorylcholine from ceramide.[9, 75] The two phenotypes are similar in the amounts of lipids stored in large "foam cells" throughout the reticuloendothelial tissues outside the brain. In both forms, hepatosplenomegaly also begins in the first year of life, and storage in the lungs detectable by x-ray film becomes prominent shortly thereafter. The form commonly called *type A,* however, is associated with psychomotor retardation that progresses to a vegetative state that is usually fatal by the third year. This is classical *Niemann-Pick disease.* In the other form, *type B,* psychic and neurologic development is normal and has continued to be in patients followed for several decades. In type A, most of the patients develop a cherry-red spot before death; there are no ocular signs in type B. These two allelic forms of sphingomyelinase deficiency thus are separated by a vital difference in central nervous system involvement. The gene for type A is of high frequency in Ashkenazi Jews; that for type B is not.

There are other forms of mild sphingomyelin excess in which hepatosplenomegaly and nervous system involvement occur, usually later. Sphingomyelinase activity may be moderately deficient, and such patients who may represent genetic compounds have been tentatively called *type C.* They may have a cherry-red spot but can have a very protracted course. A possible variant, found in children related to parents of a Nova Scotian community, has been called *type D* by Crocker.[14, 15] These patients may become blind but have normal fundi. Sphingomyelinase activity is normal or only slightly depressed. Some patients of "type C" or "D," and others with similar lipid storage and completely normal sphingomyelinase activity, are undoubtedly falsely classified under the sphingomyelinoses. Some may represent disordered metabolism of other sphingolipids.

A certain number of such patients have probably been included in a diverse collection called the *syndrome of the sea-blue histiocyte.*[76] This is not a specific diagnosis. In type A Niemann-Pick disease and other specific tissue storage diseases, like Tangier disease, there are present large histiocytes in bone marrow that stain a sea-blue color with Giemsa's or Wright's stain.

Ceramide storage. *Farber's disease (lipogranulomatosis)* is a rare disease, observed in siblings, characterized by progressive arthropathy, subcutaneous nodules, nutritional failure, and psychomotor retardation.[1] Cogan and Kuwabara[12] report one patient with this disorder who had grayish discoloration of the macula. The retinal ganglion cells were found to contain birefringent crystals that stained strongly with periodic acid–Schiff reagent. Prensky et al. have described an increased content of ceramide (Fig. 2-2) in the organs of several patients.[61, 69] Quite recently, Sugita, Dulaney, and Moser[83] have reported a pronounced decrease in activity of ceramidase, an enzyme splitting the fatty acid from sphingosine in this final product of sphingolipid degradation. The staining reactions reported in the tissues of some patients with Farber's disease indicate that other compounds having *cis*-glycol groups are also being stored, and excess gangliosides, glycolipids, and mucopolysaccharides have been detected in tissues of some patients. How the enzyme defect so far detected results in this pleomorphic lipid storage is not clearly established.

Mucopolysaccharidoses (MPS)

Two comprehensive reviews of these disorders are contained in McKusick's text[57] and a review by Dorfman and Matalon,[19] and the biochemical defects have been summarized by Neufeld.[63] Mucopolysaccharides are much more complicated structures than are sphingolipids. They consist of long glycoside polymers, some having as many as a hundred sugar residues per chain, attached to a protein core. All the classified mucopolysaccharidoses, except the Morquio syndrome, are caused by defective lysosomal catabolism of two classes of polymers, dermatan sulfate and heparan sulfate. Dermatan sulfate polymers consist of residues of uronic acid (glucuronic or L-iduronic acid, sulfated and nonsulfated) alternating with sulfated N-acetyl galactosamine. Heparan sulfate differs in the amino sugar present. It contains glucosamine, the amino group of which is either sulfated or acetylated (Fig. 2-5).

The degradation of these polymers normally begins at the terminal glycosidic residue and proceeds sequentially. An example involving only one of several enzymes involved in MPS metabolism is shown in Fig. 2-5. The initial cleavage may occur at a sulfate group or between sugars. If any of the specific enzymes required at each sequential step is not functioning normally, normal degradation stops. The resulting polymers may then be cleaved into large fragments by endoglycosidases, such as hyaluronidase. Some of these water-soluble fragments are released into the blood and secreted into the urine. In the fashion of other lysosomal disorders, many tissues may take up an excess of this undegradable material, with compromise of their structure and function.

The recent elucidation of the specific enzyme defects in the mucopolysaccharidoses has been made by taking advantage of older observations that metachromatic material is stored in cultured fibroblasts from affected patients. This

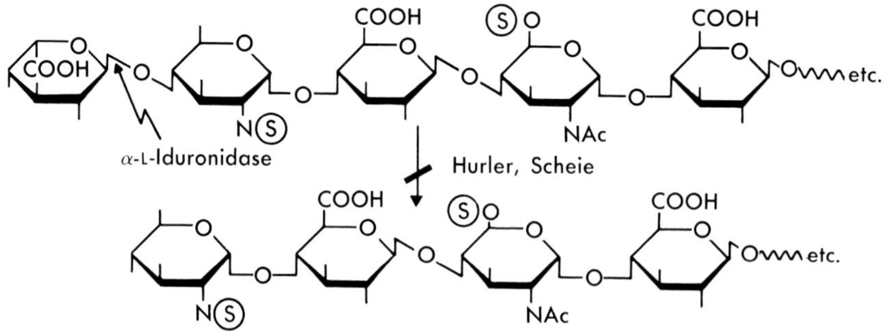

Fig. 2-5. Terminal glycosidic residues in heparan sulfate. Deficient activity of the enzyme sulfoiduronidase prevents initiation of the cleavage of the polysaccharide polymer in mucopolysaccharidosis I. Two allelic forms of enzyme deficiency, the Hurler and Scheie syndromes, are phenotypically quite distinct. (Courtesy Dr. Elizabeth Neufeld, Bethesda, Md.)

storage in tissue cultures can be reversed or prevented by addition of a "corrective factor" derived from urine or skin cultures of normal subjects or other phenotypic forms of MPS. Subsequently, the responsible enzyme in the "corrective factors" has been identified.[63] In this way, not only the normal requirement for certain lysosomal enzymes but also the chemical nature of material accumulating in MPS has been discovered. One reason that the Morquio syndrome has not yet been elucidated is the fact that it is associated with excretion of keratan sulfate, polymers of which are not made in skin fibroblasts. Neufeld has pointed out[63] that chondrocytes or perhaps corneal fibroblasts, which produce keratan sulfate, may afford the necessary opportunity for discovery of the defect.

Mucopolysaccharidosis I (Hurler and Scheie syndromes). In the 1972 classification of mucopolysaccharidoses by McKusick,[57] several older syndromes are now grouped as MPS-I, all caused by deficiency of α-L-iduronidase.[2, 3] Three phenotypic forms exist in which at least two different mutations affect the activity of this enzyme. As mentioned earlier in the discussion of allelism, the *Hurler*[42] and *Scheie*[73] syndromes are each believed to be the homozygous states of mutant alleles that are different in each disease[57] (Fig. 2-5). In addition there is a Hurler-Scheie compound in which the genotype is believed to include one H allele and one S allele. The latter was earlier suspected on clinical grounds and shown to be the case in tissue culture studies where addition of only corrective factor for S or for H failed to eliminate all MPS accumulation.

MPS-I H usually is evident within a few months of birth and is fatal by 10 years on the average, the earliest age of death for all recognized MPS. Growth, especially that of bones, is early affected; mucopolysaccharide storage causes hepatosplenomegaly and damage to vascular structures, especially the heart valves and tunica intima of the coronary arteries. Mental development is affected after the first year, partly because of meningeal involvement and resultant hydrocephalus and partly because of storage within nerve cells. The dwarfed child, with large head, enlarged tongue, widely spaced facial features, short neck, with kyphosis, protruding abdomen, and deformed joints and extremities presents a fairly classic appearance. There is excessive urinary secretion of both dermatan sulfate and heparan sulfate.

Cloudy corneas appear in all cases of MPS-I, with the opacities being located in the medial and deeper layers of the cornea. Other ocular abnormalities, not listed in Table 2-1, include possible buphthalmos and megalocornea, and there may be histopathologic changes in the retina. Cardiac failure and respiratory disease are the usual causes of death.

The Scheie syndrome (MPS-1 S) is much milder. There is corneal clouding, deformity of the hands, and aortic valve involvement with few other somatic changes and normal intelligence.[3, 57] Excess collagenous tissue and vacuolated cells are found in the skin, cornea, and conjunctiva. Excess excretion of both dermatan sulfate and heparan sulfate occurs in the urine. MPS-I H/S, the compound syndrome, represents an intermediate phenotype.

Hunter's syndrome (MPS-II). The absence of corneal clouding separates MPS-I (Hurler's) from MPS-II *(Hunter's syndrome)*. In addition, the latter patients survive longer. Both dermatan sulfate and heparan sulfate are excreted in the urine in excess, but the mucopolysaccharide patterns excreted differ in the proportion of different types of heparan sulfate compared to MPS-I. The enzyme defect is deficient activity of sulfoiduronate sulfatase.[2] Although the cornea is grossly clear in MPS-II, there is minimal involvement detectable by slit lamp, and MPS deposits on the cornea are demonstrable in adults.[36] In addition retinitis pigmentosa has been reported, on occasion leading to blindness.[57] As already noted MPS-II is the only MPS that is X linked in inheritance.

Sanfilippo syndromes (MPS-III). There are two Sanfilippo phenotypes called A and B, and they involve deficiencies of different enzymes.[57] The *Sanfilippo A* phenotype is caused by deficient heparan sulfate sulfatase.[50] The *Sanfilippo B* phenotype is related to deficient N-acetyl-α-D-glucosaminidase.[89] Both result in excretion of excess heparan sulfate in the urine. These disorders are autosomal recessive in inheritance. A pigmentary retinopathy may develop.

Morquio's syndrome (MPS-IV). One other MPS affects the eye. This is *Morquio's syndrome.*[59] The patients are dwarfed and have severe skeletal deformities. Long survival is possible, but patients frequently die of pulmonary changes related to chest deformities. There is severe corneal clouding. The MPS excreted is keratan sulfate, and the enzymatic defect is unknown.

Maroteaux-Lamy syndrome (MPS-VI A and B). This syndrome is associated only with excess excretion of dermatan sulfate. There are two forms, one milder than the other, but both associated with osseous changes, cloudy cornea, and clear intellect.[56, 57] Clinically and pathologically it combines many features of MPS-I H and MPS-I S, being distinguished from the latter by more osseous deformities and shorter survival. A corrective factor has been demonstrated in tissue-culture studies, but the enzyme or enzymes have not yet been identified. It is suspected that they may be either or both $N(SO_4)$-galactosamine sulfatase or galactosaminidase.[63]

β-Glucuronidase deficiency (MPS-VII). The basic defect in this disease was established when there was only one known example.[78] He had an unusual facies, hepatosplenomegaly, gibbus, and puffy hands and feet. Later, physical and mental development slowed. An unrelated female who had similar abnormalities but, in addition, corneal clouding, was subsequently reported. Both patients excreted particularly large amounts of dermatan sulfate. Appropriate tissues show a deficiency of β-glucuronidase. The homogeneity of the two examples is still uncertain and there is some question as to whether this is a true mucopolysaccharidosis.

Mucolipidoses

The term "mucolipidosis"[79] has been used to distinguish disorders having features of both mucopolysaccharidoses and sphingolipidoses. It includes *fucosidosis*[87] and *mannosidosis,*[46] *lipomucopolysaccharidosis,*[80] *I-cell disease,*[16] and the *pseudo-Hurler variant*[55] and may also embrace Farber's disease, the GM$_1$ gangliosidoses, and the multiple sulfatase deficiency variant of the sulfatide lipidoses, depending on the whim of the classifier.

Mucolipidosis II (I-cell disease). In mucolipidosis II, there are evident at birth, or shortly after, dislocations of the hips, thoracic deformities, hernia, and hyperplastic gums.[16] X-ray films reveal Hurler syndrome–like bony changes and joint limitation and psychomotor retardation soon appear. Mild corneal clouding is present. There is no excess MPS excretion in the urine. A striking feature is the presence of lysosomal inclusion bodies in fibroblasts in many tissues, hence the term "I," or "inclusion cell" disease. This is a lysosomal disorder of a different kind. The cultured fibroblasts from such patients show multiple enzyme deficiencies, yet the culture medium, or plasma and urine, of the patients show excess activities of many lysosomal enzymes. These enzymes have weak "corrective factor" activity in crossing experiments in tissue culture. Thus lysosomal hydrolases appear in excess extracullularly and diminished within lysosomes. Neufeld has speculated that perhaps most lysosomal enzymes are normally secreted from the cell and taken up by others through selective pinocytosis.[63] She further postulates that, in I-cell disease, lysosomal enzyme uptake is deficient, perhaps from changes in recognition markers (a sugar?) induced by mutation.

Mucolipidosis III (pseudo-Hurler polydystrophy). This disorder is clinically similar to MPS-I, but slower in evolution and lacking mucopolysacchariduria.[55] There is fine, ground-glass clouding of the corneas, and the conjunctional fibroblasts also show lysosomal inclusions.[57] The limited studies thus far indicate that this disease arises from a general defect similar to that in I-cell disease.

Other mucolipidoses. A single patient has been reported[46, 67] who died at age 4 with Hurler syndrome–like dystrophies, and cloudiness in the capsule of the lens. Cells in the central nervous system were ballooned with a polymeric material containing mannose and glucosamine. In the liver, α-mannosidase activity was deficient. This phenotype has been called *mannosidosis*.[46] The description of rare patients with deficient α-fucosidase activity includes evidence for accumulation of partially degraded glycoproteins and glycolipids in the liver. Fucose appears in keratan sulfate, but not in other mucopolysaccharides. Ocular abnormalities do not appear to be characteristic of this α-*fucosidosis*.[19]

As the chemistry of these complex polymeric substances becomes better known, enzymes required for sequential degradation of different chains will become self-evident. With this knowledge will come further subclassification of similar phenotypes and inclusion in the catalog of numerous rare examples of obscure variants of the lysosomal hydrolase deficiencies described above. Continued improvement in taxonomy is essential, of course, as prenatal screening increases and the need for definitive diagnoses becomes apparent. As important as this is, enzyme replacement has supplanted it as the major source of excitement. Given the extraordinary progress of the past decade, it would be foolish to doubt that this, too, will become a practical reality in at least some of the "lysosomal diseases."

REFERENCES

1. Abul-Haj, S. K., Martz, D. G., Douglas, W. F., and Geppert, L. J.: Farber's disease. Report of a case, with observations on its histogenesis and notes on the nature of the stored material, J. Pediat. **61**:221-232, 1962.
2. Bach, G., Eisenberg, Jr., F., Cantz, M., and Neufeld, E. F.: The defect in the Hunter syndrome: Deficiency of sulfoiduronate sulfatase, Proc. Nat. Acad. Sci. **70**:2134-2138, 1973.
3. Bach, G., Friedman, R., Weissmann, B., and Neufeld, E. F.: The defect in the Hurler and Scheie syndromes: Deficiency of α-L-iduronidase, Proc. Nat. Acad. Sci. **69**:2048-2051, 1972.
4. Bearn, A. G.: Wilson's disease. In Stanbury, J. B., Wyngaarden, J. B., and Fredrickson, D. S., editors: The metabolic basis of inherited disease, ed. 3, New York, 1972, McGraw-Hill Book Co., pp. 1033-1050.

5. Bergsma, D., editor: The second conference on the clinical delineation of birth defects. Part VIII, Eye, Baltimore, 1971, The Williams & Wilkins Co.

6. Bernheimer, H., and Seitelberger, F.: Über das Verhalten der Ganglioside im Gehirn bei 2 Fällen von spätinfantiler amaurotischer Idiotie, Wien. Klin. Wochenschr. **80:**163, 1968.

7. Bhattacharya, A. K., and Connor, W. E.: β-Sitosterolemia and xanthomatosis: A newly described lipid storage disease in two sisters, J. Clin. Invest. **52:**9a, 1973.

8. Brady, R. O.: The sphingolipidoses. Medical progress report, New Eng. J. Med. **275:** 312-318, 1966.

9. Brady, R. O., Kanfer, J. N., Mock, M. B., and Fredrickson, D. S.: The metabolism of sphingomyelin, II. Evidence of an enzymatic deficiency in Niemann-Pick disease, Proc. Nat. Acad. Sci. **55:**366-369, 1966.

10. Brady, R. O., Tallman, J. F., Johnson, W. G., Gal, A. E., Leahy, W. R., Quirk, J. M., and Dekaban, A. S.: Replacement therapy for inherited enzyme deficiency. Use of purified ceramidetrihexosidase in Fabry's disease, New Eng. J. Med. **289:**9-14, 1973.

11. Cash, R., and Berger, C. K.: Acrodermatitis enteropathica: Defective metabolism of unsaturated fatty acids, J. Pediatr. **74:**717-729, 1969.

12. Cogan, D. G., and Kuwabara, T.: The sphingolipidoses and the eye, Arch. Ophthalmol. **79:**437-452, 1968.

13. Cogan, D. G., Kuwabara, T., and Moser, H.: Metachromatic leucodystrophy, Ophthalmologica **160:**2-17, 1970.

14. Crocker, A. C.: The cerebral defect in Tay-Sachs disease and Niemann-Pick disease, J. Neurochem. **7:**69-80, 1961.

15. Crocker, A. C., and Farber, S.: Niemann-Pick disease: A review of eighteen patients, Medicine **37:**1-95, 1958.

16. De Mars, R., and Leroy, J. G.: The remarkable cells cultured from a human with Hurler's syndrome: An approach to visual selection for in vitro genetic studies, In Vitro **2:**107, 1966.

17. Desnick, R. J., Simmons, R. L., Allen, K. Y., Woods, J. E., Anderson, C. F., Najarian, J. S., and Krivit, W.: Correction of enzymatic deficiencies by renal transplantation: Fabry's disease, Surgery **72:**203-211, 1972.

18. Di Ferrante, N., Nichols, B. L., Donnelly, P. V., Neri, G., Hrgovcic, R., and Berglund, R. K.: Induced degradation of glycosaminoglycans in Hurler's and Hunter's syndromes by plasma infusion, Proc. Nat. Acad. Sci. **68:**303-307, 1971.

19. Dorfman, A., and Matalon, R.: The mucopolysaccharidoses. In Stanbury, J. B., Wyngaarden, J. B., and Fredrickson, D. S., editors: The metabolic basis of inherited disease, ed. 3, New York, 1972, McGraw-Hill Book Co., pp. 1218-1272.

20. Fabry, J.: Ein Beitrag zur Kenntnis der Purpura haemorrhagica nodularis (purpura papulosa hemorrhagica Hebrae), Arch. Derm. Syph. **43:**187, 1898.

21. Fitzpatrick, T. B., and Quevedo, Jr., W. C.: Albinism. In Stanbury, J. B., Wyngaarden, J. B., and Fredrickson, D. S., editors: The metabolic basis of inherited disease, ed. 3, New York, 1972, McGraw-Hill Book Co., pp. 326-337.

22. Franceschetti, A.: Congenital and hereditary neuro-ophthalmic diseases. In Congenital anomalies of the eye (Transactions of the New Orleans Academy of Ophthalmology, New Orleans, 1967), St. Louis, 1968, The C. V. Mosby Co., pp. 99-113.

23. François, J.: Congenital cataracts, Assen, Netherlands, 1963, Royal Van Gorcum Ltd.

24. François, J.: Ocular manifestations in certain congenital errors of metabolism. In Congenital anomalies of the eye (Transactions of the New Orleans Academy of Ophthalmology, New Orleans, 1967), St. Louis, 1968, The C. V. Mosby Co., pp. 157-198.

25. Frazier, P. D., and Wong, V. G.: Cystinosis: Histologic and crystallographic examination of crystals in eye tissues, Arch. Ophthal. **80:**87-91, 1968.

26. Fredrickson, D. S.: A physician's guide to hyperlipidemia, Mod. Concepts Cardiovasc. Dis. **XLI:**31-36, 1972.

27. Fredrickson, D. S., and Levy, R. I.: Familial hyperlipoproteinemia. In Stanbury, J. B., Wyngaarden, J. B., and Fredrickson, D. S., editors: The metabolic basis of inherited disease, ed. 3, New York, 1972, McGraw-Hill Book Co., pp. 531-614.

28. Fredrickson, D. S., and Sloan, H. R.: Glucosyl ceramide lipidoses: Gaucher's disease. In

Stanbury, J. B., Wyngaarden, J. B., and Fredrickson, D. S., editors: The metabolic basis of inherited disease, ed. 3, New York, 1972, McGraw-Hill Book Co., pp. 730-759.

29. Fredrickson, D. S., and Sloan, H. R.: Sphingomyelin lipidoses: Niemann-Pick disease, In Stanbury, J. B., Wyngaarden, J. B., and Fredrickson, D. S., editors: The metabolic basis of inherited disease, ed. 3, New York, 1972, McGraw-Hill Book Co., pp. 783-807.

30. Fredrickson, D. S., Gotto, A. M., and Levy, R. I.: Familial lipoprotein deficiency (abetalipoproteinemia, hypobetalipoproteinemia, and Tangier disease). In Stanbury, J. B., Wyngaarden, J. B., and Fredrickson, D. S., editors: The metabolic basis of inherited disease, ed. 3, New York, 1972, McGraw-Hill Book Co., pp. 493-530.

31. Fredrickson, D. S., Levy, R. I., and Lees, R. S.: Fat transport in lipoproteins: An integrated approach to mechanisms and disorders, New Eng. J. Med. **276:**34-44, 94-103, 148-156, 215-226, 273-281, 1967.

32. Garrod, A. E.: Inborn errors of metabolism (The Croonian Lectures), Lancet **2:**1-7, 73-79, 142-148, 214-220, 1908.

33. Gerritsen, T., and Waisman, H. A.: Homocystinuria. In Stanbury, J. B., Wyngaarden, J. B., and Fredrickson, D. S., editors: The metabolic basis of inherited disease, ed. 3, New York, 1972, McGraw-Hill Book Co., pp. 404-412.

34. Gjone, E., and Bergaust, B.: Corneal opacity in familial plasma cholesterol ester deficiency, Acta Ophthal. **47:**222-227, 1969.

35. Goldberg, M. F.: A review of selected inherited corneal dystrophies associated with systemic diseases. In Bergsma, D., editor: The second conference on the clinical delineation of birth defects. Part VIII, Eye, Baltimore, 1971, The Williams & Wilkins Co., pp. 13-25.

36. Goldberg, M. F., and Duke, J. R.: Ocular histopathology in Hunter's syndrome. Systemic mucopolysaccharidosis type II, Arch. Ophthal. **77:**503-512, 1967.

37. Goodman, G.: Sickle cell ocular disease. In Congenital anomalies of the eye (Transactions of the New Orleans Academy of Ophthalmology, New Orleans, 1967), St. Louis, 1968, The C. V. Mosby Co., pp. 247-271.

38. Hayman, S., and Kinoshita, J. H.: Isolation and properties of lens aldose reductase, J. Biol. Chem. **240:**877-882, 1965.

39. Hers, H. G.: Inborn lysosomal diseases, Gastroenterology **48:**625-633, 1965.

40. Hooft, C., De Laly, P., Herpol, J., Deloore, F., and Verbeeck, J.: Familial hypolidaemia and retarded development without steatorrhoea, Helv. Paediat. Acta **17:**1-23, 1962.

41. Hug, G., and Schubert, W. K.: Lysosomes in type II glycogenosis. Changes during administration of extract from *Aspergillus niger,* J. Cell Biol. **35:**C1-C6, 1967

42. Hurler, G.: Über einen Typ multipler Abartungen, vorwiegen am Skelettsystem, Z. Kinderheilk. **24:**220-234, 1919.

43. Irreverre, F., Mudd, S. H., Heizer, W. D., and Laster, L.: Sulfite oxidase deficiency: Studies of a patient with mental retardation, dislocated ocular lenses, and abnormal urinary excretion of S-sulfo-L-cysteine, sulfite, and thiosulfate, Biochem. Med. **I:**187-217, 1967.

44. Jatzkewitz, H., and Mehl, E.: Cerebroside-sulphatase and arylsulphatase A deficiency in metachromatic leukodystrophy (ML), J. Neurochem. **16:**19-28, 1969.

45. Kabak, M. M., and Zeigers, R. S.: Heterozygote detection in Tay-Sachs disease: A prototype community screening program for the prevention of recessive genetic disorders, Adv. Exper. Med. Biol. **19:**613-632, 1972.

46. Kjellman, B., Gamstorp, I., Brun, A., Öckerman, P.-A., and Palmgren, B.: Mannosidosis: A clinical and histopathologic study, J. Pediat. **75:**366-373, 1969.

47. Klintwork, G. K.: Current concepts on the ultrastructural pathogenesis of macular and lattice corneal dystrophies. In Bergsma, D., editor: The second conference on the clinical delineation of birth defects. Part VIII, Eye, Baltimore, 1971, The Williams & Wilkins Co., pp. 27-31.

48. Knox, W. E.: Phenylketonuria. In Stanbury, J. B., Wyngaarden, J. B., and Fredrickson, D.S., editors: The metabolic basis of inherited disease, ed. 3, New York, 1972, McGraw-Hill Book Co., pp. 266-295.

49. Krabbe, K.: A new familial, infantile form of diffuse brain sclerosis, Brain **39:**74, 1916.

50. Kresse, H., and Neufeld, E. F.: The Sanfilippo A corrective factor. Purification and mode of action, J. Biol. Chem. **247:**2164-2170, 1972.

51. La Du, B. N.: Alcaptonuria. In Stanbury, J. B., Wyngaarden, J. B., and Fredrickson, D. S., editors: The metabolic basis of inherited disease, ed. 3, New York, 1972, McGraw-Hill Book Co., pp. 308-325.

52. Laster, L., Irreverre, F., Mudd, S. H., and Heizer, W. D.: A previously unrecognized disorder of metabolism of sulfur-containing compounds—abnormal urinary excretion of *S*-sulfo-L-cysteine, sulfite and thiosulfate in a severely retarded child with ectopia lentis, J. Clin. Invest. **46:**1082, 1967.

53. Lauer, R. M., Mascarinas, T., Racela, A. S., and Diehl, A. M.: Administration of a mixture of fungal glucosidases to a patient with type II glycogenosis (Pompe's disease), Pediatrics **42:**672-676, 1968.

54. Mapes, C. A., Anderson, R. L., Sweeley, C. C., Desnick, R. J., and Krivit, W.: Enzyme replacement in Fabry's disease, an inborn error of metabolism, Science **169:**987-989, 1970.

55. Maroteaux, P., and Lamy, M.: La pseudo-polydystrophie de Hurler, Presse Med. **74:**2889-2892, 1966.

56. Maroteaux, P., Frézal, J., Tahbaz-Zadeh, and Lamy, M.: Une observation familiale d'oligophrénie polydystrophique, J. Genet. Hum. **15:**93-102, 1966.

57. McKusick, V. A.: Heritable disorders of connective tissue, ed. 4, St. Louis, 1972, The C. V. Mosby Co.

58. McKusick, V. A.: Mendelian inheritance in man. Catalogs of autosomal dominant, autosomal recessive, and X-linked phenotypes, ed. 3, Baltimore, 1971, The Johns Hopkins Press.

59. Morquio, L.: Sur une forme de dystrophie osseuse familiale, Bull. Soc. Pediat. Paris **27:**145, 1929.

60. Moser, H. W.: Sulfatide lipidosis: Metachromatic leukodystrophy. In Stanbury, J. B., Wyngaarden, J. B., and Fredrickson, D. S., editors: The metabolic basis of inherited disease, ed. 3, New York, 1972, McGraw-Hill Book Co., pp. 688-729.

61. Moser, H. W., Prensky, A. L., Wolfe, H. J., and Rosman, N. P.: Farber's lipogranulomatosis. Report of a case and demonstration of an excess of free ceramide and ganglioside, Am. J. Med. **47:**869-890, 1969.

62. Mudd, S. H.: Homocystinuria and homocysteine metabolism: Selected aspects. In Nyhan, W. L., editor: Hereditable disorders of amino acid metabolism, ed. 2, New York, 1974, John Wiley & Sons, Inc., pp. 429-541.

63. Neufeld, E. F.: The biochemical basis of mucopolysaccharidoses and mucolipidoses. In Steinberg, A. G., and Bearn, A. G., editors: Progress in medical genetics, New York, 1974, Grune & Stratton, Inc. (In press.)

64. Norum, K. R., Glomset, J. A., and Gjone, E.: Familial lecithin : cholesterol acyl transferase deficiency. In Stanbury, J. B., Wyngaarden, J. B., and Fredrickson, D. S., editors: The metabolic basic of inherited disease, ed. 3, New York, 1972, McGraw-Hill Book Co., pp. 531-544.

65. O'Brien, J. S.: G$_{M1}$ gangliosidoses. In Stanbury, J. B., Wyngaarden, J. B., and Fredrickson, D. S., editors. The metabolic basis of inherited disease, ed. 3, New York, 1972, McGraw-Hill Book Co., pp. 639-662.

66. O'Brien, J. S., Stern, M. B., Landing, B. H., O'Brien, J. K., and Donnell, G. N.: Generalized gangliosidosis. Another inborn error of ganglioside metabolism? Am. J. Dis. Child. **109:**338-346, 1965.

67. Öckerman, P. A.: A generalized storage disorder resembling Hurler's syndrome, Lancet **2:**239-241, 1967.

68. Pompen, A. W. M., Ruiter, M., and Wyers, H. J. G.: Angiokeratoma corporis diffusum (universale) Fabry, as a sign of an unknown internal disease: Two autopsy reports, Acta Med. Scand. **128:**234, 1947.

69. Prensky, A. L., Ferreira, G., Carr, S., and Moser, H. W.: Ceramide and ganglioside accumulation in Farber's lipogranulomatosis, Proc. Soc. Exper. Biol. Med. **126:**725-728, 1967.

70. Refsum, S.: Heredopathia atactica polyneuritiformis. A familial syndrome not hitherto described, Acta Psychiat. Scand. (suppl.) **38-39:** 9-303, 1946.

71. Salen, G., and Grundy, S. M.: The metabolism of cholestanol, cholesterol, and bile acids in cerebrotendinous xanthomatosis, J. Clin. Invest. **52:**2822-2835, 1973.

72. Sandhoff, K., Andreae, U., and Jatzkewitz, H.: Deficient hexosaminidase activity in an exceptional case of Tay-Sachs disease with additional storage of kidney globoside in visceral organs, Life Sci. **7:**283-288, 1968.

73. Scheie, H. G., Hambrick, Jr., G. W., and Barness, L. A.: A newly recognized forme fruste of Hurler's disease (gargoylism), Am. J. Ophthal. **53:**753-769, 1962.

74. Schneider, J. A., and Seegmiller, J. E.: Cystinosis and the Fanconi syndrome. In Stanbury, J. B., Wyngaarden, J. B., and Fredrickson, D. S., editors: The Metabolic basis of inherited disease, ed. 3, New York, 1972, McGraw-Hill Book Co., pp. 1581-1604.

75. Schneider, P. B., and Kennedy, E. P.: Sphingomyelinase in normal human spleens and in spleens from subjects with Niemann-Pick disease, J. Lipid Res. **8:**202-209, 1967.

76. Silverstein, M. N., Ellefson, R. D., and Ahern, E. J.: The syndrome of the sea-blue histiocyte, New Eng. J. Med. **282:**1-4, 1970.

77. Sloan, H. R., and Fredrickson, D. S.: G_{M2} gangliosidoses: Tay-Sachs disease. In Stanbury, J. B., Wyngaarden, J. B., and Fredrickson, D. S., editors: The metabolic basis of inherited disease, ed. 3, New York, 1972, McGraw-Hill Book Co., pp. 615-638.

78. Sly, W. S., Quinton, B. A., McAlister, W. H., and Rimoin, D. L.: Beta glucuronidase deficiency: Report of clinical, radiologic, and biochemical features of a new mucopolysaccharidosis, J. Pediatr. **82:**249-257, 1973.

79. Spranger, J. W., and Wiedemann, H.-R.: The genetic mucolipidoses. Diagnosis and differential diagnosis, Humangenetik **9:**113-139, 1970.

80. Spranger, J. W., Wiedemann, H.-R., Tolksdorf, M., Graucob, E., and Caesar, R.: Lipomucopolysaccharidose: Eine neue Speicherkrankheit, Z. Kinderheilk. **103:**285, 1968.

81. Stanbury, J. B., Wyngaarden, J. B., and Fredrickson, D. S., editors: The metabolic basis of inherited disease, ed. 3, New York, 1972, McGraw-Hill Book Co.

82. Steinberg, D.: Phytanic acid storage disease: Refsum's syndrome. In Stanbury, J. B., Wyngaarden, J. B., and Fredrickson, D. S., editors: The metabolic basis of inherited disease, ed. 3, New York, 1972, McGraw-Hill Book Co., pp. 833-853.

83. Sugita, M., Dulaney, J. T., and Moser, H.W.: Ceramidase deficiency in Farber's disease (lipogranulomatosis), Science **178:**1100-1102, 1972.

84. Suzuki, K., and Suzuki, Y.: Galactosyl ceramide lipidosis: Globoid cell leucodystrophy (Krebbe's disease). In Stanbury, J. B., Wyngaarden, J. B., and Fredrickson, D. S., editors: The metabolic basis of inherited disease, ed. 3, New York, 1972, McGraw-Hill Book Co., pp. 760-782.

85. Sweeley, C. C., Klinosky, B., Krivit, W., and Desnick, R. J.: Fabry's disease: Glycosphingolipid lipidosis. In Stanbury, J. B., Wyngaarden, J. B., and Fredrickson, D. S., editors: The metabolic basis of inherited disease, ed. 3, New York, 1972, McGraw-Hill Book Co., pp. 663-687.

86. Tyler, F. H.: Muscular dystrophies. In Stanbury, J. B., Wyngaarden, J. B., and Fredrickson, D. S., editors: The metabolic basis of inherited disease, ed. 3, New York, 1972, McGraw-Hill Book Co., pp. 1204-1217.

87. Van Hoof, F., and Hers, H. G.: Mucopolysaccharidosis by absence of α-fucosidase, Lancet **1:**1198, 1968.

88. Volk, B. W., Adachi, M., Schneck, L., Saifer, A., and Kleinberg, W.: G_5-ganglioside variant of systemic late infantile lipidosis. Generalized gangliosidosis, Arch. Path. **87:**393-403, 1969.

89. von Figura, K., and Kresse, H. The Sanfilippo B corrective factor: A *N*-acetyl-α-glucosaminidase, Biochem. Biophys. Res. Commun. **48:**262-269, 1972.

90. Waardenburg, P. J., Franceschetti, A., and Klein, D., editors: Genetics and ophthalmology, Oxford, 1961, Blackwell Scientific Publications Ltd.

91. Walsh, F. B.: Clinical neuro-ophthalmology, ed. 2, Baltimore, 1957, The Williams & Wilkins Co.

92. Wong, V. G., Lietman, P. S., and Seegmiller, J. E.: Alterations of pigment epithelium in cystinosis, Arch. Ophthal. **77:**361-369, 1967.

93. Zaidman, J. L., Julsary, A., Kook, A. I., Szeinberg, A., Wallis, K., and Azizi, E.: Abetalipoproteinemia in acrodermatitis enteropathica, New Eng. J. Med. **284:**1387, 1971.

3

Ophthalmic aspects of inborn errors of metabolism*

Alan Sugar**
Steven M. Podos

The inherited biochemical diseases or "inborn errors of metabolism" long have been of interest to the ophthalmologist. Although many had been viewed as rare curiosities with often devastating ocular manifestations, there increasingly has been stress on the diagnostic role of the ophthalmologist in detecting subtle, early, and occasionally pathognomonic lesions. Only a few years ago diagnosis of these diseases was of largely academic interest. The recent advances in biochemical understanding, carrier identification, and prenatal diagnosis have made possible the prevention and therapy of many of these entities.[5, 28, 101, 113, 142]

Recent reviews approach the inborn errors of metabolism from the standpoint of biochemical diagnosis[5, 28] and management.[101, 142] Others discuss eye findings in each ocular tissue.[21] This chapter is organized by biochemical grouping of diseases where possible, with emphasis on the ocular manifestations of selected entities. Each section begins with a list of the diseases and their major eye signs. In instances where categorization is not yet well understood the groupings may be arbitrary. Several large and important categories, particularly diabetes mellitus and the hemoglobinopathies, are covered in separate chapters of this book. Other entities with ill-defined biochemical bases, such as some of the inherited connective tissue disorders, are mentioned only in passing. Table 3-1 at the end of this chapter contains a partial differential diagnosis for the various ocular abnormalities associated with the inborn errors of metabolism.

*Supported in part by research grant EY-00004 from the National Eye Institute, Bethesda, Maryland.

**Department of Ophthalmology, Washington University School of Medicine, St. Louis, Missouri.

34

LIPID ABNORMALITIES

Disease	*Eye signs*
Refsum's disease	Retinal pigmentary degeneration, cataract
LCAT deficiency	Corneal deposits, corneal arcus
Cholestanolosis	Cataract
Hyperlipoproteinemias	Lipemia retinalis, xanthelasma, corneal arcus
Tangier disease	Corneal deposits
Abetalipoproteinemia	Retinal pigmentary degeneration

The diseases of lipid metabolism chiefly involve deficiency or excess of naturally occurring lipid substances. The specific enzyme anomalies are known only in a few. Many of the lipid diseases have ocular findings.

Refsum's disease results from the accumulation of a fatty acid, phytanic acid, because of the absence of phytanic acid α-hydroxylase.[163] It is recessively inherited. Intermediate enzyme levels are detectable in heterozygotes.[77] The affected patient is characterized by cerebellar ataxia, peripheral polyneuropathy with gait disturbances, tremors, nystagmus, paresis, and sensory loss. Elevated cerebrospinal fluid protein without pleocytosis is characteristic. Other manifestations include heart disease, deafness, and ichthyosis. Onset occurs from childhood to the fifth decade. Periods of exacerbation and remission are typical. Night blindness is often the earliest abnormality. It is associated with a pigmentary retinopathy of mottled, salt and pepper, or typical bone-spicule type[4] (Figs. 3-1 and 3-2). Retinal arterioles are often narrowed and the electroretinogram (ERG) may be diminished or extinct. Visual field loss is common. It is suggested that the excess phytanic acid interferes with vitamin A esterification in the rhodopsin cycle.[4] Posterior cortical or subcapsular cataracts are present in about 35% of cases.[4, 163] Pathologic examination demonstrates lipid deposition in the retinal pigment epithelium, iris, and trabecular meshwork, with degeneration of photoreceptors.[171] Dietary restric-

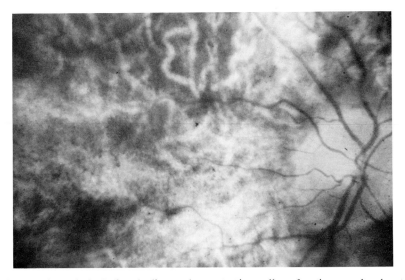

Fig. 3-1. Posterior pole in Refsum's disease demonstrating pallor of optic nerve head, arteriolar narrowing, and retinal pigmentary disease.

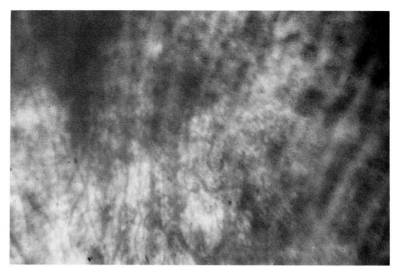

Fig. 3-2. Retinal periphery in Refsum's disease may show mottling, salt-and-pepper pattern, or bone spicule pigmentary degeneration.

tion of phytanic acid intake is being employed by some investigators, but its effect on ocular signs is unknown.[42]

Lecithin : cholesterol acyl transferase (LCAT) deficiency results in very low plasma cholesterol esters and elevated total cholesterol and triglycerides.[62] Normochromic anemia, proteinuria, and slowly progressive, mild nephropathy are the systemic manifestations of this rare autosomal recessive condition.[74] Fine grayish deposits in the central corneal stroma cause a nebulous haze that does not decrease visual acuity.[61] An annular limbal opacity suggests a prominent arcus senilis but is present at puberty. Plasma transfusions, presumably containing the deficient enzyme, are suggested as treatment for the renal disease.[122]

Cholestanolosis or cerebrotendinous xanthomatosis results from the accumulation of cholestanol and cholesterol esters in the nervous system and tendons.[135] Cerebellar ataxia, dementia, and pseudobulbar palsy progress until death. Tendinous xanthomas and premature atherosclerosis are present. Juvenile cataracts, progressive through youth and usually requiring surgery in young adulthood, are noted in two of six cases in one series and eight of twelve patients in another.[149, 158]

The *hyperlipoproteinemias,* as described by Fredrickson, et al.,[54] are summarized in the previous chapter. In type I, lipemia retinalis and palpebral eruptive xanthomas may be found. Iris xanthomas, lipid keratopathy, and adult onset Coats' disease are described less frequently.[174] Type II is the only form of hyperlipoproteinemia in which lipemia retinalis is rarely, if ever, observed. This common type is associated with arcus senilis in 10% of patients under 30 and 50% of patients under 50 years of age.[5] Xanthelasmas are common. Xanthomas may be seen on occasion in other ocular tissues. Type III hyperlipoproteinemia is associated with arcus senilis, tuberous or eruptive xanthomas of the lids, and Schnyder's crystalline corneal dystrophy. Lipemia of the limbal and retinal vessels is described.[10] In type

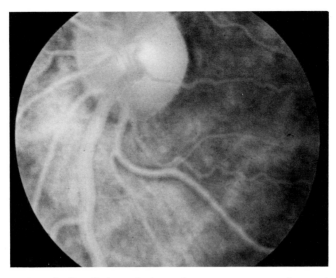

Fig. 3-3. In lipemia retinalis, all the retinal vessels appear creamy-opalescent in color and the whole fundus takes on orange hue.

IV, lipemia retinalis (Fig. 3-3) and palpebral eruptive xanthomas may be seen. Type V patients have a very high incidence of palpebral eruptive xanthomas and lipemia retinalis.

Lipemia retinalis occurs only when triglyceride levels are greater than 2500 mg.%.[174] Since types III, IV, and V of the hyperlipoproteinemias often are associated with diabetes mellitus, the protean ocular manifestations of this disease may be present. Atherosclerotic changes may be observed at an early age in types II, III, and IV.

The *hypolipoproteinemias* present with the absence of, or decrease in, a particular lipoprotein. Other lipids may be elevated. *Tangier disease,* analphalipoproteinemia, is a rare autosomal recessive trait caused by deficiency of high-density lipoproteins.[20] Cholesterol esters are deposited throughout the body, while serum cholesterol levels are low. Enlarged yellow-orange tonsils are pathognomonic. Hepatosplenomegaly and peripheral neuropathy may occur. Hazy stromal infiltrates or fine dots in the cornea are noted in four of six reported adults. Visual acuity is not affected.[53]

Bassen-Kornzweig syndrome, abetalipoproteinemia, is an autosomal recessive condition, characterized by malabsorption and steatorrhea in infancy. This results in low blood cholesterol and vitamin A levels. Ataxia and posterior column disease develop in childhood and cardiovascular disease appears in early adulthood.[89] The red blood cells are misshapen into spur forms called acanthocytes. Nystagmus, strabismus, and ptosis are common. A blue-yellow color vision defect may occur.[92] The most significant ocular finding is a retinal pigmentary degeneration with arteriolar narrowing and pigment clumping in the midperiphery or with areas of pigment atrophy (Fig. 3-4). Some patients present a picture resembling retinitis punctata albescens[73] (Fig. 3-5). Optic nerve pallor and posterior pole degenera-

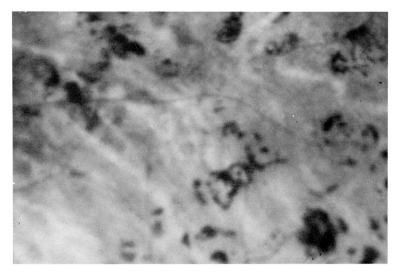

Fig. 3-4. Typical blotches and spicules of pigment in periphery of retina in patient with abetalipoproteinemia.

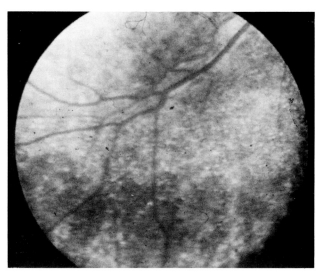

Fig. 3-5. Flecked retina similar to retinitis punctata albescens in abetalipoproteinemia. This patient demonstrated greatly reduced electroretinogram amplitude, contracted fields, and night blindness.

tion may be seen[86] (Fig. 3-6). Abnormal fields, dark adaptation, and abnormal electroretinogram findings are usually present.[162] It is significant that the administration of high doses of vitamin A may improve the ocular findings, suggesting that these manifestations are secondary to the abnormal lipid transport in this disease. This is the first inherited disease in which a vitamin A deficiency is associated with retinitis pigmentosa.[73] Histopathology shows loss of rods, cones, and

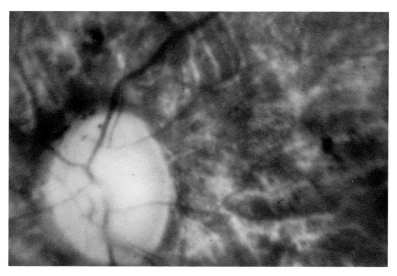

Fig. 3-6. Pale, waxy disk, and arteriolar narrowing accompany the retinal pigmentary degeneration in abetalipoproteinemia. Note pigment splotches near the macula.

the outer granular layer and deposition of rounded bodies in the optic nerve.[175]

In *Hooft's syndrome* there are decreased β-lipoproteins, retarded growth, and skin disease.[81] Tapetoretinal degeneration of the Leber's type may be a concomitant feature.

SPHINGOLIPIDOSES

Disease	*Eye signs*
Farber's disease	Gray macula
Krabbe's disease	Optic atrophy
Metachromatic leukodystrophy	Gray macula, optic atrophy
Niemann-Pick disease	Cherry-red spot
Gaucher's disease	Brown pingueculas, strabismus, cherry-red spot (rare)
Fabry's disease	Corneal whorl deposits, saccular retinal and conjunctival vessels, cataract
Lactosyl ceramidosis	Gray macula, optic atrophy
Tay-Sachs disease	Cherry-red spot, optic atrophy
GM_2 gangliosidosis (type 2)	Cherry-red spot, optic atrophy
GM_2 gangliosidosis (type 3)	Retinal pigmentary degeneration, optic atrophy

The sphingolipidoses are a group of diseases characterized by deficiency of specific lysosomal enzymes involved in the degradation of gangliosides. These lipid substances are in high concentrations in nervous tissue. Their functions in gray matter are poorly understood. The clinical description of many of these diseases prior to their biochemical definition results in an often confusing eponymic array of "amaurotic idiocies" or cerebroretinal degenerations.[39] Except where noted, these diseases are inherited in autosomal recessive fashion. The elucidation of enzyme abnormalities now permits specific diagnosis of those affected, prenatally and postnatally, and of the carrier state.[128] The multilaminated bodies, seen in these entities by electron microscopy, are believed to be distended, distorted lysosomes.[144]

In *Farber's disease,* ceramide accumulates because of ceramidase deficiency.[166] This is associated with lipogranulomas in the nervous system and lesions in the skin, joints, and larynx. A parafoveal gray retinal density and peripheral retinal pigmentation are reported in at least one case.[24]

Krabbe's disease, or globoid leukodystrophy, results primarily from galactosyl ceramide–β-galactosidase deficiency and galactocerebroside deposition in macrophages.[168] This is the only one of the storage diseases in which no lipid is increased above normal levels.[5] Myelin degeneration is diffuse.[43] Progressive mental and neurologic deterioration begin at 3 to 6 years of age, with demise within 1 to 2 years. Blindness and deafness are common. Optic atrophy is prominent.[22]

Arylsulfatase A is absent in *metachromatic leukodystrophy.* Galactocerebroside sulfate deposits in neurons and renal tubules. Myelin disintegration occurs. Paralysis, dystonia, ataxia, and dementia usually begin at 1 to 2 years, resulting in death by the age of 10. A more delayed juvenile form and a rare adult form are described.[117] Vision is affected late. Ocular signs include optic atrophy, macular grayness[23] and occasionally a subtle central red macular spot. The milder juvenile variant reflects a deficiency of all the isoenzymes of arylsulfatase and presents with skeletal and visceral abnormalities similar to those of the mucopolysaccharidoses. Corneal deposits sometimes are seen. Adding the deficient enzyme to tissue cultures of cells from patients with metachromatic leukodystrophy reverses the biochemical abnormality, but enzyme replacement appears less successful clinically.[178]

Niemann-Pick disease is an autosomal recessive disorder classically caused by sphingomyelin deposition in the brain and viscera. At least five forms of the disease are known.[52] The infantile form, the most common, is characterized by hepatosplenomegaly, psychomotor retardation, and death in infancy. Sphingomyelinase is deficient. In type B, the nervous system is spared, the life-span may be normal, and no ocular lesions are seen. Type C has neural and visceral involvement. It follows a chronic course, with death in adolescence.[44, 154] Type D is similar but occurs only in Nova Scotian families. Apparently normal patients with sphingomyelin accumulation are found in group E which may be genetically and chemically a different disease.[52]

About 50% of the Niemann-Pick type A patients have true cherry-red spots in their maculas.[22] Blindness is common. A reddish-brown macula and diminished B wave of the electroretinogram (ERG) are described in one of the chronic forms.[154] Type C usually has a normal fundus and ERG or occasionally a cherry-red spot. Ballooning of the retinal ganglion cells is described histologically,[145] in addition to the presence of membranous cytoplasmic bodies in most ocular structures.[144] Increased translucency of the sclera occurs.[44] Cherry-red spots are not noted in the Nova Scotia variant. The syndrome of the "sea-blue histiocyte" is considered to be another Niemann-Pick variant. In adults it is associated with a white perimacular opacity that produces no visual deficit.[22, 180]

Gaucher's disease, a glucocerebrosidase defect, occurs in adult, juvenile, and infantile forms. Reticuloendothelial storage of glucocerebroside results in hepatosplenomegaly, bone-marrow infiltration, and secondary hematologic complications in all types. The infantile form has central nervous system involvement. Strabismus is frequent. Yellow-brown wedge-shaped pingueculas occur in 25% of the adult patients.[101] Perimacular degeneration[25] and cherry-red spots[111] occasionally are reported. Corneal clouding is described in one case.[7]

In *Fabry's disease,* ceramide trihexoside accumulates. α-Galactosidase (ceramide trihexosidase) is either deficient or structurally altered.[80, 94] Telangiectatic skin lesions of angiokeratoma corporis diffusum, episodes of fever, and pain begin in adolescence. Death occurs in adulthood from cardiac or renal failure. Histopathologic deposits of glycolipid may be found in blood vessel endothelium, renal glomeruli, sympathetic nerves, epithelium, and smooth muscle.[47] This is a sex-linked recessive disease. Ocular manifestations occur in 90% of cases.[51] Systemic

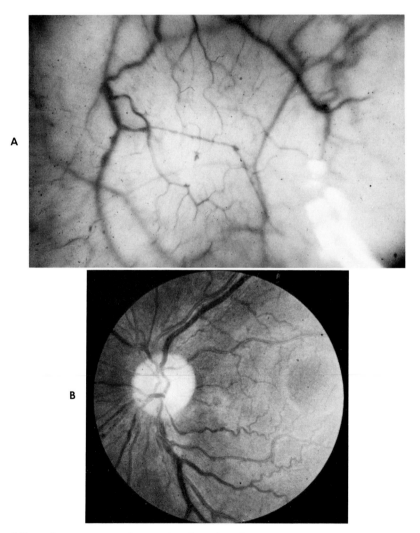

Fig. 3-7. A, Saccular tortuosity and beading of conjunctival vessels in a man with Fabry's disease. **B,** Tortuous, corkscrew retinal vessels of same patient.

and ocular manifestations are more frequently expressed in males. The Lyon hypothesis of random X-chromosome inactivation may account for the variable expression in female carriers. Decreased enzyme levels identify the female heterozygote. Her skin fibroblasts grown in tissue culture may be cloned into two distinct populations, one abnormal and one normal. Saccular tortuosity and corkscrewing of conjunctival and retinal vessels are seen in 60% of males (Fig. 3-7). It relates to ceramide trihexoside deposition in vessel walls. Retinal edema, periorbital and macular edema, and papilledema may occur, but are probably secondary to renal disease.[161] The most characteristic lesion is a bronze-colored deposit in a whorl pattern in the corneal epithelium (Fig. 3-8) associated with a gold dust corneal haze. This is similar to the corneal lesion seen in chloroquine keratopathy. Visual acuity is not impaired. The corneal lesion occurs in most female carriers also. In the past it was considered a separate entity, cornea verticillata of Fleischer.[51] The ophthalmologist's ability to identify the carrier state assumes importance in genetic counseling. These deposits are found in the basal epithelial cells of the cornea and in the associated ridges in the basement membrane.[176] Posterior subcapsular lens opacities and a star-shaped condensation of lens sutures are reported in 50% of cases[161] (Fig. 3-9).

Since Fabry's disease does not involve the central nervous system, enzyme replacement therapy is not limited by the blood-brain barrier. Infusions of normal plasma reverse the biochemical abnormalities but are limited by a short half-life.[110] A more intriguing approach is the use of renal transplantation, presumably with new enzyme production by the homograft. This relieves the symptoms and biochemical abnormalities in some cases.[37, 136] The mechanism of the correction of the basic metabolic defect by transplantation is disputed.[19]

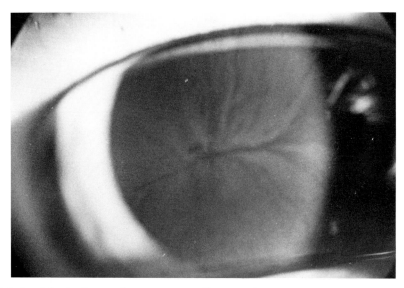

Fig. 3-8. In Fabry's disease the corneas of affected males and carrier females may demonstrate superficial, bronze-colored, whorl-like deposits resembling chloroquine keratopathy. (Courtesy Dr. H. Saul Sugar, Detroit, Mich.)

Lactosyl ceramidosis, a disease caused by a defect originally postulated to exist in the pathway between the compounds that accumulate in Fabry's and Gaucher's diseases, has recently been described in a child with cerebral degeneration, ataxia, and hepatosplenomegaly.[33] Progressive optic atrophy and mild macular grayness were seen. Deficiency of lactosyl ceramide galactosyl hydrolase was demonstrated.[34]

Several entities result from deficiency of hexosaminidase A or B or both. All involve storage of GM_2 ganglioside, Tay-Sachs ganglioside. The enzyme deficiencies are identifiable in a variety of tissues of those affected, in cultured amniotic fluid cells and, in intermediate degrees, in heterozygote carriers.[125, 131]

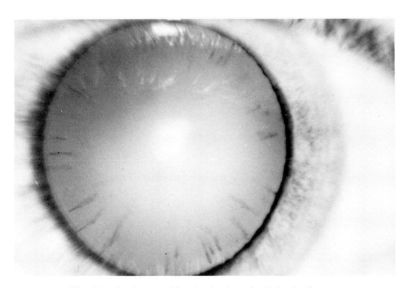

Fig. 3-9. Spoke opacities in the lens in Fabry's disease.

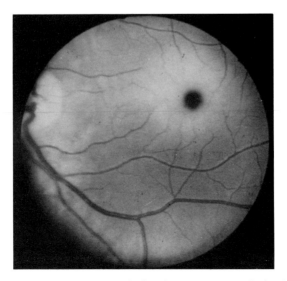

Fig. 3-10. Cherry-red spot of Tay-Sachs disease, GM_2 gangliosidosis, type I.

Tay-Sachs disease (GM₂ gangliosidosis, type 1) is the first described and the most common gangliosidosis. Hexosaminidase A is absent.[39] This defect can be detected in white blood cells, serum, tears, or cultures of amniotic fluid cells.[129] Heterozygotes can be detected by reduced enzyme levels in these tissues and even in assay of tears.[17] The enzyme defect is demonstrable in the retina.[27] About one in 30 to 50 Ashkenazi Jews and one in 300 non-Jews carry this recessive gene.[39] Affected infants are usually normal at birth. Motor weakness appears about 6 months of age followed by startle reactions to sound (hyperacusis), progressive deafness, early blindness, and convulsions. Macrocephaly develops after the first year. Death occurs usually by the age of 3. A white opacification of the macula caused by GM₂ ganglioside deposition in ganglion cells allows the choroidal vasculature to show through as the typical foveal cherry-red spot in at least 90% of cases (Fig. 3-10). Optic atrophy is present early.[39] Although patients are usually blind by 12 months, the pupillary light reflex may be intact throughout their course. Therefore, the blindness may be partially of central rather than retinal origin.[157] Strabismus and loss of following movements occur early followed by progressive decline in all oculomotor function.[87] Electron microscopy reveals characteristic cytoplasmic laminated storage bodies in nervous tissue.[144]

Sandhoff's disease (GM₂ gangliosidosis, type 2) has neurologic and ocular signs similar to those of Tay-Sachs disease. In addition, there is visceral accumulation of a number of related glycosphingolipids, including globoside. Skeletal abnormalities, coarse facies and features similar to those seen in Hurler's disease may be present.[98] These patients are of non-Jewish origin. Both the A and B forms of hexosaminidase are absent.[8]

Juvenile Tay-Sachs disease (GM₂ gangliosidosis, type 3) is differentiated by later onset, from 2 to 6 years, with death from age 5 to 15. Visual loss occurs late. Cherry-red spots are absent. Optic atrophy and pigmentary retinopathy may be present late in the course.[39] Hexosaminidase A is partially deficient in this variant,[167] which may be allelic with the disorder of Tay-Sachs.[5] This disease is often confused in the older literature with the juvenile amaurotic idiocies of Batten-Mayou and Spielmeyer-Vogt. In the latter disorders, retinitis pigmentosa, macular pigmentation, and blindness are early signs. These disorders have normal sphingolipids but accumulate ceroid-lipofuscin in neurons.[188] A deficiency of myeloperoxidase is described.

MUCOLIPIDOSES

Disease	Eye signs
GM₁ gangliosidosis (type 1)	Cherry-red spot, optic atrophy, corneal clouding
GM₁ gangliosidosis (type 2)	Retinal pigmentary degeneration, optic atrophy
Lipomucopolysaccharidosis	Cherry-red spot, corneal clouding
Pseudo-Hurler polydystrophy	Corneal opacities
Mannosidosis	Cataract
Goldberg variant	Cherry-red spot, corneal clouding

The mucolipidoses (MLS) are disorders with both ganglioside and mucopolysaccharide accumulation. Biochemically and clinically they are intermediate between the sphingolipidoses and the mucopolysaccharidoses. The most important members of this group for the ophthalmologist are the two forms of GM₁ gangliosidosis.

GM$_1$ type 1, generalized gangliosidosis, is characterized by storage of GM$_1$ ganglioside, the normal major brain ganglioside, in brain and viscera and a keratan sulfate–like substance in viscera.[156] Both vacuolated and multilaminated inclusions can be found on electron microscopy. The A, B, and C isoenzymes of β-D-galactosidase are deficient. This leads to impaired cleavage of galactose from both ganglioside and mucopolysaccharide. Severe progressive cerebral degeneration occurs from birth. The patients become convulsive, deaf, and decerebrate. They die by the age of 2 years. Frontal bossing, low-set ears, hirsutism, and macroglossia give an appearance resembling Hurler's syndrome. However, mucopolysacchariduria is absent. Hepatosplenomegaly and skeletal changes of dysostosis are prominent.[124] Ocular findings include esotropia, nystagmus, optic nerve pallor, and retinal arteriolar narrowing or tortuosity.[45, 82] Cherry-red spots are seen in the maculas of about 50% of cases. Mild corneal clouding is noted in two of 16 cases.[45]

GM$_1$ type 2, juvenile gangliosidosis, has its initial neurologic symptoms at about 1 year of age. These include locomotor ataxia and mental deterioration. Seizures, blindness, and death follow from 3 to 10 years of age.[36, 124] No visceromegaly or bony changes are present. Optic atrophy, strabismus, esotropia, and pigmentary degeneration of the retina are present in some patients.[127] Macular and corneal changes are not reported. The enzyme deficiency may be allelic to that in type 1. Only the B and C isoenzymes of β-galactosidase are deficient.[156]

Lipomucopolysaccharidosis (MLS-I) is clinically similar to the GM$_1$ diseases. It, too, is associated with cherry-red spots in the macula and corneal clouding.[69] *I-cell disease* (MLS-II) is very similar to Hurler's disease but lacks corneal clouding. *Pseudo-Hurler polydystrophy* (MLS-III) is characterized by fine corneal opacities without retinal abnormalities.[140] Goldberg et al. describe a patient with dwarfism, gargoylism, and mental retardation who had corneal clouding, and macular cherry-red spots. This represents another variant in this intermediate group of diseases.[69]

Mannosidosis is characterized by symptoms and signs similar to Hurler's syndrome but no mucopolysaccharide storage. α-Mannosidase is deficient. The only ocular finding is occasional capsular lenticular opacity.[38, 130]

MUCOPOLYSACCHARIDOSES

Disease	Eye signs
Hurler's syndrome	Corneal clouding, retinal pigmentary degeneration, optic atrophy
Hunter's syndrome	Retinal pigmentary degeneration, optic atrophy
Sanfilippo's syndrome	Retinal pigmentary degeneration, optic atrophy
Morquio's syndrome	Corneal clouding
Scheie's syndrome	Corneal clouding, retinal pigmentary degeneration
Maroteaux-Lamy syndrome	Corneal clouding
Winchester's syndrome	Peripheral corneal opacity and furrow

The mucopolysaccharidoses (MPS) are a group of diseases characterized by deposition of mucopolysaccharide in tissue and their excess urinary excretion. Several recently described syndromes and further biochemical definition suggest modification of their original classification. All are autosomal recessive in inheritance except Hunter's syndrome.

Electron microscopic studies of conjunctival biopsies and other ocular tissues

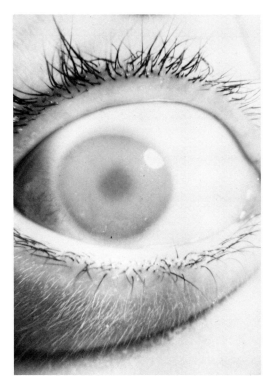

Fig. 3-11. Hazy, diffuse, ground-glass appearance of the cornea in patient with classic, late-stage Hurler's syndrome.

in the mucopolysaccharidoses demonstrate two types of cytoplasmic inclusions. Fibrillogranular vacuoles are believed to contain mucopolysaccharides. Membranous lamellar vacuoles, or zebra bodies, probably containing glycolipids are similar to those found in the sphingolipidoses.[91, 141, 170] Gangliosides may be increased in this group of diseases. Carrier detection and prenatal diagnosis are becoming possible.[113]

Hurler's syndrome (MPS-I) is the most common form of mucopolysaccharidosis. Patients present in early childhood with large heads, coarse facies, stiff joints, large tongue, skeletal abnormalities, deafness, visceromegaly, cardiac defects, and severe mental and growth retardation.[177] Ptosis, proptosis, and hypertelorism may occur.[56] The cornea is clear at birth. Characteristically, it becomes progressively opacified by fine gray stromal deposits of mucopolysaccharide, beginning peripherally and posteriorly, leading to a ground-glass appearance (Fig. 3-11).[64] Retinal pigmentary degeneration is common.[49, 56] The ERG amplitude usually decreases with increasing age and probably all patients are so affected.[104] Optic atrophy is frequently noted and may be secondary either to the retinal disease or hydrocephalus. Vacuolation of the iris pigment epithelium is present histologically. Urinary excretion of dermatan sulfate and heparan sulfate and metachromatic vacuolated intracellular inclusions suggest the diagnosis. The discovery that the supernatant fluid of fibroblast cultures from patients with one mucopolysaccharide disease produces correction of the biochemical and cellular defects in tissue culture of another, suggests the existence of different deficient corrective factors. This technique provides a means of distinguishing diseases. Such studies suggest that Hurler's syndrome and Scheie's syndrome are not mutually corrective and are biochemically identical.[177] The deficient enzyme is α-L-iduronidase in both.[3] *Scheie's syndrome* describes patients with corneal clouding, mild skeletal abnormalities, and normal intelligence.[152] The corneal haze is noted at birth or shortly after birth in all corneal layers, requiring differentiation from congenital glaucoma. The opacity is slowly progressive. It results in severe visual loss and responds poorly to corneal transplantation.[26] Night blindness, retinal perivascular pigmentation, and subnormal or nonrecordable ERGs usually are noted and may be present to some degree in all cases.[104] McKusick explains the presence of these two clinically separate entities with identical enzyme deficiencies by the hypothesis of allelism. Patients are homozygous for different alleles at the same genetic locus.[109] In other words, there may be two different defects in the production of the same enzyme, one severe and one mild.

Hunter's syndrome (MPS-II) is distinguished from the other mucopolysaccharidoses by sex-linked inheritance. Clinical features are similar to those of Hurler's syndrome but are less severe. Mixed-culture techniques readily separate these entities. Corneal clouding is usually absent although slit-lamp findings of slight stromal haze are noted at times.[56, 170] Chronic papilledema, optic atrophy, and progressive pigmentary retinopathy, documented with diminished ERG amplitude occur.[56] It is the only MPS in which some patients have normal and others have abnormal ERGs.[104] Histopathologic findings indistinguishable from typical retinitis pigmentosa are reported.[65] There is some clinical but no laboratory evidence that more than one form of Hunter's syndrome exists. Some patients appear to have very mild involvement with normal intelligence.[107] The existence of allelism can be invoked. There is a deficiency of sulfoiduronate sulfatase.[5]

In the *Sanfilippo syndrome* (MPS-III), skeletal changes and hepatosplenomegaly are mild, but mental retardation is very severe. Heparan sulfate is the predominant storage substrate. Corneal clouding does not occur. Optic atrophy and retinal pigmentary abnormalities, manifested by changes in ERG findings, are common.[56, 66, 104] Biochemically, two nonallelic forms are evident on the basis of mixed culture experiments.[96] Deficiency of N-acetyl-α-D-glucosaminidase is found in one clinical type of Sanfilippo syndrome and of heparan sulfate sulfatase in the other. The two diseases are clinically identical.[126]

The *Morquio syndrome* (MPS-IV) is distinguished by the characteristic skeletal changes of severe dwarfing, barrel chest, and crouch posture. Intelligence may or may not be affected. Fine gray peripheral corneal opacities develop late and are slowly progressive.[66] The fundi and ERG appearance are normal.[104] In contradistinction to the other mucopolysaccharidoses, keratan sulfate is the abnormally stored mucopolysaccharide. The specific enzyme deficiency is unknown.

Maroteaux-Lamy syndrome (MPS-VI) is characterized by normal intelligence and moderate visceral and skeletal changes. Two allelic forms of this syndrome may exist as well. Corneal haze develops early.[68] Histopathologically, acid mucopolysaccharide accumulates intracellularly and extracellularly in the cornea and sclera.[91] Papilledema, secondary to hydrocephalus, and optic atrophy may occur.[68]

Retinal vascular tortuosity may be present. Pigmentary retinal changes are not described and ERG appearances are normal.[91, 104]

The discovery of corrective factors in the mucopolysaccharidoses suggested that replacement therapy may be efficacious. There is experimental and early clinical evidence that plasma infusion providing the deficient enzyme might be of value in the treatment of the mucopolysaccharidoses.[3, 83, 90]

Some intermediate forms of the mucopolysaccharidoses have been described above as the mucolipidoses; other unclassified forms have been reported. Still others might represent the combination of two different allelic abnormal genes at the same genetic locus, analogous to the mixed hemoglobinopathies, such as sickle cell–hemoglobin C (SC) disease.[109] Progressive peripheral corneal opacities have been noted in two patients with *Winchester's syndrome.*[183] This disease is not a lysosomal storage disorder. These patients had features of both rheumatoid arthritis and the mucopolysaccharidoses. They were described by Brown and Kuwabara as having peripheral annular corneal furrowing with vascularization.[11] *Chondroitin-4-sulfate mucopolysaccharidosis* has been described in an adult[169] and a child[134] with peripheral corneal haze.

CARBOHYDRATE DISEASES

Disease	*Eye signs*
Galactosemia	Cataract
Galactokinase deficiency	Cataract

Although many disorders of carbohydrate metabolism including diabetes mellitus and the glycogen storage diseases exist, only two will be discussed.

Classical *galactosemia* results from deficiency of galactose-1-phosphate uridyl transferase, an enzyme in the conversion pathway from galactose to glucose. This enzyme can be measured in blood cells and tissue culture. As a result of the deficiency, galactose-1-phosphate accumulates, as does dulcitol (galactitol), its reduction product.[76] Dietary galactose is provided by the lactose of milk. Thus, after postnatal feeding, patients develop the signs and symptoms of the disease. These include failure to thrive, hepatosplenomegaly, hypoglycemic convulsions, jaundice, generalized aminoaciduria, and eventually mental retardation. They may die if untreated. Cataracts are present in 70% of cases[121, 123] (Fig. 3-12). Dulcitol deposition in the lens produces hyperosmotic swelling and altered lens permeability.[59, 93, 173] Vacuolar "oil droplet" changes are present in the lens early. The later lens changes may be anterior cortical, zonular, lamellar, or posterior cortical.[102, 182] Lens changes may be seen as early as the first week of life.[123] It is not established whether heterozygotes for this autosomal recessive condition have an increased incidence of cataracts. A number of variants of this enzyme deficiency are described. The "Duarte" variant is asymptomatic,[60] but the "Indiana" variant is associated with nuclear cataract.[18]

The treatment for all forms of galactosemia is dietary elimination of galactose. Treatment before a critical point in the early months of infancy may prevent cataract formation and progression or cause regression of early changes.[93, 123] The use of tetramethylene glutaric acid, an aldose reductase inhibitor, prevents dulcitol formation in lenses in tissue culture.[55] Experimentally, the enzyme deficiency may

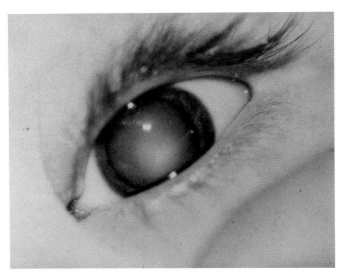

Fig. 3-12. Complete opacification of lens in patient with untreated galactosemia. (Courtesy Dr. Edward Cotlier, Lake Forest, Ill.)

be corrected in skin fibroblast cultures from galactosemic patients by transduction with a bacteriophage containing the transferase gene. Presumably, new genetic material is incorporated into the deficient cells.[112] Although not yet applicable to patients, this method suggests exciting modes of genetic engineering as a treatment for this metabolic disease.

The first step in galactose metabolism is dependent on the enzyme galacto-kinase. *Galactokinase deficiency* is associated with cataracts similar to those seen in transferase deficiency.[58, 106, 123] These patients are generally otherwise healthy although progressive neurologic disease is described in one family.[137] Early onset of cataract is noted in one out of seven heterozygotes for this enzyme deficiency.[106, 115] In another study, although children with unexplained cataracts demonstrated normal galactokinase activity, many of their mothers had low levels of this enzyme.[74b] Galactose restriction is suggested for both patients and carriers. Regression of lens changes may occur after treatment.[106]

AMINO ACID ABNORMALITIES

Disease	Eye signs
Albinism	Transilluminable iris, visible choroidal vessels, nystagmus, strabismus, photophobia
Familial dysautonomia	Alacrimia, poor corneal sensation, exotropia, corneal ulcers
Tyrosine aminotransferase deficiency	Corneal ulcers
Alkaptonuria	Scleral brown deposits
Homocystinuria	Ectopia lentis, glaucoma, peripheral retinal degeneration, myopia
Sulfite oxidase deficiency	Ectopia lentis, optic atrophy
Hyperlysinemia	Ectopia lentis, spherophakia

Disease	*Eye signs*
Hypophosphatasia	Band keratopathy, proptosis, papilledema
Lowe's syndrome	Congenital glaucoma and cataract
Cystinosis	Corneal crystals, peripheral retinal pigmentation
Wilson's disease	Kayser-Fleischer ring, chalcosis lentis
Hyperornithinemia	Gyrate chorioretinal atrophy

The amino acid disorders comprise several broad categories. One group, including albinism, involves enzyme defects in amino acid metabolism that result in deficiency of a necessary product. This first group of disorders is not associated with abnormal urinary amino acids.[41]

Albinism is a group of diseases rather than a single entity. *Oculocutaneous albinism* is an autosomal recessive disease until recently believed to be caused solely by deficiency of tyrosinase. This enzyme is responsible for conversion of the amino acid tyrosine to dopa in the biosynthetic pathway to the formation of melanin. Two forms of oculocutaneous albinism are suggested by the report of two albinotic parents having normal offspring.[120, 172, 184] This is another example of genetic heterogeneity. One form of generalized albinism manifests tyrosinase deficiency. Tyrosinase-negative albinos have white hair, pink skin, and cutaneous photosensitivity. The retinal red reflex is prominent and the pinkish-gray iris readily transmits light (Fig. 3-13). Retinal pigment and the fovea appear absent[48]; choroidal pigment is variable (Fig. 3-14, *A*). Photophobia and nystagmus are common features. Strabismus, predominantly exotropia, is present in two thirds of the cases.[46] High refractive errors, particularly hyperopia and astigmatism, are frequent. Single binocular vision is rare.[46] Vision is usually in the range of 20/200, possibly because of dazzling, pigment epithelial deficiency, or poor foveal development.[48, 101] The scotopic ERG is supernormal during the first two decades of life. It then becomes normal. The electro-oculogram (EOG) may also be supernor-

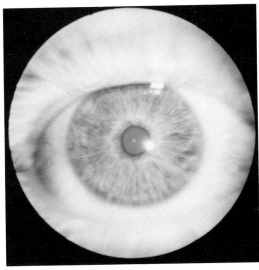

Fig. 3-13. Diaphanous iris, devoid of pigment, readily transilluminates in all forms of albinism.

mal.[97] Treatment with contact lenses from infancy, to decrease light input, is being evaluated.

In another variety of oculocutaneous albinism, tyrosinase levels are normal. Tyrosinase-positive oculocutaneous albinos have yellow hair, lightly pigmented skin, and only moderate photophobia and nystagmus.[5] They tend to develop pigmentation with age, particularly in more pigmented races. The metabolic defect appears to be in transport or utilization of tyrosine.[184] Irides tend to be blue to ochre, with a cartwheel effect on transillumination. Fundus pigmentation also increases with age. Visual acuity may improve throughout childhood.[120]

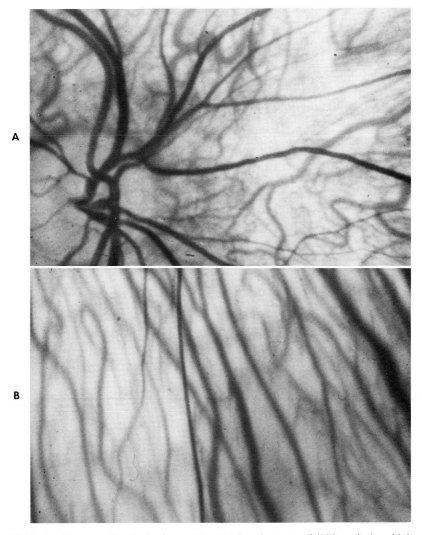

Fig. 3-14. A, Absence of retinal pigment in albinism leads to visibility of choroidal vasculature throughout fundus. **B,** Peripheral fundus of patient shown in **A.** This patient actually had the Chediak-Higashi syndrome.

The *Chediak-Higashi syndrome* includes a form of partial oculocutaneous albinism. Patients demonstrate light grayish hair, photophobia, nystagmus, and decreased uveal and retinal pigmentation[159] (Fig. 3-14, *B*). The systemic disease is characterized by hepatosplenomegaly, lymphadenopathy, and pancytopenia. Cytoplasmic inclusions in white blood cells represent giant defective lysosomes. Immune function is abnormal. The development of recurrent infections or lymphomatous malignancy, or both, lead usually to death in childhood.[88] Subcapsular lens opacities and corneal opacities are seen rarely.[48]

Ocular albinism is a sex-linked recessive condition affecting the eyes alone. The ocular signs and function are similar to that in generalized albinism, but the iris may show some pigmentation.[48] Female carriers may have diaphanous irides and macular and peripheral retinal pigment clumping.[5, 72] However, their visual function usually is normal. Here, too, the ophthalmologist has a distinct role in genetic counseling.

The *Waardenburg syndrome* is an autosomal dominant form of partial albinism. It is characterized by a white forelock, deafness, lateral displacement of the lacrimal puncta, eyebrow confluence, and heterochromia of the iris in 25% of cases.[48, 63] Patches of nonpigmented retina and bilateral anterior lenticonus are reported.[165]

Familial dysautonomia, the Riley-Day syndrome, is an autosomal recessive disorder primarily of Ashkenazi Jews. It is associated with reduced or absent plasma dopamine-β-hydroxylase activity.[179] Patients present in infancy with feeding difficulty, indifference to pain, orthostatic hypotension and absent fungiform tongue papillae. Ophthalmologic findings include alacrimia, decreased or absent corneal sensation, exotropia, and miosis after 2.5% methacholine instillation.[67] Corneal ulcers are frequent and tear substitutes or tarsorrhaphy are often necessary. Myopia and tortuosity of the retinal vessels frequently occur. Glaucoma is mentioned in one case report.[57] Absence of flare on intradermal histamine injection is diagnostic. Treatment with systemic bethanechol may be of value in increasing tear function and reducing gastrointestinal symptoms.[2]

Primary aminoacidurias

Certain amino acid abnormalities reflect specific enzyme deficiencies that lead to increased blood levels of substrate in addition to diminution of product. Depending on renal tubular capacity for resorption of that amino acid, excess urinary excretion becomes manifest.[41]

Tyrosinemia is described in two forms. The classic form presents with hepatosplenomegaly, cirrhosis, renal defects, and rickets.[5] One case report notes cataracts that developed during youth.[100] Another form is tyrosine aminotransferase (TAT) deficiency (type II). These patients show mental deficiency, palmar and plantar keratosis, and bilateral superficial stellate central corneal ulcers in infancy.[13, 14] Feeding rats large amounts of tyrosine may produce a corneal lesion.[15]

Deficiency of the enzyme homogentisic acid oxidase is the cause of *alkaptonuria.* This autosomal recessive disease is characterized by ochronosis, the deposition of brown-colored pigment in cartilaginous and fibrous tissue.[5, 99] Arthritis is a prominent sequela. This pigment is seen in the sclera near the insertion of the horizontal recti usually in patients by the age of 30 (Fig. 3-15). The conjunctiva

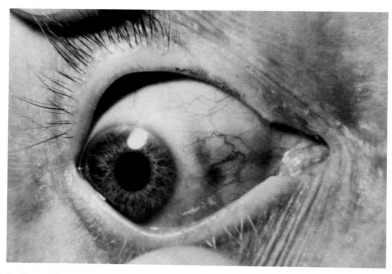

Fig. 3-15. Deposition of ochre pigment in sclera over medial rectus insertion in alkaptonuria.

may be diffusely involved by fine deposits. Golden-brown deposits may be seen in the superficial cornea near the limbus.[48]

Homocystinuria is a recently described disease. Yet it is rapidly becoming more important to the clinical opthalmologist for at least two reasons. First, it may present initially with ocular signs. Second, some patients are responsive to systemic therapy. Cystathionine synthetase activity is deficient in this disease. Homocystine accumulates in blood and urine, and methionine accumulates in the blood. Genetic heterogeneity exists.[119] In some cases, enzyme activity can be stimulated with pyridoxine, the coenzyme, and folate.[116] This leads to a biochemical cure. Follow-up studies are too short to document amelioration of signs. About half the patients with this autosomal recessive disease are mentally retarded. Most have fair hair and skin, malar flush, joint stiffness, arachnodactyly, and mild skeletal anomalies.[48] Some have seizures and hepatomegaly. There is a strong tendency to thromboembolic disease, and death is frequently the result of vascular accidents. Some patients have died during ophthalmic operations. One article suggests that a combination of 100 mg. of dipyridamole and 1 gram of aspirin daily prevents the platelet hyperutilization responsible for these vascular accidents.[71a] Ocular findings are prominent. Most patients present with dislocated lenses.[29, 85] It is estimated that the disease accounts for 5% of all patients with nontraumatic ectopia lentis. The lenses are disclocated downward or nasally in almost two thirds of the cases and frequently dislocate into the anterior chamber (Fig. 3-16) or vitreous.[29] Secondary pupillary block glaucoma is frequent.[108] Buphthalmos is described. Retinal detachment can occur either before or after surgical intervention. Although the risks of general anesthesia and vitreous loss are considerable, lens extraction when indicated has a moderately favorable prognosis.[29, 85] Other ocular features include cataracts, optic atrophy,[139] retinal artery occlusion,[108, 181] high myopia,[48] and pigmentary mottling near the ora serrata (Fig. 3-17). Histopathologic studies show peripheral retinal degneration (Fig. 3-18) and PAS-positive deposits, which are zonular fragments, on the ciliary body.[143] These may be progressive changes.

Because patients with homocystinuria may have an appearance similar to cases of *Marfan's syndrome,* a few differentiating features should be mentioned. Marfan's syndrome is dominantly transmitted and is not associated with mental retardation. Lens dislocation is slightly less frequent, occurs later in life, and is directed superi-

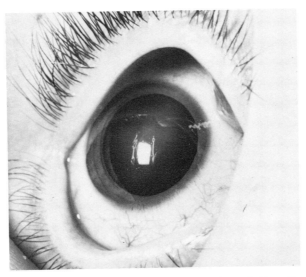

Fig. 3-16. Lens is dislocated down and into anterior chamber of this patient with homocystinuria.

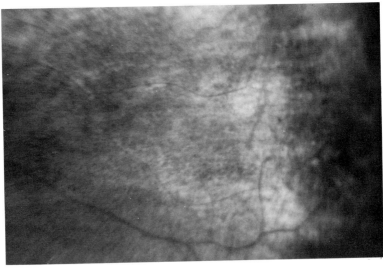

Fig. 3-17. Pigmentary mottling near ora serrata in a young girl with homocystinuria.

orly in two thirds of the cases[29] (Fig. 3-19). Patients with homocystinuria are best distinguished by the easily accomplished urinary cyanide nitroprusside screening test, analysis of urinary amino acids, or enzyme assays.[5, 71, 146] All patients with nontraumatic ectopia lentis should be screened biochemically.

Sulfite oxidase deficiency was reported in a patient with severe psychomotor retardation, muscular ridigity, and death in infancy. The lenses were bilaterally

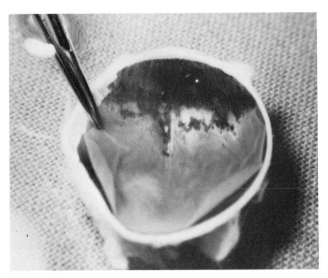

Fig. 3-18. Gross pathologic demonstration of peripheral retinal degeneration in homocystinuria. (Courtesy Dr. Myron Yanoff, Philadelphia, Penn.)

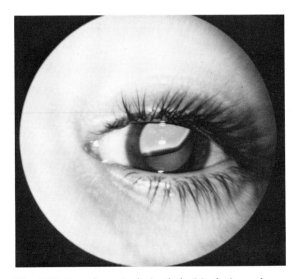

Fig. 3-19. Superior ectopia lentis in Marfan's syndrome.

dislocated. Blindness and nystagmus were present.[84] Like homocystinuria, this defect involved the metabolism of sulfur-containing amino acids.[118] It might provide a clue about zonular biochemistry.

Hyperlysinemia has been associated with bilateral lens dislocation in one case and spherophakia in another, in addition to retarded growth and joint laxity.[160]

Hypophosphatasia is distinguished by low serum alkaline phosphatase and urinary excretion of phosphoethanolamine. Skeletal deformities similar to rickets, craniostenosis, and hypercalcemia may be present.[5] Ocular findings may include band keratopathy, conjunctival calcification, orbital malformations, blue scleras, cataracts, proptosis, and papilledema.[9, 103]

Other metabolic aminoacidurias are less frequently associated with eye disease. *Phenylketonuria* is a common amino acid defect. Its signs include mental retardation and an albinoid appearance. The only ocular findings are light-colored irides and very rarely lamellar congenital cataracts.[133] In *maple-syrup urine disease*, delayed optic nerve maturation, nystagmus, ptosis, strabismus, and lens opacities are reported.[48, 147] Choreoathetoid ocular movements are noted in a case of *hyperalaninemia with hyperpyruvicemia*.[138]

Recently, 15 patients were described with gyrate atrophy of the retina and choroid and hyperornithinemia.[168a] These patients demonstrated extinguished electroretinograms, abnormal electro-oculograms, various degrees of night blindness, cataracts, myopia, and increased plasma, aqueous humor, and cerebrospinal fluid ornithine levels. Glittering crystals were seen in areas of fundus pigmentation.

Secondary aminoacidurias

The amino acid abnormalities in this group of diseases are secondary to renal tubular defects. These renal defects may be specific, with excretion of defined groups of amino acids, or nonspecific, leading to generalized aminoaciduria.[41]

The *oculocerebrorenal syndrome of Lowe* is believed to be a sex-linked recessive disorder. Severe psychomotor retardation, rickets, muscular hypotonia, generalized aminoaciduria, proteinuria, and acidosis occur in young, blond males.[1, 78] Bilateral cataracts are present at birth in almost all cases. These are dense nuclear, zonular, or polar opacities.[1, 48] Glaucoma occurs congenitally in about two thirds of the cases, often with typical buphthalmos (Fig. 3-20) and optic nerve changes. Posterior synechias, strabismus, nystagmus, and microphthalmos are reported.[1, 48] The patients often are enophthalmic and demonstrate the oculodigital sign. The visual prognosis is generally poor. Histologic specimens reveal angle anomalies and a thin, small lens with warty excrescences.[30] The clinical presence of lens opacities may indicate the carrier state in females,[132] but this is refuted in some studies.[79] The rare occurrence of Lowe's syndrome in females[75] suggests genetic heterogeneity, but it may be a manifestation of the Lyon hypothesis.

Cystinosis is an autosomal recessive disease. A number of forms of this disease exist. Cystine deposition occurs in white blood cells and most tissues.[151] The classic infantile or nephropathic variety includes polyuria, fever, growth retardation, rickets, and progressive renal failure. Demise is often in childhood. An anatomic renal tubular defect results in generalized aminoaciduria, phosphaturia, and glucosuria. The ocular findings are of diagnostic importance but cause no functional deficit.[48] On slit-lamp examination, cystine crystals can be seen in the cornea (Fig.

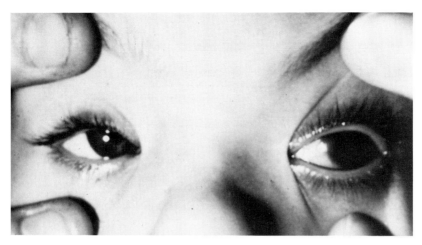

Fig. 3-20. Lowe's syndrome frequently presents with congenital glaucoma. Note buphthalmic left eye.

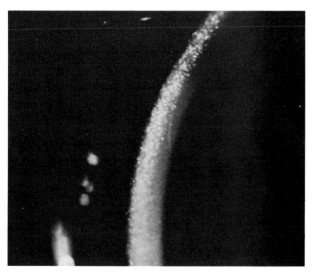

Fig. 3-21. Slit-beam view of cornea in cystinosis. Cystine deposits are predominantly superficial.

3-21) and conjunctiva. Crystals may dust the iris. Myriads of fine, refractile, birefringent, polychromatic deposits are present (Fig. 3-22) in the anterior corneal stroma. The greatest concentration is in the corneal periphery. These are to be differentiated from the corneal crystalline deposits in gout, dysproteinemia, and Bietti's dystrophy. Photophobia may occur although the epithelium is intact.[48, 50] Peripheral pigmentary retinal degeneration with a mottled appearance is a frequent occurrence[50, 150, 185] (Figs. 3-23 and 3-24). Maculopathy is reported.[148] Conjunctival biopsy is a relatively easy method to confirm the diagnosis.[153, 186] The results

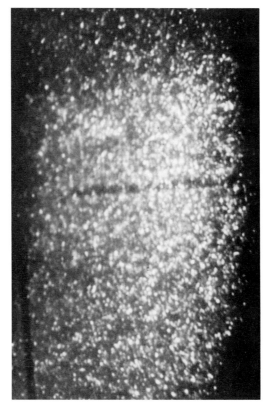

Fig. 3-22. High-power view of multiple, refractile, birefringent cystine crystals in cornea of patient with infantile cystinosis.

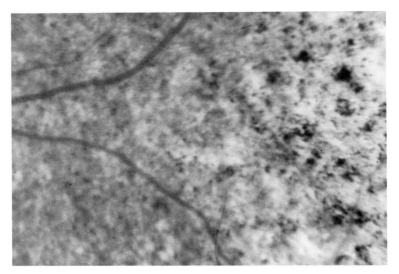

Fig. 3-23. In cystinosis, peripheral retinal pigment splotches and mottling are a frequent occurrence. (Courtesy Dr. Vernon Wong, Washington, D. C.)

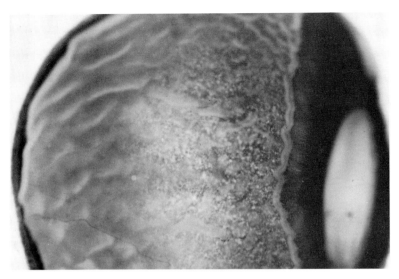

Fig. 3-24. Gross pathologic demonstration of cystinotic eye with peripheral pigmentary disturbance. (Courtesy Dr. Vernon Wong, Washington, D. C.)

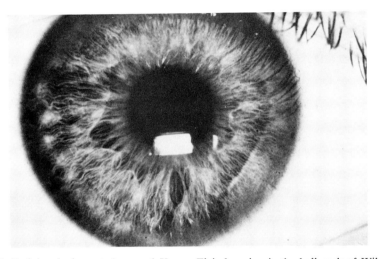

Fig. 3-25. Peripheral pigmented corneal Kayser-Fleischer ring is the hallmark of Wilson's disease.

of tissue examination suggest a lysosomal disorder.[187] The adult benign form of cystinosis is asymptomatic and lacks the renal and retinal changes.[12, 95] A few cases in juveniles or adolescents, with findings intermediate between the other forms, are described.[70] Cystinosis is not to be confused with cystinuria. The latter is a relatively benign disease with no ocular signs.[6]

Wilson's disease, hepatolenticular degeneration, is an autosomal recessive disorder of copper metabolism. There is a deficiency of the copper-binding protein ceruloplasmin. The copper deposition has a predilection for the basal ganglia and liver. Progressive neurologic deterioration, with extrapyramidal signs, and cirrhosis, with hepatic insufficiency, are characteristic. Chorioathetosis with tremor or dystonia with muscle rigidity may ensue. A renal tubular defect leads to generalized aminoaciduria. The ocular lesions are pathognomonic. Copper deposits in Descemet's membrane in the corneal periphery. This produces a complete or incomplete brown to green ring near the limbus known as the Kayser-Fleischer ring (Fig. 3-25). The deposition is most noticeable superiorly and inferiorly. It is seen best in the early stages with the gonioprism.[48] Radiating brownish spokes of copper carbonate on the anterior or posterior lens capsule form the characteristic "sunflower cataract," chalcosis lentis.[16] Both the ocular and systemic signs may regress after

Table 3-1. Inborn errors of metabolism associated with various ocular abnormalities

	Lipid	*Sphingolipid*	*Mucolipid*
Corneal opacity	LCAT deficiency Tangier disease Hyperlipoproteinemias (types I, II, III)	Fabry's disease Niemann-Pick disease (type A)	GM_1 gangliosidosis (type I) Lipomucopolysaccharidosis Pseudo-Hurler polydystrophy Goldberg variant Juvenile metachromatic leukodystrophy
Cataract	Cholestanolosis Refsum's disease	Fabry's disease	Mannosidosis
Ectopia lentis			
Infantile glaucoma			
Cherry-red spot		Tay-Sachs disease GM_2 gangliosidosis (type II) Niemann-Pick disease (type A) Gaucher's disease	GM_1 gangliosidosis (type I) Lipomucopolysaccharidosis Goldberg variant
Gray macula		Farber's disease Metachromatic leukodystrophy Lactosyl ceramidosis	
Retinal pigmentary disease	Refsum's disease Bassen-Kornzweig disease Hooft's syndrome	GM_2 gangliosidosis (type III) Farber's disease (?)	GM_1 gangliosidosis (type II)
Optic atrophy	Refsum's disease Bassen-Kornzweig disease Hooft's syndrome	GM_2 gangliosidoses Krabbe's disease Metachromatic leukodystrophy Lactosyl ceramidosis	GM_1 gangliosidoses

therapy with systemic penicillamine, a drug that chelates copper and leads to its excretion.[35, 114] Treatment in asymptomatic patients to prevent disease is proposed.[164] It is reported that liver transplantation has been attempted in late-stage cirrhosis of Wilson's disease.[40]

Menkes' kinky-hair disease is not an amino acid disorder but is mentioned here because it is caused by a copper defect. The deficiency of copper is secondary to an absorption defect.[31] This sex-linked recessive disease presents with mental retardation, failure to thrive, depigmented steely hair, and arterial lesions.[32, 155] Microcysts of the iris pigment epithelium and decreased retinal ganglion cells are seen. Decreased visual evoked responses document functional abnormalities.[105]

Mucopolysaccharide	Carbohydrate	Amino acid	Miscellaneous
Hurler's syndrome Scheie's syndrome Morquio's syndrome Maroteaux-Lamy syndrome Winchester variant Chondroitin-4-sulfate disease		Hypophosphatasia Wilson's disease Tyrosinemia (type II) Cystinosis	
	Galactosemia Galactokinase deficiency Infantile hypoglycemia Diabetes mellitus	Lowe's syndrome Wilson's disease	Infantile hypopara- thyroidism Pseudohypoparathy- roidism
		Homocystinuria Sulfite oxidase defi- ciency Hyperlysinemia (?)	Marfan's syndrome Marchesani syndrome
	Infantile hypoglycemia	Lowe's syndrome Homocystinuria	Marfan's syndrome Zellwegger's syndrome
Hurler's syndrome Hunter's syndrome Sanfilippo's syndrome Scheie's syndrome		Cystinosis Homocystinuria Hyperornithinemia	Juvenile cerebromacu- lar degenerations
Hurler's syndrome Hunter's syndrome Sanfilippo's syndrome Maroteaux-Lamy syndrome		Hypophosphatasia	Juvenile cerebromacu- lar degenerations Menkes' disease Osteopetrosis

ACKNOWLEDGMENT

Dr. Bernard Becker made helpful suggestions and Thelma Williams provided technical assistance.

GENERAL SOURCES

1. Stanbury, J. B., Wyngaarden, J. B., and Fredrickson, D. S., editors: The metabolic basis of inherited disease, ed. 3, New York, 1972, McGraw-Hill Book Co.
2. McKusick, V. A.: Heritable disorders of connective tissue, ed. 4, St. Louis, 1972, The C. V. Mosby Co.
3. Goldberg, M. F., editor: Genetic and metabolic eye disease, Boston, 1974, Little, Brown & Co.

REFERENCES

1. Abbassi, V., Lowe, C., and Calcagno, P. L.: Oculo-cerebro-renal syndrome—a review, Am. J. Dis. Child. **115:**145, 1968.
2. Axelrod, F. B., Branom, N., Becker, M., Nachtigall, R., and Dancis, J.: Treatment of familial dysautonomia with bethanechol (Urecholine), J. Pediatr. **81:**573, 1972.
3. Bach, G., Friedman, R., Weissmann, B., and Neufeld, E. F.: The defect in the Hurler and Scheie syndromes: Deficiency of α-L-iduronidase, Proc. Nat. Acad. Sci. U.S.A. **69:** 2048, 1972.
4. Baum, J. L., Tannenbaum, M., and Kolodny, E. H.: Refsum's syndrome with corneal involvement, Am. J. Ophthalmol. **60:**699, 1965.
5. Berman, E. R.: Biochemical diagnostic tests in genetic and metabolic eye diseases. In Goldberg, M., editor: Genetic and metabolic eye disease, Boston, 1974, Little, Brown & Co.
6. Bigger, J. F.: Retinal hemorrhages during penicillamine therapy of cystinuria, Am. J. Ophthalmol. **66:**954, 1968.
7. Boudet, M. M., Costeau, J., and Raynaud, J. M.: Opacités cornéennes et maladie de Gaucher, Bull. Soc. Ophtalmol. France **66:**443, 1966.
8. Brady, R. L., and Kolodny, E. H.: Disorders of ganglioside metabolism, Progr. Med. Genet. **8:**225, 1972.
9. Brenner, R. L., Smith, J. L., Cleveland, W. W., Bejar, R. L., and Lockhart, W. S.: Eye signs of hypophosphatasia, Arch. Ophthalmol. **81:**614, 1969.
10. Bron, A. J., and Williams, H. P.: Lipaemia of the limbal vessels, Br. J. Ophthalmol. **56:** 343, 1972.
11. Brown, S. I., and Kuwabara, T.: Peripheral corneal opacification and skeletal deformities, Arch. Ophthalmol. **83:**667, 1970.
12. Brubaker, R. F., Wong, V. G., Schulman, J. D., Seegmiller, J. E., and Kuwabara, T.: Benign cystinosis, Am. J. Med. **49:**546, 1970.
13. Buist, N. R., Kennaway, N. G., and Burns, R. P.: Eye and skin lesions in tyrosinaemia, Lancet **1:**620, 1973.
14. Burns, R. P.: Soluble tyrosine aminotransferase deficiency: An unusual cause of corneal ulcers, Am. J. Ophthalmol. **73:**400, 1972.
15. Burns, R. P., Beard, M., and Squires, E.: Modification of tyrosine-induced keratopathy by adrenal corticosteroid. Read at A.R.V.O. meeting, Sarasota, Florida, May 1973.
16. Cairns, J. E., Williams, H. P., and Walshe, J. M.: "Sunflower cataract" in Wilson's disease, Br. Med. J. **3:**95, 1969.
17. Carmody, P. J., Rattazzi, M. C., and Davidson, R. G.: Tay-Sachs disease: The use of tears for the detection of heterozygotes, Am. J. Hum. Genet. **24:**30A, 1972.
18. Chacko, C. M., Christian, J. C., and Nadler, H. L.: Unstable galactose-1-phosphate uridyltransferase: A new variant of galactosemia, J. Pediatr. **78:**454, 1971.
19. Clarke, J. T., Guttmann, R. T., Wolfe, L. S., Beaudoin, J. G., and Morehouse, D. D.: Enzyme replacement therapy by renal allotransplantation in Fabry's disease, New Eng. J. Med. **287:**1215, 1972.

20. Clifton-Bligh, P., Nestel, P. F., and Whyte, H. M.: Tangier disease, report of a case and studies of lipid metabolism, New Eng. J. Med. **286:**567, 1972.
21. Cogan, D. G.: Ocular correlates of inborn metabolic defects, Can. Med. Assoc. J. **95:** 1055, 1966.
22. Cogan, D. G., and Kuwabara, T.: The sphingolipidoses and the eye, Arch. Ophthalmol. **79:**437, 1968.
23. Cogan, D. G., Kuwabara, T., and Moser, H.: Metachromatic leucodystrophy, Ophthalmologica **160:**2, 1970.
24. Cogan, D. G., Kuwabara, T., Moser, H., and Hazard, G. W.: Retinopathy in a case of Farber's lipogranulomatosis, Arch. Ophthalmol. **75:**752, 1966.
25. Collier, M. M.: Dégénérescence maculaire d'un type spécial dans un cas de maladie de Gaucher, Bull. Soc. Ophtal. France **6:**497, 1961.
26. Constantopoulos, G., Dekaban, A. S., and Scheie, H. G.: Heterogeneity of disorders in patients with corneal clouding, normal intellect, and mucopolysaccharidosis, Am. J. Ophthalmol. **72:**1106, 1971.
27. Cotlier, E.: Tay-Sachs retina: Deficiency of acetyl hexosaminidase A, Arch. Ophthalmol. **86:**352, 1971.
28. Cotlier, E.: Biochemical detection of inborn errors of metabolism affecting the eye, Trans. Am. Acad. Ophthalmol. Otolaryngol. **76:**1165, 1972.
29. Cross, H. E., and Jensen, A. D.: Ocular manifestations in the Marfan syndrome and homocystinuria, Am. J. Ophthalmol. **75:**405, 1973.
30. Curtin, V. T., Joyce, E. E., and Ballin, N.: Ocular pathology in the oculo-cerebro-renal syndrome of Lowe, Am. J. Ophthalmol. **64:**533, 1967.
31. Danks, D. M., Cartwright, E., and Stevens, B. J.: Menkes' steely-hair (kinky-hair) disease, Lancet **1:**891, 1973.
32. Danks, D. M., Stevens, B. J., Campbell, P. E., Gillespie, J. M., Walker-Smith, J., Blomfield, J., and Turner, B.: Menkes' kinky-hair syndrome, Lancet **1:**1100, 1972.
33. Dawson, G., and Stein, A. O.: Lactosyl ceramidosis: Catabolic enzyme defect of glycosphingolipid metabolism, Science **170:**556, 1970.
34. Dawson, G., Matalon, R., and Stein, A. O.: Lactosylceramidosis: Lactosylceramide galactosyl hydrolase deficiency and accumulation of lactosylceramide in cultured skin fibroblasts, J. Pediatr. **79:**423, 1971.
35. Deiss, A., Lynch, R. E., Lee, G. R., and Cartwright, G. E.: Long-term therapy of Wilson's disease, Ann. Intern. Med. **75:**57, 1971.
36. Derry, D. M., Fawcett, J. S., Andermann, F., and Wolfe, L. S.: Late infantile systemic lipidosis, Neurology **18:**340, 1968.
37. Desnick, R. J., Bernlohr, R. W., Simmons, R. L., Najarian, J. S., Sharp, H. L., and Krivit, W.: Enzyme therapy for Fabry's disease, Am. J. Hum. Genet. **24:**23A, 1972.
38. Dorfman, A., and Matalon, R.: The mucopolysaccharidoses. In Stanbury, J. B., Wyngaarden, J. B., and Fredrickson, D. S., editors: The metabolic basis of inherited disease, ed. 3, New York, 1972, McGraw-Hill Book Co., p. 1244.
39. Editorial: Amaurotic family idiocy, Lancet **1:**469, 1973.
40. Editorial: Enzyme transplants, Lancet **2:**1235, 1972.
41. Efron, M. L.: Aminoaciduria, New Eng. J. Med. **272:**1058, 1965.
42. Eldjarn, L., Try, K., Stokke, O., Munthe-Kass, A. W., Refsum, S., Steinberg, D., Avigan, J., and Mize, C.: Dietary effects of serum-phytanic-acid levels and on clinical manifestations in heredopathia atactica polyneuritiformis, Lancet **1:**691, 1966.
43. Emery, J. M., Green, W. R., and Huff, D. S.: Krabbe's disease, histopathology and ultrastructure of the eye, Am. J. Ophthalmol. **74:**400, 1972.
44. Emery, J. M., Green, W. R., Huff, D. S., and Sloan, H. R.: Niemann-Pick disease (type C), Am. J. Ophthalmol. **74:**1144, 1972.
45. Emery, J. M., Green, W. R., Wyllie, R. G., and Howell, R. R.: GM_1-gangliosidosis, ocular and pathological manifestations, Arch. Ophthalmol. **85:**177, 1971.
46. Fonda, G.: Characteristics and low-vision corrections in albinism, Arch. Ophthalmol. **68:**754, 1962.
47. Font, R. L., and Fine, B. S.: Ocular pathology in Fabry's disease, Am. J. Ophthalmol. **73:**419, 1972.

48. François, J.: Ocular manifestations in aminoacidopathies, Adv. Ophthalmol. **25:**28, 1972.
49. François, J., and DeRouck, A.: L'électro-rétino-encéphalographie dans la maladie de Hurler, Ophthalmologica **139:**45, 1960.
50. François, J., Hanssens, M., Coppieters, R., and Evens, L.: Cystinosis—a clinical and histopathologic study, Am. J. Ophthalmol. **73:**643, 1972.
51. François, J., Snacken, J., and Stockmans, L.: Fabry's disease (glycolipid lipidosis), Pathol. Eur. **3:**347, 1968.
52. Fredrickson, D. S., and Sloan, H. R.: Sphingomyelin lipidoses: Niemann-Pick disease. In Stanbury, J. B., Wyngaarden, J. B., and Fredrickson, D. S., editors: The metabolic basis of inherited disease, ed. 3, New York, 1972, McGraw-Hill Book Co., p. 783.
53. Fredrickson, D. S., Gotto, A. M., and Levy, R. I.: Familial lipoprotein deficiency. In Stanbury, J. B., Wyngaarden, J. B., and Fredrickson, D. S., editors: The metabolic basis of inherited disease, ed. 3, New York, 1972, McGraw-Hill Book Co., p. 493.
54. Fredrickson, D. S., Levy, R. I., and Lees, R. S.: Fat transport in lipoproteins—an integrated approach to mechanisms and disorders, New Eng. J. Med. **276:**34, 94, 148, 215, 273, 1967.
55. Gabbay, K. H.: The sorbitol pathway and the complications of diabetes, New Eng. J. Med. **288:**831, 1973.
56. Gills, J. P., Hobson, R., Hanley, W. B., and McKusick, V. A.: Electroretinography and fundus oculi findings in Hurler's disease and allied mucopolysaccharidoses, Arch. Ophthalmol. **74:**596, 1965.
57. Ginsberg, S. P., Polack, F. M., Ravin, M. B., and Smith, M. D.: Autonomic dysfunction syndrome, Am. J. Ophthalmol. **74:**1121, 1972.
58. Gitzelmann, R.: Hereditary galactokinase deficiency, a newly recognized cause of juvenile cataracts, Pediat. Res. **1:**14, 1967.
59. Gitzelmann, R., Curtius, H., and Schneller, I.: Galactitol and galactose-1-phosphate in the lens of a galactosemic infant, Exp. Eye Res. **6:**1, 1967.
60. Gitzelmann, R., Poley, J. R., and Prader, A.: Partial galactose-1-phosphate uridyltransferase deficiency due to a variant enzyme, Helv. Paediatr. Acta **22:**252, 1967.
61. Gjone, E., and Bergaust, B.: Corneal opacity in familial plasma cholesterol ester deficiency, Acta Ophthalmol. **47:**222, 1969.
62. Gjone, E., and Norum, K. R.: Familial serum cholesterol ester deficiency, Acta Med. Scand. **183:**107, 1968.
63. Goldberg, M. F.: Waardenburg's syndrome with fundus and other anomalies, Arch. Ophthalmol. **76:**797, 1966.
64. Goldberg, M. F.: A review of selected inherited corneal dystrophies associated with systemic diseases, Birth Defects: Original Article Series, **VII**(3):13, 1971.
65. Goldberg, M. F., and Duke, J. R.: Ocular histopathology in Hunter's syndrome, Arch. Ophthalmol. **77:**503, 1967.
66. Goldberg, M. F., Maumenee, A. E., and McKusick, V. A.: Corneal dystrophies associated with abnormalities of mucopolysaccharide metabolism, Arch. Ophthalmol. **74:**516, 1965.
67. Goldberg, M. F., Payne, J. W., and Brunt, P. W.: Ophthalmologic studies of familial dysautonomia, Arch. Ophthalmol. **80:**732, 1968.
68. Goldberg, M. F., Scott, C. I., and McKusick, V. A.: Hydrocephalus and papilledema in the Maroteaux-Lamy syndrome (mucopolysaccharidosis type VI), Am. J. Ophthalmol. **69:**969, 1970.
69. Goldberg, M. F., Cotlier, E., Fichenscher, L. G., Kenyon, K., Enat, R., and Borowsky, S.: Macular cherry-red spot, corneal clouding, and β-galactosidase deficiency, Arch. Intern. Med. **128:**387, 1971.
70. Goldman, H., Scriver, C. R., Aaron, K., Delvin, E., and Canlas, Z.: Adolescent cystinosis: Comparison with infantile and adult forms, Pediatrics **47:**979, 1971.
71. Goldstein, J. L., Campbell, B. K., and Gartler, S. M.: Homocystinuria: Heterozygote detection using phytohemagglutinin-stimulated lymphocytes, J. Clin. Invest. **52:**218, 1973.
72. Goodman, G.: Clinical diagnosis of sex-linked ocular disorders. In Congenital anomalies

of the eye (Transactions of the New Orleans Academy of Ophthalmology), St. Louis, 1968, The C. V. Mosby Co., p. 272.

73. Gouras, P., Carr, R. E., and Gunkel, R. D.: Retinitis pigmentosa in abetalipoproteinemia: Effects of vitamin A, Invest. Ophthalmol. **10:**784, 1971.
74. Hamnstrom, B., Gjone, E., and Norum, K. R.: Familial plasma lecithin:cholesterol acyltransferase deficiency, Br. Med. J. **2:**283, 1969.
74a. Harker, L. A., Slichter, S. J., Scott, C. R., and Ross, R.: Homocystinemia, vascular injury and arterial thrombosis, New Eng. J. Med. **291:**538, 1974.
74b. Harley, J. D., Irvine, S., Mutton, P., and Gupta, J. D.: Maternal enzymes of galactose metabolism and the inexplicable infantile cataract, Lancet **2:**259, 1974.
75. Harris, L. S., Gitter, K. A., Galin, M. A., and Plechaty, G. P.: Oculo-cerebro-renal syndrome—report of a case in a baby girl, Br. J. Ophthalmol. **54:**278, 1970.
76. Hill, H. Z., and Puck, T. T.: Errors of metabolism: Galactosemia, Science **179:**1136, 1973.
77. Herndon, J. H., Steinberg, D., and Uhlendorf, B. W.: Refsum's disease: Defective oxidation of phytanic acid in tissue derived cultures from homozygotes and heterozygotes, New Eng. J. Med. **281:**1034, 1969.
78. Holmes, G. E., and Tucker, V.: Oculo-cerebro-renal syndrome, a four generation family study and case reports of two living children, Clin. Pediatr. **11:**119, 1972.
79. Holmes, L. B., McGowan, B. L., and Efron, M. L.: Lowe's syndrome: A search for the carrier state, Pediatrics **44:**358, 1969.
80. Ho, M. W., Beutler, S., Tennant, L., and O'Brien, J. S.: Fabry's disease: Evidence for a physically altered α-galactosidase, Am. J. Hum. Genet. **24:**256, 1972.
81. Hooft, C., Delaey, P., Herpol, J., DeLoore, F., and Verbeeck, J.: Familial hypolipidaemia and retarded development without steatorrhoea, Helv. Paediatr. Acta **17:**1, 1962.
82. Hooft, C., Senesael, L., Delbeke, M. J., Kint, J., and Dacremont, G.: The GM₁ gangliosidosis (Landing disease), Eur. Neurol. **2:**225, 1969.
83. Hussels, I. E., Eikman, E. A., Kenyon, K. R., and McKusick, V. A.: Treatment of mucopolysaccharidoses, Am. J. Hum. Genet. **24:**32A, 1972 (abstract).
84. Irreverre, F., Mudd, S. H., Heizer, W. D., and Laster, L.: Sulfite oxidase deficiency: Studies of a patient with mental retardation, dislocated ocular lenses, and abnormal urinary excretion of *S*-sulfo-L-cysteine, sulfite, and thiosulfate, Biochem. Med. **1:**187, 1967.
85. Jensen, A. D., and Cross, H. E.: Surgical treatment of dislocated lenses in the Marfan syndrome and homocystinuria, Trans. Am. Acad. Ophthalmol. Otolaryngol. **76:**1491, 1972.
86. Jampel, R. S., and Falls, H. F.: Atypical retinitis pigmentosa, acanthocytosis, and heredodegenerative neuromuscular disease, Arch. Ophthalmol. **59:**818, 1958.
87. Jampel, R. S., and Quaglio, N. D.: Eye movements in Tay-Sachs disease, Neurology **14:**1013, 1964.
88. Johnson, D. L., Jacobson, L. W., Toyama, R., and Monahan, R. M.: Histopathology of eyes in Chediak-Higashi syndrome, Arch. Ophthalmol. **75:**84, 1966.
89. Kayden, H. J.: Abetalipoproteinemia, Ann. Rev. Med. **23:**285, 1972.
90. Kenyon, K. R., and Maumenee, I. H.: Effects of plasma infusion on conjunctival ultrastructure in the systemic mucopolysaccharidoses. Read at A.R.V.O. Meeting, Sarasota, Florida, May 1973.
91. Kenyon, K. R., Topping, T. M., Green, W. R., and Maumenee, A. E.: Ocular pathology of the Maroteaux-Lamy syndrome (systemic mucopolysaccharidosis type VI), Am. J. Ophthalmol. **73:**718, 1972.
92. Khachadurian, K., Freyha, R., Mamma'a, M. M., and Baghdassarian, S. A.: A-β-lipoproteinemia and colour-blindness, Arch. Dis. Child. **46:**871, 1971.
93. Kinoshita, J. H.: Cataracts in galactosemia, Invest. Ophthalmol. **4:**786, 1965.
94. Kint, J. A.: Fabry's disease: Alpha-galactosidase deficiency, Science **167:**1268, 1970.
95. Kraus, E., and Lutz, P.: Ocular cystine deposits in an adult, Arch. Ophthalmol. **85:**690, 1971.
96. Kresse, H., and Neufeld, E. F.: The Sanfilippo A corrective factor, J. Biol. Chem. **247:**2164, 1972.

97. Krill, A. E.: Hereditary retinal and choroidal diseases, Hagerstown, Md., 1972, Harper & Row, Publishers, vol. I, p. 258.

98. Krivit, W., Desnick, R. J., Lee, J., Moller, J., Wright, F., Sweeley, C. C., Snyder, P. D., and Sharp, H. L.: Generalized accumulation of neutral glycosphingolipids with GM₂ ganglioside accumulation in the brain, Sandhoff's disease, Am. J. Med. **52:**763, 1972.

99. LaDu, B. N.: Alcaptonuria. In Stanbury, J. B., Wyngaarden, J. B., and Fredrickson, D. S., editors: The metabolic basis of inherited disease, ed. 3, New York, 1972, McGraw-Hill Book Co., p. 308.

100. LaDu, B. N., and Gjessing, L. R.: Tyrosinosis and tyrosinemia. In Stanbury, J. B., Wyngaarden, J. B., and Fredrickson, D. S., editors: The metabolic basis of inherited disease, ed. 3, New York, 1972, McGraw-Hill Book Co., p. 296.

101. Leopold, I. H., and Schwartz, A. L.: Management of inborn errors of metabolism with ocular involvement. In Leopold, I. H., editor: Symposium on ocular therapy, St. Louis, 1972, The C. V. Mosby Co., vol. 5, pp. 1-29.

102. Lerman, S.: The lens in congenital galactosemia, Arch. Ophthalmol. **61:**88, 1959.

103. Lessell, S., and Norton, E. W. D.: Band keratopathy and conjunctival calcification in hypophosphatasia, Arch. Ophthalmol. **71:**497, 1964.

104. Leung, L. E., Weinstein, G. W., and Hobson, R. R.: Further electroretinographic studies of patients with mucopolysaccharidoses, Birth Defects: Original Article Series **VII**(3): 32, 1971.

105. Levy, N. S., and Dawson, W. W.: Electrophysiological abnormalities associated with Menkes' kinky-hair syndrome. Read at A.R.V.O. meeting, Sarasota, Florida, May 1973.

106. Levy, N. S., Krill, A. E., and Beutler, E.: Galactokinase deficiency and cataracts, Am. J. Ophthalmol. **74:**41, 1972.

107. Lichtenstein, J. R., Bilbrey, G. L., and McKusick, V. A.: Clinical and probable genetic heterogeneity within mucopolysaccharidosis II. Report of a family with a mild form, Johns Hopkins Med. J. **131:**425, 1972.

108. Lieberman, T. W., Podos, S. M., and Hartstein, J.: Acute glaucoma, ectopia lentis and homocystinuria, Am. J. Ophthalmol. **61:**252, 1966.

109. McKusick, V. A., Howell, R. R., Hussels, I. E., Neufeld, E. F., and Stevenson, R. E.: Allelism, non-allelism, and genetic compounds among the mucopolysaccharidoses, Lancet **1:**993, 1972.

110. Mapes, C. A., Anderson, R. L., Sweeley, C. C., Desnick, R. J., and Krivit, W.: Enzyme replacement in Fabry's disease, an inborn error of metabolism, Science **169:**987, 1970.

111. Menkes, J. M., Andrews, J. M., and Cancilla, P. A.: The cerebroretinal degenerations, J. Pediatr. **79:**183, 1971.

112. Merril, C. R., Geier, M. R., and Petricciani, J. C.: Bacterial virus gene expression in human cells, Nature **233:**398, 1971.

113. Milunsky, A., and Littlefield, J. W.: The prenatal diagnosis of inborn errors of metabolism, Ann. Rev. Med. **23:**57, 1972.

114. Mitchell, A. M., and Heller, G. L.: Changes in Kayser-Fleischer ring during treatment of hepatolenticular degeneration, Arch. Ophthalmol. **80:**622, 1968.

115. Monteleone, J. A., Bentles, E., Monteleone, P. L., Utz, C. C., and Casey, E. C.: Cataracts, galactosuria, and hypergalactosemia due to galactokinase deficiency in a child, Am. J. Med. **50:**403, 1971.

116. Morrow, G., and Barness, L. A.: Combined vitamin responsiveness in homocystinuria, J. Pediatr. **81:**946, 1972.

117. Moser, H. W.: Sulfatide lipidosis: Metachromatic leukodystrophy. In Stanbury, J. B., Wyngaarden, J. B., and Fredrickson, D. S., editors: The metabolic basis of inherited disease, ed. 3, New York, 1972, McGraw-Hill Book Co., p. 688.

118. Mudd, S. H., Irreverre, F., and Laster, L.: Sulfite oxidase deficiency in man: Demonstration of enzymatic defect, Science **156:**1599, 1967.

119. Mudd, S. H., Levy, H. L., and Morrow, G.: Deranged B-12 metabolism: Effects on sulfur amino acid metabolism, Biochem. Med. **4:**193, 1970.

120. Nance, W. E., Witkop, C. J., and Rawls, R. F.: Genetic and biochemical evidence for two forms of oculocutaneous albinism in man, Birth Defects: Original Article Series **VII**(3):125, 1971.

21. Nordmann, J.: L'Oculiste et la détection préventive systématique de la galactosémie, Ophthalmologica **163:**129, 1971.
122. Norum, K. R., Glomset, J. A., and Gjone, E.: Familial lecithin:cholesterol acyltransferase deficiency. In Stanbury, J. B., Wyngaarden, J. B., and Fredrickson, D. S., editors: The metabolic basis of inherited disease, ed. 3, New York, 1972, McGraw-Hill Book Co., p. 531.
123. Oberman, A. E., Wilson, W. A., Frasier, S. D., Donnell, G. N., and Bergren, W. R.: Galactokinase-deficiency cataracts in identical twins, Am. J. Ophthalmol. **74:**887, 1972.
124. O'Brien, J.: Generalized gangliosidosis, J. Pediatr. **75:**167, 1969.
125. O'Brien, J. S.: Current concepts: Ganglioside storage disease, New Eng. J. Med. **284:** 893, 1971.
126. O'Brien, J. S.: Sanfilippo syndrome: Profound deficiency of alpha-acetylglucosaminidase activity in organs and skin fibroblasts from type-B patients, Proc. Nat. Acad. Sci. U.S.A. **69:**1720, 1972.
127. O'Brien, J.: GM_1 gangliosidoses. In Stanbury, J. B., Wyngaarden, J. B., and Fredrickson, D. S., editors: The metabolic basis of inherited disease, ed. 3, New York, 1972, Mc-Graw-Hill Book Co., p. 639.
128. O'Brien, J. S., Okada, S., Ho, M. W., Fillerup, D. L., Veath, M. L., and Adams, K.: Ganglioside storage diseases, Fed. Proc. **30:**956, 1971.
129. O'Brien, J. S., Okada, S., Fillerup, D. L., Veath, M. L., Adornato, B., Brenner, P. H., and Leroy, J. G.: Tay-Sachs disease: Prenatal diagnosis, Science **172:**61, 1971.
130. Ockerman, P., Autio, S., and Norden, N.: Diagnosis of mannosidosis, Lancet **1:**207, 1973.
131. Okada, S., Veath, M. L., Leroy, J., and O'Brien, J. S.: Ganglioside GM_2 storage diseases: Hexosaminidase deficiencies in cultured fibroblasts, Am. J. Hum. Genet. **23:**55, 1971.
132. Pallisgaard, G., and Goldschmidt, E.: The oculo-cerebro-renal syndrome of Lowe in four generations of one family, Acta Paediatr. Scand. **60:**146, 1971.
133. Parks, M. M., and Schwilk, N. F.: Bilateral lamellar type cataracts in a case of phenylketonuria, Am. J. Ophthalmol. **56:**140, 1963.
134. Philippart, M., and Sugarman, G. I.: Chondroitin-4-sulfate mucopolysaccharidosis—a new variant of Hurler's syndrome, Lancet **2:**854, 1969.
135. Philippart, M., and Van Bogaert, L.: Cholestanolosis (cerebrotendinous xanthomatosis), Arch. Neurol. **21:**603, 1969.
136. Philippart, M., Franklin, S., and Gordon, A.: Reversal of an inborn sphingolipidosis (Fabry's disease) by kidney transplantation, Ann. Intern. Med. **77:**195, 1972.
137. Pickering, W. R., and Howell, R. R.: Galactokinase deficiency: Clinical and biochemical findings in a new kindred, J. Pediatr. **81:**50, 1972.
138. Podos, S. M.: Hyperpyruvicemia with hyper-alpha-alaninemia, Arch. Ophthalmol. **83:** 504, 1970.
139. Presley, G. D., Stinson, I. N., and Sidbury, J. B.: Ocular defects associated with homocystinuria, Southern Med. J. **62:**944, 1969.
140. Quigley, H. A., and Goldberg, M. F.: Conjunctival ultrastructure in mucolipidosis III (pseudo-Hurler polydystrophy), Invest. Ophthalmol. **10:**568, 1971.
141. Quigley, H. A., and Goldberg, M. F.: Scheie syndrome and macular corneal dystrophy: An ultrastructural comparison of conjunctiva and skin, Arch. Ophthalmol. **85:**553, 1971.
142. Raine, D. N.: Management of inherited metabolic disease, Br. Med. J. **2:**329, 1972.
143. Ramsey, M. S., Yanoff, M., and Fine, B. S.: The ocular histopathology of homocystinuria, Am. J. Ophthalmol. **74:**377, 1972.
144. Robb, R. M., and Kuwabara, T.: The ocular pathology of type A Niemann-Pick disease, Invest. Ophthalmol. **12:**366, 1973.
145. Robinowicz, T., Klein, D., and Tchicaloff, M.: Juvenile form of Niemann-Pick disease, Pathol. Eur. **3:**347, 1968.
146. Rosenthal, A. F., and Yaseen, A.: Improved qualitative screening test for cystinuria and homocystinuria, Clin. Chim. Acta **26:**363, 1969.
147. Roy, F. H., and Kelly, M. L.: Maple syrup urine disease, J. Pediatr. Ophthalmol. **10:**70, 1973.

148. Sanderson, P. O., Kuwabara, T., and Stark, W. J.: Cystinosis. Read at A.R.V.O. meeting, Sarasota, Florida, May 1973.
149. Salen, G.: Cholestanol deposition in cerebrotendinous xanthomatosis, Ann. Intern. Med. **75:**843, 1971.
150. Schneider, J. A., Wong, V., and Seegmiller, J. E.: The early diagnosis of cystinosis, J. Pediatr. **74:**114, 1969.
151. Schneider, J. A., Wong, V., Bradley, K., and Seegmiller, J. E.: Biochemical comparisons of the adult and childhood forms of cystinosis, New Eng. J. Med. **279:**1253, 1968.
152. Scheie, H. G., Hambrick, G. W., and Barness, L. A.: A newly recognized forme fruste of Hurler's disease (gargoylism), Am. J. Ophthalmol. **53:**753, 1962.
153. Schulman, J. D., Wong, V. G., Bradley, K. H., and Seegmiller, J. E.: A simple technique for the biochemical diagnosis of cystinosis, J. Pediatr. **76:**289, 1970.
154. Sebestyen, J., and Galfi, I.: Retinal functions in Niemann-Pick lipidosis, Ophthalmologica **157:**349, 1969.
155. Seelenfreund, M. H., Gartner, S., and Vinger, P. F.: The ocular pathology of Menkes' disease, Arch. Ophthalmol. **80:**718, 1968.
156. Singer, H. S., and Schafer, I. A.: Clinical and enzymatic variations in GM_1 generalized gangliosidosis, Am. J. Hum. Genet. **24:**454, 1972.
157. Sloan, H. R., and Fredrickson, D. S.: GM_2 gangliosidoses: Tay-Sachs disease. In Stanbury, J. B., Wyngaarden, J. B., and Fredrickson, D. S., editors: The metabolic basis of inherited disease, ed. 3, New York, 1972, McGraw-Hill Book Co., p. 615.
158. Sloan, M. R., and Fredrickson, D. S.: Rare familial diseases with neutral lipid storage. In Stanbury, J. B., Wyngaarden, J. B., and Fredrickson, D. S., editors: The metabolic basis of inherited disease, ed. 3, New York, 1972, McGraw-Hill Book Co., p. 825.
159. Smith, D. W.: Recognizable patterns of human malformations, Philadelphia, 1970, W. B. Saunders Co., p. 276.
160. Smith, T. H., Holland, M. G., and Woody, N. C.: Ocular manifestations of familial hyperlysinemia, Trans. Am. Acad. Ophthalmol. Otolaryngol. **75:**355, 1971.
161. Spaeth, G. L., and Frost, P.: Fabry's disease, its ocular manifestations, Arch. Ophthalmol. **74:**760, 1965.
162. Sperling, M. A., Hiles, D. A., and Kennerdell, J. S.: Electroretinographic responses following vitamin A therapy in a-beta-lipoproteinemia, Am. J. Ophthalmol. **73:**342, 1972.
163. Steinberg, D.: Phytanic acid storage disease: Refsum's syndrome. In Stanbury, J. B., Wyngaarden, J. B., and Fredrickson, D. S., editors: The metabolic basis of inherited disease, ed. 3, New York, 1972, McGraw-Hill Book Co., p. 833.
164. Sternlieb, I., and Scheinberg, I. H.: Prevention of Wilson's disease in asymptomatic patients, New Eng. J. Med. **278:**352, 1968.
165. Stevens, P. R.: Anterior lenticonus and the Waardenburg syndrome, Br. J. Ophthalmol. **54:**621, 1970.
166. Sugita, M., Dulaney, J. T., and Moser, H. W.: Ceramidase deficiency in Farber's disease (lipogranulomatosis), Science **178:**1100, 1972.
167. Suzuki, Y., and Suzuki, K.: Partial deficiency of hexosaminidase component A in juvenile GM_2-gangliosidosis, Neurology **20:**848, 1970.
168. Suzuki, K., and Suzuki, Y.: Galactosyl ceramide lipidosis: Globoid cell leucodystrophy (Krabbe's disease). In Stanbury, J. B., Wyngaarden, J. B., and Fredrickson, D. S., editors: The metabolic basis of inherited disease, ed. 3, New York, 1972, McGraw-Hill Book Co., p. 760.
168a. Takki, K.: Gyrate atrophy of the choroid and retina associated with hyperornithinaemia, Br. J. Ophthalmol. **58:**3, 1974.
169. Thompson, G. R., Nelson, N. A., Castor, C. W., and Grobelny, S. L.: A mucopolysaccharidosis with increased urinary excretion of chondroitin-4-sulfate, Ann. Intern. Med. **75:**421, 1971.
170. Topping, T. M., Kenyon, K. R., Goldberg, M. F., and Maumenee, A. E.: Ultrastructural ocular pathology of Hunter's syndrome, Arch. Ophthalmol. **86:**164, 1971.
171. Toussaint, D., and Danis, P.: An ocular pathologic study of Refsum's syndrome, Am. J. Ophthalmol. **72:**342, 1971.

172. Trevor-Roper, P. D.: Marriage of two complete albinos with normally pigmented offspring, Br. J. Ophthalmol. **36:**107, 1952.
173. Van Heyningen, R.: Galactose cataract: A review, Exp. Eye Res. **11:**415, 1971.
174. Vinger, P. F., and Sachs, B. A.: Ocular manifestations of hyperlipoproteinemia, Am. J. Ophthalmol. **70:**563, 1970.
175. Von Sallmann, L., Gelderman, A. H., and Laster, L.: Ocular histopathologic changes in a case of a-beta-lipoproteinemia, Doc. Ophthalmol. **26:**451, 1969.
176. Weingeist, T. A., and Blodi, F. C.: Fabry's disease: Ocular findings in a female carrier, Arch. Ophthalmol. **85:**169, 1971.
177. Wiesmann, U., and Neufeld, E. F.: Scheie and Hurler syndromes: Apparent identity of the biochemical defect, Science **169:**72, 1970.
178. Wiesmann, U. N., Rossi, E. E., and Herschkowitz, N. N.: Treatment of metachromatic leukodystrophy in fibroblasts by enzyme replacement, New Eng. J. Med. **284:**672, 1971.
179. Weinshilboum, R. M., and Axelrod, J.: Reduced plasma dopamine-β-hydroxylase activity in familial dysautonomia, New Eng. J. Med. **285:**938, 1971.
180. Wewalkar, F. G.: Syndrome of the sea-blue histiocyte, Lancet **2:**1248, 1970.
181. Wilson, R. S., and Ruiz, R. S.: Bilateral central retinal artery occlusion in homocystinuria, Arch. Ophthalmol. **82:**267, 1969.
182. Wilson, W. A., and Donnell, G. N.: Cataracts in galactosemia, Arch. Ophthalmol. **60:**215, 1958.
183. Winchester, P., Grossman, H., Lim, W. N., and Danes, B. S.: A new acid mucopolysaccharidosis with skeletal deformities simulating rheumatoid arthritis, Am. J. Roentgenol. Radium Ther. Nucl. Med. **106:**121, 1969.
184. Witkop, C. J., Nance, W. E., Rawls, R. F., and White, J. G.: Autosomal recessive oculocutaneous albinism in man: Evidence for genetic heterogeneity, Am. J. Hum. Genet. **11:**55, 1970.
185. Wong, V. G., Lietman, P. S., and Seegmiller, J. E.: Alterations of pigment epithelium in cystinosis, Arch. Ophthalmol. **77:**361, 1967.
186. Wong, V. G., Schulman, J. D., and Seegmiller, J. E.: Conjunctival biopsy for the biochemical diagnosis of cystinosis, Am. J. Ophthalmol. **70:**278, 1970.
187. Wong, V. G., Kuwabara, T., Brubaker, R., Olson, W., Schulman, J., and Seegmiller, J. E.: Intralysosomal cystine crystals in cystinosis, Invest. Ophthalmol. **9:**83, 1970.
188. Zeman, W., and Dyken, P.: Neuronal ceroid lipofuscinosis (Batten's disease), Relationship to amaurotic family idiocy? Pediatrics **44:**570, 1969.

Ocular involvement in metabolic disease

CHAIRMAN: **Charles D. Phelps***

Dr. Phelps: For those of you who have been out of medical school for 20 and 30 years, I have only been out for 10 years but also find it rather difficult to keep up with these complex metabolic problems. Are there any questions from the the audience? Please send them forward. To start off, Dr. Fredrickson, what tests should we as ophthalmologists order when we have a patient with either an arcus juvenilis or a xanthelasma, and what will our yield be in finding systemic lipoprotein disease?

Dr. Fredrickson: Patients with xanthelasma are said to have hyperlipidemia about 50% of the time, but there has been no extensive survey made on that particular point for nearly 20 years. The presence of arcus before about age 40 is said to be rather highly associated with hyperlipidemia, but the more experience I get, the more frequently I see patients who do not have hyperlipidemia. But the answer as to what tests one should do is very simple. Patients with either of those lesions should have a measurement of both plasma cholesterol and plasma triglyceride concentration. These two tests are available now in practically every large laboratory. The blood need not be taken in a fasting state for cholesterol, but it must be for triglyceride. What is hyperlipidemia? Well, without extending my time in answering this question, I would say today, with the fact that most methods being used are automated, that most patients or any patient up to about age 55 whose cholesterol is over 240 and whose triglyceride is over 200 (this is in milligrams per 100 ml.) or both has hyperlipidemia of clinical significance enough to require further explanation.

Dr. Phelps: Once you find hyperlipidemia, in how many instances are you going to be able to do something about it?

Dr. Fredrickson: Well, in most instances you can do something about hyperlipidemia. The first thing you do is to exclude secondary hyperlipidemia in insulin-deficient diabetes that is not properly treated, patients with hyperthyroidism, paraproteinemias, lupus, or multiple myeloma, or the nephrotic syndrome. Do not treat the hyperlipidemia because it will go away when the primary disease is properly managed. But for the majority of patients, who

*Department of Ophthalmology, University of Iowa College of Medicine, Iowa City, Iowa.

have primary hyperlipoproteinemia one can, in most instances, have some reasonable effect. And there are now a whole range of drugs that can be used for treating some of these more energetically and somewhat more specifically. You can do something about hyperlipidemia in most patients.

Dr. Phelps: I have a question directed to Dr. Podos. Is it possible to prevent thromboembolic phenomena in homocystinuria?

Dr. Podos: There have been some suggestions in the literature that heparinizing these patients will prevent the thromboembolic phenomena. The one case I know of in which that was done resulted in more complications than one could imagine both in terms of the eye where there were hemorrhages throughout the fundus and systemically. I do not think at this time there is anything one can do for homocystinuria in terms of the thromboembolic phenomena except to be very careful. Obviously, if one has to operate on these patients and the intraocular pressure is elevated, it would be judicious to be careful with giving hyperosmotic agents intravenously because these can precipitate thromboembolic phenomena in and by themselves. Other than that there is no treatment for this particular aspect of the disease except possibly in those individuals who appear pyridoxine responsive. It has been suggested in the literature that there is some difficulty in enhanced platelet aggregation in patients because of the elevated levels of homocystine, and although it has not been proved, it is certainly that in those pyridoxine responsive individuals where enough enzyme is generated in order to take care of the homocystine as the biochemical levels of homocystine come down, one may have decreased platelet aggregation or thromboembolic phenomena, or both.

Dr. Phelps: Perhaps Dr. Cogan would like to field this question. It is in regard to patients with cataracts that come on early in life. Should we screen all these patients for galactosemia of one of the two varieties? What will be our yield if we do that? And, finally, could you explain how a cataract occurs in galactokinase deficiency?

Dr. Cogan: There was a very informative article within the past few months by Beutler and his group from California that was in the *New England Journal of Medicine* (**288**:1203, 1973) showing the difference in cataract formation in the two types of galactose abnormality. The transferase abnormality, characteristically as Dr. Podos showed, comes on within a few weeks after birth and is associated with a mental deficiency and poor feeding, but the significant thing I think is that in galactokinase deficiency there may be no other systemic abnormality evident in these patients except for the cataracts, and the cataracts may not come on until much later in life, even in adults, as I recall. I think it is very important from our point of view to distinguish these two types of galactose cataracts. The one that would be called congenital although I suppose if it is not present at birth we should not call it congenital, but at least it is a neonatal cataract where the other can be easily missed because the cataract does not come on till later and it is the only deficiency. In answer to your questions specifically, then, yes, I think all patients with cataracts at least before the senile period should have their tests for galactokinase deficiency or transferase deficiency. I do not think that is yet available in most laboratories though Dr. Fredrickson could answer that better than I.

Dr. Fredrickson: I think that is certainly true. It is not widely available.

Dr. Cogan: Will there be a possibility that that is forthcoming in the near future that we can do this?

Dr. Fredrickson: I think so. I do not know specifically when or where, but I think that is certainly possible.

Dr. Phelps: I was just wondering a little bit about the mechanism of cataract-formation galactokinase deficiency.

Dr. Cogan: Well, the mechanism has been beautifully demonstrated by Dr. Kinoshita. Galactose, sucrose, or other sugars diffuse into the lens and are reduced there to the alcohol form and get trapped in the cells and then cause a cataract because they cannot get out in the alcohol form. They are retained there and cause swelling of the individual lens fibers, ultimately bursting the fibers and producing disruption of the pump mechanism that keeps the fibers of reasonable size. I think it is a beautiful demonstration of clinical biochemistry and I do not know that there is any better example, at least in ophthalmology, of the application of biochemistry to clinical medicine.

Dr. Fredrickson: In addition, Dr. Kinoshita, as I understand, has some chemicals that can be used to block the enzyme and I believe it is the aldose reductase that is responsible for the production of dulcitol. There is hope that in addition to the dietary therapy that prevents the cataracts there may be an actual form of drug therapy that may eventually prevent the cataracts.

Dr. Newell: I would like to comment on the yield in testing for galactokinase. We participated in Beutler's study and in some 50 specimens from youngsters with cataract there were 3 positive for galactokinase from our place and I think 6% is fairly high. I do not think Dr. Beutler would welcome specimens from each of you, but I think for the moment in observing a minor lens opacity developing after the first or second year of life and before the tenth it might be well to put these children on a galactose-free diet and see if one can reverse it just in the hopes that it is a galactokinase type in the absence of any other obvious etiologic factor.

Dr. Phelps: Dr. Fredrickson, could the efficacy of plasma infusions of enzymes in conditions of enzyme deficiency be improved if the enzymes were packaged in envelopes that could be recognized by the appropriate cells?

Dr. Fredrickson: They might be. I did not get a chance to talk about the mucolipidoses and I would like to take that opportunity for just one moment because they deal with this very problam. The mucolipidoses are rare diseases, as you heard, that lie between the sphingolipidoses and mucopolysaccharidoses. The two best known are I-cell disease; I is for "inclusion" because one of the striking features of this disease, which is somewhat like Hurler's syndrome in its manifestations, is the presence particularly in cultured fibroblasts of very large inclusion bodies. The other is a pseudo-Hurler polydystrophy, which is also similar. But these two disorders are different from the others that I mentioned because it is not a deficiency of activity of the lysosomal enzymes that is at fault, but it appears to be a failure of these enzymes to enter the cell. And thus, these disorders provide several very important and exciting lessons. One is the apparent requirement for lysosomal enzymes to be transported from one cell to another, that is, each cell does not elaborate its own complement of these acid hydrolases, but many cells must take them up from others. And this uptake seems to be deficient in the mucolipidoses and work today is based on the determination of just what it is that makes a cell recognize a lysosomal hydrolase and therefore receive it. So it may very well be that the recognition sites on the enzymes may be as simple as a particular sugar or acid. It may not be the lipid envelope that eventually will make lysosomal enzymes welcome in the cell, but it may be other recognition sites, yet part of the whole problem of enzyme replacement is to determine just what makes an enzyme a welcome entry into the cell.

Dr. Phelps: I have another question from the audience for you, which relates to an earlier question. A busy clinical ophthalmologist in private practice will likely see one to three or more patients every single day with xanthelasma. Should we order plasma cholesterol and triglyceride tests on each patient? These are very expensive tests. I think the extension of the question is, if something is found, is there something that can be done to prevent other systemic complications of these conditions?

Dr. Fredrickson: Well, it is a fair question. Let me say this, if the patient is under 50, you may not order the tests, but you should ask if his internist or his other referring physician has done the same. Repetition of measurements of cholesterol and triglyceride will usually not change the general average value so that a patient who has had a normal cholesterol and triglyceride test within the past year or even in the past 5 years, if his weight has not changed, or his way of life, will not need to have that repeated. But, if you can find that the patient does have hyperlipidemia and he was unaware of it, I think that from a general standpoint you would be doing him a favor. I wanted to stress that with regard to your earlier question; it is unlikely that you will be able to do anything about xanthelasma or about arcus by either dietary or drug treatment, the real question is what you may be doing for his vascular status by at least energizing him or moving him into a pathway of reasonable management of hyperlipidemia.

Dr. Phelps: Dr. Saunders, I understand you have some new information on eye-motility problems in Niemann-Pick disease.

Dr. Saunders: It is important for ophthalmologists to be aware that certain neurolipidoses may have specific ocular motor defects. A vertical supranuclear palsy has recently been described as a diagnostic sign in chronic forms of Niemann-Pick disease, with a diagnostic foam cell found in the bone marrow the "sea-blue histiocyte" (Sanders and Wybar, 1969; Neville et al., 1973). These patients have initial difficulty with performing vertical saccadic movements for which they substitute compensatory head thrusts. In the later stages there is a complete vertical gaze palsy, and horizontal movements may also show impaired saccadic velocites.

A horizontal supranuclear gaze palsy has also recently been seen at The National Hospital in association with juvenile Gaucher's disease.

Dr. Phelps: What is our batting average on amniocentesis when looking for inborn errors of metabolism?

Dr. Fredrickson: Well, roughly it's about 1 in 4, since you are only looking for these autosomal recessive defects in the main. Dr. Neufeld has looked at the amniotic cell fluid cells in 35 patients for a mucopolysaccharidosis, and she found nine, which is pretty close to the average you might expect. What is it in the sphingolipidoses? I have no idea, but it must be fairly close to that because almost invariably these parents have already had one affected child with these recessive defects. The question is not what the batting average is, of course, but the difficult one of maintaining the most strict quality control of the enzyme measurements and, in some of these newer disorders, the knowing what the cell enzymes are at the particular stage of cell growth so that, although one may believe that enzyme measurements become reasonably standardized in a couple of these defects, it still is a problem that requires the greatest circumspection in the main. But certainly it is here to stay and is the only mode of preventing the birth of these fatal or semilethal defects that have been extraordinarily severe and not compatible with any kind of normal life.

4

Collagen and rheumatic diseases: systemic aspects

Giles G. Bole, Jr.

During the past 2 years several major works and reviews dealing with the rheumatic diseases have appeared or been published in new editions.* The current classification of the rheumatic diseases encompasses over 100 diseases or syndromes.[37] Our discussion is restricted to the major forms of polyarthritis of unknown etiology, Sjögren's syndrome, and the acquired "connective tissue" disorders. Other diseases or syndromes that can be associated with eye involvement include the inherited disorders of connective tissue (mucopolysaccharidoses), gout, Behçet's syndrome, relapsing polychondritis, and the arthropathy of inflammatory intestinal disease.

It is important to comment upon the term "diffuse collagen diseases" originally proposed by Klemperer and associates.[23] The name was derived from the tinctorial appearance of the histopathologic changes observed in the connective tissue constituents of joints, serosal membranes, blood vessel walls, and viscera. Currently, the term "collagen" designates a specific structural protein found in several specialized forms of connective tissue. There is little evidence that defects in collagen formation or metabolism are involved primarily in the pathogenesis of the acquired diseases of connective tissue. It has been recommended that the term "collagen diseases" be abandoned and that the term "acquired diseases of connective tissue" be used to designate the several disorders included in this group of rheumatic diseases.

MEDIATORS AND MECHANISMS RESPONSIBLE FOR INFLAMMATION
Immune mechanisms

The intensive investigations in progress in the field of immunology have been stimulated in many instances by clinical or pathologic findings in the connective tissue diseases. The classic studies of Rich[35] on experimental drug hypersensitivity found an apparent counterpart in the lesions noted in polyarterteritis (PAr),

---

*See additional readings at the end of this chapter.

rheumatic fever, systemic lupus erythematosus (SLE), and rheumatoid arthritis (RA). The observations of Dixon[9] and others on experimental serum sickness have contributed greatly to our understanding of disease processes responsible for human glomerulonephritis and the nephritis of SLE. Many other examples could be cited and are enumerated in today's texts dealing with immunology and immunopathology.[16, 26, 39] The presence of hypergammaglobulinemia in patients with RA, SLE, or other connective tissue disorders and the detection of a spectrum of "autoantibody" reactions led MacKay and Burnet[26] to classify the acquired connective tissue diseases as autoimmune disorders. Current information indicates that "autoimmunity" may play an important part in the pathogenesis of several of the connective disorders. The defects in host defense mechanisms responsible for these aberrations, that is, the primary etiologic events, remain unknown. Infectious particles (viruses) are envisioned as possible precipitating agents. They could modify cell structure or functions such that "self" is recognized as "nonself" and they could stimulate autoantibody formation. During the past 5 years, many reports have dealt with the isolation of infectious agents of bacterial, mycoplasmal or viral origin from patients with rheumatic disorders.[44, 55] Currently, the nature and significance of the microtubular structures found on electron microscopic study of cells from patients with SLE as well as other rheumatic and nonrheumatic disorders illustrate the complexity of this problem.[55]

It is beyond the scope of this discussion to deal with the progress made in the structural study of the immunoglobulins, cellular events involved in initiation of an immune response, or the chemical reactions critical to activation of the complement system.[42] Progress in these areas has contributed to a better understanding of immunologic reactions that are responsible for initiation and perpetuation of inflammatory processes. The mechanisms by which antibodies interact with antigens to produce immunopathologic tissue damage may involve anaphylaxis, cytolytic reactions, toxic complex formation, or delayed hypersensitivity.[16, 39, 53] More than one of these immune mechanisms often operate simultaneously to produce certain of the pathologic changes observed in the acquired connective tissue diseases. Bioactive substances formed by activation of the complement system can mediate a local immunoinflammatory reaction and lead to tissue destruction. This destruction is believed to be produced in several instances by release of lysosomal (hydrolytic) enzymes from exudative cells, such as the polymorphonuclear leukocyte. The fourth general type of immune reaction—delayed hypersensitivity (cellular immunity)—operates as a normal part of the host defense system. Direct experimental confirmation that major deficiencies in cellular immunity occur in the several connective tissue diseases remains controversial.[50, 55] However, the histopathology of many of the lesions and the clinical responses of some rheumatic patients to cytotoxic (immunosuppressive) drug regimens support the concept that altered cellular immunity plays a role in the pathogenesis of these disorders.

Nonimmune mechanisms

It has been emphasized repeatedly that the chemical and cellular events involved in the inflammatory response are by first priority a host defense system. The local response to any noxious stimulus can be described morphologically as including a vascular phase, followed by exudation and cell differentiation. Under normal circumstances the process is terminated by a reparative response. The distinction between "wound repair" and the destructive effect (local and systemic) of a chronic inflammatory reaction represents defective operation of host defense systems and can be recognized as a pathologic lesion or process. As noted in the description of cellular immunity, failure to "regulate" this phenomenon can lead to the production of an inflammatory lesion.

Recent investigations have demonstrated a complex series of interactions between immune factors, the kinin system, the coagulation sequence, and chemical substances (lymphokines, "activators," chemotactic factors) that affect the function of inflammatory cells.[14] The regulation of subcellular events involved in polymorphonuclear and macrophage phagocytosis (including the release of lysosomal enzymes) has been recognized as critical to the evolution and perpetuation of an inflammatory response.[14, 25] This is another example of a host defense mechanism (phagocytosis) that can be subverted so as to participate in the propagation rather than the modulation and control of an inflammatory response.

When the histopathology of chronic inflammatory disorders such as rheumatoid arthritis is examined, lesions compatible with immunologic injury are easily identified. The subsynovial location of immunocompetent cells has been demonstrated[45] and is recognized as a classic histopathologic feature of this disease. However, it is difficult to explain fully the formation of granulation tissue (pannus) and the destructive changes encountered on the articular hyaline cartilage surfaces of the joints. Progress in the biochemical identification of the structural constituents of cartilage and, in particular, collagen[41] make it apparent that the action of relatively nonspecific lysosomal hydrolases could not explain completely the destructive effect of chronic inflammatory cells present in articular pannus. More detailed study of the spectrum of lysosomal enzymes and the isolation of specific collagenases[14] appears to offer an explanation of the mechanism of destruction of cartilage matrix and other constituents of fibrous supporting structures, including bone.

Great progress has been made in identifying important immune and nonimmune mechanisms that contribute to the histopathology of each of the rheumatic or connective tissue disorders. Much of this information has contributed to an improved understanding of other human disease states, including several that affect the eye.

CLINICAL MANIFESTATIONS OF THE INFLAMMATORY DISEASES OF CONNECTIVE TISSUE

The diseases to be discussed have been selected on the basis of the reported frequency of occurrence of eye involvement.[18] Prevalence data for the rheumatic diseases have been obtained from clinical and population studies but are still incomplete. The frequency of occurrence of ocular complications can only be estimated, since almost all of the data have been derived from retrospective studies.[18, 22, 40] It is difficult to determine whether some of the reported associations between rheumatic and ocular diseases are simply chance occurrence of two common clinical disorders, such as the spectrum of eye disease in patients with osteoarthritis.[22]

Before dealing with the major clinical manifestations found in the several forms of polyarthritis and the acquired diseases of connective tissue, I should make a brief comment on the information contained in Tables 4-1 to 4-3. In Tables 4-1 and 4-2, the relative value of the most common clinical laboratory procedures used in confirming the clinical diagnosis in each of these diseases has been sum-

Table 4-1. Laboratory studies used in differential diagnosis of connective tissue disease*

Procedure	Most value	Usually abnormal	Occasional abnormality
Complete blood counts	SLE, SS		All others
Urine	SLE, PAr		RA, JRA, SS, RS, PSS
Erythrocyte sedimentation rate	PMR	All others	
Acute-phase reactants (C-reactive protein)		All	
Serological test for syphilis	SLE		
Rheumatoid factor	RA	SS	JRA, SLE, PSS, PDM
Lupus erythematosus cell	SLE		RA, SS, PSS, PDM, PAr
Antinuclear antibodies	SLE	SS, PSS	RA, JRA, PDM, PAr
Anti-DNA antibodies	SLE		
Complement (serum for SLE, synovial fluid for RA)	SLE, RA		SS, PAr
Coombs' antibodies	SLE		RA, SS
Serum protein electrophoresis	SLE, SS	RA, JRA	PSS, PDM, PAr
Immunoglobulin measurements	SLE, JRA	SS	RA, PSS, PDM, PAr
Cryoglobulins	SLE, SS		RA, PSS
Muscle enzymes (SGOT, creatine phosphokinase, aldolase)	PDM		RA, SS, SLE, PSS
Renal function studies	SLE, PSS, PAr		RA, SS

*AS, Ankylosing spondylitis; JRA, juvenile rheumatoid arthritis; PAr, polyarteritis and variants; PDM, polymyositis and dermatomyositis; PMR, polymyalgia rheumatica; PsA, psoriatic arthritis; PSS, progressive systemic sclerosis; RA, rheumatoid arthritis; RS, Reiter's syndrome; SLE, systemic lupus erythematosus; SS, Sjögren's syndrome.

Table 4-2. Other procedures of value in diagnosis of connective tissue disease*

Procedure	Most value	Individual cases
Synovianalysis	RA, JRA	RS, PsA, AS
Biopsy:		
Synovium	RA, JRA	RS, PsA, AS, PSS
Kidney	SLE, PAr	PSS, SS
Muscle	PDM, PAr	RA, SS, SLE, PSS
Vessel	PAr, PMR	
Nodule	RA, PSS	JRA, SLE
Other	PSS (skin)	SLE (skin), SS (salivary)
Electrocardiography	AS, RS, PAr	RA, SS, JRA, SLE, PSS
Electromyography and nerve-conduction studies	PDM, PAr	SS, RA, PSS, SLE
Electroencephalography	SLE, PAr	
Pulmonary function studies	PSS, PDM	RA, AS, PAr
Radiologic:		
Joint	AS + others	
Chest	All	
Gastrointestinal studies	PSS, PDM	PAr, SLE
Vascular	PAr	PMR, PSS
Special		SS (sialography)

*Abbreviation for each disease is the same as that used in Table 4-1.

Table 4-3. Summary of major therapeutic approaches to treatment of connective tissue diseases

Disease	Conservative measures*	Other drugs	Gold salts	Other agents	Corticosteroids‡			Cytotoxic or immunosuppressive drugs		Surgical procedures
					Intra-articular	Low oral	High oral	Alkylating agents	Anti-metabolites	
Rheumatoid arthritis	+	Antimalarials, phenylbutazone, indomethacin	+	Analgesics	+	+		+	‡	Synovectomy, arthroplasty, joint prostheses
Sjögren's syndrome	+			Wetting agents					‡	
Juvenile rheumatoid arthritis	+		‡		‡	+	‡	‡	‡	As for rheumatoid arthritis
Ankylosing spondylitis	+	Phenylbutazone, indomethacin		"Muscle" relaxants	‡	+	‡	‡		Joint prostheses Spinal osteotomy
Psoriatic arthritis	+	Phenylbutazone, indomethacin		Dermatologic	+	+			‡	
Reiter's syndrome	+	Phenylbutazone, indomethacin		?Tetracycline	+	+	‡	‡		
Systemic lupus erythematosus	+	Antimalarials				+	+	+	+	Joint prostheses ?Renal transplant
Progressive systemic sclerosis	+			Potassium para-aminobenzoate Vasodilators		‡		‡		
Polymyositis and dermatomyositis	+						+	‡		
Polyarteritis and variants	+			?Anticoagulants		+	+	‡		
Polymyalgia rheumatica	+					+	‡			

*Includes the use of aspirin and appropriate physical therapeutic measures.
†Low dose oral < 10 mg, and high dose oral 60 mg. prednisone (or equivalent) per day.
+Commonly employed agents.
‡Use has been reported, or is used, in severe, progressive disease.

marized. In Table 4-3, drug therapy, use of physical therapeutic measures, and notation of some of the major surgical approaches to treatment have been listed. This table has been arranged so that therapeutic alternatives (left to right) proceed from the initial or more conservative alternatives to those considered appropriate in treatment of severe or progressive disease activity. I emphasize that the use of the so-called cytotoxic (immunosuppressive) drugs must at this time be considered a clinical investigative approach to treatment. Modifications and exceptions to these diagnostic and therapeutic generalizations will be discussed as a part of the clinical description of each disease.

ACUTE AND CHRONIC FORMS OF POLYARTHRITIS
Rheumatoid arthritis (RA)

Standard criteria for the diagnosis of rheumatoid arthritis have been established by the American Rheumatism Association.[38] These criteria are useful in establishing the diagnosis in individual cases, but they are most frequently employed in epidemiologic and clinical studies. Rheumatoid arthritis is the most common form of inflammatory articular disease. It can occur at any age, but is noted with highest frequency in females who are in the childbearing years (third to fifth decades of life). The ratio of females to males in most studies remains remarkably constant at approximately 3:1. Some of the pathogenetic mechanisms found to be important in this disorder have been discussed briefly in the section dealing with the inflammatory response.

Clinical findings. The criteria for diagnosis of rheumatoid arthritis[38] emphasize the joint abnormalities that are the hallmark of this disease. Typically the onset is insidious with stiffness and aching in the small joints of the hands and feet. Objective signs of synovitis (swelling, pain, and redness) in the involved joints may be of gradual or occasionally abrupt onset. Symmetric involvement of small joints (proximal interphalangeal, metacarpophalangeal or metatarsophalangeal) as well as large joints (wrists, knees, ankles, elbows, shoulders, hips) is a typical feature of the disease. The clinical appearance of the hands of a patient with definite rheumatoid arthritis is depicted in Fig. 4-1. This disease can affect any diarthrodial joint, including the cervical spine. Involvement is typically progressive in number and severity of joint disease; however, population surveys[30] have shown that the remission rate may be much higher than predicted from study of hospitalized cases.

Constitutional symptoms, including morning stiffness, fatigue, weight loss, fever, malaise, and tachycardia, can occasionally be severe and lead to confusion regarding diagnosis. The systemic nature of rheumatoid arthritis is apparent when one examines the number of extra-articular lesions associated with this disease (see outline below). Subcutaneous rheumatoid nodules (granulomas) can be found in approximately 20% of patients with rheumatoid arthritis. Most commonly they occur in patients with seropositive (rheumatoid factor–positive) disease and those with active or progressive rheumatoid arthritis. The ocular complications of rheumatoid arthritis will be dealt with in more detail elsewhere. Iatrogenic ocular complications from the therapeutic use of antimalarials, gold salts, or corticosteroids can induce pathologic changes in the eye.[18]

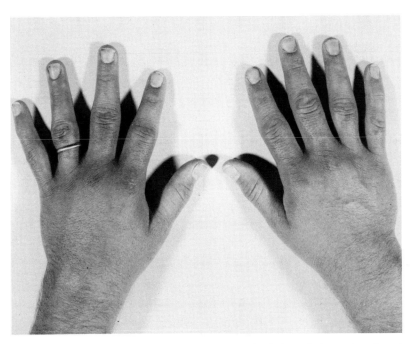

Fig. 4-1. Symmetric chronic active synovitis of proximal interphalangeal and metacarpophalangeal joints in a 22-year-old male with rheumatoid arthritis of 3 year's duration.

Extra-articular involvement in rheumatoid arthritis

Cutaneous	Subcutaneous rheumatoid nodules, ulcers, and purpura
Ocular	Scleritis and episcleritis
	Scleromalacia performans
	Keratoconjunctivitis sicca
	Iatrogenic
Cardiac	Pericarditis
	Conduction defects
	Valve lesions (aortic, ?mitral)
Pulmonary	Pleurisy
	Nodules (rheumatoid)
	Caplan's syndrome
	Diffuse interstitial fibrosis
	Cricoarytenoid dysfunction
Neuromuscular	Peripheral neuropathy
	Compression neuropathies
	Myositis or myopathy
Hematologic	Anemia
	Lymphadenopathy
	Felty's syndrome
Vascular	Vasculitis
	Necrotizing arteritis
	Raynaud's phenomenon
Miscellaneous	Amyloidosis
	Generalized osteoporosis
	Constitutional

Cardiac abnormalities associated with rheumatoid arthritis include pericarditis and "rheumatoid" heart disease.[19] Granulomatous lesions similar to subcutaneous nodules can occur in the heart (epicardium, myocardium, and valves). Conduction defects, valvular incompetence (aortic more than mitral) are the most common clinical manifestations of this lesion. Inflammation in the pleura can lead to pleuritis with or without effusion. Rheumatoid fluid has certain distinctive characteristics, in that there are low glucose, complement components, and multinucleate giant cells.[19, 37] Rheumatoid nodules in the lung and pleura most commonly occur in seropositive males. These lesions may cavitate and often require biopsy to differentiate them from neoplasms or specific granulomas. A distinctive form of pneumoconiosis *(Caplan's syndrome)* has also been described.[4] In other seropositive patients, diffuse interstitial pulmonary fibrosis has been reported to occur in higher frequency than in the general population. Hoarseness, dyspnea, or stridor have been related to rheumatoid involvement of the cricoarytenoid joints and may be found in 50% of autopsy cases.

Neuromuscular complications are often difficult to differentiate from the secondary effects produced on these structures by articular disease. The most common neurologic lesion is a mild distal sensory neuropathy. This is most frequent in seropositive patients and may abruptly change to a more severe sensorimotor neuropathy including foot or wrist drop (mononeuritis multiplex). In the more severe cases, other signs of a diffuse vasculitis or necrotizing arteritis are apparent. Nerve compression syndromes occur as a direct or indirect complication of articular disease (carpal tunnel or peroneal syndrome). Rheumatoid involvement of the cervical spine can produce atlantoaxial (C1-C2) or C3-C4 subluxation, and in some cases, if unrecognized, it can lead to cord compression. Clinical and electromyographic abnormalities consistent with myositis or myopathy can be observed.

A normochromic and normocytic anemia is common and related to disordered ferrokinetics and abnormal sequestration of iron stores. Lymphadenopathy also correlates with disease activity and in some series with seropositivity. It is now recognized that lymph-node hyperplasia is related to the immune diathesis present in this disease. *Felty's syndrome* is observed in some patients with rheumatoid arthritis and indicates the presence of splenomegaly, leukopenia, and pigmented chronic leg ulcers.[19, 37] In some cases, increased susceptibility to infection is found.

As noted in the description of several of the extra-articular manifestations of rheumatoid arthritis, the presence of inflammation (vasculitis) in and about small blood vessels can be detected at biopsy or autopsy. Rheumatoid arteritis (1% to 2% of cases) can express itself as a necrotizing angiitis with clinical findings of peripheral neuropathy, skin ulcers, gangrene, and visceral lesions. This "malignant" form of rheumatoid disease was noted prior to the use of steroids and can be confused with polyarteritis nodosa. Some authors[24] observed an increased incidence of this disorder during the first decade of corticosteroid use. Patients with advanced disease who are seropositive and have rheumatoid nodules are most prone to development of rheumatoid arteritis. The condition appears to be more common in males and, in severe form, can be life threatening or cause death. Raynaud's phenomenon occurs in approximately 10% of rheumatoid patients and is usually caused by occlusive rather than vasospastic disease in the digital arteries.

Amyloidosis associated with rheumatoid arthritis is of secondary type and has been reported to occur in 20% of autopsy cases. In addition to juxta-articular osteoporosis associated with synovitis, generalized osteopenia is a common finding.

Laboratory findings. There is no specific test for rheumatoid arthritis. Several clinical laboratory procedures should be performed routinely to assist in the evaluation of a patient's disease (Tables 4-1 and 4-2). Seropositivity (rheumatoid factors) in patients tends to suggest the potential for more active or aggressive disease as contrasted to consistent seronegativity.[16] The tests for rheumatoid factor are frequently negative in early or minimal disease. Lupus erythematosus cells are present in approximately 5% to 10% of cases. Tests for antinuclear antibodies are positive in 25% to 30% of patients with active or progressive disease. An important finding (in contrast to patients with active systemic lupus erythematosus) is the presence of normal serum complement levels with low values in synovial fluid; the value is also reduced in rheumatoid pleural effusions. A typical synovial fluid analysis demonstrates a turbid inflammatory (group II) effusion.[21] Biopsy of a subcutaneous nodule with demonstration of the classic histopathologic condition of a rheumatoid granuloma is an important diagnostic aid. Synovial biopsy will commonly reveal a chronic nonspecific synovitis. However, the presence of synovial villus formation caused by synovial cell hyperplasia and hypertrophy with subsynovial accumulations of lymphocytes and plasma cells is typical of rheumatoid arthritis and helps to exclude other forms of synovitis. Joint roentgenograms in early disease may be normal or demonstrate only soft tissue swellings and effusions. Marginal erosions at the site of synovia-cartilage reflections are the first definitive signs of destructive inflammatory disease. Serial joint films are helpful in evaluation of the patient's clinical status and response to treatment. A more detailed description of the radiology of rheumatoid disease can be found elsewhere.[27]

Treatment. Therapeutic decisions made during treatment of a patient with rheumatoid arthritis depend on a series of variables. The general approach to treatment of this disease is outlined in Table 4-3. In a young adult, sustained inflammation in the joints, progressive joint involvement, positive tests for rheumatoid factor and extra-articular complications suggest a poor prognosis. Under these circumstances, an orderly addition or modification in the use of therapeutic modalities is well advised. Full ophthalmologic evaluation should be performed before and every 3 months during treatment with the antimalarials (chloroquine, or preferably hydroxychloroquine). Fortunately, ocular and visual complications are rare, but the threat of retinal damage is real, even at low daily dosage (hydroxychloroquine, 200 mg. per day). Failure to control rheumatoid activity after an adequate trial of conservative measures (including one or more of the nonsteroidal drugs) indicates that a course of gold therapy is justified (aurothioglucose or aurothiomalate). An alternative approach to the treatment of poorly controlled rheumatoid activity is the use of low daily doses of corticosteroids (10 mg. prednisone or less per day). Selective use of intra-articular corticosteroid therapy is an effective adjunct to conservative management and during the early phase of gold or systemic steroid treatment. In properly selected cases, surgical treatment can lead to impressive rehabilitation of patients with joint deformities.

The use of cytotoxic (immunosuppressive) drugs should be restricted to those patients with uncontrolled progressive disease who have failed to respond to conventional modes of therapy. At the present time, cyclophosphamide is the drug most frequently used in this circumstance. It has been shown to be effective in a controlled clinical trial.[8] The threat of serious drug toxicity is real even under careful clinical observation. The complete spectrum of complications (including the development of neoplasms) from use of this or similar agents remains to be defined.

Sjögren's syndrome (SS)

The cardinal features of this disorder are the occurrence of keratoconjunctivitis sicca and xerostomia (sicca complex) secondary to chronic inflammatory cell infiltration of the lacrimal and salivary glands. In addition, over half of the patients have rheumatoid arthritis (10% to 15% of patients with rheumatoid arthritis) or one of the other connective tissue diseases (SLE, progressive systemic sclerosis, polymyositis). It is now appreciated that this syndrome is a multisystem disorder with numerous autoimmune abnormalities. It occurs most frequently in females beyond the fifth decade of life.[48]

Clinical findings. The spectrum of clinical abnormalities found in patients with Sjögren's syndrome is listed in the outline below. In cases in which the sicca complex coexists with rheumatoid arthritis or one of the other connective tissue diseases, the additional clinical features can be assumed to be manifestations of the latter. In some cases, a constellation of findings such as sialadenitis, lymph-node enlargement, purpura, vasculitis, splenomegaly, and leukopenia occur in the absence of rheumatoid arthritis. During long-term follow-up of some patients, the development of "pseudolymphoma," primary macroglobulinemia or overt reticulum cell sarcoma has been described.[49]

Clinical features associated with Sjögren's syndrome

Sicca complex (dry mouth, dry eye)
    Salivary gland swelling
    Mucous membrane ulcers
    Dysphagia, dysphonia
    Polydipsia
    Respiratory infections
Chronic arthritis (rheumatoid)   Renal tubular acidosis
Raynaud's phenomenon   Vasculitis and purpura
Hashimoto's thyroiditis   Myositis and myopathy
Chronic hepatitis   Lymphadenopathy
Pancreatitis   Pseudolymphoma
Gastric achlorhydria   Lymphoma
Felty's syndrome

Laboratory findings. Demonstration of the sicca complex as it involves the eye is described elsewhere. Salivary (parotid) gland involvement can be determined by measurement of salivary flow rates, sialography, scintography, or more simply by lower-lip biopsy. Laboratory findings are listed in Tables 4-1 and 4-2. Poly-clonal hypergammaglobulinemia is common, and over 90% of patients have positive tests for rheumatoid factor. Positive lupus erythematosus cell and anti-nuclear antibody reactions occur frequently. Tests for organ-specific autoanti-bodies (thyroid, salivary cells, gastric cells, and so forth) are positive in many patients. Lymph node or other tissue biopsies may demonstrate extraglandular lymphoid proliferation and lead to the diagnosis of "pseudolymphoma" or malignant lymphoma.

Treatment. In most cases treatment is directed at palliation of the symptoms related to the sicca complex. Treatment of a coexistent rheumatic disorder follows the usual pattern of therapy for that disease. It has been proposed that corticosteroids or immunosuppressive drugs are useful in patients with visceral organ involvement or "pseudolymphoma."[48]

Juvenile rheumatoid arthritis (JRA)

This disease cannot be considered a mirror image of adult onset rheumatoid arthritis. Although the two diseases have common clinical and histopathologic features, there are notable differences in the mode of onset, course, degree of joint involvement and incidence of seropositivity (IgM rheumatoid factor). Criteria for diagnosis of the disease have been published.[2] Iridocyclitis is a frequent and serious problem in patients with JRA in contrast to its apparent chance occurrence in patients with the adult form of the disease.[40] Ocular involvement occurs most commonly in patients with monoarticular or oligoarticular disease and requires prophylactic ophthalmologic evaluation and follow-up even when the signs of arthritis are minimal or absent.[5, 40]

Clinical findings. Three patterns of disease onset and progression are found in JRA. The disease may develop before the age of 1 year. Peak incidence in boys and girls is observed at 2 to 3 and 9 to 10 years of age. The ratio of males to females and patterns of disease presentation or progression appear to differ in the two sexes.[5, 40] At present the *systemic form* of disease (20% of cases) occurs most commonly in boys and is the entity originally described by Still. High-spiking fever and extra-articular lesions without evidence of joint involvement make the diagnosis difficult. The extra-articular manifestations may include weight loss, fatigue, lymphadenopathy, and hepatosplenomegaly. A transient morbilliform rash has characteristic features and, if noted, may suggest the correct diagnosis. Pleuritis, pericarditis, and vasculitis occur. Less commonly, myocarditis or encephalitis are encountered. Ocular involvement rarely occurs in this form of JRA.

The most common presentation includes joint involvement from the onset and represents the *polyarticular form* of the disease (approximately 50% of cases). In these patients the disease course may be variable, but they represent the group that most frequently develop deformity and major crippling from their arthritis. In the *monoarticular form* of disease the knee is most frequently involved. These patients may subsequently develop oligoarticular (less than four joints) disease or less frequently polyarticular disease.[5] It is this group who most often demonstrate Still's ocular triad: iridocyclitis, band keratopathy, and cataracts.

Differential diagnosis is influenced by the mode of onset. Systemic onset requires exclusion of infections, neoplasms, and diverse causes of fever. Polyarticular and oligoarticular (pauciarticular) diseases require exclusion of rheumatic fever and other juvenile rheumatic disorders. Monoarticular disease requires exclusion of traumatic lesions or specific infections (tuberculosis). In these cases synovial fluid analysis, culture, and biopsy are necessary to clarify the diagnosis.

Laboratory findings. Routine tests for rheumatoid factor (IgM) are negative in the younger child but seropositivity increases with age.[2] Positive tests for anti-nuclear antibodies may reflect systemic involvement. It is important to determine immunoglobulin levels since children with agammaglobulinemia may present with synovitis indistinguishable from JRA. Tuberculin skin tests should be given. Roentgenograms may demonstrate nonspecific soft-tissue changes and juxta-articular osteoporosis. Erosive changes appear late especially in monoarticular cases. The effects of synovitis on the joint in the developing child lead to growth abnormalities both in the direction of accelerated maturation and premature closure of epiphyseal centers. Subperiosteal bone apposition is frequently noted in films of involved joints.[27]

Treatment. Prognosis is favorable in over 75% of patients and at 10 years approximately two thirds of the patients are in remission.[3] Aspirin in appropriate dosage for the child effectively controls fever and synovitis in most cases. Other conservative measures are employed as in adult rheumatoid arthritis. Nonsteroidal agents are employed infrequently because of their potential to produce serious side effects. Gold salts are occasionally employed in cases with progressive joint disease. Corticosteroids may be required in patients with severe or life-threatening systemic manifestations. In addition to the usual complications from their use, growth abnormalities can be accentuated in the child with JRA.

Ankylosing spondylitis (AS)

This inflammatory disease[28] of the spinal articulations demonstrates a striking predilection for young adult males. Ocular involvement is a frequent complication. The male to female ratio is approximately 9:1. There is a greater tendency to fibrosis, bony ankylosis, ossification of spinal ligaments, and bony bridging (syndesmophytes) in this disease than found in the lesions of peripheral rheumatoid arthritis. The disease onset most commonly occurs between 20 and 40 years. It may occur in late adolescence but is extremely rare after 50 years of age.

Clinical findings. The onset is usually insidious with the most common complaint being low back pain, which reflects involvement of the sacroiliac joints. This pain occurs with or without radiation into the buttocks or thighs. Generalized aching and stiffness are frequently noted along with constitutional symptoms. Restricted motion of the lumbar spine with progressive involvement of the dorsal and cervical segments occurs over a variable period of time (months to years). Peripheral joint involvement may be found in slightly less than half the cases. Except for the "root joints," that is, hips and shoulders, peripheral joint synovitis is transient and benign. As the upper segments of the spine are involved, respiratory excursion is restricted and radicular thoracic or cervical pain may be quite severe. Unless vigorous efforts are expended by the patient, thoracolumbar kyphosis, anterior flexion of the cervical spine, and flexion contractures of the hips will produce the classic deformed spondylitic posture.

Extra-articular involvement includes iridocyclitis, spondylitic aortitis with aortic insufficiency (approximately 5% of cases), and cardiac conduction abnormalities. Pulmonary complications may occur because of restriction in chest expansion. A cauda equina syndrome may develop as a late manifestation of advanced spondylitis.

Laboratory findings. The sedimentation rate is elevated in active disease.

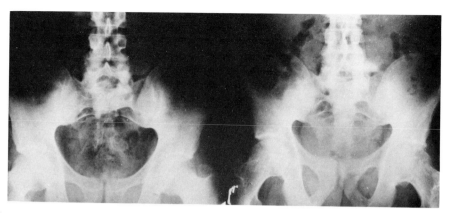

Fig. 4-2. Progressive sacroiliac and lumbar spine changes in young male with ankylosing spondylitis. In *left* roentgenogram there is blurring, erosive widening, and marginal sclerosis of sacroiliac joints. Two years later (*right* roentgenogram), sacroiliac joints are fused and syndesmophyte formation has produced bony bridging of lower lumbar vertebrae. Erosive arthritis has progressed in left hip joint.

Rheumatoid factor is absent and other standard immunologic parameters are normal. The most important diagnostic findings are the changes observed in initial or serial roentgenograms of the sacroiliac joints and upper spine (Fig. 4-2). Blurring, erosions, and marginal sclerosis are followed by fusion of the sacroiliac joints. Syndesmophyte formation, noted first at the dorsolumbar junction, coupled with erosive remodeling of the involved vertebrae are additional diagnostic signs. Atlantoaxial subluxation is identified in some cases.[27]

Treatment. Aspirin therapy and a rigorously enforced program of supervised physical therapy can provide significant relief of symptoms. Despite spinal fusion, physical therapy can diminish postural deformity. The nonsteroidal agents (phenylbutazone or indomethacin) are useful in this disease and more effective than in certain of the other rheumatic diseases. Corticosteroids may be required in severe cases. Surgical approaches to hip disease can yield gratifying results in selected cases.

Psoriatic arthritis (PsA)

The occurrence of inflammatory joint disease in patients with psoriasis is now recognized as a distinct clinical entity. It most frequently occurs in patients with overt skin disease. In some cases, arthritis develops before skin involvement or coincident with its appearance. The chance association of two common diseases, psoriasis and rheumatoid arthritis, has led to confusion as to the true incidence of psoriatic arthritis.[54] Some believe that psoriatic arthritis and Reiter's syndrome are indistinguishable because of the similarity of skin and ocular and radiologic features. Approximately 5% of patients with psoriasis will develop joint involvement typical of psoriatic arthritis.

Clinical findings. A history of psoriasis in the patient or a relative can be an important clue to the proper diagnosis. Common or typical findings in patients with psoriatic arthritis are listed in the outline below. One clinical expression of the disease is inflammatory involvement of the distal interphalangeal joints of the fingers and toes. There may also be nail pitting and onycholysis of involved or adjacent digits. In other cases, asymmetric involvement of a limited number of peripheral joints may occur. The synovitis can be intermittent or persistent and commonly affects the small joints of the hands and feet. In a few patients, severe destructive disease occurs in multiple peripheral joints and is referred to as "arthritis mutilans." These latter patients frequently demontrate sacroiliac and spinal involvement. Sacroiliac changes may remain unilateral, and syndesmophyte formation can arise from the marginal and nonmarginal surfaces of the vertebral margins. This radiologic feature also occurs in Reiter's syndrome, but not in ankylosing spondylitis.[28] Symmetric seropositive polyarthritis is believed to represent the chance association of rheumatoid arthritis and psoriasis.

> *Psoriatic arthritis, common or essential features*
>   Synovitis, distal interphalangeal joints
>   Asymmetric involvement
>   Nail pitting, onycholysis
>   Concurrence of skin and joint flares
>   "Atypical" spondylitis
>   Absence of rheumatoid factor or nodules
>   Characteristic radiologic features
>   Destructive erosions
>   Subperiosteal bone apposition
>   Marginal and nonmarginal syndesmophytes

Laboratory findings. Patients with psoriatic arthritis have negative tests for rheumatoid factor. The histopathologic features of the synovitis are indistinguishable from those of rheumatoid arthritis. Roentgenographic changes[27] reflect the clinical findings but also demonstrate characteristic features. These features are destructive erosive changes affecting isolated small joints, osteolysis of terminal phalanges, subperiosteal bone apposition (a fluffy form of periostitis), and atypical spondylitic changes as described above.

Treatment. The conservative measures (aspirin and physical therapy) may be adequate. In more severe cases, intra-articular steroids and nonsteroidal anti-inflammatory drugs may be helpful. Gold therapy is ineffective and contra-indicated, since its use may lead to a flare of the psoriasis. The same is true for the use of antimalarial drugs. Corticosteroids improve the skin and joint disease, but serious complications including flare of the skin lesions during withdrawal tend to outweigh any short-term benefits. Treatment of the psoriasis may, in some cases, ameliorate the arthritis. In severe cases, antimetabolites, especially methotrexate,[52] are employed, but hepatic damage from this agent dictates cautious usage and careful follow-up of these patients.

Reiter's syndrome

The syndrome describes the association of nonbacterial (nongonococcal) urethritis, arthritis, and conjunctivitis. Most commonly, it affects young adult males after venereal exposure, but it has been reported in males and females after epidemics of dysentery. Reiter's case was apparently of the latter type. Although the triad of symptoms remains as originally defined, it is now recognized that mucocutaneous lesions are as typical as the triad and that individual manifestations of the disease may be temporally separated by weeks or months. The correct diagnosis in the latter cases can only be recognized in retrospect. Infectious agents have been isolated from the urethral discharge or tissue exudates obtained from these patients. Mycoplasmal species (T strain) and a chlamydial organism (trachoma-psittacosis group) have been reported to occur with high frequency in specific groups of patients subjected to intensive investigation. Confirmation of these findings with consistent isolation of the same agent or agents by other investigators has not, to date, been accomplished.[13] Some authors now review Reiter's syndrome as a venereal disease–associated arthropathy in which an unusual host response to infectious agents occurs.

Clinical findings. The initial attack of the disease usually follows a self-limited course. Urethritis and conjunctivitis occur and are followed by the appearance of an asymmetric acute polyarthritis. The weight-bearing joints (knees, ankles, metatarsophalangeal areas) are more commonly involved than those of the upper extremities. Weight loss and fever may be present during the acute attack. Gonococcal urethritis may occur simultaneously in some cases and require prompt recognition and treatment with penicillin. The spectrum of clinical findings observed in the acute or protracted course of Reiter's syndrome is presented in the outline below.

Reiter's syndrome, common or essential features
>   Venereal exposure common—males
>   Sequelae of dysentery—males and females
>   Nonbacterial urethritis
>   Mucopurulent conjunctivitis
>   Asymmetric polyarthritis
>   Mucocutaneous lesions
>   Circinate balanitis
>   Keratodermia blennorrhagica
>   Orolingual ulcers
>   Keratotic nails
>   Sacroilitis and atypical spondylitis
>   Cardiac abnormalities

The mucocutaneous manifestations (buccal or penile) can be minor or prominent features of the disorder. Keratodermia blennorrhagica may be confused with pustular psoriasis and some believe that the lesions are psoriatic in origin (Fig. 4-3). The keratotic nail lesions can persist for months, but in most cases the skin and nail changes heal without residua.

Joint involvement frequently subsides in a few weeks, although destructive changes can occur in some patients. Heel pain (from calcaneal periostitis) and back symptoms can persist or progress over a period of years. Recurrences have been observed in over 50% of patients subjected to long-term follow-up.[51] Sacroiliac joint changes and spondylitis may predominate in the chronic course of the disease. Clinical and radiologic features of spinal involvement differ from those of ankylosing spondylitis, but are similar to those found in psoriatic arthritis.[27, 28] Cardiac involvement has been documented in a small percentage of cases.[32]

Laboratory findings. The history of veneral exposure requires prompt bacteriologic investigation of exudative lesions. Aspiration of synovial fluid will commonly demonstrate high total call counts (30-50,000 per mm.[3], 95% polymorpho-

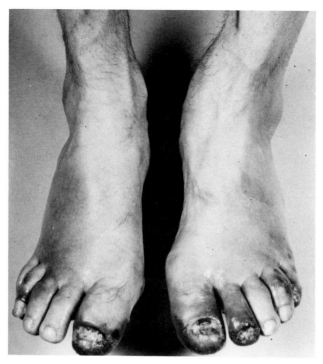

Fig. 4-3. Acute skin, nail, and joint changes in patient with Reiter's syndrome. Synovitis is present in metatarsophalangeal joints, left midtarsal joint, and left ankle joint.

nuclear neutrophil leukocytes) and joint fluid cultures are needed to exclude specific infection. High joint fluid complement levels are found in many cases of acute synovitis. Joint roentgenograms in progressive disease demonstrate certain characteristic features that differ from rheumatoid arthritis. They are similar to those found in psoriatic arthritis.[27]

    Treatment. During the acute attack, aspirin and nonsteroidal anti-inflammatory drugs are useful. Physical therapy can provide symptomatic relief and retard or prevent soft-tissue deformities. Some physicians favor the prompt use of oral tetracycline, but evidence for its usefulness is questionable. During severe attacks, intra-articular or oral corticosteroids may be required in selected patients.

ACQUIRED CONNECTIVE TISSUE DISORDERS
Systemic lupus erythematosus (SLE)

    In this disease well-defined immunopathogenic processes can account for several of the major histopathologic lesions. These include immune-complex nephritis, vasculitis, autoimmune hemolytic anemia, thrombocytopenia, and leukopenia. Precision of diagnosis improved after recognition of the "LE cell" phenomenon by Hargraves in 1948 and has been further improved by recognition of the universal occurrence of antinuclear antibodies in SLE patients' serum. More diagnostic specificity has been conferred by testing for the presence of antideoxyribonucleic acid antibodies (anti-DNA antibodies) and detection of serum complement depletion during active disease. The latter two measurements are also useful in evaluation of the effectiveness of therapeutic agents in suppressing disease activity.

The acute fulminating form of systemic disease was recognized over 80 years ago; the indolent, incipient cases with single organ involvement are now recognized much earlier than previously because of improvements in laboratory diagnosis. SLE affects females in over 80% of cases and occurs most frequently in the late adolescent and childbearing years. However, no age group is spared, and SLE has been diagnosed in both males and females in each decade of life.

Clinical findings. Preliminary criteria for diagnosis of SLE have been proposed and are useful in differentiating cases of SLE from other disorders.[7] The onset is usually insidious and attended by constitutional symptoms. The major multisystem manifestations of this disease are listed in the outline below.

Clinicopathologic features of systemic lupus erythematosus

Musculoskeletal	Polyarthritis, arthralgia, tenosynovitis, myopathy, osteonecrosis
Cutaneous	Erythematous "butterfly" rash, discord lupus, periungual lesions, photosensitive mucosal ulcers, alopecia
Pulmonary	Pleurisy, pneumonitis, discoid atelectasis
Cardiovascular	Pericarditis, myocarditis, endocarditis (Libman-Sacks disease), hypertension, vasculitis, Raynaud's phenomenon
Renal	Focal, diffuse, membranous, glomerulonephritis; nephrotic syndrome; uremia
Hematologic	Anemia, leukopenia, thrombocytopenia, lymphadenopathy
Neurologic	Seizures, psychosis, chorea, cerebrovascular accients, polyneuritis, peripheral neuropathy, cranial nerve palsies
Gastrointestinal	Abdominal crisis, esophageal dysfunction, splenomegaly, colitis
Ocular	Retinopathy (disease related and iatrogenic)

The most frequent initial manifestation of SLE and one that occurs at some time in 90% of patients is polyarthritis and polyarthralgias. Arthritis is rarely erosive, although soft-tissue deformities, such as synovitis and ulnar deviation of the fingers, can mimic those found in rheumatoid arthritis. Frequently, a history of episodic tenosynovitis of brief duration (hours) is obtained. Subcutaneous rheumatoid nodules have been identified in some patients but are rare. Aseptic (avascular) necrosis of bone (osteonecrosis) and myopathy occur in some patients. In most instances these complications are observed in patients receiving steroids (in osteonecrosis) or chloroquine (in myopathy).

The classical "butterfly" rash involving the central facial areas is uncommon (Fig. 4-4). However, cutaneous erythematosus eruptions are common and occur in most cases during some phase of the illness. An erythematous rash involving the exposed parts (face, neck, extremities) and a distinctive periungual erythema are typical lesions. Cutaneous eruptions may be photosensitive, but this is far less common than popular impressions imply. Superficial ulcerations of the oropharyngeal or genital membranes and chronic discoid lesions also occur. Alopecia (temporal baldness) and broken scalp hair is a classic and common finding.

The most common cardiopulmonary manifestations are pleuritis, pericarditis, or pleuropericarditis. A history of pleurisy or pleurisy with effusion is reported to occur in at least 50% of cases. Aseptic pneumonitis, basal discoid atelectasis, or pleuropericarditis are observed in some patients. Endocarditis originally described by Libman and Sacks (1924) is an infrequent pathologic finding of little clinical

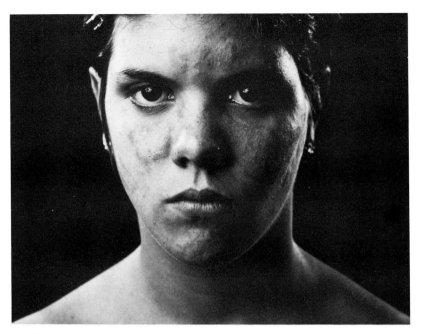

Fig. 4-4. Classic erythematous "butterfly" rash in central facial areas of young woman with active systemic lupus erythematosus.

significance. Hypertension is in most instances secondary to renal involvement. Vasculitis produces a spectrum of cutaneous signs similar to those found in rheumatoid arthritis. Raynaud's phenomenon has been reported to occur in 15% to 25% of patients.

Renal disease occurs in approximately 50% of patients and remains the leading cause of death, although other causes now rival it in frequency.[10] The use of renal biopsy has defined three histopathologic forms of glomerulitis (focal, diffuse-proliferative, or membranous). The course, progression to renal failure, and incidence of nephrotic syndrome and response to corticosteroid therapy differ in each of these subtypes of glomerulitis.[1] Most agree that local proliferative nephritis carries a better prognosis than cases with severe diffuse-proliferative, or membrano-proliferative disease.[1, 10]

Anemia is a frequent finding, whereas autoimmune hemolytic anemia and thrombocytopenia are far less common. Lymphadenopathy may be detected in 20% to 30% of patients and splenomegaly in approximately one half this number of cases. Central nervous system involvement may present a confusing array of signs and symptoms as enumerated in the preceding outline. During the early days of use of corticosteroids, psychologic aberrations were believed to be induced by these agents. Most neurologic abnormalities, including peripheral neuropathy or neuritis, are now recognized as manifestations of active disease. Severe irreversible central nervous system involvement now accounts for a number of the deaths that occur in SLE.[10] Abdominal crises may simulate an acute surgical abdomen and be traced to aseptic peritonitis, pancreatitis, or colitis. In other instances vascular lesions can produce gastrointestinal hemorrhage or dysfunction. The ocular manifestations of this disease will be dealt with elsewhere is this volume. Iatrogenic disease is an important cause of ocular abnormalities.

Laboratory findings. The laboratory procedures of value in diagnosis of SLE are listed in Tables 4-1 and 4-2. The Coombs reaction is positive more frequently than one finds evidence of hemolysis by other hemolytic indices. Initially, detection of renal involvement depends on careful evaluation of the routine urinalysis and performance of renal function tests. Renal biopsy is essential to determine the nature and extent of histopathologic changes. Serum complement and anti-DNA antibody measurements are useful in evaluation of renal involvement. The LE cell test (positive 50% to 70%) is the classic procedure used to confirm the diagnosis, although the detection of antinuclear antibodies (positive 95% to 100%) is a more sensitive procedure. Neither test is specific for SLE. Current information suggests that detection of antibodies to double-stranded DNA (anti-DNA) occurs only in active SLE. Detection of antinuclear antibodies is usually performed by use of an indirect immunofluorescent procedure. Nuclear staining patterns observed when this method is used depend on the predominate species of antinuclear antibodies present in the patient's serum. No pattern is specific for SLE although "homogeneous" (anti-DNA nucleoprotein) is most common and a "peripheral" (anti-DNA) pattern is associated with active disease.[37] Pronounced elevation in serum immunoglobulin levels (especially the IgG class) are common in SLE. Rheumatoid factor activity is detected in 15% to 20% of patients and particularly in those with hypergammaglobulinemia. A biologically false positive (BFP) serologic reaction is noted in as many as 20% of patients with SLE and may long predate other disease manifestations.

Other antinuclear antibodies directed against single-stranded DNA or nuclear or cytoplasmic ribonucleic acid can be found in SLE serum. It has been reported that one of these extractable nuclear antigen (ENA) correlates with a distinctive subtype of SLE or condition referred to as mixed connective tissue disease.[43] An antibody to double-stranded RNA has also been found in high frequency. Since this chemical moiety is unusual in mammalian tissue but common RNA virus infections, this finding is of special interest. Ultramicroscopic studies of renal tissues and skin have demonstrated cytoplasmic inclusions similar to the nucleocapsid of paramyxovirus. These inclusions have not proved to be specific for SLE.[55]

Treatment. In the absence of overt renal, hematologic, or central nervous system involvement, therapeutic doses of aspirin will often control musculoskeletal and constitutional symptoms (see Table 4-3). Antimalarial drugs used with close ophthalmologic follow-up exert a beneficial effect on cutaneous and serosal lesions. At our institution hydroxychloroquine is used in low dosage (200 to 400 mg. per day) in preference to chloroquine. Acute systemic disease or exacerbations require the use of corticosteroids and these drugs are effective in suppression of acute symptomology in a majority of cases. Hematologic, renal, or neurologic manifestations are most commonly treated with 60 mg. of prednisone per day or its equivalent. Treatment regimens and manipulation of the daily dosage require individualization. In severe multisystem disease much higher daily doses of corticosteroids are required (prednisone, 120 mg. per day).

In patients with serious corticosteroid side effects or those with steroid unresponsive disease, the administration of immunosuppressive drugs is justified. Currently, azathioprine (2.5 mg. per kilogram per day) or cyclophosphamide (1 to 2 mg. per kilogram per day) are most frequently used in conjunction with prednisone. Limited control trials and studies in the experimental animal model (NZB/NZW mouse) support the use of these agents in severe disease.[47] Serious complications can occur from the use of immunosuppressive drug regimens, and deaths from their use have been reported.[10, 47] Nevertheless, all major studies reported in the last 3 to 5 years document major improvement in longevity for SLE patients.[1, 10]

Progressive systemic sclerosis (PSS)

This is now the preferred name for the systemic disorder in which the term "scleroderma" describes the external manifestations. The connective tissues of the body undergo inflammatory, sclerotic, and degenerative changes. These alterations include a vasculitic component that affects the skin, the joints, and internal organs. The disease is most common in the 30 to 50 year age group and affects females two or three times more frequently than males. Immunologic abnormalities occur in a significant number of patients and imply that immunopathologic processes contribute to the genesis of this disease. At the same time there is morphologic and biochemical evidence indicative of defective collagen metabolism.[36] The course of

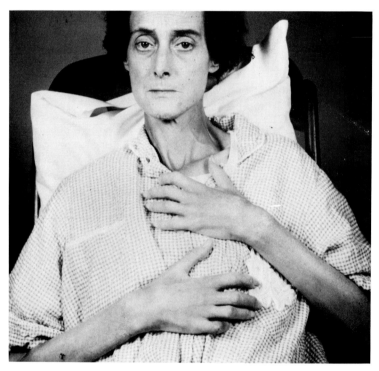

Fig. 4-5. Patient with moderately advanced progressive systemic sclerosis. Skin changes are apparent on face, neck, and upper extremities. Soft-tissue changes have produced flexion deformities in hands and wrists. Note pigmentary changes in sclerodermatous skin over hands and lower arms.

the disease may be protracted, but occasionally it is fulminate, with death occurring from renal, cardiac, or multiple systemic complications. Localized forms of scleroderma unrelated to PSS are recognized and include morphea and linear and nodular scleroderma. A variant form of PSS is referred to as Thibierge-Weissenbach or *CRST syndrome* (subcutaneous calcinosis, Raynaud's phenomenon, sclerodactyly, and telangiectasia).

Clinical findings. The major clinical manifestations noted during the course of PSS are listed in the outline below; the appearance of a patient with moderately advanced disease is shown in Fig. 4-5. Raynaud's phenomenon is the initial finding in 50% of cases and is reported to occur in most patients. Early skin changes tend to appear edematous and proceed to the thickened hide-bound appearance defined as scleroderma. The terms "acrosclerosis" and "sclerodactyly" define anatomic variants of distal extremity involvement. Loss of accessory skin structures, pigmentary changes, epidermal atrophy, telangiectasia, and dystropic circumscribed subcutaneous calcinosis describe the spectrum of integumentary changes. Progression of the disease involves symmetric areas on the upper and lower extremities, upper trunk, abdomen, face, and back. Synovitis may occur as an early manifestation and mimic rheumatoid arthritis. Joint stiffness is usually more characteristic than is articular pain. Soft-tissue fibrosis may produce severe digital and peripheral joint deformities. Clinical and laboratory findings of myositis can occur in PSS.

Clinical features of progressive systemic sclerosis

    Raynaud's phenomenon
    Skin lesions
        Acrosclerosis
        Sclerodactyly
        Scleroderma
        Telangiectasia
        Hypopigmentation
        Hyperpigmentation
        Calcinosis circumscripta
    Polyarthralgia and polyarthritis
    Osteolysis of terminal phalanges
    Polymyositis
    Esophageal dysfunction
    Pulmonary fibrosis and hypertension
    Cardiomyopathy
    Intestinal hypomotility, steatorrhea, pseudodiverticula
    Scleroderma kidney
    Malignant hypertension

Visceral lesions ordinarily appear as the disease progresses but occasionally occur before skin or musculoskeletal signs. Pathologic involvement of the lower esophagus produces dysphagia. Esophageal motility studies are abnormal in 75% to 80% of patients. Disturbance in gastrointestinal motility can produce distension, steatorrhea, and malabsorption. Dyspnea and other cardiopulmonary symptoms reflect the degree of interstitial fibrosis that occurs in the lungs and heart. Pulmonary changes are found in most patients. Cardiac abnormalities include conduction defects and signs of myocardial failure. Cardiopulmonary complications are a major cause of death in PSS. Renal changes have been referred to as the "scleroderma kidney." Some authors have associated the onset of renal failure and malignant hypertension with the use of corticosteroids. It is clear, however, that this lethal complication may occur regardless of whether the patient has or is receiving these drugs. Pathologically the kidney demonstrates local necrotizing angiitis in intralobular arteries and afferent arterioles.

Laboratory findings. Diagnosis depends on the identification of typical histopathologic changes in the skin or other tissue biopsies. As noted in Tables 4-1 and 4-2, positive tests for antinuclear antibodies occur in approximately 80% of patients. Immunofluorescent nuclear staining patterns are most commonly of speckled or nucleolar type. These patterns are not specific for PSS. Hypergammaglobulinemia and positive tests for rheumatoid factor and for LE cells may also occur. Distinctive radiologic changes occur in the chest roentgenogram, gastrointestinal tract, and distal phalanges.[27] Angiographic studies may demonstrate digital artery occlusions or obstructions in the renal vasculature. Pulmonary function and esophageal motility studies should be accomplished to document or detect preclinical involvement of these organs.

Treatment. There is no generally accepted therapeutic regimen currently employed in the treatment of patients with PSS (Table 4-3). Potassium *para*-aminobenzoate in divided daily doses of 12 to 20 grams is recommended by some physicians. The efficacy of this agent remains a matter of controversy. Corticosteroids are of questionable benefit in treating the cutaneous or visceral manifestations of PSS. Currently, reports (uncontrolled studies) on the use of immunosuppressive agents, especially the alkylating agents chlorambucil and cyclophosphamide, are encouraging.

Polymyositis and dermatomyositis (PDM)

These disorders are characterized by acute and chronic inflammatory involvement of striated muscle groups (polymyositis). Dermal involvement is more commonly seen in children and in those adult cases associated with malignant neoplasms (dermatomyositis). Myositis also occurs in several of the other connective tissue diseases. The age of onset, association with malignancy, acuity of muscle damage, and association with other rheumatic disorders can influence prognosis and the approach to treatment. This had led to the identification of several subgroups (types I to VI) in this disorder.[33] As observed in PSS, females are affected approximately twice as frequently as males. In cases associated with malignancy, males are affected as frequently as females.

Clinical findings. A summary of signs and symptoms is presented in the outline below. Cases with acute onset may manifest severe constitutional symptoms. Muscle weakness is progressive and affects the proximal pelvic girdle and then the proximal muscles of the upper extremities. In severe or chronic cases distal muscles may be involved. Cervical flexors are commonly involved, whereas facial and extraocular muscles are less frequently affected. The voluntary musculature of the pharynx can be involved and lead to dysphagia and dysphonia of variable severity. The degree of pain and tenderness of involved muscle groups usually varies in a direct relationship to the acuteness of the disease process. Atrophy and contractures of muscle are late complications. Calcinosis is a sequela of severe muscle inflammation and is observed in advanced stages of the disease, especially in children or adolescents.

Clinical findings in polymyositis and dermatomyositis

Muscle weakness
  Proximal pelvic girdle
  Proximal shoulder girdle
  Neck (flexors)
  Pharyngeal (dysphagia and dysphonia)
  Facial and extraocular areas
Muscle pain and tenderness
Muscle atrophy and contractures
Skin lesions
  Erythematous rash
  Heliotrope rash
  Periugual and articular rash
  Subcutaneous edema
Calcinosis universalis
Raynaud's phenomenon
Acute synovitis and arthralgias
Pulmonary fibrosis
Gastrointestinal symptoms

The rash observed in dermatomyositis is typically a dark, erythematous, mildly hyperkeratotic plaque-like eruption. It occurs over the face, neck, upper trunk, and arms and has a special predilection for the knuckles and periungual areas. A dusky iliac suffusion of the eyelids is referred to as a heliotrope rash. During acute disease, significant facial and subcutaneous edema may occur at the sites of inflammatory involvement. Raynaud's phenomenon has been reported to occur in one third of the cases and is noted frequently in patients with mild acrosclerotic skin changes. Synovitis may occur in the peripheral joints (fingers, wrists, knees). Pulmonary function may be compromised in acute disease because of weakness of the intercostal muscles. Some patients develop interstitual pulmonary fibrosis or aspiration pneumonitis. Dysfunction of the lower esophagus (as in PSS) is not uncommon. In the childhood form of the disease severe abdominal pain and gastrointestinal ulcerations may occur.

The association of this disease with malignancy is of considerable interest and has therapeutic implications. Successful eradication of the neoplasm usually leads to remission of the signs of dermatomyositis. When adult forms of the disease (in patients over 40 years of age) are segregated from the childhood form, the incidence of malignancy is approximately 20%.

Laboratory findings. The diagnosis is established by examination of biopsy material from an involved muscle (Fig. 4-6). Of equal importance is the measurement of "muscle enzymes" (serum glutamic oxaloacetic transminase [SGOT], creatine phosphokinase [CPK], and aldolase) levels in serum and electromyographic studies that will demonstrate the presence of muscle damage. Other laboratory abnormalities found in these patients are listed in Tables 4-1 and 4-2.

Treatment. Rest is of critical importance during active disease. Corticosteroids (60 mg. per day, prednisone or equivalent) effectively suppress disease activity in most cases. Reductions or adjustment in dosage can be evaluated by muscle testing and measuring serum levels of the "muscle" enzymes. Tapering of the dose should be gradual and some patients require long-term maintenance therapy. In refractory or corticosteroid-unresponsive patients, immunosuppressive agents (methotrexate

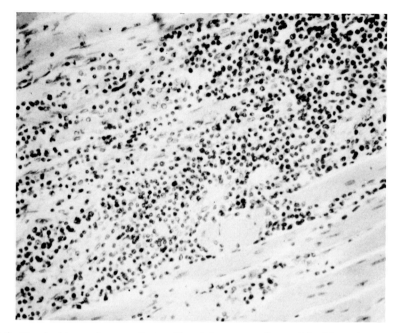

Fig. 4-6. Muscle biopsy from patient with adult onset polymyositis. There is muscle fiber degeneration, loss of cross-striations, muscle fiber necrosis, and centralization of muscle nuclei. The extensive inflammatory cell infiltrate contains lymphocytes, plasma cells, and polymorphonuclear leukocytes. There is also evidence of muscle fiber phagocytosis.

and cyclophosphamide) have been reported to provide benefit, although experience with these agents is limited. Children and young adults have a better prognosis than do adults over the age of 50 years.[29]

Necrotizing arteritis and other forms of vasculitis (PAr)

Classification of polyarteritis and its clinical variants is difficult. Confusion develops when one attempts to subdivide these diseases by the pathologic changes observed in blood vessels and ignore the clinical findings that seem to identify separate disease states. A revised classification of these disorders has been presented.[37] In this discussion the clinical disorders in which eye involvement occurs most frequently will be emphasized. Inflammatory destruction of the vessel wall (Fig. 4-7) can be associated in some instances with immune-complex deposition. Recently, occurrence of hepatitis-associated antigen and immune-complex formation has been reported in some cases of polyarteritis.[5] In giant cell arteritis, the histopathologic picture differs from that seen in experimental or clinical examples of immune-complex vasculitis or necrotizing arteritis.

Polyarteritis (nodosa). The so-called true or classic form of the disease demonstrates necrotizing arteritis of medium-sized and small muscular arteries. This disease affects predominantly males in the 30 to 50 year age group. The onset and multisystem progression is highly variable and often confused with other conditions. The major features of this disorder are listed in the general order of decreasing frequency in the outline below. The course may or may not be influenced by

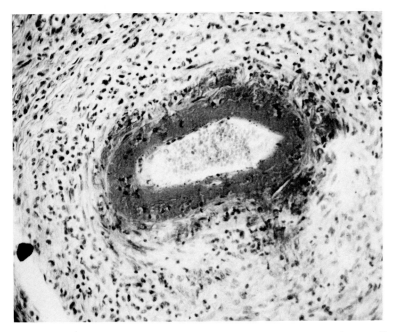

Fig. 4-7. Necrotizing vasculitis. Subacute inflammatory cell infiltrate throughout wall of small muscular artery with fibrinoid necrosis of intimal layer of vessel wall. These changes can be found in any one of the clinical variants of polyarteritis in which acute vessel necrosis is the predominate lesion.

treatment with corticosteroids. Death from renal failure or hypertensive cardiovascular complications commonly occurs. Abdominal crises with severe pain and gastrointestinal hemorrhage may require surgical intervention. Pathologic examination of abdominal lesions removed at the time of surgery may be the basis for initial recognition of the disorder. Pulmonary involvement is attended by pronounced peripheral eosinophilia (more than 50% total white cell count). Lung involvement is characterized by a granulomatous response. Some classify the latter condition as the polyarteritis of Churg and Strauss. These authors referred to the condition as *allergic granulomatous angiitis* and felt that it was distinct from true polyarteritis and represented an extreme form of *Loeffler's syndrome.* In true polyarteritis, peripheral and central nervous system involvement is eventually noted in 50% to 70% of cases. Organic psychosis, seizures, and focal neurologic defects (including unilateral blindness) are found. Peripheral neuritis is usually severe and of symmetric type. *Cogan's syndrome,*[6] which includes nonsyphilitic interstitual keratitis and inner ear disease (deafness, vertigo, tinnitus), occurs in young adults and appears to be a localized manifestation of polyarteritis or one of its variants.

Major clinicopathologic features in classical polyarteritis (nodosa)

Constitutional—fever, weight loss	Myocardial infarction and failure
Renal vascular disease	Focal CNS lesions
Hypertension (renovascular)	Peripheral neuritus
Abdominal crises	Arthralgias and myalgias
Bronchial asthma (hypereosinophilia)	Dermal lesions

Hypersensitivity angiitis. The pathologic lesions contain large numbers of eosinophils, occur in smaller vessels (than polyarteritis), and are of similar age. In this disorder a clear-cut history of drug provocation (penicillin, sulfa drugs, or antithyroid drugs) should be evident in the majority of cases. Pulmonary and cutaneous lesions are common in this condition. Removal of the offending drug and corticosteroid treatment may limit and suppress this disorder. Some consider allergic granulomatous angiitis a variant of this condition in which the offending agent (drug) cannot be identified.

Wegener's granulomatosis. Wegener's granulomatosis or granuloma is now considered a variant of polyarteritis[37] because the classic lesions found in the sinuses and lungs are produced by a necrotizing granulomatous angiitis. A focal or diffuse form of necrotizing granulomatosis is found in the kidney. When the angiitic component is minimal or the lesions are limited to the upper respiratory passages, the condition may present as lethal midline granuloma. On occasion, Wegener's granuloma may be more widely disseminated and involve the central nervous system, heart, gastrointestinal tract, and joints. The disease affects males and females most commonly in the 20 to 50 year age group and can cause death in a few months. Granulomatous lesions produce destructive changes in the facial sinuses and may invade the orbital region, leading to exophthalmos and ptosis. Peripheral leukocytosis is common and hypereosinophilia (50% to 80%) is a frequent finding in this disorder. Corticosteroid therapy is variably effective. Recent reports suggest that immunosuppressive drugs may be more uniformly effective in suppressing the disease.[12]

Giant cell arteritis. In Fig. 4-8 a relationship between giant cell arteritis, temporal or cranial arteritis, and Takayasu's arteritis is depicted. In addition, the clinical disorder of polymyalgia rheumatica is included, since these patients may have temporal arteritis. They may also on occasion develop signs of a partial or complete aortic arch syndrome because of giant cell arteritis.[17] The constellation of clinical findings, course, location, and extent of granulomatous arteritis form the basis on which these conditions are separated from each other. Involvement of the arterial supply to the eye resulting in blindness can occur in giant cell arteritis, temporal arteritis, and polymyalgia rheumatica (with temporal arteritis). The reported frequency of visual complications in each of these disorders varies widely.

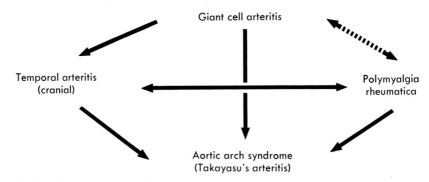

Fig. 4-8. Possible interrelationships between polyarteritis variants and polymyalgia rheumatica.

SYSTEMIC FORM. Pathologically this condition can affect branches or segments of the aorta at single or multiple sites. The arterial wall is infiltrated with inflammatory cells including numerous giant cells. Vessel occlusions occur because of proliferative changes or thrombosis, or both. Recanalization of the diseased segment can occur. The disorder is uncommon below the age range of 50 to 55 years and the female to male ratio is approximately 3:1. Constitutional symptoms are usually present. Other clinical manifestations depend on the sites of arterial disease. Temporal arteritis and cranial arteritis may be viewed as localized manifestations of this disorder. It shares with these disorders the potential for sudden unilateral or bilateral loss of vision. It can produce a clinical aortic arch syndrome in the elderly patient similar to that described as Takayasu's disease in young females. The syndrome of polymyalgia rheumatica can be the clinical expression of this disorder. Corticosteroid therapy is effective in suppressing disease manifestations.

TEMPORAL (CRANIAL) ARTERITIS. This condition is a localized variant of giant cell arteritis that is commonly associated with polymyalgia rheumatica. Pain is present over the temporal vessels and may radiate to other parts of the face and to the jaw. This may be described as a headache. Tender nodulations of the temporal artery may occur but are not always palpable. Involvement of the ophthalmic arteries leads to blindness as discussed above. This complication makes early diagnosis and treatment extremely important. The diagnosis is established by arterial biopsy[11] with or without prior arteriographic study.[20]

Takayasu's arteritis. This disorder produces an aortic arch syndrome and is also referred to as "pulseless disease," reversed coarctation of the aorta, or giant cell arteritis of the aorta.[31] The histopathologic lesion is similar to the other forms of giant cell arteritis, although the inflammatory reaction tends to be more medial and involve the vasa vasorum. In contrast to the other forms of giant cell arteritis, this disease affects females during the second to fifth decades of life. The efficiency of the development of collateral circulation influences the severity of ocular, central nervous system, and musculoskeletal signs and symptoms. Absence of peripheral pulses and bruits in the neck and upper extremities may be noted, with the patient complaining only of transient visual defects, syncopal attacks, faintness, or vertigo. Deaths occur from major uncompensated occlusions of arterial trunks. Hypergammaglobulinemia, positive tests for LE cells, and antinuclear antibodies suggest that immunopathogenic mechanisms are operable in these patients. Angiographic studies will detect the sites and extent of disease as well as the degree of collateral circulation. Corticosteroids and anticoagulant therapy are employed in these patients.

Polymyalgia rheumatica (PMR)

This clinical entity has a well-established cross relationship with giant cell arteritis and temporal arteritis. Although described many years ago, Barber was the first to use the term "polymyalgia rheumatica" (1957). Only in the past decade have detailed descriptions of the disorder appeared in the American literature.[17, 34] This is a disorder of elderly patients over the age of 50 years, with females more commonly affected than males. Onset of disabling muscle pains in the trunk and proximal extremities may occur gradually or quite abruptly. Constitutional symptoms may be severe. Pain and stiffness can make locomotion difficult, but on being tested, the muscles are not weak or tender. Later one may find signs of temporal arteritis or arterial bruits and pulse abnormalities indicative of aortic giant cell arteritis. The cardinal laboratory finding is a pronounced elevation of the sedimentation rate (Westergren method, 50 to 100 mm. per hour). All other laboratory tests used in routine differential diagnosis of rheumatic disease should be negative. Temporal artery biopsy may be positive even in the absence of local symptoms.[11] It is not routinely performed[34] unless the diagnosis is unclear or prodromal symptoms of ocular involvement (headache, temporal pain, visual symptoms) are present. Because of the unpredictable occurrence of blindness and the prompt clinical response to oral corticosteroids, this has become the preferred mode of therapy. Treatment may be initiated with suppressive doses of prednisone (or equivalent) 40 to 60 mg. per day and tapered promptly to more tolerable levels of 10 to 15 mg. per day. In some cases suppression of symptoms and a normal sedimentation rate allow withdrawal of the drug in 3 to 6 months. Ocular or systemic signs of giant cell arteritis require prompt recognition and resumption of higher daily doses of corticosteroids. Steroid complications accumulate rapidly in these elderly patients and close follow-up is required. In the absence of signs suggestive of temporal arteritis, therapeutic doses of aspirin have been shown to be effective in reducing the musculoskeletal symptoms.[34]

REFERENCES

1. Baldwin, D. S., Lowenstein, J., Rothfield, N. F., Gallo, G., and McClusky, R. T.: The clinical course of the proliferative and membranous forms of lupus nephritis, Ann. Intern. Med. **73:**929-942, Dec. 1970.
2. Brewer, E. J., et. al.: Criteria for the classification of juvenile rheumatoid arthritis, Bull. Rheum. Dis. **23:**712-719, 1972.
3. Calabro, J. J.: Juvenile rheumatoid arthritis. In Hollander, J. H., and McCarthy, D. J., editors: Arthritis and allied conditions, ed. 8, Philadelphia, 1972, Lea & Febiger, pp. 387-402.
4. Caplan, A., Payne, R. B., and Withey, J. L.: A broader concept of Caplan's syndrome related to rheumatoid factors, Thorax **17:**205-212, Sept. 1962.
5. Cassidy, J. T., Brody, G. L., and Martel, W.: Monoarticular juvenile rheumatoid arthritis, J. Pediatr. **70:**867-875, June 1967.
6. Cogan, D. G., and Dickersin, G. R.: Nonsyphilitic interstitial keratitis with vestibulo-auditory symptoms: A case with fatal aortitis, Arch. Ophthalmol. **71:**172-175, Feb. 1964.
7. Cohen, A. S., et al.: Preliminary criteria for the classification of systemic lupus erythematosus, Bull. Rheum. Dis. **21:**643-648, May 1971.
8. Cooperating Clinics Committee of the American Rheumatism Association: A controlled trial of cyclophosphamide in rheumatoid arthritis, New Eng. J. Med. **283:**883-889, Oct. 1970.
9. Dixon, F. J.: The immunopathology of glomerulonephritis. In Immunological diseases, ed. 2, Boston, 1971, Little, Brown & Co., pp. 1125-1133.
10. Estes, D., and Christian, C. L.: The natural history of systemic lupus erythematosus by prospective analysis, Medicine **50:**85-95, March 1971.
11. Fauchald, P., Rygvold, O., and Oystese, B.: Temporal arteritis and polymyalgia rheumatica, Ann. Intern. Med. **77:**845-852, Dec. 1972.
12. Fauci, A. S., Wolff, S., and Johnson, J. S.: Effect of cyclophosphamide upon the immune response in Wegener's granulomatosis, New Eng. J. Med. **285:**1493-1496, Dec. 1971.
13. Ford, D. K.: Reiter's syndrome, Bull. Rheum. Dis. **20:**588-591, Jan. 1970.
14. Forscher, B. K., and Houck, J. C.: Immunopathology of inflammation, Amsterdam, 1971, Excerpta Medica.
15. Gocke, D. J., Hsu, C., Morgan, C., Bombardieri, S., Lockshin, M., and Christian, C.: Association between polyarteritis and Australia antigen, Lancet **2:**1149-1153, Dec. 1970.

16. Good, R. A., and Fisher, D. W.: Immunobiology, Stamford, Conn., 1971, Sinauer Associates, Inc.
17. Healey, L. A.: Polymyalgia rheumatica. In Hollander, J. H., and McCarthy, D. J., editors: Arthritis and allied conditions, ed. 8, Philadelphia, 1972, Lea & Febiger, pp. 885-889.
18. Henkind, P., and Gold, D. H.: Ocular manifestations of rheumatic disorders, Rheumatology **4:**13-59, 1973.
19. Hollingsworth, J. W.: Local and systemic complications of rheumatoid arthritis, Philadelphia, 1968, W. B. Saunders Co.
20. Hunder, G. G., Baker, H. L., Rhoton, A. L., Sheps, S. G., and Ward, L. E.: Superficial temporal arteriography in patients suspected of having temporal arteritis, Arthritis Rheum. **15:**561-570, Nov. 1972.
21. Jessar, R. A.: The study of synovial fluid. In Hollander, J. H., and McCarthy, D. J., editors: Arthritis and allied conditions, ed. 8, Philadelphia, 1972, Lea & Febiger, pp. 67-81.
22. Kimura, S. A., Hogan, M. J., O'Connor, G. R., and Epstein, W. V.: Uveitis and joint diseases, Arch. Ophthalmol. **77:**309-316, March 1967.
23. Klemperer, P., Pollack, A. D., and Baehr, G.: Diffuse collagen disease: Acute disseminated lupus erythematosus and diffuse scleroderma, J.A.M.A. **119:**331-332, May 1942.
24. Kulka, J. P.: The vascular lesions associated with rheumatoid arthritis, Bull. Rheum. Dis. **10:**201-202, Dec. 1959.
25. Lepow, I. H., and Ward, P. A.: Inflammation mechanisms and control, New York, 1972, Academic Press Inc.
26. MacKay, I. R., and Burnet, F. M.: Autoimmune diseases: Pathogenesis, chemistry and therapy, Springfield, Ill., 1963, Charles C Thomas, Publisher.
27. Martel, W.: Radiology of the rheumatic diseases. In Hollander, J. H., and McCarthy, D. J., editors: Arthritis and allied conditions, ed. 8, Philadelphia, 1972, Lea & Febiger, pp. 82-135.
28. McEwen, C., DiTata, D., Ling, C., Porini, A., Good, A., and Rankin, T.: Ankylosing spondylitis and spondylitis accompanying ulcerative colitis, regional enteritis, psoriasis, and Reiter's disease, Arthritis Rheum. **14:**291-318, May 1971.
29. Medsger, T. A., Robinson, H., and Masi, A. T.: Factors affecting survivorship in polymyositis: A life-table study of 124 patients, Arthritis Rheum. **14:**249-258, March 1971.
30. Mikkelsen, W. M., and Dodge, H.: A four year follow-up of suspected rheumatoid arthritis: The Tecumseh, Michigan, Community Health Study, Arthritis Rheum. **12:**87-91, 1969.
31. Nakao, K., Ikeda, M., Kimata, S., Niitani, H., Miyahara, M., Ishimi, Z., Hashiba, K., Takeda, Y., Ozawa, T., Matsushita, S., and Kuramochi, M.: Takayasu's arteritis: Clinical report of 84 cases and immunological studies of seven cases, Circulation **35:**1141-1155, June 1967.
32. Paulus, H. E., Pearson, C. M., and Pitts, W.: Aortic insufficiency in five patients with Reiter's syndrome, Am. J. Med. **53:**464-472, Oct. 1972.
33. Pearson, C. M.: Polymyositis, Annu. Rev. Med. **17:**63-82, 1966.
34. Plotz, C. M., and Spiera, H.: Polymyalgia rheumatica, Bull. Rheum. Dis. **20:**578-581, Nov. 1969.
35. Rich, A. R.: Hypersensitivity in disease with especial reference to periarteritis nodosa, rheumatic fever, disseminated lupus erythematosus and rheumatoid arthritis, Harvey Lectures **42:**106-147, 1946-1947.
36. Rodnan, G. P.: Progressive systemic sclerosis (scleroderma). In Hollander, J. H., and McCarthy, D. J., editors: Arthritis and allied conditions, ed. 8, Philadelphia, 1972, Lea & Febiger, pp. 962-1005.
37. Rodnan, G. P., McEwen, C., and Wallace, S. L.: Primer on the rheumatic diseases, J.A.M.A. **224:**662-812, April 30, 1973.
38. Ropes, M. W., Bennett, G. A., Cobb, S., Jacox, R. F., and Jessar, R. A.: 1958 Revision of diagnostic criteria for rheumatoid arthritis, Bull. Rheum. Dis. **9:**175-176, Dec. 1958.
39. Samter, M.: Immunological diseases, ed. 2, Boston, 1971, Little, Brown & Co.
40. Schaller, J., Kupfer, C., and Wedgewood, R. J.: Iridocyclitis in juvenile rheumatoid arthritis, Pediatrics **44:**92-100, July 1969.

41. Schubert, M., and Hamerman, D.: A primer on connective tissue biochemistry, Philadelphia, 1968, Lea & Febiger.

42. Schur, P. H., and Austen, K. F.: Complement in the rheumatic diseases, Bull. Rheum. Dis. **22:**666-673, 1971-72.

43. Sharp, G. C., Irwin, W. S., Tan, E. M., Gould, R. G., and Holman, H. R.: Mixed connective tissue disease, Am. J. Med. **52:**148-159, Feb. 1972.

44. Sharp, J. T.: Mycoplasmas and arthritis, Arthritis Rheum. **13:**263-271, May 1970.

45. Smiley, D. J., Sachs, C., and Ziff, M.: In vitro synthesis of immunoglobulin by rheumatoid synovial membrane, J. Clin. Invest. **47:**624-632, March 1968.

46. Stage, D. E., and Mannik, M.: Rheumatoid factors in rheumatoid arthritis, Bull. Rheum. Dis. **23:**720-725, 1972-1973.

47. Steinberg, A. D., Kaltreider, H. B., Staples, P. J., Goetzl, E. J., Talal, N., and Decker, J. L.: Cyclophosphamide in lupus nephritis: A controlled trial, Ann. Intern. Med. **75:** 165-171, Aug. 1971.

48. Talal, N.: Sjögren's syndrome and connective tissue disease with other immunologic disorders. In Hollander, J. H., and McCarthy, D. J., editors: Arthritis and allied conditions, ed. 8, Philadelphia, 1972, Lea & Febiger, pp. 849-859.

49. Talal, N., Sokoloff, L., and Barth, W. F.: Extrasalivary lymphoid abnormalities in Sjögren's syndrome (reticulum cell sarcoma, "pseudolymphoma," macroglobulinemia), Am. J. Med. **43:**50-65, July 1967.

50. Waxman, J., Lockshin, M. D., Schnapp, J. J., and Doneson, I. N.: Cellular immunity in rheumatic diseases, Arthritis Rheum. **16:**499-506, July 1973.

51. Weinberger, H. W., Ropes, M. W., Kulka, J. P., and Bauer, W.: Reiter's syndrome, clinical and pathologic observations, Medicine **41:**35-91, Feb. 1962.

52. Weinstein, G. D., and Frost, P.: Methotrexate for psoriasis: A new therapeutic schedule, Arch. Dermatol. **103:**33-38, Jan. 1971.

53. Winkelstein, A.: Principles of immunosuppressive therapy, Bull. Rheum. Dis. **21:**627-634, Feb. 1971.

54. Wright, V., and Moll, J. M. H.: Psoriatic arthritis, Bull. Rheum. Dis. **21:**627-631, Jan. 1971.

55. Ziff, M.: Viruses and the connective tissue diseases, Ann. Intern. Med. **75:**951-958, Dec. 1971.

ADDITIONAL READINGS

Boyle, J. A., and Buchanan, W. W.: Clinical rheumatology, Philadelphia, 1971, F. A. Davis Co.

Hollander, J. H., and McCarty, D. J.: Arthritis and allied conditions, Philadelphia, 1972, Lea & Febiger.

Mason, M., and Currey, H. L. F.: Clinical rheumatology, Philadelphia, 1970, J. B. Lippincott Co.

Mikkelsen, W. M., et al.: Twenty-first rheumatism review, New York, 1974, The Arthritis Foundation.

5

Collagen and rheumatic diseases: ophthalmic aspects

Thomas P. Kearns

Shortly after my arrival at the Mayo Clinic, Drs. Kendall and Hench shared a Nobel Prize for their work with compound E. I recall the excitement that spread through the institution as word-of-mouth announcement proclaimed this event. I recall too that I was aware that this work with steroids was of major importance; however, neither I nor the others could have realized then the significance of these discoveries and their impact on the future of medicine in general, or on rheumatology and ophthalmology in particular.

I mention this historic event not only to introduce my subject but also to delineate my years of association as an ophthalmologist working closely with the rheumatologists in this clinic. This association was, and continues to be, a most pleasant one. Over these years, the Division of Rheumatology has allowed me and my colleagues in ophthalmology to share in the responsibility of diagnosis and treatment of their patients. They never hesitate to call for an ophthalmologic consultation on either an outpatient or a hospitalized patient when it appears that such will be beneficial to the patient. I have also found them most ready to consult with the ophthalmologists when we have problems. I have found them to be especially helpful with advice regarding the management of long-term steroid therapy. This close association has been not only enjoyable and instructive to me but also beneficial to our mutual patients.

I am amazed at the number of rheumatic and connective tissue diseases that may affect the eye. As I look at the classification of polyarthritis of undetermined etiology and of connective tissue disorders, I am struck by the idea that all of these diseases rather frequently have ophthalmic involvement. The following classification represents the first two sections of the "Classification of Rheumatic Disease," proposed by the Nomenclature and Classification Committee of the American Rheumatic Association and was officially adopted by that society in 1963. The latest modification of this classification appeared in the April 30, 1973, issue of the *Journal of the American Medical Association*.[15]

CLASSIFICATION OF THE RHEUMATIC DISEASES

I. Polyarthritis of unknown etiology
    A. Rheumatoid arthritis
    B. Juvenile rheumatoid arthritis (including Still's disease)
    C. Ankylosing spondylitis
    D. Psoriatic arthritis
    E. Reiter's syndrome
    F. Others
II. "Connective tissue" disorders (acquired)
    A. Systemic lupus erythematosus
    B. Progressive systemic sclerosis (scleroderma)
    C. Polymyositis and dermatomyositis
    D. Necrotizing arteritis and other forms of vasculitis
        1. Polyarteritis nodosa
        2. Hypersensitivity angiitis
        3. Wegener's granulomatosis
        4. Takayasu's (pulseless) disease
        5. Cogan's syndrome
        6. Giant cell arteritis (including polymyalgia rheumatica)
    E. Amyloidosis
    F. Others

RHEUMATOID ARTHRITIS

Scleritis and keratoconjunctivitis sicca are the two major ophthalmologic complications accompanying rheumatoid arthritis. True iritis is seen infrequently and most authorities believe that its association with the adult form of rheumatoid arthritis is only coincidental. Iritis, however, is encountered rather frequently with the juvenile form of rheumatoid arthritis (Still's disease). As we shall see, it is also commonly associated with ankylosing spondylitis.

Watson and Lobascher,[23] in a study from London, found that 26 of their 35 patients with scleritis (73%) had some form of rheumatic disease. Eighteen or slightly more than half of their patients had rheumatoid arthritis. On the other hand, they rarely found a systemic disease in patients with simple episcleritis.

The onset of scleritis is usually insidious, and pain is not a problem in the early stages. In later stages, when the sclera is more involved, the patient may have generalized discomfort or even true pain in and around the eye. Often only one section of the globe is affected initially, and one may have to lift the lid and have the patient look down in order to see the inflamed portion of the sclera. Shortly thereafter, multiple sectors of the globes of both eyes become involved. In severe scleritis, the vision will be decreased, and examination with the slit lamp will reveal cells and flare in the anterior chamber. Occasionally, secondary glaucoma will occur, even without the effect from topical use of steroids.

In long-standing scleritis or that which is refractive to treatment, thinning and bulging of the inflamed sclera develop and can lead to the serious complication of scleromalacia perforans. The areas of thinning appear blue because of the unmasking effect on the underlying uvea. Even in the absence of perforations, these areas are unsightly and are cosmetically disturbing to the patient (Fig. 5-1).

Although topical use of steroids usually will control episcleritis, it rarely will control scleritis. Systemic dosages are often necessary to control and suppress this inflammation. Because of the frequent association of scleritis with rheumatoid arthritis, most of the patients are already taking small doses of steroids. After a conference with the rheumatologist, the dosage is usually increased to or maintained

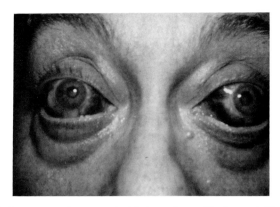

Fig. 5-1. Late stage of severe scleritis in patient with rheumatoid arthritis.

at the level required to suppress the scleritis. Topical application and at times an injection of steroids under Tenon's capsule are also used as adjuncts. Surgical intervention may become necessary when perforation threatens, but I believe, as do most others, that, if possible, such surgery should be avoided.

Keratitis sicca is usually not the severe eye disease that scleritis may be. Often, however, the patient is very uncomfortable and is most grateful when relief is obtained. Jones and Coop[10] stated in 1965 that 15% of all patients with rheumatoid arthritis have some degree of keratitis sicca. They also noted that 75% of all patients having keratitis sicca had some evidence of rheumatoid disease.

Keratitis sicca is generally easy to diagnose. In fact, I find that the diagnosis usually is made or strongly suspected on the basis of the history obtained by the referring rheumatologist. The symptoms of dry eyes, sandy feeling, stringy discharge, and inability to shed tears are so monotonously similar in all patients that it is difficult to mistake this diagnosis. It is often associated with dryness of the mouth. This combination is often referred to as "Sjögren's syndrome," named after Henrik Sjögren,[18] who first classified the disorder in a monograph in 1933. Arthritis is not a prerequisite to the diagnosis of Sjögren's syndrome, although it is present in most instances. The syndrome is a multisystem disorder with diverse features. Like other connective tissue diseases, few organs escape injury. In its complete form, Sjögren's syndrome is typified not only by dryness of the eyes and mouth but also by dryness of the nose, pharynx, tracheobronchial tree, vagina, and stomach, as well as enlargement of the salivary and occasionally of the lacrimal glands. The syndrome also may include dry skin, pancreatitis, interstitial nephritis, hepatobiliary disease, vasculitis, thyroid abnormalities, and lymphoma.[17]

Two clinical aids in the diagnosis of keratitis sicca are Schirmer's test of tearing and rose bengal staining to demonstrate the presence of the typical conjunctival and corneal lesions. After more than 10 years' experience with Schirmer's test, I abandoned it. I hope I am not alone when I say I have not used Schirmer's test in 15 years. I should add that I have not felt the need to use it in 15 years either. False-positive results to this test and the fact that negative results to Schirmer's test do not exclude keratitis sicca led to my disenchantment. Since I do rose bengal staining on all patients with symptoms or signs pointing to keratitis sicca, I see no reason to waste my time or the patient's time with Schirmer's test.

I like to instill proparacaine hydrochloride (Ophthaine) into the conjunctival sac before using rose bengal, which often causes considerable discomfort without such protection. I have not found that the use of Ophthaine gives rise to any false-positive results. I have noted many of our younger ophthalmologists applying a small amount of rose bengal to the conjunctival sac by means of a sterile toothpick or cotton applicator. Perhaps I am old fashioned, but I prefer to pour it on and wash it out with saline solution. At least, if the eye does not stain, it is not because of a lack of available dye.

The frequent use of one of the artificial tear preparations usually brings about improvement in the appearance of the corneal epithelium and reduces the patient's ocular symptoms. I like to tell my patients to use the preparation as they would a hand lotion. The principle is the same—to correct dryness by moistening and protecting. In this way, they are better able to adjust the frequency of instillation to their symptoms. I have found that, as in many other likes and dislikes, some patients prefer one type, whereas others, for unexplained reasons, prefer another type. Therefore, it is often necessary to try several different types and brands, until one satisfies the patient.

At this clinic, we have given up the procedure of closing off the lacrimal puncta. Some patients will have a remission of symptoms, and it is much more difficult to reopen the canaliculi than it is to occlude them. Also, some patients do not benefit from such occlusive therapy. Jones and Coop[10] consider occlusion most beneficial in selected patients. They do point out that a trial of occlusion using gelatin rods described by Professor Foulds of Glasgow is very helpful in deciding which patients will benefit from permanent occlusive procedures.

Cataracts frequently are seen in patients with long-standing rheumatoid arthritis. However, they are usually secondary to the steroid therapy rather than to the disease itself. These cataracts are of the posterior subcapsular type and are likely to produce visual symptoms in a relatively earlier stage of development. Progression of the cataracts is the general rule, as many of the severely arthritic patients find it impossible to discontinue or even reduce their steroid dosage. In such a situation, I have found it important to discuss the cataract problem with the patient and together weigh the risks of continued long-term usage of steroids. Such patients should be, and usually are, willing to share the responsibility of assuming the risks of cataract progression induced by steroids.

JUVENILE RHEUMATOID ARTHRITIS

Iridocyclitis is a serious manifestation of juvenile rheumatoid arthritis and may at times lead to blindness. The incidence of iridocyclitis in these patients varies from 5% to 15%.[2, 3, 11, 16, 19, 20] The incidence is even higher among patients with a monarticular onset of arthritis than among those with a polyarticular onset. Schaller, Kupfer, and Wedgwood[16] found iridocyclitis in 29% of their juvenile patients with monarticular rheumatoid disease but in only 2% of those children with polyarticular disease.

The onset of the iridocyclitis in these children may be insidious. It will smolder along undetected for many months until decreasing vision calls attention to its

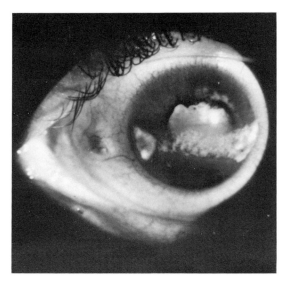

Fig. 5-2. Band keratopathy in patient with juvenile rheumatoid arthritis.

presence. Therefore, all children with juvenile rheumatoid arthritis should have an initial eye examination and periodic recheck examinations by an ophthalmologist.

Calcific band keratopathy is an almost universal feature accompanying chronic iridocyclitis in children with juvenile rheumatoid arthritis. O'Connor[14] found this complication in 35 of 36 patients with uveitis associated with Still's disease. The band keratopathy is found in the intrapalpebral area of the cornea. It begins near but not at the limbus; a clear area separates it from the limbus. Another characteristic is the presence of holes forming a Swiss-cheese pattern. These holes are believed to occur where the corneal nerves penetrate Bowman's membrane. The band meets in the center of the cornea as it progresses from either side (Fig. 5-2).

Cataracts secondary to chronic uveitis, and perhaps aggravated by steroids, soon follow. The iridocyclitis, the band keratopathy, and the cataracts form the characteristic ocular triad of juvenile rheumatoid arthritis.

The acute form of iridocyclitis is relatively easy to control with mydriatics and topical use of steroids. The chronic form is a different matter, and, like the control of scleritis in adults, systemic administration of steroids is usually necessary. Subconjunctival injection of steroids may be effective, but since many of the patients are young children, it is necessary to use a general anesthetic to carry out the procedure and, despite all attempts at therapy, serious visual handicaps and even blindness often develop.

ANKYLOSING SPONDYLITIS

Like juvenile rheumatoid arthritis, ankylosing spondylitis frequently has an associated iridocyclitis as a manifestation. In a report[13] from Montreal in 1966, a 12% incidence (11 of 92 patients) of iridocyclitis was noted in ankylosing spondylitis. Kimura and associates,[12] in a report from San Francisco that same year, noted that ankylosing spondylitis was the most frequently found joint disease causing uveitis. Ankylosing spondylitis was established in 41 of 191 (21.5%) individuals with uveitis. In other words, a fifth of all patients with uveitis can be expected to have ankylosing spondylitis.

The iridocyclitis is usually acute, bilateral, and recurrent. It is not unusual for the ocular disease to precede the other manifestations of ankylosing spondylitis. Therefore, any patient presenting with iritis deserves, as part of his general examination, roentgenographic studies of his sacroiliac joints for evidence of the characteristic changes of ankylosing spondylitis.

PSORIATIC ARTHRITIS

Psoriasis and arthritis have been known to be associated for many years, but only in recent years has psoriatic arthritis been considered as a distinct clinical entity. Duke-Elder[5] pointed out the similarity of the ocular findings in psoriatic arthritis and those in Reiter's syndrome. Both diseases may be associated with uveitis and conjunctivitis. Although my experience is limited, I have found that iritis is more common in psoriatic arthritis, whereas conjunctivitis is more common in Reiter's syndrome.

The treatment of the iritis in patients having psoriatic arthritis is the same as in patients having other rheumatic disorders. Chloroquine should be avoided by patients with psoriasis, since it often aggravates the skin lesions.

REITER'S SYNDROME

Hans Reiter died Nov. 25, 1969, at 88 years of age. His description in 1916 of an acute febrile illness characterized by urethritis, conjunctivitis, arthritis, and diarrhea in a German soldier was one of the earliest published reports of a syndrome that since then has been recognized with increasing frequency almost exclusively in young men.[21]

The disease usually starts as a nonbacterial urethritis and sometimes with colitis (especially in women). Arthritis and ocular complications usually develop later. Most patients recover from the initial episode in 6 weeks to 6 months. Recurrences, however, are common, and the clinical features of the recurrence may vary from a single manifestation to the complete triad with its complications.

Conjunctivitis is the usual ocular manifestation, although iritis, keratitis, episcleritis, retinitis, and optic neuritis are encountered less frequently. Conjunctivitis is usually bilateral and mucopurulent in type.

In a report on clinical and pathologic observations, 16 patients with Reiter's syndrome had bilateral purulent conjunctivitis.[24] The authors described the triad of Reiter's syndrome as urethritis, arthritis, and conjunctivitis. Only one of these 16 patients had iritis as the predominant ocular feature of his disease.

The treatment of the eye disease consists of steroids used topically or systemically and most patients respond to such treatment. Only rarely do such complications as cataract or secondary glaucoma develop.

SYSTEMIC LUPUS ERYTHEMATOSUS

The retinopathy of lupus erythematosus is often believed to be a distinct entity, which should allow the ophthalmoscopist to diagnose this condition with unfailing accuracy. This is certainly not true. Retinopathy appearing in patients with lupus

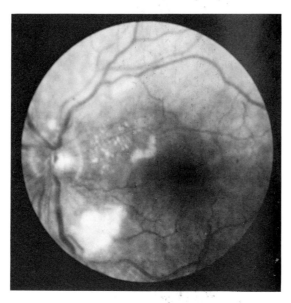

Fig. 5-3. Retinopathy of lupus erythematosus.

consists of soft exudates (Fig. 5-3), which may also be seen in various other conditions.

These exudates are really small infarcts in the nerve fiber layer of the retina. The histopathologic counterpart is the cytoid body, a swelling of the terminal nerve fiber resulting from degenerative changes in the nerve fiber.

The term "cotton-wool patch" is often used synonymously to refer to these lesions. Since this term is used so frequently to describe lesions associated with hypertension, in my opinion much confusion would be avoided if its use were restricted to hypertensive retinopathy.

In addition to hypertension, these lesions may be seen in a variety of conditions. They may be seen in any patient with a highly elevated sedimentation rate, and hence they appear in patients with malignancy, severe infections, and diabetes, as well as in patients having various rheumatic and connective tissue diseases.

I have frequently used the term "toxic retinopathy" to refer to the presence of these exudates. Although the term may not be scientific, it is a useful descriptive term when the cause for retinopathy cannot be determined with certainty from the ophthalmoscopic examination alone.

The soft exudates in lupus erythematosus are often small and tend to be distributed in the peripapillary areas of the retina. This may be of some help in differentiating lupus retinopathy from the retinopathy of the aforementioned conditions. However, these same characteristics may occur in the retinopathy, sometimes with scleroderma and dermatomyositis.

Retinopathy of lupus is seen much less frequently now than in previous years. I had believed this to be true in my experience, and it is confirmed by a recent study from England.[6] This study of the ocular findings in lupus was based on an analysis of 61 patients (51 females and 10 males). It was shown that the high incidence of ocular manifestations in this disease is no longer valid. This finding is attributed to the more effective treatment afforded today's patients. In fact, the authors of this article found that patients with lupus rarely have ocular signs or symptoms. They found retinopathy in only two patients (3.3%) as compared to previously reported incidences as high as 28%. None of their patients had retinal hemorrhage, retinal edema, or papilledema, all of which have been reported in most earlier studies.

This same study points out another changing pattern of symptomatology and ocular findings in lupus. A number of their patients had "macular pigment mottling," and four of the group had advanced chloroquine retinopathy. Apparently, therefore, the ophthalmologist's role in relation to lupus has shifted from the detection of retinopathy to monitoring for signs of retinal toxicity from treatment.

Chloroquine retinopathy, although rarely blinding, may produce severe visual impairment. The incidence of this complication has decreased since this retinal toxicity was recognized. Sporadic examples however are, and will continue to be, seen. Contrary to a number of reports, my colleagues and I have not found any way to detect this complication until the retinopathy is well established. Fluorescein angiography has been of some help in verifying early examples and in excluding other suspected examples. The characteristic bull's-eye pattern is enhanced by the

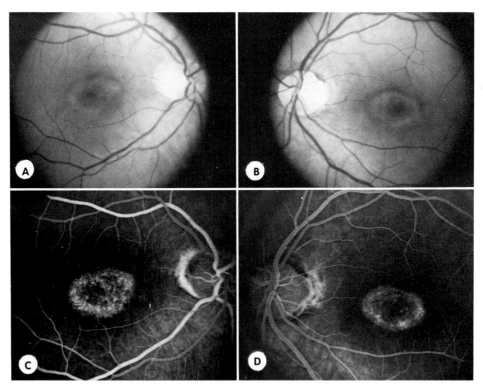

Fig. 5-4. Chloroquine retinopathy. **A** and **B,** Fundus photographs of right and left eyes. **C** and **D,** Fluorescein angiogram of right and left eyes.

use of fluorescein, since the depigmentation of the pigmented epithelium is more readily visualized (Fig. 5-4).

The problems related to this toxic effect of chloroquine are complicated further by the fact that retinopathy has continued to progress even though use of the drug has been stopped. At this clinic it is our opinion that patients taking chloroquine should have a base-line ophthalmoscopic examination as well as periodic reexaminations. However, we must admit that we are unable to predict impending trouble and, as the saying goes, we usually lock the barn door after the horse is gone.

The answer to this dilemma is obviously in controlling the dosage of chloroquine. I have found it most helpful to follow what I call "O'Duffy's rule." Dr. John D. O'Duffy is a consultant in the Division of Rheumatology of the Mayo Clinic. His rule states that it is usually safe to use 250 mg. of chloroquine a day for 3 years or a total of 250 grams. So far, I have not found retinopathy in any patient on this dosage for 3 years. Chloroquine retinopathy, in my experience, has developed in patients who had been using much higher doses for much longer periods—5 to 10 years. It certainly is not possible to set exact limits on any potentially toxic drug, but this rule gives me a guideline that I have found most useful.

Patients who are to be given chloroquine should be advised initially of the potential risk to the eye. However, chloroquine is a valuable drug, and they should not be so frightened that they will refuse therapy. I usually tell them that it is, in my mind, not as potentially toxic as steroids. When the patient has taken the drug for 3 years, it is wise to review again with him the danger of continued usage. As with the use of steroids, the patient must agree to share with the physician the risks of such side effects.

If toxic retinopathy develops there should be no basis for medicolegal actions against the physician, hospital, or pharmaceutical companies if the patient has been informed and knows that he shares the responsibility. It is wise to make a note to the effect that such discussion with the patient has taken place. In previous lawsuits arising from this complication in which I have testified or given deposition, the real liability appeared to be the lack of the physician's discussion of the risks with the patient.

PROGRESSIVE SYSTEMIC SCLEROSIS (SCLERODERMA)

Ophthalmoscopic changes may occur in scleroderma, but they are usually of little diagnostic value, since they are nonspecific. A toxic retinopathy may be seen, such as in lupus erythematosus, and consists of soft exudates. Since renal disease is an important component of scleroderma, hypertensive retinopathy may be seen in more advanced examples of this disorder. Nothing is unique about this hypertensive retinopathy to indicate to the ophthalmoscopist that the hypertension is a manifestation of scleroderma.

The ocular manifestations of scleroderma usually are limited to the more superficial ocular tissues. Skin changes are a major manifestation of this disease, as the name "scleroderma" suggests, and the lids do not escape involvement. The thickening and tightening of the skin of the lids are readily detected when the physician attempts to evert either the lower or upper lid. This induration is symmetric in both eyes and is merely a part of the generalized skin abnormality. I have often diagnosed scleroderma on finding these characteristic lid changes, but rarely have I made the initial diagnosis. The patient usually has other skin changes, often involving the fingers and hands, and his general physician has already made the diagnosis. Whenever I suspect scleroderma on the basis of lid changes, I shift my examination to the patient's fingers in order to confirm the diagnosis.

Small telangiectases may appear in the eyelids just as they do on other areas of the face. Perhaps my nondermatologic eye has not been trained to see these, since I have not noted them as often as the literature indicates that they occur. A recent publication, again from the British literature, reports the ocular findings in 23 patients with scleroderma.[8] Tight skin of the eyelids was noted in 15 patients, and telangiectases of the lids were noted in four patients. Eleven of the patients had decreased formation of tears and seven had keratitis sicca. Five patients had shallow conjunctival fornices, a result of the dermatologic effect on the lids. One patient had recurrent nodular episcleritis. The author of this article mentioned that cataract is often said to be a frequent ocular manifestation of scleroderma. However, only one patient in his series had cataract, and this was believed to be of the senile variety and unrelated to the scleroderma. None of these patients had retinopathy, although one patient did have a small retinal hemorrhage.

POLYMYOSITIS AND DERMATOMYOSITIS

These two disorders usually are grouped together because of their similar clinical and pathologic features. Although ocular involvement is not rare, examination of the eye is of little help in the diagnosis.

Walsh and Hoyt[22] stated that swelling of the eyelids and periorbital edema undoubtedly are the most common ocular lesions, and heliotrope eyelids should immediately suggest the diagnosis of dermatomyositis.

Conjunctivitis, iritis, ptosis, and paralysis of the extraocular muscles may be seen in dermatomyositis, as pointed out by Bruce[1] in 1938. All three of his patients had severe retinopathy, consisting of distended veins and numerous grayish yellow exudates. Hollenhorst and Henderson[7] found that retinopathy was the most frequent ocular finding in their 1951 study of Mayo Clinic cases. I would suspect that the incidence of retinopathy is much less today than it was previously. Just as has occurred with lupus, better and more effective treatment should tend to lower the incidence of ocular complications.

NECROTIZING ARTERITIS (CRANIAL ARTERITIS)

Since giant cell arteritis (cranial arteritis) is such an important disorder from the ophthalmic standpoint, I will confine my discussion to it. It may represent only the most superficial manifestation in a more widespread form of giant cell arteritis. More recently a clinical syndrome termed "polymyalgia rheumatica" has been recognized frequently among patients with giant cell arteritis.[9] These patients have had not only cranial arteritis but also widespread chronic inflammation of medium and large arteries with the addition of pain and stiffness of the trunk and extremities. A recent report[1] from the Mayo Clinic illustrates the close relationship of these two disorders. Nine patients with polymyalgia rheumatica had biopsy-proved giant cell arteritis. Eight of these nine patients had headaches. From the ophthalmic standpoint, these two disorders may be considered as the same entity. Serious loss of vision may develop as a result of either disorder. One should be especially fearful that ocular involvement may occur in polymyalgia rheumatica if headache, signaling cranial involvement, is present.

Cranial arteritis ranks as the prime medical emergency in ophthalmology, there being no other disease in which the prevention of blindness depends so much on prompt recognition and early treatment. Loss of vision, either unilateral or bilateral, is the most serious sequela of cranial arteritis. For this reason, the ophthalmologist should be thoroughly familiar with this disease process and aware of his important role in its diagnosis if the incidence of blindness from this cause is to be reduced.

The onset of ocular involvement is usually catastrophic and without warning. Occasionally, the patient will notice an increased light sensitivity preceding the actual loss of vision. Often such a history is obtained only in retrospect, but it is a grave prognostic sign in any patient known to have cranial arteritis.

The actual loss of vision may be preceded a day or so by visual symptoms not unlike the amaurosis fugax of occlusive disease of the carotid artery. Again, this symptom usually is mentioned only in retrospect, and a patient describes it as a symptom leading to his loss of vision.

Ischemic optic neuritis is the characteristic ophthalmoscopic finding in patients with loss of vision from cranial arteritis (Fig. 5-5). Like that of most optic neuritis, the visual loss is often greater than would be expected from the appearance of the optic nerve head. Unlike its appearance in most optic neuritis, the optic nerve head will be pale (ischemic) and not hyperemic. This pallor appears immediately, before any secondary optic atrophy occurs. The disk is only slightly elevated and the margins are blurred by edema. Generally, some hemorrhage is apparent on or near the disk. The arterioles of the affected eye are narrowed and often exhibit focal irregularity. Occasionally, actual occlusion of arterioles occurs and fragmentation of the blood columns may be visible.

Rarely, one may see evidence of ischemic optic neuritis in an elderly patient who does not have cranial arteritis. Almost always associated with such an idiopathic ischemic optic neuritis is a high degree of hypertensive sclerosis of the retinal arterioles and often evidence of retinal vascular disease. Therefore, the

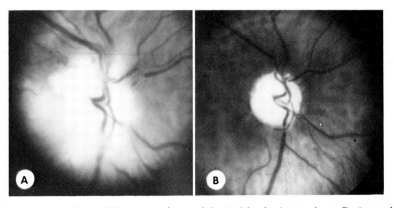

Fig. 5-5. Ischemic optic neuritis, as seen in cranial arteritis. **A,** Acute phase. **B,** 6 months later.

presence of ischemic optic neuritis in the absence of such retinal changes is typical of cranial arteritis.

The edema of the disk gradually disappears a week or so after the onset of ischemic optic neuritis. The hemorrhage then absorbs, and the pallor of second-ary optic atrophy appears. The narrowing and focal irregularity of the arterioles remain. No improvement in vision can be expected.

A few patients with cranial arteritis present with typical closure of the central retinal artery instead of ischemic optic neuritis. Such an occurrence can be a diag-nostic danger for the ophthalmologist, since the lesion may be regarded as an ordinary and idiopathic closure of the retinal artery and its full significance will not become apparent until visual loss occurs in the other eye. All patients who are 60 years of age or over and who have closure of the central retinal artery should be suspected of having cranial arteritis, and the symptoms and signs should be sought. The sedimentation rate probably should be determined in all such patients to rule out any possibility of cranial arteritis.

Approximately 5% of all patients with cranial arteritis exhibit mild extra-ocular nerve paralysis. Any muscle may be affected but generally the weakness is minimal. Often, the patient will give a history of vague diplopia, although on examination nothing is found to explain this.

Cotton-wool patches (soft exudates or toxic exudates) are seen at times in patients with cranial arteritis. Two mechanisms may be responsible for their ap-pearance. The first mechanism is toxic retinopathy and the soft exudates merely reflect the elevation of the sedimentation rate encountered in other diseases dis-cussed previously. The second mechanism is ischemic retinopathy representing more widespread retinal infarction with edema and occlusion of retinal arterioles. This is a more serious problem, and in a small percentage of patients it produces a serious loss of vision.

There is no question that steroids are effective in the treatment of cranial arteritis. The patient will always feel much better, and his headache will disappear or at least lessen within 48 hours after initiating such treatment. Furthermore, the sedimentation rate will begin to decrease after a few days and will gradually return to normal. It is usually wise to give 40 to 60 mg. of prednisone per day initially and to reduce the dosage as the sedimentation rate decreases.

The patient should be forewarned that no improvement in vision can be ex-pected. This lack of improvement in vision has led some ophthalmologists to believe that steroid therapy has no value in the treatment of cranial arteritis. The value of steroid therapy insofar as the visual problem is concerned is one of prophylaxis and not of cure, and it is this factor that necessitates prompt and early diagnosis. It is impossible to say which patient will or will not lose vision without steroid therapy, but it is obvious that if the systemic disease process can be suppressed before the visual loss occurs, the incidence of such loss will be reduced.

It does not seem proper for the ophthalmologist to manage the treatment of cranial arteritis alone. Consequently, he should participate in a joint effort with the general physician in the management of this disease and its related problems. By such cooperation, the patient's best interests are served.

Several rules of thumb for the ophthalmologist regarding cranial arteritis may be postulated.

CRANIAL ARTERITIS

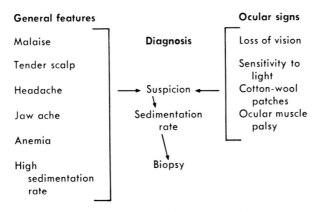

Fig. 5-6. The main general and ocular features of cranial arteritis.

1. Headache in any patient more than 60 years of age should be considered as a manifestation of cranial arteritis until proved otherwise by history, laboratory findings, and biopsy, if necessary. The ophthalmologist will not see many patients in this category.
2. Loss of vision from optic neuritis, retrobulbar neuritis, closure of the central retinal artery, or ischemic retinopathy in any patient more than 60 years of age should be considered a manifestation of cranial arteritis until proved otherwise. Such patients usually are seen by the ophthalmologist.
3. Any patient with a diagnosis of cranial arteritis, or strongly suspected of having it, should be hospitalized as an emergency measure and steroid therapy should be started immediately. The only exception, perhaps, is the patient who is already blind in both eyes, but even such a patient needs relief from the headache, malaise, and other symptoms.

With knowledge of the systemic as well as the ocular aspects of cranial arteritis, and with constant alertness for its possible existence in the older age group of patients, the ophthalmologist can play an important role in the prevention of blindness from cranial arteritis (Fig. 5-6).

CONCLUSION

Because of the frequent ocular manifestations of rheumatic and connective tissue diseases, the ophthalmologist should play an important role in the diagnosis and treatment of such diseases. The close cooperation of the ophthalmologist and the rheumatologist is most important in the diagnosis and management of the many patients with rheumatic and connective tissue diseases.

REFERENCES

1. Bruce, G. M.: Retinitis in dermatomyositis, Trans. Am. Ophthalmol. Soc. **36**:282-297, 1938.
2. Calabro, J. J., Parrino, G. R., Atchoo, P. D., et al.: Chronic iridocyclitis in juvenile rheumatoid arthritis, Arthritis Rheum. **13**:406-413, July-Aug. 1970.
3. Cassidy, J. T., Brody, G. L., and Martel, W.: Monarticular juvenile rheumatoid arthritis, J. Pediatr. **70**:867-875, June 1967.

4. Dickson, E. R., Maldonado, J. E., Sheps, S. G., and Cain, J. A.: Systemic giant-cell arteritis with polymyalgia rheumatica: Reversible abnormalities of liver function, J.A.M.A.
224:1496-1498, June 1973.

5. Duke-Elder, S.: System of ophthalmology. Vol. 9, Diseases of the uveal tract, St. Louis,
1966, The C. V. Mosby Co.

6. Gold, D. H., Morris, D. A., and Henkind, P.: Ocular findings in systemic lupus erythematosus, Br. J. Ophthalmol. **56:**800-804, 1972.

7. Hollenhorst, R. W., and Henderson, J. W.: The ocular manifestations of the diffuse collagen diseases, Am. J. Med. Sci. **221:**211-222, 1951.

8. Horan, E. C.: Ophthalmic manifestations of progressive systemic sclerosis, Br. J. Ophthalmol. **53:**388-392, June 1969.

9. Hunder, G. G., Disney, T. F., and Ward, L. E.: Polymyalgia rheumatica, Mayo Clin.
Proc. **44:**849-875, Dec. 1969.

10. Jones, B. R., and Coop, H. V.: The management of keratoconjunctivitis sicca, Trans.
Ophthalmol. Soc. U.K. **85:**379-389, 1965.

11. Kazdan, J. J., McCulloch, J. C., and Crawford, J. S.: Uveitis in children, Can. Med.
Assoc. J. **96:**385-391, Feb. 1967.

12. Kimura, S. J., Hogan, M. J., O'Connor, G. R., et al.: Uveitis and joint disease: A review
of 191 cases, Trans. Am. Ophthalmol. Soc. **64:**291-310, 1966.

13. Kinsella, T. D., MacDonald, F. R., and Johnson, L. G.: Ankylosing spondylitis: A later
re-evaluation of 92 cases, Can. Med. Assoc. J. **95:**1-9, July 1966.

14. O'Connor, G. R.: Calcific band keratopathy, Trans. Am. Ophthalmol. Soc. **70:**58-79, 1972.

15. Rodman, G. P., McEwen, C., and Wallace, S. L.: Primer on the rheumatic diseases.
Section 4: Classification of rheumatic disease, J.A.M.A. **224:**678-679, April 30, 1973.

16. Schaller, J., Kupfer, C., and Wedgwood, R. J.: Iridocyclitis in juvenile rheumatoid arthritis, Pediatrics **44:**92-100, July 1969.

17. Shearn, M. A.: Sjögren's syndrome, Major Problems Intern. Med. **2:**1-262, 1971.

18. Sjögren, H.: Zur Kenntnis der Keratoconjunctivitis sicca (Keratitis filiformis bei Hypo-
funktion der Tränendrüsen), Acta Ophthalmol. (suppl.) **2:**1-151, 1933.

19. Smiley, W. K.: The visual prognosis in Still's disease with eye involvement, Proc. R. Soc.
Med. **53:**196, 1960.

20. Smiley, W. K.: Iridocyclitis in Still's disease, Trans. Ophthalmol. Soc. U. K. **85:**351-356,
1965.

21. Twentieth rheumatism review: Review of American and English literature for the years
1969 and 1970, New York, 1973, Arthritis Foundation, Inc.

22. Walsh, F. B., and Hoyt, W. F.: Clinical neuro-ophthalmology, ed. 3, Baltimore, 1969,
The Williams & Wilkins Co.

23. Watson, P. G., and Lobascher, D.: The diagnosis and management of episcleritis and
scleritis, Trans. Ophthalmol. Soc. U.K. **85:**369-375, 1965.

24. Weinberger, H. W., Ropes, M. W., Kulka, J. P., and Bauer, W.: Reiter's syndrome,
clinical and pathologic observations, Medicine (Baltimore) **41:**35-91, Feb. 1962.

Ocular involvement in collagen and rheumatic diseases

CHAIRMAN: **P. J. Leinfelder***

Dr. Leinfelder: We have heard a very complete discussion of the various forms of a wide spectrum of diseases under the heading of rheumatoid and collagen diseases. It seems at first thought that some of these relationships are accidental, for some of the components of the syndromes exist independently without evidence of rheumatoid or collagen disease. This occurs frequently with uveitis and keratitis sicca. Similarly we frequently see rheumatoid arthritis without keratitis sicca or uveitis. For a number of years I have observed an apparent change in the incidence and severity of uveitis. Prior to the introduction of cortisone we saw many very severe cases of iridocyclitis, patients who required hospitalization for days and often weeks, but now we very rarely see that type of situation. I wonder if Dr. Bole has an explanation for this? Is it corticosteroid related?

Dr. Bole: Well, I should first mention that steroids is the anathema of the rheumatologist when we speak about rheumatoid arthritis. I believe that in attempting to respond to your question first I would say that in the several forms of acquired connective tissue disease (lupus and the others that we discussed today) we can be fairly convinced that the balance of effectiveness and suppression and inflammatory signs against the awesome complications that we all recognize can occur in individual patients is a well calculated and justified risk. In rheumatoid arthritis I believe that one is not on as firm gound unless one is dealing with a patient with severe progressive disease with the many systemic signs that occur. I agree with your premise that perhaps even in medical school the rheumatologist does a poor job in underscoring other approaches to the treatment of rheumatoid arthritis and perhaps all too often the patients who could probably do well with other forms of therapy will have had their experience with steroids. I would like to take off on your question, if I can have one more minute, and suggest that the battery of admittedly nonspecific but highly sensitive serologic studies we can use in the differential diagnosis of rheumatic disease has expanded greatly in the last several years

*Department of Ophthalmology, University of Iowa College of Medicine, Iowa City, Iowa.

and I am quite convinced that in lupus, for instance, we are diagnosing this disease far earlier when a single system may be involved than the classic description of the young female with the rash. Therefore in addition to therapy earlier recognition and then appropriate application of therapeutic modalities probably both underscore the changing percent instance of some of the classic systemic signs.

I would like to make a few comments. In over 120 systemic lupus patients that I personally followed some for as long as 14 years, I have only seen one outpatient with retinopathy. On the other hand, I have seen hospitalized lupus patients who had never previously been diagnosed, presenting in crisis. One with bilateral central artery occlusion, and one with bilateral central retinal vein occlusion. Its almost as if they are two different diseases, yet you can make the diagnosis in either by positive testing; so there is something different about the critically ill lupus patient. They do certainly have a vasculopathy and I believe they get the retinopathy irrespective of whether they have hypertension. Another thing that is rather striking to me is that I have never seen it in a rheumatoid arthritic patient and that one presented with an acute iritis, and yet in Still's disease with the monarticular form we have seen quite a number of cases. The patient with rheumatoid arthritis who gets ocular complaints generally has multiple articular involvement often in an active phase and often with lung or cardiac signs. I would bring up a point that Dr. Kearns did not bring up in his otherwise very excellent discussion. During the past 3 years we have seen the corneas with severe ulceration that were not bacterial, but were a melting away of a portion of the lower third of the cornea. Two of these went on to perforate, being treated by our own residents who had not recognized this. I know of at least 15 such cases of a sort of keratomalacia-like picture in rheumatoid arthritis.

Dr. Leinfelder: Would they have arteritis as well?

Dr. Henkind: No arteritis and no scleritis, and I believe this has been pointed out in the literature amply. Another thing that is terribly striking to me is that we have had a patient with an expulsive hemorrhage not, thank God, on our service, but in one of our attendings of a rheumatoid arthritic patient. The reason I bring it up is that I believe it is terribly important because you will operate on arthritic patients. Almost all of them are on aspirin, and you normally do not do bleeding work-ups on your patients. It's very illustrative to do a bleeding work-up on a rheumatoid arthritic patient who is on aspirin. When we had to operate on the second eye of this unfortunate lady when her vision was about 20/800, I got a bleeding work-up and I was amazed to find that, though she was off her cortisone and off phenylbutazone and her bleeding work-up was poor because she was still on aspirin, the rheumatologist took her off aspirin for a minimum of 10 days before her bleeding work-up came back to normal. I do not know whether that had anything to do with her original expulsive hemorrhage, but she did all right on her second lens extraction. The other thing that I learned in England is that subconjunctival steroids given to patients with rheumatoid arthritis particularly in the face of scleritis or episcleritis are more prone to perforate their scleras. I have not realized this, but apparently scleromalacia perforans really does not perforate.

It gets thin, and if you give them steroids, the scleras can perforate. Now I have never personally had a patient perforate with scleromalacia who had not been treated with steroids, and this was told to me by Mike Saunders. He might remember we had a conference in England and there were two cases of patients given sub-Tenon's injections and both perforated at the site of the injection months or years later. People with wide experience in England had never seen a true perforation from scleromalacia until this. Maybe they saw one or two, but it was rare, and as soon as they started giving steroids, the sclera would melt away and more perforations resulted. There is another thing I would like to ask a small question on. We had a 63-year-old lady with sudden loss of vision in one eye. We always get sedimentation rates; it was 125 mm per hour. We repeated it five times over a period of 5 days and got biopsies of both temporal arteries, both perfectly normal. Would you treat a woman on the basis of this high sedimentation rate? We have had this on a number of occasions—high sedimentation rates and loss of vision in older people. Do they treat these patients in the Mayo Clinic with steroids?

Dr. Kearns: Yes, as I said I do not believe we can say this is temporal arteritis, cranial arteritis or polymyalgia rheumatica. You cannot biopsy the arteries that cause a loss of vision. In the face of a negative biopsy, if the patient is 60 years of age or older and has a sedimentation rate of twice her age, maybe that is diagnosed as cranial arteritis.

Dr. Henkind: She has severe diabetes.

Dr. Kearns: Well, that makes it more complicated, but this is a risk that the rheumatologist and people that are working with us on this disease agree has to be taken. Why don't we go back a minute. I was very upset when I had not seen your article that came out in the *Journal of Rheumatology*. That paper was exactly the paper that I gave here today. I wished I had seen it earlier because I could have just copied it. As a matter of fact, I thought we should have traded lectures, except that I do not know enough about diabetes to trade with you, but I recommend this article. Dr. Bole has it in his bibliography. It was in the *Journal of Rheumatology*; I believe April of this year. Do you use Schirmer's test still?

Dr. Henkind: I use Schirmer's test. I use rose bengal a lot, but I find that it is so painful that I start with the Schirmer test. You know there is an interesting thing about the Schirmer test. It is positive; that is, you get very little tearing in so many old people and yet they do not have any symptoms. Now I do not know what that means, I do not treat patients unless their corneas are starting to break down. I do have one problem though. I do not do my rose bengal test with Ophthaine. I find I have an occasional patient who will start having his cornea break down from one drop of Ophthaine. I believe some of you must have had this, and if you then put on the rose bengal, the cornea stains, and the only way I can tell the difference is that the conjunctival epithelium does not break down as readily as the corneal epithelium does with Ophthaine.

There is an article by Norn in *Acta Ophthalmologica* in which he shows you can dilute the rose bengal. Dave Knox says that usually it is the preservative that causes the pain. I do not know. We have been lucky enough to burn almost every patient we have had to the point where I will get calls sometimes late at night. "Doctor, what have you done to me?" and I tell them to put a cold compress on it.

Dr. Cogan: I would like to point out that therapeutic occlusion of the puncta is beneficial for dry eyes. It helps conserve not only what tears the patient has but also whatever artificial tears are administered. Temporary occlusion may be obtained by use of a hot wire cautery or by a Hildreth cautery. The procedure may be repeated or the puncta may be surgically excised for permanent effect.

Dr. Leinfelder: Dr. Hayreh has asked to express a viewpoint on this from research that he has done.

Dr. Hayreh: I was involved in the running of the scleritis clinic at Moorfields for years and we had just completed compiling our results of over 400 cases of scleritis and episcleritis. We found that as regards to therapy we should give subconjunctival steroid to all the patients whose scleras were perforated. We found the oxyphenbutazone did help significantly. In our series we found that corticosteroids in 100% of the cases resulted in a regression of the disease, but some of the cases required a very long-term maintenance, as much as years, and the moment we took them off, the whole thing recurred. If you get a recurrence of scleritis, then just going back to the previous dose does not help. You have to start right from the beginning from a high dose if you want a good response. Otherwise it keeps smoldering. And this has been our experience based on quite a large series. I believe it is the largest series ever reported.

Dr. Wolfe: Nobody has mentioned it, but I find all these tests mentioned for diagnosing conjunctivitis sicca offensive. I think that if you have a lady with a white dress on and you get rose bengal on her dress you are going to buy her a new dress because the stain is not going to come out. Schirmer's test is so time consuming. I have done a test that I think I learned from Louis Girard that I find highly satisfactory and that is the fluorescein test, which you can do very easily when you are taking the patient's tension by applanation. I do not put any anesthetic in the eye, and I put a generous amount of fluorescein in the eye and then watch the fragmentation of that tear film. Now a person who has dry eyes will not let you hold his eye open very long. You can see that just as that tear film fragments, he blinks, and you can hardly keep him from blinking, and I find this is a very valuable test, and this is all I do. I see a lot of old ladies in my practice and most of them complain not of dry eyes, but of their eyes watering. My first test on a patient who complains of his eyes watering is this fluorescein test, followed by irrigation of his lacrimal canaliculi. I find this fluorescein test very worthwhile.

Dr. Bietti: In regard to the treatment of Sjögren's disease, I do not know if you here in America are familiar with two substances: one is called physalemine (extracted from the skin of *Physalemus,* an amphibian of South America) and the other is called eledoisin (extracted from the salivary glands of *Eledone moschata,* an octopus of the Mediterranean Sea). We have tried these two substances in the form of eye drops; they are chemically very close to the cerebral P substance, and they have shown the capacity to stimulate the lacrimal secretion. This stimulation produces an increase of three to five times the amount of tears that are normally produced. Of course, this is not a persistent effect, but by the use of drops three or four times a day, the majority of the patients are relieved from their symptoms. Our experience with the eledoisin is based on about 30 cases and with physalemine 12 cases. These two substances are not on the market yet, and you cannot even buy them in Italy, but they are worthy of consideration, and in the near future they will be sold because they are extremely effective. I believe that they are the most effective substances you can use in keratoconjunctivitis sicca.

6

Systemic aspects of nutritional eye disease

Donald S. McLaren

DEFINITION AND CONCEPTS OF NUTRITION AND ITS DISORDERS

The teaching of nutrition usually receives very little attention in the medical school. I therefore propose to make a few general remarks that I hope will help us to understand the part played by nutritional factors in disease processes.

Nutrition may be defined as the "process whereby food is utilized by the body." The study of nutrition related to the individual comprises the nutritive value of food, the nutritional requirements of the body, and the processes of ingestion, elimination, and utilization for the maintenance of life, production of energy, function of organs, growth, and reproduction in health and disease. At the community, national, or global level nutrition is concerned with such matters as quantity and quality of food supply in relation to the special needs of various population groups under varying circumstances.

I have found it helpful[20] to visualize the scope of nutrition in the context of the agent-host-environment interaction system as shown in Fig. 6-1. The part of the environment that we eat is called food, which may be defined as "edible mixtures." The agent of nutrition found within food is the part of food that nourishes and may be termed "nutriment." Food and nutriment are not synonymous because much in food does not nourish the body. Some is beneficial, like the indigestible fiber or roughage; some is harmful, like toxins of various kinds, natural or added.

Fig. 6-2 sets out in the same interaction scheme an outline of the content and scope of normal nutrition. Nutriment may be divided into two classes of dietary substances—aliments and nutrients. *Aliments* consist of carbohydrate, fat, and protein, which are consumed in large amounts, give rise to the liberation of energy, and for which there are no special requirements under normal conditions. Exceptions are nitrogen from protein and small amounts of essential fatty acids. *Nutrients* cannot be made by the body and therefore must be present in the diet in small amounts for health. At present nutrients are comprised of nearly 50 chemical substances—14 vitamins, many elements, and nine essential

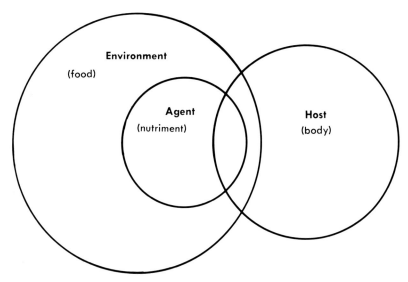

Fig. 6-1. Agent-host-environment concept applied to nutrition. (From McLaren, D. S.: Nutrition and its disorders, Edinburgh, 1972, Churchill Livingstone.)

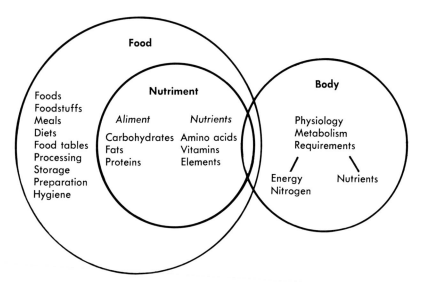

Fig. 6-2. The content of normal nutrition. (From McLaren, D. S.: Nutrition and its disorders, Edinburgh, 1972, Churchill Livingstone.)

amino acids. *Malnutrition* is disordered nutrition. Disordered nutrition may be classified according to the following four ways:

1. *Cause.* Primary or secondary, or perhaps better exogenous or endogenous, depending on whether the defect is in the agent (nutriment) or the body
2. *Kind.* Affecting energy, protein, vitamins, minerals, or most commonly a combination

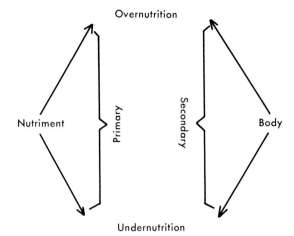

Fig. 6-3. Forms of nutritional disorders. (From McLaren, D. S.: Nutrition and its disorders, Edinburgh, 1972, Churchill Livingstone.)

Table 6-1. Secondary or endogenous malnutrition

Defect in	*Examples*
Digestion	Pancreatic disease, intestinal surgery
Absorption	Malabsorption syndromes
Transport	Abetalipoproteinemia
Storage	Cirrhosis, hemochromatosis
Metabolism	Inborn errors (phenylketonuria, galactosemia, etc.), vitamin dependency (B_6, B_{12}), ?obesity
Elimination	Trauma, renal failure, protein-losing enteropathy
Requirements (increased)	Pyrexia, injury, thyrotoxicosis

3. *Type.* Undernutrition or overnutrition; deficiency or excess

4. *Degree.* Mild, moderate, or severe

Some of these interrelationships are shown in Fig. 6-3. Finally, the endogenous cause of malnutrition is multiple and there are several possible kinds of defects as shown in Table 6-1.

Against this background we will now consider systemic aspects of the two major nutritional deficiencies related to ocular disease in man. Deficiency of vitamin A causes most serious and widespread ocular damage, which Dr. Halasa discusses in detail in Chapter 7. Vitamin B_{12} is linked with cyanide intoxication in the causation of amblyopia in several clinical entities.

VITAMIN A (RETINOL)
Physiology

This alcohol, $C_{20}H_{30}O$, results from the biodegradation of the highly unsaturated hydrocarbon β-carotene or seven or eight others of the nearly 100 carotenoid pigments to be found in nature, commonly in dark-green leafy vegetables (Fig. 6-4). In the mucosa of the small intestine, esterification, mainly as

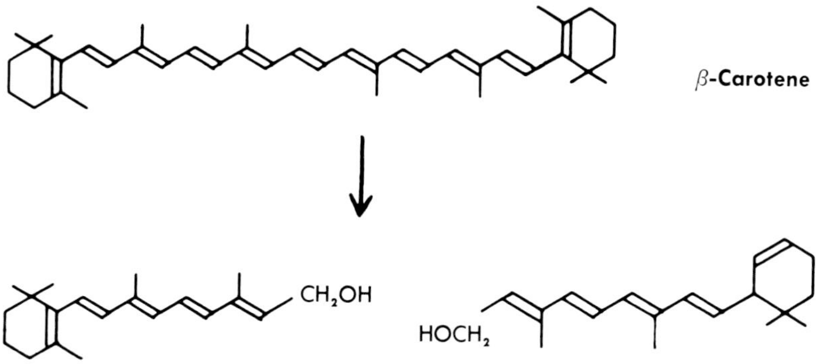

Fig. 6-4. Relationship of retinol to β-carotene.

palmitate, takes place and is followed by incorporation into chylomicrons. It is carried in the postabsorptive plasma attached to β-lipoprotein and stored in the liver, mostly as palmitate and mainly in lipocytes rather than in Kupffer cells as previously supposed.[38]

In the resting state most of the vitamin A in the circulation is in the form of retinol with a normal level in man of 20 to 50 μg. per 100 ml. It is attached to one molecule of retinol-binding protein (RBP of molecular weight 21,000) and one molecule of tryptophan-rich prealbumin of molecular weight 64,000 and binding also thyroxine.[14] In kidney diseases resulting in tubular proteinuria RBP and retinol have been found together in large amounts in urine. A free form of RBP has also been detected in plasma with a low content of retinol and one amino acid residue less of arginine.[26] It is probably a transitory form that is rapidly degraded by the kidney. During experimental deficiency of vitamin A in the rat both RBP and vitamin A in plasma declined; however the liver content of RBP of deficient animals was four times that of controls.[32] When vitamin A was given, serum RBP rose rapidly. It appears that vitamin A deficiency in some way interferes with secretion rather than synthesis of RBP by the liver. Protein deficiency also interferes to some extent with RBP synthesis by the liver.[10]

Circulating levels of vitamin A, RBP, and prealbumin (PA) are affected by different diseases.[24, 33] In liver disease all were depressed, and with recovery from acute hepatitis, levels of all rose. Molecular ratios of RBP:PA and RBP:vitamin A were normal. In renal disease RBP and vitamin A were distinctly raised; PA was normal. Molecular ratios of RBP:PA and RBP:vitamin A were distinctly raised. Much of the RBP was free. The normal process of catabolism of RBP by the kidney is impaired in renal disease, and so RBP in serum rises.

Function

Apart from our detailed understanding of the role of vitamin A in visual processes, our knowledge of the function of the vitamin in the body is still very limited. Vitamin A is of special importance in growth, possibly through its action on appetite. Deficient rats rapidly become anorexic, probably as a result of the loss of the sense of taste.[3] The well-known role of vitamin A in reproduction remains unexplained. The claim that there is a decrease in Δ^5-3β-hydroxysteroid dehydrogenase in deficient rats[13] could not be confirmed in pair-fed animals.[29]

Present evidence suggests that vitamin A probably does not have coenzyme function as was once believed, although it may stabilize certain enzymes. The membrane action of vitamin A is now well established. In particular it causes rapid release of lysosomal enzymes, with lysosomes remaining intact. This effect is specific to compounds with vitamin A activity, but the mechanism is not fully understood. The effect also takes place in vivo with both hyper- and hypovitaminosis A. Addition of RBP prevents these effects.[9] The red cell membrane is distorted in hypovitaminosis A, and bound ATPase is more readily released.[1]

Several pieces of evidence suggest a role for vitamin A in protein synthesis, either direct or indirect, with depression of some enzymes involved in facilitation of incorporation of precursors into RNA.[7] The same group has more recently shown that vitamin A is necessary for the biosynthesis of a specific glycopeptide from the goblet cells of rat small-intestine mucosa and that retinol acts as a carrier for monosaccharides in the biosynthesis of glycoproteins.[8] However, other workers have reported protein synthesis by liver ribosomes enhanced in vitamin A deficiency.[36]

Recent work suggests an important role for vitamin A in the immune process. Retinol appears to be the only naturally occurring enhancer discovered so far.[34] We have shown in our laboratory that retinal is equally active.[4] Other studies showed that vitamin A, in aqueous or oily form, inhibits circulating hemolytic complement in mice. The concomitant administration of a tolerance-inducing dose of antigen failed to produce unresponsiveness, and mice became immune.[2] Further, mice receiving vitamin A and a tolerance-inducing dose of antigen regularly developed immunity instead of the expected tolerance.[17] Possibly related to the effect it has on the immune response is the inhibitory effect of vitamin A during chemical carcinogenesis[27] and its determination of the state of differentiation of tracheal epithelium.[15] Retinyl acetate and retinol reduced tumors from DMBA (7,12-dimethylbenz[α]anthracene). Filipin, also a lysosome labilizer like retinol, reduced tumor formation, whereas the lysosome stabilizers chloroquine and hydrocortisone increased tumor incidence.[30]

Epidemiology of xerophthalmia

In regard to clinical aspects of vitamin A deficiency there is little new to report and it is discouraging to realise that despite considerable advances in our knowledge of the function and physiology of vitamin A, xerophthalmia remains a scourge of childhood in many developing countries, being responsible for blindness and death in thousands of children every year. Several autopsy studies from Canada and the United States[28] suggest that subclinical deficiency may be widespread even in affluent communities.

Fig. 6-5, showing the global distribution of xerophthalmia, was drawn more than 10 years ago, but it remains essentially correct today. Xerophthalmia is primarily a problem of public health magnitude in the rice-eating countries of south and east Asia, where 1% or more of all pre-school age children may be affected. The reason is that rice is devoid of carotenoid precursors of vitamin A,

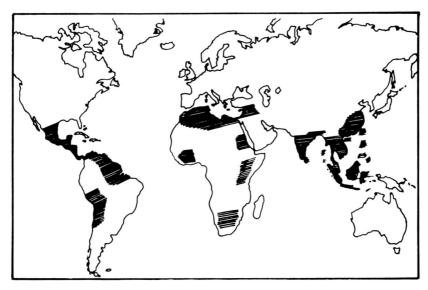

Fig. 6-5. Global occurrence of xerophthalmia. (From McLaren, D. S.: Xerophthalmia, Am. J. Clin. Nutr. **11**:603, 1962.)

milk is a relatively poor source, and green leaves, although abundant, are not incorporated into the young child's diet. The situation would be transformed if a carotene-containing variety of rice could be developed.

Treatment

Large doses of about 100,000 I.U. daily of vitamin A palmitate in aqueous solution are effective if given early in the disease. However, in practice the child is often not brought to the doctor until irreversible blindness from keratomalacia has supervened. These advanced cases frequently die, perhaps because a point of "no return" has been reached with disruption of lysosome membranes and release of hydrolyzing enzymes.[21]

Some instances of failure to respond to treatment are attributable to the use of oily injections. These are not mobilized from the site of injection and should be banned.

Prevention

Prevention clearly remains the ultimate objective, but little progress has been made recently. It is probably true that xerophthalmia is now being recognized earlier and being given more attention by governments and United Nations agencies. Incorporation of green leafy vegetables into the weanling child's diet should always be emphasized as the keystone of nutrition education concerning vitamin A. Fortification of sugar is being implemented in Central America and of tea in India, and results are awaited with interest. Massive prophylactic dosing is being introduced in India, Indonesia, and Bangladesh and should certainly prove effective where and when it is applied fully. Unfortunately such a measure is expensive of manpower, requires well-organized clinics, is limited in the numbers it can reach, and has to be constantly repeated.

VITAMIN B$_{12}$ (THE COBALAMINS)
Physiology

The cobalamins have in common with the folates their action as coenzymes in DNA synthesis and their use as therapeutic agents in the treatment of megaloblastic anemia. However, for our present purpose vitamin B$_{12}$ can largely be considered on its own.

The molecular structure consists of a nucleotide, 5,6-dimethylbenziminazole, linked at right angles to a four-pyrrol ring, similar to a porphyrin with a cobalt atom attached—a corrin group (Fig. 6-6). Several interconvertible cobalamins occur in nature, differing only in the ligand attached to the cobalt atom. Neither hydroxocobalamin nor cyanocobalamin is active, but two coenzyme forms of vitamin B$_{12}$, methylcobalamin the major form in plasma and deoxyadenosylcobalamin, are.[16, 35] The various forms in plasma have been separated by thin-layer chromatography and the individual cobalamins identified by a B$_{12}$-dependent organism's growth response.[18] Cobalamins arise in nature from synthesis by microorganisms in soil, water, and the intestine but are not absorbed from the colon

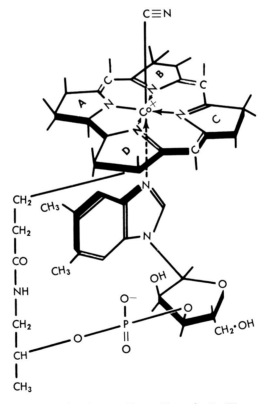

Fig. 6-6. Molecular structure of vitamin B$_{12}$. (From Chanarin, I.: The megaloblastic anaemias, Oxford, 1969, Blackwell Scientific Publications Ltd.)

in man. Strict vegetarians tend to develop deficiency but may derive their requirements (about 5 μg. per day) in the form of 5-deoxyadenosylcobalamin, which is synthesized by microorganisms in legume nodules of root vegetables and is present in tap water.

Peptide bonds binding cobalamin in food to protein are dissociated by cooking, digestion at acid pH in the stomach, or digestion by intestinal enzymes, and free cobalamin is bound to intrinsic factor secreted by the parietal cells of the gastric mucosa. Intrinsic factor probably has two receptor sites, one for vitamin B_{12} and the other for ileal microvilli, which specifically requires a neutral pH and the presence of free calcium. Very little vitamin B_{12} is absorbed passively.

There are at least two vitamin B_{12}–transport proteins; transcorrin I and II, which bind methyl-5'-deoxyadenosylcobalamin and hydroxocobalamin. Total plasma level in healthy subjects is 140 to 750 picograms per ml., representing only about a thousandth of the body content. The main route of excretion is in bile, with most of the 40 μg. reaching the jejunum per day, since it is reabsorbed by the intrinsic factor mechanism. Much less (up to 0.25 μg. per day) is lost in the urine.

Function

Vitamin B_{12} and folic acid are both involved in nucleoprotein synthesis. The exact role of vitamin B_{12} has not yet been defined, but it centers around the reduction of the ribose moiety of uridylic acid, which probably precedes the methylation of uracil to thymine (5-methyluracil) in the synthesis of DNA.

Methylcobalamin passes on a methyl group for the conversion of homocysteine into methionine, which it gets from tetrahydromethyl folate. 5'-Deoxyadenosylcobalamin acts as coenzyme in the conversion of methylmalonate to succinate. Methylmalonic acid excretion in the urine is increased in vitamin B_{12} deficiency.

Deficiency of vitamin B_{12} may rise in a multitude of ways and Herbert has classified the various conditions under five headings[12]: inadequate ingestion, inadequate digestion, inadequate utilization, increased requirement, and increased excretion. See outline* below:

1. *Primary deficiency*
    a. *Inadequate diet.* Vegetarianism, chronic alcoholism (rare), dietary faddism
2. *Secondary deficiency*
    a. *Inadequate absorption.* Lack of intrinsic factors (pernicious anemia, destruction of gastric mucosa, endocrinopathy), intrinsic factor inhibition, small intestine disorders (celiac disease, sprue, malignancy, drugs, specific malabsorption for vitamin B_{12}), competition for vitamin B_{12} (fish tapeworm, blind loop syndrome)
    b. *Inadequate utilization.* Antagonists, enzyme deficiencies, organ disease (liver, kidney, malignancy, malnutrition), transport protein abnormality
    c. *Increased requirement.* Hyperthyroidism, infancy, parasitization
    d. *Increased excretion.* Inadequate binding in serum, liver disease, renal disease

*From Herbert, V.: Am. J. Clin. Nutr. **26**:77, 1973.

Amblyopia, cyanide, and vitamin B_{12} deficiency

Amblyopia denotes "dimness of vision without detectable organic lesion of the eye" and early accounts frequently associated it with nutritional deficiency, especially beriberi or pellagra.[19] In more recent times hundreds of cases occurred among prisoners of war in the Far East during World War II where it was known as "camp eyes," and endemic foci have been reported in parts of West Africa[22] and the Caribbean.[6] Frequently the eyes have been affected only as a part of a multiple neuropathy, in which exaggerated reflexes and sensory loss affecting the posterior columns were prominent features.[19]

Amblyopia of a similar nature has also been described in alcoholism but is more commonly associated with heavy smoking, usually by the pipe, and sometimes there is a combination of both tobacco and alcohol amblyopia. Finally there is a group of conditions in which optic atrophy is a feature. These include pernicious anemia, Leber's hereditary optic atrophy, dominantly inherited optic atrophy, and optic atrophy of obscure origin.

For all of these disorders in which amblyopia features more or less prominently, there is a very incomplete understanding of the etiology at the present time. The situation is reminiscent of the early years of the present century when there were rival theories of the cause of such diseases as beriberi, pellagra, and rickets. The earlier favored a toxic origin, only to be superseded by deficiency as the cause when the vitamins were discovered. In the case of amblyopia the deficiency theory was first in the field, with the B vitamins, especially thiamine or riboflavin, being mainly implicated. Later cyanide, either from foodstuffs or smoking, was incriminated, and for reasons that will appear shortly, this is usually linked with deficiency of vitamin B_{12}.

In 1958 significant lowering of plasma vitamin B_{12} in tobacco amblyopia was reported.[11] Good response was obtained with parenteral vitamin B_{12} therapy. In 1961 Smith[31] suggested that tobacco amblyopia might be caused by the conversion of serum hydroxocobalamin to cyanocobalamin by the cyanide in tobacco smoke.

There is evidence to suggest that vitamin B_{12} is an important intermediary on one of the pathways of cyanide detoxication, through the ready conversion of hydroxocobalamin to cyanocobalamin. Wilson and Langman[10] proposed a

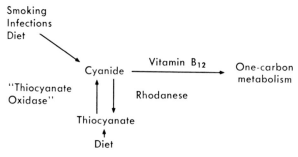

Fig. 6-7. Hypothesis to explain neurologic complications in vitamin B_{12} deficiency. (From Wells, D. G., Langman, M. J. S., and Wilson, J.: Thiocyanate metabolism in human vitamin B_{12} deficiency, Br. Med. J. 4:588, 1972).

general hypothesis that could account for the occurrence of neurologic complications in a minority of patients with vitamin B_{12} deficiency. This is summarized in Fig. 6-7. Cyanide and thiocyanate are in metabolic equilibrium. Cyanide concentration is determined (1) by conversion to thiocyanate by the enzyme rhodanase present in liver and kidney, (2) by incorporation into the one-carbon pool through the intermediary action of vitamin B_{12}, (3) by exposure to exogenous sources of cyanide or cyanogens from smoking, infections, or diet, and (4) by the formation of cyanide from thiocyanate by "thiocyanate oxidase" present in red blood cells. Possible dietary sources include performed thiocyanate from brassicas or milk and several plant foodstuffs in common use in the tropics, such as lima beans, yams, and cassava, which contain cyanide, either as glycosides or nitriles.[23]

The red cell mass that determines "thiocyanate oxidase" activity might be expected to be a rate-limiting factor in this system, and the known inverse relationship between the occurrence of neurologic complications in pernicious anemia and the degree of anemia might be accounted for in this way.[39]

At the present time certain facts are well established, but we are far from a complete understanding of the relationships between cyanide and thiocyanate, and vitamin B_{12} and the neuropathy. Several investigations have demonstrated that plasma concentrations of cyanide and thiocyanate rise with smoking[39] or cassava eating[25] and vitamin B_{12} levels fall. Under these circumstances amblyopia and other neurologic disorders have sometimes been found to occur[41] and at other times have been absent.[37]

The frequency of heavy smoking in patients with the neurologic complications of pernicious anemia is well documented. Recently however, Wells, Langman, and Wilson[39] found that patients with subacute combined degeneration of the cord who smoked had significantly lower plasma thiocyanate levels than did healthy smokers. Furthermore, plasma thiocyanate values in nonsmoking patients were not significantly different from control values.

Estimation of the separate cobalamins in plasma by Matthews has shown that cyanocobalamin is considerably raised in tobacco amblyopia, Leber's optic atrophy, and some other cases of amblyopia of obscure origin.[18] He believes that the primary defect is in cyanide metabolism and that the changes in cobalamins are only secondary. Now that a method is available for the separate estimation of the different cobalamins in plasma there is need for the development of a method for the measurement of the small amounts of free cyanide levels in plasma normally circulating. Meanwhile treatment should consist of withdrawal of the possible toxin, in the form of smoking or cyanide in the diet and large doses of vitamin B_{12} preferably in the form of hydroxocobalamin.[5]

At the time of the meeting I was not aware of the penetrating review of tobacco amblyopia recently published by Dr. Albert M. Potts (*Survey of Ophthalmology* 17:313-339, 1973). I find his case for the nutritional-deficiency etiology of the condition most convincing.

REFERENCES

1. Anderson, O. R., Pfister, R., and Roels, O. A.: Dietary retinol and alpha-tocopherol and erythrocyte structure in rats, Nature **213:**47, 1967.
2. Azar, M. M., and Good, R. A.: The inhibitory effect of vitamin A on complement levels and tolerance production, J. Immunol. **106:**241, 1971.

3. Bernard, R. A., and Halpern, B. P.: Taste changes in vitamin A deficiency, J. Gen. Physiol. **52:**444, 1968.
4. Charabati, M., and McLaren, D. S.: Action des différentes formes actives de la vitamin A sur le mécanisme immunitaire chez le rat, Experientia **29:**343, 1973.
5. Chisholm, I. A., Bronte-Stewart, J., and Foulds, W. S.: Hydroxocobalamin versus cyanocobalamin in the treatment of tobacco amblyopia, Lancet **2:**450, 1967.
6. Cruickshank, E. K.: Neuromuscular disease in relation to nutrition, Fed. Proc. Suppl. No. 7, p. 345, 1961.
7. DeLuca L., Schumaker, M., and Wolf, G.: Biosynthesis of a fucose-containing glycopeptide from rat small intestine in normal and vitamin A deficient conditions, J. Biol. Chem. **245:**4551, 1970.
8. DeLuca, L., and Wolf, G.: The mechanism of action of vitamin A, Proc. IX Intern. Congr. Nutr., Mexico City Abstracts, p. 60, 1972.
9. Dingle, J., Fell, H. B., and Goodman, D. S.: The effect of retinol and of retinol-binding protein on embryonic skeletal tissue in organ culture, J. Cell. Sci. **11:**393, 1972.
10. Glover, J.: Effect of vitamin A status on retinol-binding protein (RBP) in the rat on normal and low protein diets, Proc. Eur. Nutr. Conf., Abstract No. 54, Cambridge, England, July 1973.
11. Heaton, J. M., McCormick, A. J. A., and Freeman, A. G.: Tobacco amblyopia—a clinical manifestation of vitamin B_{12} deficiency, Lancet **2:**286, 1958.
12. Herbert, V.: The five possible causes of all nutrient deficiency: Illustrated by deficiency of vitamin B_{12} and folic acid, Am. J. Clin. Nutr. **26:**77, 1973.
13. Juneja, H. S., Murthy, S. K., and Ganguly, J.: The effect of vitamin A deficiency on the biosynthesis of steroid hormones in rats, Biochem. J. **99:**138, 1966.
14. Kanai, M., Raz, A., and Goodman, D. S.: Retinol binding protein: The transport protein for vitamin A in human plasma, J. Clin. Invest. **47:**2025, 1968.
15. Kaufman, D. G., Baker, M. S., Smith, J. M., Henderson, W. R., Harris, C. C., Sporn, M. B., and Saffiotti, U.: RNA metabolism in tracheal epithelium: Alteration in hamsters deficient in vitamin A, Science **177:**1105, 1972.
16. Lindstrand, K., and Ståhlberg, K. G.: On vitamin B_{12} forms in human plasma, Acta Med. Scand. **174:**665, 1963.
17. Major, P. C., Westfall, S. S., and Wirtz, G. H.: Vitamin A: Probe of immune complement reactions, Immunochemistry **6:**527, 1969.
18. Matthews, D. M.: Experimental approach in chemical pathology, Br. Med. J. **3:**659, 1971.
19. McLaren, D. S.: Malnutrition and the eye, New York, 1963, Academic Press Inc.
20. McLaren, D. S.: Nutrition and its disorders, Edinburgh, 1972, Churchill Livingstone.
21. McLaren, D. S., Shirajian, E., Tchalian, M., and Khoury, G.: Xerophthalmia in Jordan, Am. J. Clin. Nutr. **17:**117, 1965.
22. Money, G. L.: Endemic neuropathies in the Epe District of southern Nigeria. West Afr. Med. J. **7:**58, 1958.
23. Montgomery, R. D.: The medical significance of cyanogen in plant foodstuffs, Am. J. Clin. Nutr. **17:**103, 1965.
24. Muto, Y., Smith, J. E., Milch, P. O., and Goodman, D. S.: Regulation of retinol-binding protein metabolism by vitamin A status in the rat, J. Biol. Chem. **247:**2542, 1972.
25. Osuntokun, B. O., Monekosso, G. L., and Wilson, J.: Relationship of degenerative tropical neuropathy to diet: Report of a field survey, Br. Med. J. **1:**547, 1969.
26. Peterson, P. A.: Characteristics of a vitamin A–transporting protein complex occurring in human serum, J. Biol. Chem. **246:**34, 1971.
27. Polliack, A., and Ben-Sasson, Z.: Increased incidence of Rous sarcomas in response to excess vitamin A, Nature **234:**547, 1971.
28. Raica, N., Jr., Scott, J., Lowry, L., and Sauberlich, H. E.: Vitamin A concentration in human tissues collected from five areas in the U.S., Am. J. Clin. Nutr. **25:**291, 1972.
29. Rogers, W. E., Jr., and Bieri, J. G.: Adrenal Δ^5-3β-hydroxysteroid dehydrogenase as related to vitamin A, J. Biol. Chem. **243:**3404, 1968.

30. Shamberger, R. J.: Inhibitory effect of vitamin A on carcinogenesis, J. Natl. Cancer Inst. **47:**667, 1971.
31. Smith, A. D. M.: Retrobulbar neuritis in addisonian pernicious anaemia, Lancet **1:**1001, 1961.
32. Smith, F. R., and Goodman, D. S.: The effects of diseases of the liver, thyroid, and kidneys on the transport of vitamin A in human plasma, J. Clin. Invest. **50:**2426, 1971.
33. Smith, F. R., Raz, A., Goodman, D. S.: Radioimmunoassay of human plasma retinol-binding protein, J. Clin. Invest. **49:**1754, 1970.
34. Spitznagel, J. K., and Allison, A. C.: Mode of action of adjuvants: Retinol and other lysosome-labilizing agents as adjuvants, J. Immunol. **104:**119, 1970.
35. Toohey, J. I., and Barker, H. A.: Isolation of coenzyme B_{12} from liver, J. Biol. Chem. **236:**560, 1961.
36. Tryfiates, G. P., Krause, R. F., and Shuler, J. K.: Transfer ribonucleic acid of vitamin A–deficient rats, Am. J. Clin. Nutr. **26:**41, 1973.
37. Wadia, N. H., Desai, M. M., Quadros, E. V., and Dastur, D. K.: Role of vegetarianism, smoking and hydroxocobalamin in optic neuritis, Br. Med. J. **3:**264, 1972.
38. Wake, K.: "Sternzellen" in the liver: Perisinusoidal cells with special reference to storage of vitamin A, Am. J. Anat. **132:**429, 1971.
39. Wells, D. G., Langman, M. J. S., and Wilson, J.: Thiocyanate metabolism in human vitamin B_{12} deficiency, Br. Med. J. **4:**588, 1972.
40. Wilson, J., and Langman, M. J. S.: Relation of sub-acute combined degeneration of the cord to vitamin B_{12} deficiency, Nature **212:**787, 1966.
41. Wilson, J., and Matthews, D. M.: Metabolic inter-relationships between cyanide, thiocyanate and vitamin B_{12} in smokers and non-smokers, Clin. Sci. **31:**1, 1966.

7

Ocular manifestations of nutritional diseases

Adnan H. Halasa

Malnutrition as a cause of blindness has been and still is much underestimated.[15] Vitamin A deficiency with its complications of xerophthalmia and keratomalacia is well recognized as a leading cause of blindness throughout the world, especially in young children. The onset is often insidious and difficult to diagnose and the later stages proceed rapidly to irreversible damage. Ocular manifestations of nutritional deficiency are among the oldest signs and symptoms of disease known to man. Night blindness and its cure by liver is mentioned in the Ebers papyrus (1600 B.C.), in Chinese writings of the same period, and later by Hippocrates and Roman writers.[16] It was not until the nineteenth century that xerophthalmia began to emerge as a clinical entity with its characteristic pathology, symptomatology, and etiologic relationship to dietary deficiency.

The discovery of the fat soluble vitamin A and the demonstration of its efficacy in the Danish outbreak during the World War I as well as in induced deficiency in experimental animals proved that the early retinal dysfunction and later corneal damage were caused by vitamin A deficiency.[15] Of shorter history and less well-defined etiology is nutritional amblyopia, resulting from deficiency of vitamins of the B complex. This reached epidemic proportions in the camps of some Far Eastern prisons of war during World War II. Deficiency of other nutrients may produce serious ocular complications.

Deficiency of vitamin C producing clinical scurvy may result in hemorrhages in the lids, conjunctivae, orbit, and retina. Cataracts associated with tetany from vitamin D deficiency are well known. Deficiency of vitamin K in the newborn is a common cause of retinal hemorrhages.

However this presentation will be confined to discussing in more detail the ocular manifestations of the deficiency of vitamin A and vitamins of the B complex, together with the role of malnutrition in certain other eye diseases.

HYPOVITAMINOSIS A

"Hypovitaminosis A" is an explicit term used to encompass all manifestations of the deficiency state. "Xerophthalmia" is a descriptive clinical term implying serious affection of the eyes and often associated with an advanced state of general

136

hypovitaminosis A. The more specific terms "xerosis conjunctivae" and "xerosis corneae" are used to describe the state of the eye itself. "Keratomalacia" implies an advanced and largely irreversible corneal damage.

Hypovitaminosis A can be primary or secondary. Primary hypovitaminosis A occurs through dietary lack of the vitamin or the provitamins, the carotenes. Secondary deficiency may be a feature of diseases in which absorption or storage of the vitamin is affected as in the various malabsorption syndromes and certain liver disorders. It also occurs in diseases such as hypothyroidism and diabetes mellitus, which interfere with the conversion of carotene to vitamin A, and in conditions causing rapid destruction or loss of vitamin A, such as sustained fever and renal disease.

Secondary vitamin A deficiency may also be secondary to failure of enzymatic cleavage of β-carotene[18] and in abetalipoproteinemia[26] (Bassen-Kornzweig syndrome), which is characterized by malabsorption, atypical retinitis pigmentosa with nonrecordable electroretinogram, acanthocytosis, and mild neurologic disease similar to Friedrich's ataxia.

OCULAR MANIFESTATIONS OF HYPOVITAMINOSIS A

These manifestations may be divided into affections of the anterior segment and affections of the posterior segment.

Affections of the anterior segment

Children of 9 months to 4 years of age are most commonly affected. We have seen a child a few weeks old with keratomalacia (Fig. 7-1). Childhood infections, particularly measles, play an all important role in precipitating the eye lesions in patients in whom vitamin A levels are already low. The corneal affection in measles makes this disease of special significance in predisposing to keratomalacia.

Conjunctival xerosis and Bitot's spot. The bulbar conjunctiva shows the first changes especially noticeable in the interpalpebral fissure. Dryness of the conjunctiva precedes any changes in the cornea. There is loss of transparency, unwettability, wrinkling, pigmentation of the conjunctiva, and accumulation of debris (Fig. 7-2). Conjunctival biopsies usually reveal pronounced epidermalization of the conjunctival epithelium with total absence of goblet cells.[27]

Bitot's spot is an integral part of the conjunctival pathologic condition already mentioned. It is a small silvery gray plaque usually with a foamy surface and usually found in the interpalpebral fissure. It is frequently bilateral and temporal in location and less often nasal (Fig. 7-3, *A*). It is usually unaltered by rubbing over the closed lid, but if it is scraped directly with a spatula, most of the foam can be removed leaving a wrinkled chalky bed. The relationship of Bitot's spot to vitamin A deficiency is slightly confused in the literature. Broadly speaking, there appears to be two types of Bitot's spot from the point of view of etiology.[15]

One type consists of small isolated spots occurring in older children and adults with good dietary histories and with normal levels of vitamin A. This type does not respond to vitamin A therapy and appears to result from local factors, with exposure playing a prominent role (Fig. 7-3, *B*).

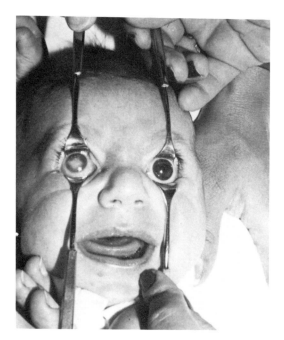

Fig. 7-1. Child few weeks old with keratomalacia.

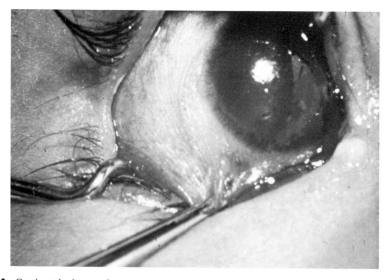

Fig. 7-2. Conjunctival xerosis; note wrinkling and pigmentation of the conjunctiva. (From McLaren, D. S., Shirajian, E., Tchalian, M., and Khoury, G.: Xerophthalmia in Jordan, Am. J. Clin. Nutr. **17:**117, 1965.)

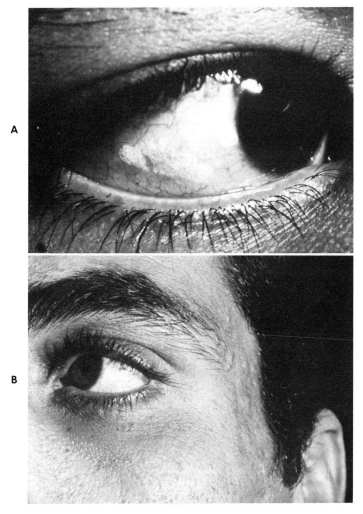

Fig. 7-3. A, Bitot's spot caused by vitamin A deficiency; note foamy surface and temporal location. **B,** Bitot's spot occurring in an adult and not associated with vitamin A deficiency. (From McLaren, D. S., Shirajian, E., Tchalian, M., and Khoury, G.: Xerophthalmia in Jordan, Am. J. Clin. Nutr. **17:**117, 1965.)

The other type consists of more diffuse spots or patches occurring in young children with other evidence of xerophthalmia and low levels of vitamin A in the plasma. These usually respond to treatment with vitamin A (see Fig. 7-3, *A*).

Corneal xerosis and keratomalacia. Xerosis of the cornea has the same characteristics as xerosis of the conjunctiva and is indicative of a more advanced stage of the disease. There is infiltration of the corneal stroma, giving it a bluish, hazy appearance (see Fig. 7-2). Before long, loss of substance of the cornea commences. At this stage a characteristic liquifactive process known as "colliquative necrosis" is responsible for the irreversible corneal damage (Fig. 7-4, *A*). At first an excavation of ulcer occurs in the central part of the cornea. As the

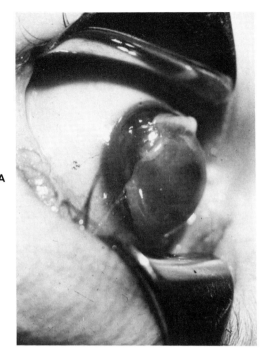

Fig. 7-4. Keratomalacia. **A,** Colliquative necrosis of the cornea. **B,** Corneal perforation with lens and vitreous prolapse. **C,** Complicated by endophthalmitis. (**A** from McLaren, D. S., Malnutrition and the eye, New York, 1963, Academic Press Inc.; **C** from McLaren, D. S., Shirajian, E., Tchalian, M., and Khoury, G.: Xerophthalmia in Jordan, Am. J. Clin. Nutr. **17:**117, 1965.)

disease progresses, corneal perforation, iris prolapse, and even loss of vitreous and extrusion of the lens may result (Fig. 7-4, *B*). When this process involves the whole cornea, it is called keratomalacia. The disease progresses very rapidly, characteristically without any reaction or inflammation because the corneal structure melts into a cloudy gelatinous mass.

In untreated cases, endophthalmitis not infrequently supervenes (Fig. 7-4, *C*). If the patient survives and treatment is started early, there may be a combination in the two eyes of a whole range of residual damage, from very fine nebulae to dense partial or total leukoma to phthisis bulbi or anterior staphyloma (Fig. 7-5). The minimal vascularization of the corneal scar is usually a striking feature of the clinical picture.

Treatment. We recommend that vitamin A be given by mouth and by intramuscular injection. By both routes aqueous dispersions are better utilized. By each route one should calculate the dose on the basis of actual body weight and should give 5000 I.U. per kilogram per day by each route for 3 days, thereafter continuing with cod-liver oil by mouth.

Affections of the posterior segment

Impairment of dark adaptation. Impairment of dark adaptation, resulting eventually in night blindness is the first symptom of vitamin A deficiency. In the

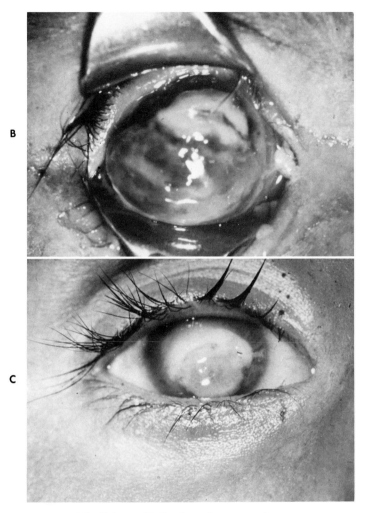

Fig. 7-4, cont'd. For legend see opposite page.

experiments of Dowling and Wald[4] dark adaptation became defective after rats had been deprived of vitamin A for 6 weeks. At this point the retina remained normal in structure. More prolonged deficiency however caused deterioration of the retinal tissue with disintegration of the outer rod segments.

To understand the role of vitamin A in dark adaptation, we need a brief review of the molecular basis of vision. A schematic representation of the major chemical events occurring in the outer segments of the rods when these receptors are stimulated by light is shown in this diagram[31] (Fig. 7-6).

As soon as light is absorbed by a visual pigment there is an immediate isomerization of the 11-*cis* form of retinal (vitamin A aldehyde) to the all-*trans* isomer.

None of the remaining reactions requires light energy. Stereochemically 11-*cis*-retinal is the most hindered of all the possible isomers of vitamin A aldehydes,

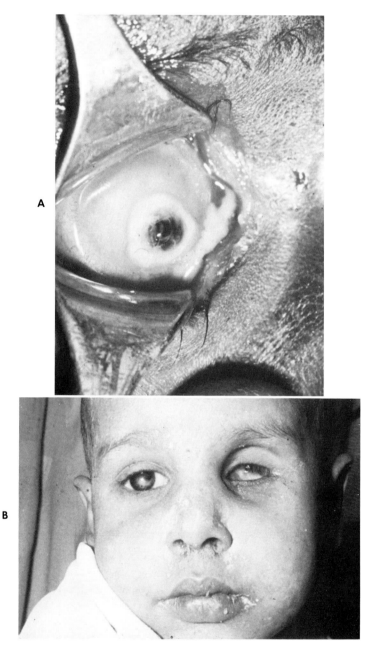

Fig. 7-5. End result of keratomalacia. **A,** Phthisis bulbi. **B,** Central leukoma O.D. and phthisis bulbi O.S. (**B** from McLaren, D. S.: Malnutrition and the eye, New York, 1963, Academic Press Inc.)

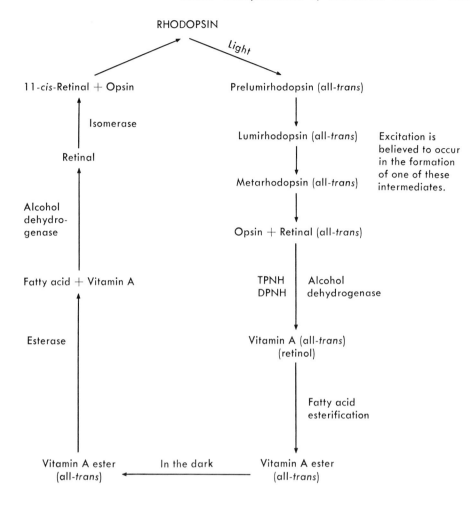

RHODOPSIN

Light

11-*cis*-Retinal + Opsin   Prelumirhodopsin (all-*trans*)

Isomerase

Retinal   Lumirhodopsin (all-*trans*)   Excitation is
                                                                   believed to occur
                                                                   in the formation
                                 Metarhodopsin (all-*trans*)   of one of these
                                                                   intermediates.

Alcohol
dehydro-
genase

                                 Opsin + Retinal (all-*trans*)

Fatty acid + Vitamin A   TPNH   Alcohol
                                 DPNH   dehydrogenase

Esterase   Vitamin A (all-*trans*)
                                      (retinol)

                                      Fatty acid
                                      esterification

Vitamin A ester   In the dark   Vitamin A ester
(all-*trans*)   ←   (all-*trans*)

Ester flows back to retina, from storage in
the pigment epithelium, where
isomerization to 11-*cis* form may partially occur.

Fig. 7-6. Scheme of major chemical events occurring in rod outer segment when these are stimulated by light. (From Wald, G.: Molecular basis of visual excitation, Science **162**:230, 1968.)

but according to Wald[32] it is the one that would fit best into the space provided for it within the protein portion of the visual pigment (opsin).

The all-*trans*-retinal is only partially released from the opsin molecule and still appears to be bound to the protein by means of a linkage between the carbonyl group of retinal and a nitrogen from one of the amino acid residues of the protein. Before resynthesis of rhodopsin can occur, vitamin A aldehyde (retinal) must undergo isomerization to the 11-*cis* form. The isomerization occurs both in the retina and pigment epithelium, but not elsewhere in the body.

Since the propagation of a nerve impulse can be ' recorded almost as soon as the light has been absorbed by the rhodopsin molecule, this would indicate that nervous excitation occurs prior to the bleaching step. The studies of Heller[13] represent a preliminary step in attempting to elucidate the molecular changes occurring in the protein portion of the rhodopsin molecule that might account for the initiation and propagation of the nerve impulse. According to Heller the protein portion of rhodopsin is held in a compact configuration in its native state. Heller proposes that this protein is held in the compact shape because the retinal portion of the molecule is attached to two areas of the protein by means of specific chemical bonds. When the rhodopsin molecule absorbs light, one of these chemical bonds is broken and the retinal portion of the rhodopsin isomerizes to the *trans* form. At the same time the protein changes its shape and takes on a different more expanded configuration (Fig. 7-7).

Recent autoradiographic studies on normal rod outer segments containing labeled amino acids have demonstrated that a continual balance exists between photoreceptor renewal and phagocytosis of the outer segment lamellae by the pigment epithelium.[25] This balance has been shown to be disturbed if there is interference with rhodopsin synthesis.

A lack of the precursor of retinal, vitamin A, eventually leads to loss of the protein portion of the visual receptor cells and finally to complete atrophy and disappearance of these cells. This fact would explain the findings of Dowling and Wald in rats that developed deterioration of retinal tissue after prolonged vitamin A deficiency. This will also explain the impairment of dark adaptation that I have already alluded to.

It should not be surmised that there is always a simple relationship between the vitamin A status as judged by plasma level and dark adaptation. The visual threshold may remain unchanged for periods ranging from several months to 2 years.[20] This discrepancy may probably be explained by the great variation in the concentration of vitamin A stored in the liver.

All authors agree that the male is more susceptible to night blindness, although Bietti states that this difference does not hold after the age of 45 years.[1]

Electroretinographic changes. Dowling[5] experimentally produced vitamin A–depleted rats, and reported the early loss of the a-wave and loss of the rod outer segments. Somewhat later the rest of the visual cell degenerates, accompanied by the disappearance of the rest of the electroretinogram.

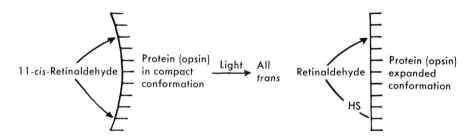

Fig. 7-7. Protein portion of rhodopsin expands when light hits rod outer segment, and retinal portion isomerizes to *trans* form.

Fundus changes

All descriptions of fundus changes associated with vitamin A deficiency have come from Japan and Indonesia where vitamin A deficiency was very prevalent.[29] They consist of a collection of small white dots in the horizontal meridian of the retina, resembling the appearance seen in retinitis punctata albescens (Fig. 7-8).

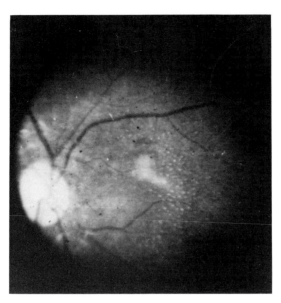

Fig. 7-8. Fundus changes in vitamin A deficiency; note collection of small white dots in horizontal meridian of retina. (From Dr. Teng-Khoen-Hing, personal communication to Dr. D. S. McLaren.)

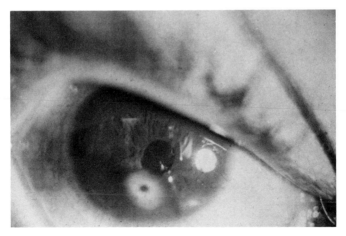

Fig. 7-9. Discrete colliquative keratopathy; note quiet and discrete dissolution of one small part of cornea.

We have not observed these fundus changes in 110 severely marasmic infants, many of whom were very deficient in vitamin A.[10]

DISCRETE COLLIQUATIVE KERATOPATHY

"Discrete colliquative keratopathy" is a term coined by McLaren to describe a mysterious disease of the cornea described originally in malnourished children in South Africa.[21] In the typical case there is a quiet and discrete dissolution of one small part of the cornea followed by prolapse of the iris (Fig. 7-9). Although investigators have maintained that this is a separate entity and distinct from keratomalacia of vitamin A deficiency, we wonder whether both might not turn out to be one and the same condition once a thorough nutritional evaluation is made of the African cases.

REFRACTIVE ERRORS OF MALNOURISHED CHILDREN

Sorsby, Sheridan, and Leary[24] have shown that the refractive state of the eye is genetically controlled. But there is evidence that environmental factors have some influence. We[10] have shown that marasmic infants tend to be myopic and that after recovery their refraction returns to normal.

DEFICIENCY OF VITAMINS OF THE B COMPLEX

Vitamins of the B complex are usually found together in nature and therefore diseases caused by their deficiency are always multiple in cause. Here again affections of the eye are divided into affections of the anterior and affections of the posterior segment.

Affections of the anterior segment

Corneal vascularization. Vascularization of the cornea as a result of riboflavin deficiency has been observed in some animal species, notably the rat, dog, and rabbit. Corneal vascularization as a feature of riboflavin deficiency was first mentioned by Kruse[14] and later by Sydenstricker.[28] The work of Gregory[9] and others has shown that vascularization of the cornea of the type observed in riboflavin-deficient subjects is not in any way specific and that the original description of corneal vascularization was attributable to misunderstanding of the normal variation in the vascular pattern of the limbic plexus. There appear to be very few well-documented cases of corneal vascularization responding to riboflavin from other areas of the world where riboflavin deficiency is widespread. Further support for the idea that corneal vascularization is not a constant or even prominent feature of riboflavin deficiency in man comes from several human experimental studies. Gordon and Vail[8] carried out a carefully controlled study of mental patients kept on a diet severely restricted in riboflavin for 15 months. None showed corneal vascularization.

Corneal epithelial dystrophy. A superficial keratitis, observed in malnourished individuals to which the name "corneal epithelial dystrophy" was given, has also been attributed to deficiency of the B vitamins.[23]

There is good evidence to suggest that corneal epithelial dystrophy is nothing more than epidemic keratoconjunctivitis possibly modified by a deficiency of the vitamins of the B complex.[22]

Affections of the posterior segment

Nutritional amblyopia. "Nutritional amblyopia" is a general term used to describe an endemic condition in certain parts of the world reaching epidemic proportions in the Far East in prisoners of war camps during World War II.

The clinical features of this syndrome are identical with the amblyopia associated with chronic alcoholism. The visual loss is usually gradual; objects are hazy at first, but when the disease is well established the scotoma may become positive in character. Carroll[2] estimated that this type of amblyopia is present in 0.3% to 0.5% of all new patients in the eye clinic of the Massachusetts Eye and Ear infirmary. Among 55 patients of his, only two were females; their average age was 55.6 years.

The characteristic visual-field defect is a central scotoma that is usually slightly irregular in shape, varying in size from 2 to 5 degrees and in density from a relative defect that requires a 1 mm. test object for its detection to an absolute loss. The margins of the scotoma are usually steep and are larger for red than for white targets. Harrington[11] stresses the central location of the scotoma in contradistinction to the centrocecal location of the scotoma in tobacco amblyopia. The scotomas are always bilateral. Ophthalmoscopy often reveals temporal pallor of the nerve head. Victor and Dreyfus[30] studied the pathologic changes in the retina, optic nerve, chiasm tracts, and lateral geniculate body in a malnourished alcoholic patient. They reported prominent loss of ganglion cells of both maculas, and symmetric loss of myelinated fibers in the optic nerves, chiasm, and tracts, accompanied by secondary gliosis and fibrosis.

They also reported diffuse loss of the small neurons of the dorsal layer in the lateral geniculate body. These authors believe that the earliest lesions are bilaterally symmetric areas of demyelination restricted to the papillomacular bundles within the retro-orbital parts of the optic nerves and that these lesions subsequently spread in a centrifugal manner to involve an ever-increasing number of fibers.

The precise etiology of nutritional amblyopia is not definite, although one can say it almost certainly involves deficiency of vitamins of the B complex.

Dreyfus[6] reported on whole blood transketolase (a thiamine-dependent enzyme) assays in two alcoholic patients suffering from untreated amblyopia.

His results indicated low levels of transketolase that point to a specific deficiency of thiamine. Dreyfus speculates on how thiamine deficiency is related to the selective localization of the pathologic changes observed in alcohol amblyopia. Animal experiments have revealed that transketolase activity is highest in those parts of the nervous system that are heavily myelinated and that during progressive thiamine depletion a decrease in enzymatic activity occurs in the areas of the central nervous system that show the most striking lesions.

However, the histologic findings in Wernicke's encephalopathy, which is caused by acute deficiency of thiamine, are against this suggestion of Dreyfus. In Wernicke's encephalopathy the brain shows capillary damage with endothelial proliferation and microscopic hemorrhages located characteristically in the mamillary bodies, walls of the third ventricle, aqueduct, and tegmentum of the medulla.[33] The eyes are commonly affected in Wernicke's encephalopathy; nystagmus, paralysis of the lateral rectus and conjugate lateral gaze, loss of vision, and papilledema are some of the eye signs.

Tobacco amblyopia and its relation to deficiency of vitamin B$_{12}$. True tobacco amblyopia is an uncommon condition. It usually develops in males over 40 years of age who are heavy pipe smokers. The most characteristic clinical finding in true tobacco amblyopia is a bilateral centrocecal scotoma.[11]

Trouble with reading is a frequently early complaint, and as Carroll[2] has remarked, less difficulty is experienced in using the left eye for reading than in using the right because the centrocecal scotoma in the left visual field does not interfere with fixation to the extent that it does in the right field. In 1958 Heaton et al.[12] suggested that tobacco amblyopia and the retrobulbar neuritis associated with pernicious anemia might be one and the same thing, both caused by low vitamin B$_{12}$ levels in the serum. In favor of this suggestion were the findings of Foulds et al.[7] who reported a high incidence of pernicious anemia among patients presenting with tobacco amblyopia.

In 1967 Chisholm et al.[3] reported that therapy with hydroxocobalamin produced more improvement in tobacco amblyopia than did therapy with cyanocobalamin.

These findings support the view initially proposed by Wokes[34] that tobacco amblyopia might be a manifestation of chronic cyanide toxicity caused by a failure of detoxification of cyanide derived from tobacco smoke. The cure of tobacco amblyopia and of the optic neuropathy of pernicious anemia with hydroxycobalamin may be attributable to detoxification of cyanide by its conversion to cyanocobalamin, a conversion that cannot occur if treatment with cyanocobalamin alone is given.

REFERENCES

1. Bietti, G. B.: Le vitamine in oftalmologia, Bologna, 1940, Casa Editrice Licinio Cappelli.
2. Carroll, F. D.: Analysis of 55 cases of tobacco-alcohol amblyopia, Arch. Ophthalmol. **14:**421, 1935.
3. Chisholm, I. S., Bronte-Stewart, J., and Foulds, W. S.: Hydroxocobalamin versus cyanocobalamin in the treatment of tobacco amblyopia, Lancet **2:**450, 1967.
4. Dowling, J. E., and Wald, G.: Vitamin A deficiency and night blindness, Proc. Nat. Acad. Sci. **44:**648, 1958.
5. Dowling, J. E.: Night blindness, dark adaptation and the electroretinogram, Am. J. Ophthalmol. **50:**875, 1960.
6. Dreyfus, P. M.: Blood transketolase levels in tobacco-alcohol amblyopia, Arch. Ophthalmol. **74:**617, 1965.
7. Foulds, W. S., Chisholm, I. S., Stewart, J. B., and Wilson, T. M.: The optic neuropathy of pernicious anemia, Arch. Ophthalmol. **82:**427, 1969.
8. Gordon, O. E., and Vail, D.: Quoted by McLaren, D. S.: Malnutrition and the eye, New York, 1963, Academic Press Inc., p. 237.
9. Gregory, M. K.: Quoted by McLaren, D. S.: Malnutrition and the eye, New York, 1963, Academic Press Inc., p. 235.
10. Halasa, A. H., and McLaren, D. S.: Refractive state of malnourished children, Arch. Ophthalmol. **71:**827, 1964.
11. Harrington, D. O.: Amblyopia due to tobacco, alcohol and nutritional deficiency, Am. J. Ophthalmol. **53:**967, 1962.
12. Heaton, J. M., McCormick, A. J. A., and Freeman, A. G.: Tobacco amblyopia—a clinical manifestation of vitamin B$_{12}$ deficiency, Lancet **2:**286, 1958.
13. Heller, J.: Structure of visual pigments: II. Binding of retinal and conformational changes on light exposure in bovine visual pigment, Biochemistry **7:**2914, 1968.

14. Kruse, H. D., Sydenstricker, V. P., Sebrell, W. H., and Cleckley, H. M.: Ocular manifestations of ariboflavinosis, Public Health Rep. **55:**157, 1940.
15. McLaren, D. S., and Halasa, A. H.: The ocular manifestations of nutritional diseases, Postgrad. Med. J. **40:**711, 1964.
16. McLaren, D. S.: Nutritional diseases and the eye, Bordens Rev. Nutr. Res. **25:**1-5, March 1964.
17. McLaren, D. S.: Malnutrition and the eye, New York, 1963, Academic Press Inc., p. 162.
18. McLaren, D. S., and Zekian, B.: Failure of enzymatic cleavage of β-carotene, Am. J. Dis. Child. **121:**278, 1971.
19. McLaren, D. S.: Malnutrition and the eye, New York, 1963, Academic Press Inc., p. 183.
20. McLaren, D. S.: Malnutrition and the eye, New York, 1963, Academic Press Inc., p. 187.
21. McLaren, D. S.: World Rev. Nutr. Diet. **2:**27, 1961.
22. McLaren, D. S.: Malnutrition and the eye, New York, 1963, Academic Press Inc., p. 241.
23. Metivier, V. M.: Eye disease due to vitamin deficiency in Trinidad; tropical nutritional amblyopia; essential corneal epithelial dystrophy; conjunctival bleeding in the newborn, Am. J. Ophthalmol. **24:**1265, 1941.
24. Sorsby, A., Sheridan, M., and Leary, S. A.: Refraction and its components in twins, Med. Res. Counc. Spec. Rep. Ser. (London) **303:**1, 1962.
25. Spencer, W. H.: Renaissance of the pigment epithelium, Arch. Ophthalmol. **88:**1, 1972.
26. Sperling, M. A., Hiles, D. A., and Kennerdell, J. S.: Electroetinographic responses following vitamin A therapy in a-beta-lipoproteinemia, Am. J. Ophthalmol. **73:**342, 1972.
27. Sullivan, W. R., McCulley, J. P., and Dohlman, C. H.: Return of goblet cells after vitamin A therapy in xerosis of the conjunctiva, Am. J. Ophthalmol. **75:**720, 1973.
28. Sydenstricker, V. P., Sebrell, W. H., Cleckley, H. M., and Kruse, H. D.: The ocular manifestations of ariboflavinosis, J.A.M.A. **114:**2437, 1940.
29. Teng-Khoen-Hing: Fundus changes in hypovitaminosis A, Ophthalmologica (Basel) **137:** 81, 1959.
30. Victor, M., and Dreyfus, P. M.: Tobacco, alcohol amblyopia, Arch. Ophthalmol. **74:** 649, 1965.
31. Wald, G.: Molecular basis of visual excitation, Science **162:**230, 1968.
32. Wald, G.: Visual systems and the vitamin A. In Biological Symposia **7:**43, Lancaster, Penn., 1942, The Jacques Cettell Press.
33. Walsh, F. B., and Hoyt, W. F.: Clinical neurophthalmology, ed. 3, Baltimore, 1969, The Williams & Wilkins Co., p. 1226.
34. Wokes, S.: Tobacco amblyopia, Lancet **2:**526, 1958.

Ocular involvement in nutritional disease

CHAIRMAN: **Hansjoerg Kolder***

Dr. Kolder: The influence of a nutritional deficiency on a child is different from that on an adult. This is obvious when measuring the height of people who grew up in an environment with limited or unbalanced food supply. I met recently middle-aged nuns in the northwestern part of Brazil who were about 135 cm. tall. The influence of malnutrition on the development of the visual system is not so evident. We know that formed vision is necessary for development of optimal macular function or binocular vision. Would it not be conceivable that poor nutrition during the critical period could stunt development of certain visual functions? Minimal brain damage was believed to be associated with malnutrition.

During the last year of World War II the food supply in Holland was deficient. After the war an investigation was initiated on minimum brain damage to find out whether a nutritional deficiency during early life may be followed by brain damage. No statistically significant evidence for a correlation between malnutrition and minimal brain damage has been found, but enough evidence has been accumulated to make such a correlation appear possible. The nutritional needs for maintaining an ocular structure are very much different from those for maintaining function. For example, if the intraocular pressure is raised, pressure amaurosis ensues in a few seconds. On the other hand, if the intraocular pressure is maintained at 200 mm. of mercury for up to 2 hours and then released, the visual function and ERG responses will return. We have here a dissociation between energy necessary to maintain the structure intact and energy necessary to maintain the function. At the present time the importance of vitamin A transcends what we used to ascribe to it in terms of keratomalacia and night blindness. There is evidence that the development of structural proteins other than opsin is dependent on vitamin A.

Dr. Berman: I'd like to ask a question and then offer a few points based on some experimental work from our laboratory. First off, not being a clinical person I would like to ask whether xerophthalmia, which means "dry eye condition," implies necessarily a deficiency of aqueous tears?

*Department of Ophthalmology, University of Iowa College of Medicine, Iowa City, Iowa.

Dr. Halasa: Yes, there is absence of goblet cells in conjunctival biopsies from patients with hypovitaminosis A.

Dr. Berman: No, excuse me. I didn't say goblet cells. I asked whether there was a deficiency of aqueous tears.

Dr. Halasa: No.

Dr. Berman: Well, this brings me to the next set of points. The work from our lab and other places has indicated in recent years that in the presence of sufficient aqueous tears one can still have a dry eye, which is then associated with various severe problems. I'd like to bring together some information Dr. McLaren provided with work that Dr. Hollings and his colleagues did in our laboratory. It is true that in some unknown way vitamin A stimulates certain kinds of epithelial cells to the production of mucins or keratin. This appears also to be true in the eye. I would like to suggest, because it hasn't been mentioned here, that at least one of the roles of vitamin A in the eye has to do with the stimulation of goblet cells in the conjunctiva for the production of mucins, which then act to coat the normally very hydrophobic surface of the cornea and allow spreading of the tear film. I'd also like to make another point. I don't think that it does very much good to describe what is going on in the cornea as colliquative necrosis. There is a tendency to put a label like that on an enzymatic process, but this does not explain what is going on. I'd like to relate this to some work that we have done with collagenases and proteases in the cornea and propose this for consideration with regard to neovascularization and possible lack of permeability change in such eyes. Dr. Halasa pointed out that these keratomalacia eyes are minimally inflamed. We have recently been making collagenase preparations from human corneal tissues (keratoplasty material). We have been very interested in the role of serum proteins for collagenase activity in joint disease or in skin diseases. Collagenase is implicated in the erosion of collagen. Now what we have seen is interesting to us. The major collagenase inhibitor in serum is α-chymoantitrypsin, which inhibits various proteases. This antiprotease, although present in the human cornea as determined by fluorescent methods does not inhibit a collagenase made from noninflammatory cells derived from cultures of human corneas. On the other hand, the serum antiprotease that inhibits human corneal collagenase from noninflammatory cells is an α-globulin at a very large molecular weight, which we see to be present in very small quantities using fluorescent techniques in the cornea. I would like to raise the possibility that at least one component of the very rapid structural matrix degradation is in fact related on the one hand to the lack of what acts as a wetting agent on the cornea, a natural wetting agent, and on the other to the fact that in the absence of vascularization normal controls of proteolytic activity have difficulties in getting into the cornea.

Dr. Halasa: To confirm what you are saying, in the few cases of keratomalacia that we have seen recently we have been giving them anticollagenase (L-cystine), in addition to vitamin A, and this seemed to help the reparative process.

Dr. Berman: I am glad to hear that. I think relatively few people are impressed with the use of collagenase inhibitors in any ulcerative problem. If that's true, it's very nice to know. I think you're fighting a real uphill battle.

Dr. Bietti: If I may tell you some curious facts about an avitaminosis that I notice. As you know, we had pellagra in northern Italy, but now it has disappeared completely, as I believe in the United States too. However, it was found, and I was called for consultation because some people in the area of the delta of the Po River developed night blindness connected with pellagra or just a mild form of pellagra. It was not so, because the test of the nicotinic acid in the blood of these pellagra people was low, but there were people without pellagra who had night blindness and a high level of nicotinic acid but had a low vitamin A level (carotene level) in the blood. What had happened? It happened that the people instead of using this yellow corn shifted to white corn because it was sweeter. And therefore they didn't get enough carotene in the corn they were using because this is very scarce in the white corn. They didn't have enough vitamins and they developed night blindness with Bitot's spots. Another fact that you have spoken about concerns these goblet cells. Actually, Bitot's spots are found not only in vitamin A deficiencies, but they are also found on other occasions and I have studied this point. You can find them in Rieger's disease (dysgenesis mesodermalis), in hydrophthalmus, in posterior embryotoxon of Axenfeld's syndrome. And why? Because these malformations are accompanied by a diminution of the goblet cells on the surface of the bulbar conjunctiva, this part of the conjunctiva is therefore more exposed to external factors, producing a Bitot spot without a low level of vitamin A in the blood. And finally, another curious thing that was observed in northern Italy was in the production of apples. It was especially in the German-speaking area of northern Italy, which we call South Tirol, that the peasants had developed very often toxic tobacco-alcohol amblyopia, and you know what was the first sign? They didn't recognize ripe apples, which are red, from green apples.

Dr. Berman: On the subject of nutrition, I want to share with you briefly the tragic irony of this whole question. We were discussing at our laboratory keratomalacia and vitamin A deficiencies when an experience was reported from India. People there heard that Westerners eat milled rice, and so they wanted milled rice also and, when they had an opportunity, would feed the husks to the animals.

Dr. McLaren: What people in developing countries want to eat is hardly relevant to the problem. Xerophthalmia is virtually confined to very young children who have absolutely no choice as to what they are given to eat, usually rice devoid of carotene.

In East Africa some years ago we carried out detailed eye examinations on various ethnic groups. These included a number of related Bantu tribes and also a group of people whose forebears had migrated there about 100 years ago from the eastern part of India. Among the Bantu tribes those who had not passed through a period of famine were found to have a normal incidence of refractive errors comparable to that found in the general population in Britain and elsewhere. However, one tribe, the Gogo of central Tanzania had suffered from severe famine some years previously. Among more than 1000 school children examined in this tribe who were of such an age that they would have been infants or very young children during the famine, we found the highest incidence of high myopia, anisometropia, and other forms of refractive error ever reported (Johnstone, W., and McLaren, D. S.: Refraction anomalies in Tanganyikan children, Br. J. Ophthalmol. **47**:95-108, 1963).

The Indian group of school children were studied for their refraction and weight and height. It was possible to compare the results with those obtained by G. S. Pendse (Refraction and body-growth, Indian Med. Res. Mem. No. 38, 1954) on a similar group living in the part of India from which those in East Africa had originally come. The refraction of the East African Indians was much closer to normal and their heights and their weights were closer to North American standards; thus these findings suggest that the improvement that had occurred was a result of better nutrition consequent upon a rise in their standard of living with emigration (McLaren, D. S.: The refraction of Indian school children: A comparison of data from East Africa and India, Br. J. Ophthalmol. **45**:604-613, 1961).

Dr. Knox: I'd like to report on some of my experiences with the entity we call "nutritional amblyopia," or "tobacco-alcohol amblyopia." If you go back to Frank Carroll's work where he had a group of heavy smoking–heavy drinking people whom he kept in the hospital and gave a good diet, their vision came back to normal on just a good diet. We have to wonder about the role of tobacco-induced cyanide in this group of patients. I believe that also in alcoholism there is much evidence that alcohol has a bad effect on the intestinal mucosa and the absorption of both folic acid and vitamin B_{12} and that with liver toxicity there are changes in the transport and storage of B_{12} and, as Dr. McLaren mentioned earlier, folic acid. I have one experience recently of a man who was wealthy enough to own his own small horse-racing farm. He was educated enough to be an electrical engineer and to maintain the tote boards at race tracks, but he came with a bilateral visual failure of acuity down to the 20/100's range. He had bilateral centrocecal scotomas; he had one drink a day and maybe one cigar a day. He'd lost his stomach 20 years before because of a peptic ulcer disease, and I thought he had pernicious anemia secondary to a loss of stomach and had a visual failure as a result of it. Well, his Schilling test was entirely normal. His B_{12} assays were entirely normal. The internist who helped me asked his wife, "Did he eat a normal diet." "Yes, he did." Well, we gave him hydroxocobalamin injections and after about 6 weeks he did not improve. I became desperate and admitted him to the hospital to do an arteriogram examination and air studies in order to find a lesion around the chiasm. Before he came to the hospital I gave him a prescription for a multivitamin preparation and folic acid. By the time he got into the hospital he told me an interesting story. We had done the arteriogram examination and we were waiting to do the air studies, and he said, "You know, Doc, something is happening. I looked at the *TV Guide* and that little box in the upper right-hand corner is red now, and it hasn't been red for the last 3 months. The next thing that happened is that my wife walked into the room today and I said, 'What a pretty color dress you've got on!' She said, 'Clarence, this is the same gray dress that I have been wearing for the last

5 years!' " The first thing he observed was that he looked at the walls of his room and he said, "You know, there are pretty colors on the walls." I said, "Are they the same with each eye?" He said, "No, there are different colors in a certain pattern with each eye." Well, we found nothing by neurodiagnostic studies, and his vision steadily improved and all we had been giving him were multivitamins, B_{12} injections, and folic acid. We began to ask him a few more questions about his diet, and it turned out that 5 days a week he was at his horse farm and all he ate was steaks and potatoes. "Do you eat many vegetables?" "None!" "Do you eat salads?" "None!" We asked his wife the same. "Well, I put them on his plate when he comes home on weekends, but he said 'Yeh, but I don't eat them.' " This is a single case in America today. Individuals from the upper middle class with plenty of social economic advantages have dietary fads or peculiar predilections for not eating certain things that can lead to a nutritional amblyopia. It doesn't have to be from alcohol and it doesn't have to be from heavy smoking. I personally think that folic acid is mixed up with vitamin A in this disease in some way.

8

The eye in endocrine diseases, especially Graves' ophthalmopathy

David H. Solomon

Among endocrine diseases, the eye is a target organ of major significance in diabetes mellitus and in Graves' disease, whereas involvement of the eye is less frequent or less important in other endocrine conditions. Diabetes is dealt with in Chapters 10 and 11. This paper focuses on the ophthalmopathy of Graves' disease because of its importance and because of my wish to confine myself to a disease of which I have at least some minimal firsthand knowledge.

For the sake of completeness, a list of endocrine conditions affecting the eye is presented in Table 8-1. Many of the listed ocular abnormalities are either extremely rare or of no clinical consequence. A few deserve comment. Internists frequently speak of the presence of band keratopathy in hyperparathyroidism. However, only an incomplete form of the band lesion is seen in this disease; it is confined to the area just inside the limbus at 3 and 9 o'clock, rather than traversing the entire exposed area of the cornea in an equatorial pattern as is the case in full-blown band keratopathy of other causes.

Ptosis and edema of the lids and periorbital areas are common in hypothyroidism, whereas the abnormalities of the lens, uvea, and muscles listed in Table 8-1 are rare. The ptosis is interesting. Its cause is partly edema of the upper lids; this responds to the diuresis that accompanies treatment with thyroid hormone. Another factor, however, is quite probably a diminished effectiveness of catecholamines when thyroid hormones are deficient.[21] The ptosis may be corrected by the instillation of phenylephrine into the conjunctival sac.[27] This response suggests that the tone of Müller's muscles is dependent on activation of sympathetic α-adrenergic receptors and that thyroid hormones, though necessary for the maintenance of normal tone, are not obligatory to sustain the response to pharmacologic levels of an α-adrenergic agent. This is compatible with the latest act in the long play on thyroid-catecholamine interactions, namely, the studies of Levey et al. showing that thyroid and catecholamine effects on the heart are additive, rather than mutually permissive or synergistic.[28]

Generally, lenticular opacities in hypothyroidism are small, punctate, and of

Table 8-1. Ocular features of endocrine disease

Gland	Disease	Ocular abnormality
Adrenal medulla	Pheochromocytoma	Hypertensive retinopathy
Adrenal cortex	Addison's disease	Pigmentation of conjunctiva and uvea
	Cushing's syndrome	Hypertensive retinopathy
		Exophthalmos
	Primary hyperaldo- steronism	Hypertensive retinopathy
Hypothalamus	Suprasellar tumors	Hemianopsia
		Papilledema
Pancreas	Diabetes mellitus	Retinopathy
		Lens: swelling, opacities, cataract
		Iritis
		Ophthalmoplegia
		Lipemia retinalis
Parathyroid	Hyperparathyroidism	Calcium deposits in conjunctiva
		Incomplete band keratopathy
	Hypoparathyroidism	Keratoconjunctivitis
		Blepharospasm
		Lens: opacities, cataract
		Papilledema
Pituitary	Tumors of anterior lobe	Hemianopsia
		Optic atrophy
		Ophthalmoplegia
Thyroid	Graves' disease	Edema
		Proptosis
		Ophthalmoplegia
		Keratitis
		Optic-nerve damage
		Papilledema
	Hypothyroidism	Edema
		Ptosis
		Lens: opacities, cataract
		Keratoconjunctivitis sicca
		Myotonia of extraocular muscles

little clinical significance. Occasionally, however, cretinism is accompanied by full-blown cataract formation. The syndrome of keratoconjunctivitis sicca is said to occur with some frequency in hypothyroidism.[38] I have never seen this, except in a patient with hypothyroidism from chronic autoimmune thyroiditis who also suffered from Sjögren's syndrome. The syndrome of keratoconjunctivitis sicca in this instance seemed to be part of classic Sjögren's syndrome, unrelated to the coincidental hypothyroidism.

OPHTHALMOPATHY OF GRAVES' DISEASE

Physicians have found it difficult to describe the abnormalities that afflict the eyes in Graves' disease in terms that other physicians can unambiguously understand. This is curious, since the condition produces such a dramatic appearance. The fault lies largely in a dogged effort to use language implying pathogenesis or thyroid functional state. Thus endocrine exophthalmos, thyrotoxic exophthalmos, and thyrotropic exophthalmos are terms that have caused confusion. We would do far better to use language that describes what we see in the patient or under the microscope and then add a separate notation as to the patient's state of thyroid function. For example, thyrotoxic exophthalmos has been used as a description of the mild, noninfiltrative eye changes of Graves' disease, principally lid retraction and lid lag, with or without mild proptosis. However, such noninfiltrative changes not infrequently occur in patients who are not thyrotoxic and may never have been thyrotoxic! An even more contorted example is the following quotation from a current edition of a prominent textbook: "Exophthalmic ophthalmoplegia is a term used to describe the progressive exophthalmos which occurs in the euthyroid state or after thyrotoxicosis has been controlled, although sometimes it is used erroneously to describe any type of endocrine exophthalmos."[2] On the contrary, if the term "exophthalmic ophthalmoplegia" were to be used, and I would prefer that it were not, it should obviously be used to describe a set of physical signs, namely, ophthalmoplegia accompanying exophthalmos, regardless of cause or state of thyroid function.

The American Thyroid Association has adopted a classification designed by Werner that allows simple and accurate description of the eye changes of Graves' disease.[46] Each of the characteristics of ophthalmopathy listed in Table 8-1 is graded, where appropriate, either *o,* absent; *a,* minimal; *b,* moderate; or *c,* marked, based on criteria spelled out in the original publication.[46] In a general way, class 1 corresponds to what has been called noninfiltrative ophthalmopathy, whereas classes 2 to 6 describe the various characteristics of infiltrative ophthalmopathy. There are no pathogenetic implications, nor can inferences regarding thyroid function be drawn. Furthermore, this classification emphasizes only that class 1 differs dramatically from class 6 in *degree* of pathologic involvement, but it neither implies nor denies that class 1 changes have the same pathogenesis as class 6. As discussed below, this is, in fact, an unsettled question. The criticism has been raised that class 3, for example, does not necessarily imply worse disease than does class 2. This is perfectly true, and furthermore a patient may suffer blindness, class 6c, and have no corneal involvement at all, that is, class 5o. Thus, the numbering of the classes does not imply an invariable sequence of progression from milder to more severe disease, and full description of Graves' ophthalmopathy requires listing of a grading for every applicable class. Nevertheless, applied in a consistent manner, the classification is quite useful and improves communication considerably.

The ophthalmopathy (or oculopathy, or "eye changes") we are describing is one of the cardinal features of Graves' disease, which, in turn, is defined today as a multisystem disease of unknown etiology, characterized by one or more of three pathognomonic clinical entities: (1) hyperthyroidism associated with diffuse hyperplasia of the thyroid gland, (2) infiltrative ophthalmopathy, and (3) infiltrative dermopathy (localized pretibial myxedema). Thyroid acropachy is a rare extrapolation of the last. Thus, a full diagnostic description of a patient should consist of the overall eponymic term (Graves' disease in the U.S.A. and Parry's or Basedow's in some other countries), followed by a statement as to thyroid status, ophthalmopathic involvement, and skin involvement. For example, a patient might have Graves' disease with hyperthyroidism, ophthalmopathy (2b, 3b, 4a, 5o, 6o), and no dermopathy. Finally, the term "euthyroid Graves' disease," or "euthyroid ophthalmopathy," has recently begun to evoke confusion rather than clarity, because some investigators have included under these headings patients who *were hyperthyroid* at one time and are currently euthyroid as a result of treatment directed at the thyroid. Pathogenetically, this is a far different situation from that of the patients originally described by Werner and others under this or similar terms[32] who *never* had been hyperthyroid.

Etiology and pathogenesis

The underlying cause of Graves' disease is still unknown. The discovery[1] of the long-acting thyroid stimulator (LATS) in the serum of patients with Graves' disease in 1956 radically changed the direction in which speculations flow. Since 1964, when two groups identified LATS as an immunoglobulin, IgG,[23, 33] the prevailing hypothesis has been that Graves' disease is an autoimmune disorder.[11] However, later studies have cast great doubt on the seemingly foregone conclusion that circulating LATS is *the* cause of the hyperthyroidism,[11] nor has LATS stood up as a reasonable cause of the ophthalmopathy.[31] Furthermore, recent work has, on the one hand, solidified the foundation underlying the autoimmune hypothesis,[18, 43] while other workers have uncovered surprising, but readily confirmable, evidence that the pituitary gland's response to thyrotropin-releasing hormone (TRH) is abnormal in Graves' disease.[12, 19] Thus, a role for the hypothalamo-pituitary unit in the origin of the disease has been resurrected at the very time when a seemingly contrary hypothesis had gained strength. Perhaps an amalgam of these hypotheses is possible; in other words, it could evolve that a hypothalamo-pituitary disorder is responsible for initially triggering both hyperthyroidism and ophthalmopathy, whereas autoimmune mechanisms (antibodies and lymphocyte-bred mediators) sustain these processes, at least in their more severe forms. The outline below lists hypotheses of the pathogenesis of Graves' disease currently under intensive investigation in various laboratories:

Theories of pathogenesis of Graves' disease
1. Autoimmune abnormality
   a. Inherited defect in immunologic surveillance[43]
   b. Acquired because of thyroid injury[24]
2. Immune abnormality: response to an exogenous agent, possibly a virus[47]
3. Intrinsic thyroid abnormality
   a. Universal hyperfunction[41]
   b. Failure of autoregulatory mechanisms[22]
4. Hypothalamopituitary dysregulation[11]
5. Combinations

Certain of these hypotheses as to the fundamental nature of Graves' disease attempt to explain the pathogenesis of ophthalmopathy. Clearly, the final answer must successfully explain hyperthyroidism, ophthalmopathy, and dermopathy as well. The outline below lists currently viable theories about ophthalmopathy:

Theories of pathogenesis of ophthalmopathy in Graves' disease
1. Autoimmune abnormality
   a. Inherited defect in immunologic surveillance[34]

  b. Cross-reaction with thyroid, accompanied by accessibility of thyroid
   antigens and lymphocytes to retro-orbital tissues[25]
 2. Hypothalamopituitary dysregulation[50]
 3. Combination[49]

A very attractive hypothesis stems from the work of Volpe and co-workers in Toronto. They have found that certain lymphocytes in the blood of patients with Graves' disease secrete migration-inhibiting factor (MIF) in response to the presence of a crude antigen made from thyroid tissue or from retro-orbital muscle.[26, 34] In a general way, the tissue that triggers this in vitro response correlates with the clinical picture; i.e., the presence of ophthalmopathy predicts a higher frequency of lymphocytes responsive to exposure to retro-orbital muscle antigen, whereas hyperthyroidism is associated with thyroid-responsive lymphocytes. If both hyperthyroidism and ophthalmopathy are present, the lymphocytes are prone to be responsive to both antigens. The general concept of Volpe's group is that patients with Graves' disease have an inherited defect in immunosurveillance resulting in their inability to eradicate abnormal clones of thymic or T-lymphocytes, arising by random mutation. The defect is visualized as less than global, confined to certain lymphocytes, including those capable of responding abnormally to thyroid or retro-orbital muscle antigens and thereby presumably causing hyperthyroidism and ophthalmopathy by cell-to-cell interactions and by producing humoral antibodies.[43] In the case of the thyroid, the activated T-lymphocytes may stimulate thyroid function,[17] whereas bursal or B-lymphocytes produce LATS and perhaps also a species-specific human thyroid stimulator.[36] In the case of the even more mysterious ocular lesion, it is possible that activated lymphocytes, which densely infiltrate retro-orbital muscles,[14] in some way alter sulfate metabolism and thus lead to the noxious accumulation of glycosaminoglycans in retro-orbital muscle. There is also at least preliminary evidence that the serum of patients with ophthalmopathy carries a unique IgG that has exophthalmogenic activity.[48] In summary, the hypothesis of abnormal ("forbidden") clones causing hyperthyroidism and ophthalmopathy is tenable at present but requires far more evidence than now available, both of the actual presence of such clones of immunocompetent cells and of their ability to cause hyperthyroidism and swelling of retro-orbital structures, particularly the muscles.

The second hypothesis involving autoimmune mechanisms in Graves' ophthalmopathy approaches it from a thyrocentric point of view. Kriss has proposed that thyroid injury leads to activation of immunocytes, production of LATS, and hyperthyroidism.[24] Although this now seems at best an incomplete explanation for hyperthyroidism,[11] its ocular corollary is of interest. Kriss and co-workers[25] have shown (both in published and unpublished observations) that there are direct lymphatic connections between the thyroid and the orbits and have postulated that thyroid antigens or thyroid lymphocytes might reach the orbits and in some way trigger the ocular disease. This anatomic approach would nicely explain the frequent asymmetry of ophthalmic involvement, but it has great difficulty in assimilating the fact that most workers do not find that thyroid ablation cures ophthalmopathy.[37, 42, 45] Direct evidence of immunologic cross reaction between thyroid and retro-orbital muscle is still lacking and is a necesary link in the chain of this hypothesis.

For many years, evidence has continued to accumulate that the pituitary gland of many species contains an exophthalmogenic factor (EF). Professor Dardenne will review this matter in detail, and I will therefore skirt it in this chapter. A few general comments may be worthwhile, to put these data into perspective in relation to the autoimmune hypotheses. The notion that pituitary secretion of an EF might cause the ophthalmopathy of Graves' disease has been encouraged by the observation that psychologic stress seems to trigger the onset of ophthalmopathy in some cases.[29] However, it has been severely weakened by the frequent failure of complete hypophysectomy to prevent or cure[20] Graves' ophthalmopathy, even though occasional patients did seem to undergo dramatic improvement.[36] Recently, the pituitary EF concept has been reinvigorated by diverse observations. Winand and Kohn have provided a possible answer to one previously nagging question: Why does the pituitary secrete a hormone whose only function is to cause exophthalmos and even destruction of the visual system? They have shown that a fragment of bovine TSH (the β-chain plus the N-terminal portion of the α-chain) possesses EF activity without detectable thyroid-stimulating activity.[50] Thus, it becomes possible that EF is a metabolite or an abnormal perversion of a vital hormone. Further, the Winand group has shown an interaction between TSH and the exophthalmogenic IgG that they had found in patients' sera,[49] thus possibly tying together the autoimmune and the hypothalamopituitary hypotheses. We have already pointed out that recent work in the thyroid area suggests that, whatever autoimmune stigmas may be present, there is also a peculiarity in the setting of the hypothalamopituitary thyrostat in Graves' disease.[12] Thus an efferent neuro-effector mechanism may be abnormal, and this might make it understandable why psychologic stress often triggers the onset of hyperthyroidism,[29] at least more easily understandable than the autoimmune hypothesis, although such an explanation has also been offered.[43]

My personal bias, unadorned by solid evidence of any kind, is that both hyperthyroidism and ophthalmopathy may originate with an abnormality in the hypothalamus or pituitary gland, just as is true in Cushing's syndrome. In the case of Graves' disease, the resultant hypersecretion or distorted secretion of TSH in some way initiates an autoimmune process affecting the thyroid, the eyes, or both. This, in turn, becomes self-perpetuating, and after a time the process can no longer be halted by even complete hypophysectomy. Although these notions are at present wildly speculative, they are subject to experimental study and therefore perhaps of some utility.

Clinical features

Ophthalmopathy in Graves' disease ranges from nonexistent to devastating. Approximately 50% of patients with hyperthyroidism have no detectable ocular abnormalities.[14] The commonest feature is widening of the palpebral fissure caused by retraction of the upper lid, which is also revealed by lid lag. This sign is attributable in some cases to the effect of hyperthyroninemia (that is, increased thyroxine, T_4, and triiodothyronine, T_3) on the adrenergic-mediated tone of Müller's muscles. It is pertinent that instillation of phentolamine[27] or guanethidine[13] has been shown to decrease transiently the widening of the palpebral fissure in some cases of Graves' disease. However, as mentioned earlier, pronounced lid retraction may be present in euthyroid patients; so either another nonthyroid factor is causing contraction of Müller's muscles, or the upper lid retraction in these cases is caused by shortening of the fibers of the levator palpebrae superiors, that is, part of the generalized infiltrative involvement of the retro-orbital (skeletal) muscles. Thus, when lid retraction occurs in the euthyroid subject, one can probably conclude that this is a mild form of the same process that can destroy vision, whereas in the hyperthyroid subject one is unsure as to its interpretation. If lid retraction is severe and fixed, it may itself threaten vision by predisposing to keratitis as a result of exposure of the cornea. However, serious consequences of exposure of the cornea rarely occur unless there is concomitant ophthalmoplegia limiting upward rotation of the eye. The reason is that Bell's phenomenon, upward rotation of the globe when the eyelids are closed, normally protects the cornea, even when the upper lid is greatly retracted.

In most series, about 20% of patients with Graves' disease exhibit proptosis.[4] Usually this reflects retro-orbital infiltration and heightened retro-orbital tension. However, at times, palpatory estimation of the resistance to retrodisplacement, a useful physical sign, reveals absolutely no indication of supranormal retro-orbital tension, despite the presence of proptosis. This paradox has never been fully resolved, although investigators have sometimes suggested that lid retraction alone may allow forward movement of the globe or that weakness of the muscles may, at a certain stage in the process, loosen the moorings of the globe to the orbital walls.

Not all patients with proptosis suffer from other signs of the infiltrative lesion involving retro-orbital tissues; such signs are soft-tissue swelling (periorbital edema, lid edema, chemosis), ophthalmoplegia, or evidence of pressure on the optic nerve or its blood supply (decrease in visual acuity, excavation of visual fields, papilledema). These phenomena, characteristic of so-called malignant or progressive exophthalmos, are fortunately quite uncommon. The exact incidence is difficult to state, because (1) the validity of most published series is negated by the fact that patients were referred to the investigators *because of* the ophthalmopathy, (2) the criteria for the diagnosis of "malignant exophthalmos" have never been codified, and (3) severe ophthalmopathy may occur years after hyperthyroidism has been treated[5] and therefore may be missed if hyperthyroidism is the criterion for inclusion in the study. If the criterion for inclusion is either severe soft-tissue swelling, 2c; severe proptosis, 3c; severe ophthalmopathy, 4c; or visual loss, 6a, b, or c; or any combination of these findings, then my guess would be that the incidence is about 5% of all patients with Graves' disease. Solid data on this point would be valuable.

The symptoms of Graves' ophthalmopathy afford a useful indication of the severity of the process. Thus soft-tissue swelling, indicative of interference with orbital drainage, is often reflected by lacrimation, grittiness, and anterior ocular discomfort. Proptosis, on the other hand, does not cause symptoms at all, except insofar as a patient's self-image is damaged and psychologic stability is upset. Diplopia is, of course, a very reliable reflection of significant infiltration—and, later, fibrosis—of retro-orbital muscles. Characteristically, diplopia is altitudinal as well as lateral and it is almost invariably less noticeable when one looks below the horizontal than at it or above. The reason is that upward rotation is impaired much earlier and more often than is downward rotation. Thus the patient frequently learns to tilt the head backward in order to unify visual images. The first complaint may actually be cervical pain or stiffness! Deep ocular pain suggests strongly heightened orbital tension, raises the question of glaucoma, and enhances the fear of optic nerve damage. Blurring of vision in either eye is, of course, an alarming symptom. It may, however, mean many different things: lacrimation, keratitis, exudative conjunctivitis, glaucoma, or optic nerve compression.

Although there are obviously many different hazards to vision, the most important to bear in mind is the effect of compression of the optic nerve as it emerges from the optic foramen. This is of great concern because of its propensity to develop suddenly and without external signs and, of course, because of the partial or complete irreversibility of optic nerve damage. Thus, visual acuity must be checked frequently in patients with any of the severe signs of Graves' ophthalmopathy previously listed. Also, the signs of optic nerve compression take precedence over all others in assessing urgency of the need for treatment, the choice of treatment, and the quality of response to treatment. Thus sequential measurements of actual proptosis mean very little indeed if their message is not consistent with the inference drawn from measurements of visual acuity.

Course

Bartels and Irie[5] beautifully documented the random character of the association between ophthalmopathy and hyperthyroidism in Graves' disease (Table 8-2). Many reviewers have stressed the onset of ophthalmopathy while hyperthyroidism is under treatment.[14] However, this is clearly only one of many possible occasions for this disorder to begin (Table 8-2). The occurrence in the months after treatment of hyperthyroidism with radioiodine has been emphasized by Kriss.[24] There is no doubt that this phenomenon occurs and that it is accompanied by a rise in serum LATS and antithyroid antibodies. However, its significance is still obscure, and its frequency may not be uniquely great as compared to other periods in the history of the patient's disease. Another question is, Does treatment with radioiodine precipitate worsening of Graves' ophthalmopathy more often than does treatment by subtotal thyroidectomy or antithyroid drugs? The general impression among thyroidologists is in the affirmative. However, no prospective

Table 8-2. Relationship of onset of exophthalmos to presence of hyperthyroidism*

Period		Number of patients
Before hyperthyroidism		9
Simultaneous with hyperthyroidism		48
After hyperthyroidism is established		32
After hyperthyroidism is treated		23
Hypothyroid	22	
Euthyroid	1	
Unassociated with hyperthyroidism		5
Total		117

*From Bartels, E. C., and Irie, M.: Thyroid function in patients with progressive exophthalmos: Study of 117 cases requiring orbital decompression. In Pitt-Rivers, R.: Advances in thyroid research, New York, 1961, Pergamon Press, Inc., pp. 163 to 170.

clinical trial, blinded or unblinded, has ever compared these forms of treatment. The results of retrospective analysis have been very suggestive, but even in such a study the difference in ocular outcome after the three forms of treatment of hyperthyroidism has not been significant.[4] This is an extremely important matter, since antithyroid drugs, subtotal thyroidectomy, and radioiodine are all satisfactory methods to control hyperthyroidism. If a clear difference in the incidence of worsening of ophthalmopathy could be demonstrated, it might become the supervening element in dictating a choice among these therapies.

Meanwhile, the question arises as to whether there is any other way to prevent or reduce the incidence of ophthalmopathy. Perhaps the avoidance of hypo-

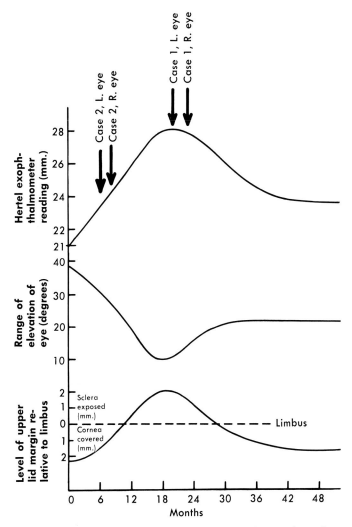

Fig. 8-1. Schematic representation of the course of ocular changes in patients with Graves' disease. (From Rundle, F. F.: Management of exophthalmos and related ocular changes in Graves' disease, Metabolism **6:**36-48, 1957.)

thyroidism is important[3]; again, no hard data are available. Catz and Perzik have suggested that total thyroidectomy, as contrasted with subtotal removal, prevents ophthalmopathy.[10] The evaluation of the course of their patients after operation is hampered by a paucity of presented data. No other group has tested this hypothesis.

Once Graves' ophthalmopathy has started to progress, it runs a somewhat predictable course. In the majority of cases, it follows the pattern summarized so nicely by Rundle in 1957[39] (Fig. 8-1). It grows steadily worse over a matter of months and then reaches a plateau, after which it slowly subsides over a period of years. Unfortunately, one cannot predict in the individual case how severe it will grow, when it will level off, whether subsidence will mean mere stabilization of abnormalities already fixed, or whether there will be actual regression. Rarely, unfortunately, is there a complete return to the normal premorbid state and position of the eyes, once severe ophthalmopathy has occurred. Mild or moderate abnormalities not infrequently do disappear entirely.

Treatment

Dr. Dardenne also discusses aspects of the treatment of Graves' ophthalmopathy in Chapter 9; so my review will be brief. The reader may wish to refer to a more detailed summary of my thoughts about treatment, which was published in 1969.[40]

Mild ophthalmopathy requires relatively simple treatment or none at all. Moderate ophthalmopathy may result in photophobia, for which dark glasses are indicated, or lacrimation, which may call for side shields. Elevation of the head of the bed, the use of a porous eyepatch, or the instillation of 1% methylcellulose drops may be useful. If chemosis and periorbital edema are prominent, diuretics are often prescribed. This therapy is of temporary value, at best, and usually is discontinued after a short trial. Guanethidine eye drops have been recommended, but they are irritating to the conjunctiva.

Over the years, a number of forms of treatment have been recommended for severe ophthalmopathy. Although each has been reported upon favorably and some still have proponents, I do not believe that any of the following significantly alters the course of the disease: (1) thyroid hormones, (2) thyroid hormone analogs, (3) irradiation of the pituitary gland, (4) ablation of the pituitary gland by various means, (5) pituitary stalk section, (6) hyaluronidase, (7) estrogens and androgens, (8) iodine, and (9) azathioprine. There are four forms of treatment of current interest, and these require somewhat more detailed comments: (1) total thyroid ablation, (2) supervoltage retro-orbital irradiation, (3) adrenal glucocorticoid therapy, and (4) orbital decompression.

Total thyroid ablation has already been noted as a suggested approach to the prevention of ophthalmopathy.[10] It has also been proposed as treatment for the established ocular disease.[6, 9] Once again, the clinical data are incomplete, making its value difficult to judge. In addition, three groups of workers have failed to confirm the original study.[37, 42, 45] For these reasons, as well as the hazards of either high-dose radioiodine therapy or total thyroidectomy, I cannot recommend this approach to the treatment of severe ophthalmopathy, until a controlled study demonstrates unequivocal advantages over treatment methods whose ability to cause improvement is well established.

Orbital irradiation was employed in the 1930s and 1940s with somewhat equivocal results.[7] Recently, Donaldson, Bagshaw, and Kriss have reintroduced this approach, using supervoltage equipment and modern techniques for collimation.[16] The results they reported are quite encouraging, with two thirds of the patients experiencing excellent or good responses. Significant improvement usually occurred either during the 2-week period of treatment or very shortly thereafter. There was no evidence of damage to the lens or retina. Other groups have shown interest in this form of treatment, and a controlled comparison of steroids and orbital irradiation might now be possible to design.

The only established pharmacologic treatment for severe ophthalmopathy of Graves' disease (malignant exophthalmos) is the administration of large doses of adrenal glucocorticoids such as prednisone. The major lesson from experience thus far has been that prednisone, if given at all, must be given in large doses. Forty milligrams per day will occasionally suffice, but generally an initial dose of 60 to 80 mg. per day or more is required to initiate improvement. As in the case of supervoltage orbital irradiation, about two thirds of the patients experience an excellent or good response[8] and improvement begins within 2 weeks of initiation of treatment. If there has been no improvement by that time, prednisone should be discontinued by a rapidly tapered reduction in dose. If improvement has occurred, the effects of hypercortisolism can be minimized by transfer to an alternate-day treatment plan or by gradual reduction in dose or both. Ultimately, it is frequently possible to discontinue prednisone without relapse; this observation suggests that the underlying disease process has become less active and that the patient's illness is now on the descending limb of Rundle's curve (Fig. 8-1).

The mainstay of surgical treatment of severe ophthalmopathy is orbital decompression. This has been accomplished by many different routes. The transantral approach, introduced by Ogura in 1947, appears to be the most successful operation up to now.[15, 35] It is more effective than the Kronlein operation and less hazardous than the Naffziger procedure, which has largely fallen into disuse.

The most difficult problem is to state the indications for each form of treatment, in the absence of controlled clinical trials. All reports have indicated better results, whatever the form of treatment, if ophthalmopathy is of short duration, preferably less than 1 year. Thus a decision should be made early, if the disease appears to be progressing, even though spontaneous abatement might occur in many instances if one waited. Clearly, this is a difficult dilemma, particularly when the forms of treatment are hazardous. However, an activistic approach is probably advisable, since there is no way to predict at what level of damage the progression of the disease will stop. I should emphasize that proptosis per se is not a valid indication for either steroids or orbital decompression. Severe soft-tissue swelling calls for either radiotherapy or prednisone. Ophthalmoplegia sufficient to cause diplopia is an indication for treatment; radiotherapy or prednisone has been reported to be effective for this symptom, whereas decompression ordinarily is not effective. If corneal exposure is the main problem, a brief trial of prednisone may be worthwhile, but usually orbital decompression will be required. A decrease in visual acuity or development of a visual-field cut is a clear indication for emergent treatment. High-dose prednisone may be given, but if no improvement is seen in 1 week or, at the most, 2 weeks, orbital decompression should be performed. In general, my present inclination is to recommend supervoltage orbital radiotherapy in moderate disease (progressive, but not yet in the "severe" category) and steroids in severe disease. Orbital decompression has its major place in the treatment of radiotherapy failures, steroid failures, and patients in whom steroids are contraindicated for other reasons. Until controlled clinical studies are performed, all recommendations must be couched in uncertain terms and represent merely inferences from individual experience. Such is the context in which the above advice should be taken.

REFERENCES

1. Adams, D. D., and Purves, H. D.: Abnormal responses in the assay of thyrotropin, Proc. Univ. Otaga Med. School **34:**11-12, 1956.
2. Allen, J. H.: May's Manual of the diseases of the eye, ed. 24, Baltimore, 1968, The Williams & Wilkins Co., pp. 378-379.
3. Aranow, H., Jr., and Day, R. M.: Management of thyrotoxicosis in patients with ophthalmopathy: Antithyroid regimen determined primarily by ocular manifestations, J. Clin. Endocrinol. Metab. **25:**1-10, 1965.
4. Barbosa, J., Wong, E., and Doe, R. P.: Ophthalmopathy of Graves' disease: Outcome after treatment with radioactive iodine, surgery, or antithyroid drugs, Arch. Intern. Med. **130:**111-113, 1972.
5. Bartels, E. C., and Irie, M.: Thyroid function in patients with progressive exophthalmos: Study of 117 cases requiring orbital decompression, Advances in Thyroid Research, New York, 1961, Pergamon Press, Inc., pp. 163-170.
6. Bauer, F. K., and Catz, B.: Radioactive iodine therapy for progressive malignant exophthalmos, Acta Endocrinol. **51:**15-22, 1966.
7. Beierwaltes, W. H.: X-ray treatment of malignant exophthalmos: A report on 28 patients, J. Clin. Endocrinol. Metab. **13:**1090-1100, 1953.
8. Brown, J., Coburn, J. W., Wigod, R. A., Hiss, J. M., Jr., and Dowling, J. T.: Adrenal steroid therapy of severe infiltrative ophthalmopathy of Graves' disease, Am. J. Med. **34:**786-795, 1963.
9. Catz, B., and Perzik, S. L.: Subtotal vs. surgical ablation of the thyroid, malignant exophthalmos, and its relation to remnant thyroid: Current topics in thyroid research, Proceedings of the International Thyroid Conference, 5th, Rome, 1965, New York, 1965, Academic Press, Inc., pp. 1183-1199.
10. Catz, B., and Perzik, S. L.: Total thyroidectomy in the management of thyrotoxic and euthyroid Graves' disease, Am. J. Surg. **118:**434-438, 1969.
11. Chopra, I. J., Solomon, D. H., Johnson, D. E., and Chopra, U.: Thyroid gland in Graves' disease: Victim or culprit? Metabolism **19:**760-772, 1970.
12. Chopra, I. J., Chopra, U., and Orgiazzi, J.: Abnormalities of hypothalamo-hypophyseal-thyroid axis in patients with Graves' ophthalmopathy, J. Clin. Endocrinol. Metab. **37:**955-967, 1973.
13. Crombie, A. L., and Lawson, A. A. H.: Long-term trial of local guanethidine in treatment of eye signs of thyroid dysfunction and idiopathic lid retraction, Br. Med. J. **4:**592-595, 1967.
14. Day, R. M., in Werner, S. C., and Ingbar, S. H.: The thyroid, a fundamental and clinical text, ed. 3, New York, 1971, Harper & Row, Publishers, pp. 535-543.
15. De Santo, L. W.: Surgical palliation of ophthalmopathy of Graves' disease; transantral approach, Mayo Clin. Proc. **47:**989-992, 1972.
16. Donaldson, S. S., Bagshaw, M. A., and Kriss, J. P.: Supervoltage orbital radiotherapy for Graves' ophthalmopathy, J. Clin. Endocrinol. Metab. **37:**276-285, 1973.
17. Edmonds, M. W., Row, V. V., and Volpe, R.: Action of globulin and lymphocytes from peripheral blood of patients with Graves' disease on isolated bovine thyroid cells, J. Clin. Endocrinol. Metab. **31:**480-490, 1970.
18. Farid, N. R., Munro, R. E., Row, V. V., and Volpe, R.: Peripheral thymus-dependent (T) lymphocytes in Graves' disease and Hashimoto's thyroiditis, New Eng. J. Med. **288:**1313-1317, 1973.

19. Franco, P. S., Hershman, J. M., Haigler, E. D., Jr., and Pittman, J. A., Jr.: Response to thyrotropin-releasing hormone compared with thyroid suppression tests in euthyroid Graves' disease, Metabolism **22:**1357-1365, 1973.
20. Furth, E. D., Becker, D. V., Ray, B. S., and Kane, J. W.: Appearance of unilateral infiltrative exophthalmos of Graves' disease after the successful treatment of the same process in the contralateral eye by apparently total surgical hypophysectomy, J. Clin. Endocrinol. Metab. **22:**518-524, 1962.
21. Harrison, T. S.: Adrenal medullary and thyroid relationships, Physiol. Rev. **44:**161-185, 1964.
22. Ingbar, S.: Autoregulation of the thyroid. Response to iodide excess and depletion, Mayo Clin. Proc. **47:**814-823, 1972.
23. Kriss, J. P., Pleshakov, V., and Chien, J. R.: Isolation and identification of the long-acting thyroid stimulator and its relation to hyperthyroidism and circumscribed pretibial myxedema, J. Clin. Endocrinol. Metab. **24:**1005-1028, 1964.
24. Kriss, J. P., Pleshakov, V., Rosenblum, A. L., Holderness, M., Sharp, G., and Utiger, R.: Studies on the pathogenesis of the ophthalmopathy of Graves' disease, J. Clin. Endocrinol. Metab. **27:**582-593, 1967.
25. Kriss, J. P.: Radioisotopic thyroidolymphography in patients with Graves' disease, J. Clin. Endocrinol. Metab. **31:**315-324, 1970.
26. Lamki, L., Row, V. V., and Volpe, R.: Cell-mediated immunity in Graves' disease and in Hashimoto's thyroiditis as shown by the demonstration of migration inhibition factor (MIF), J. Clin. Endocrinol. Metab. **36:**358-364, 1973.
27. Lee, W. H., Morimoto, P. K., Bronsky, D., and Waldstein, S. S.: Studies of thyroid and sympathetic nervous system interrelationships. I. The blepharoptosis of myxedema, J. Clin. Endocrinol. Metab. **21:**1402-1412, 1961.
28. Levey, G. S., Skelton, C. L., and Epstein, S. E.: Influence of hyperthyroidism on the effects of norepinephrine on myocardial adenyl cyclase activity and contractile state, Endocrinology **85:**1004-1009, 1969.
29. Lidz, T., and Cohn, G. L.: Hyperthyroidism: Emotional factors. In Werner, S. C., and Ingbar, S. H.: The thyroid, a fundamental and clinical text, ed. 3, New York, 1971, Harper & Row, Publishers, pp. 511-514.
30. McCullagh, E. P., Clamen, M., and Gardner, W. J.: Clinical progress in treatment of exophthalmos of Graves' disease: Effect of pituitary surgery, J. Clin. Endocrinol. Metab. **17:**1277-1292, 1957.
31. McKenzie, J. M., and McCullagh, E. P.: Observations against a casual relationship between the long-acting thyroid stimulator and ophthalmopathy in Graves' disease, J. Clin. Endocrinol. Metab. **28:**1177-1182, 1968.
32. Means, J. H.: Hyperophthalmopathic Graves' disease, Ann. Intern. Med. **23:**779-789, 1945.
33. Meek, J. C., Jones, A. E., Lewis, U. J., and Vanderlaan, W. P.: Characterization of the long-acting thyroid stimulator of Graves' disease, Proc. Natl. Acad. Sci. U.S.A. **52:**342-349, 1964.
34. Munro, R. E., Lamki, L., Row, V. V., and Volpe, R.: Cell-mediated immunity in the exophthalmos of Graves' disease as demonstrated by the migration inhibition factor (MIF) test, J. Clin. Endocrinol. Metab. **37:**286-292, 1973.
35. Ogura, J. H.: Transantral orbital decompression for progressive exophthalmos. A follow-up of 54 cases, Med. Clin. North Am. **52:**399-407, 1968.
36. Onaya, T., Kotana, M., Yamada, T., and Ochi, Y.: New in vitro tests to detect the thyroid stimulator in serum from hyperthyroid patients by measuring colloid droplet formation and cyclic AMP in human thyroid slices, J. Clin. Endocrinol. Metab. **36:**859-866, 1973.
37. Pequegnat, E. P., Mayberry, W. E., McConahey, W. M., and Wyse, E. P.: Large doses of radioiodide in Graves' disease: Effect on ophthalmopathy and long-acting thyroid stimulator, Mayo Clin. Proc. **42:**802-811, 1967.
38. Rodger, F. C., and Sinclair, H. M.: Metabolic and nutritional eye diseases, Springfield, Ill., 1969, Charles C Thomas, Publisher, p. 312.

39. Rundle, F. F.: Management of exophthalmos and related ocular changes in Graves' disease, Metabolism **6:**36-48, 1957.
40. Solomon, D. H.: Treatment of extrathyroidal manifestations of Graves' disease, Mod. Treat. **6:**516-533, 1969.
41. Solomon, D. H., and Chopra, I. J.: Graves' disease—1972, Mayo Clin. Proc. **47:**803-813, 1972.
42. Volpe, R., Desbarats-Schonbaum, M. L., Schonbaum, E., Row, V. V., and Ezrin, C.: The effect of radioablation of the thyroid gland in Graves' disease with high levels of long-acting thyroid stimulator (LATS), Am. J. Med. **46:**217-226, 1969.
43. Volpe, R., Edmonds, M., Lamki, L., Clarke, P. V., and Row, V. V.: The pathogenesis of Graves' disease. A disorder of delayed hypersensitivity? Mayo Clin. Proc. **47:**824-834, 1972.
44. Werner, S. C.: Euthyroid patients with early eye signs of Graves' disease; their responses to L-triiodothyronine and thyrotropin, Am. J. Med. **18:**608-612, 1955.
45. Werner, S. C., Feind, C. R., and Aida, M.: Graves' disease and total thyroidectomy. Progression of severe eye changes and decrease in serum long-acting thyroid stimulator after operation, New Eng. J. Med. **276:**132-138, 1967.
46. Werner, S. C.: Classification of the eye changes of Graves' disease, J. Clin. Endocrinol. Metab. **29:**982-984, 1969.
47. Werner, S. C., Wegelius, O., and Hsu, K. C.: Immune responses in stroma and basement membranes of the Graves' disease thyroid (IgM, IgE, IgG, and complement), Trans. Assoc. Am. Physicians **84:**139-142, 1971.
48. Winand, R. J., Salmon, J., and Lambert, P. H.: Characterization of the exophthalmogenic factor isolated from the serum of patients with malignant exophthalmos. In Fellinger, K., and Hofer, R.: Further advances in thyroid research, Vienna, 1971, Verlag der Wiener Medizinischen Akademie, pp. 583-593.
49. Winand, R. J., and Kohn, L. D.: The binding of 3H-thyrotropin and a 3H-labeled exophthalmogenic factor by plasma membranes of retroorbital tissues, Proc. Natl. Acad. Sci. U.S.A. **69:**1711-1715, 1972.
50. Winand, R. J., and Kohn, L. D.: Retrobulbar modifications in experimental exophthalmos: The effect of thyrotropin and an exophthalmos-producing substance derived from thyrotropin on the $^{35}SO_4$ incorporation and glycosaminoglycan content of Harderian glands, Endocrinology **93:**670-680, 1973.

9

Endocrine diseases (excluding diabetes): ophthalmic aspects

M. Ulrich Dardenne

Even when one excludes diabetes, the field of endocrine diseases of the eye is so large that I choose to limit it still further. I was requested to speak chiefly about the disease of the eye that occurs in connection with thyroid disease called "endocrine orbitopathy." Sometimes it is called "endocrine ophthalmopathy," but I believe the name "endocrine orbitopathy" is better because the pathologic changes are situated in the orbit. The symptoms of this disease are generally well known. But it seems to me that the very serious cases have become quite rare in the last 15 to 20 years. We discussed this once in a meeting in Germany. The cause for this, if it is really true, is not clear. Perhaps the treatment offered by the internists is now better. At the present time, we see mostly cases with minor chemosis of the conjunctiva. The primary course of the endocrine orbitopathy is situated, as far as is now known, in the hypothalamus-hypophysis area. A hypersecretion of a hormone that is secreted by the anterior nuclei of the hypothalamus occurs in cases with disturbance of different hormones, especially of thyroid hormones and also in cases of serious stress situations such as psychologic stress situations, and is called "thyrotropin-releasing hormone." This hormone is regulated by the thyroxin in the blood. After this secretion the hypophysis together with the thyrostimulating hormone secretes a different substance, the exophthalmos-producing substance (EPS) or exophthalmogenic factor (EF), which causes the endocrine orbitopathy. There are probably many other complex immunologic interactions at work in this situation.

PROBLEMS OF DIAGNOSIS OF ENDOCRINE ORBITOPATHY

For an exact diagnosis of endocrine orbitopathy, it seems only to be necessary to demonstrate, in the blood of a patient, the presence of the exophthalmos-producing substance. We tried to improve the method for the detection of this substance in the blood, and we did the following experimental work.

First, there were histologic investigations in experimental fish orbitopathy. Second, there were experiments to determine more quantitively the EPS content in human blood serum. Third, there was an attempt to treat or influence the experimental orbitopathy with other hormones, and fourth, there were experiments to try to separate the exophthalmos-producing substance from the various somatotropic hormones. But above all it is of decisive importance to know whether, in the commonly used fish test, the exophthalmos is caused by the same changes in the fish orbit as in the human orbit.

Because of the investigations of Smelser and his co-workers, Asboe and Hansen, Ten Groot, Kane and Kuwabara, and many others, the following alterations in the human orbit are well known. First, an increase of tissue up to 40% occurs. This tissue shows typical alterations for the endocrine orbitopathy. Second, the whole retrobulbar tissue shows edema. There is a considerable increase of water not only in the connective tissue but also in the lipid tissue and muscles. Third, the percentage of connective tissue in the retrobular tissue is increased. In advanced cases one can find a complete fibrosis of the tissue. Fourth, a clear infiltration of leukocytes, especially with mast cells, can be seen. Fifth, there is a clear increase of the acid mucopolysaccharide, theolone acid, and chondroitin sulfate acid in the orbital tissues as well as in the connective tissues and muscles. Sixth, the external eye muscles demonstrate lipid degeneration as well as interstitial edema and infiltration of leukocytes. In addition, the eye muscles appear pale and atrophic. The muscle tissues also show disappearance of nuclei and degeneration of fibrils. What could be the reason for the edema of the retrobulbar tissue? Venous obstruction is not the reason for the edema. This was shown by Day and Werner in their investigations with radioactive sodium. It is possible that the reason for the edema is an increase of permeability of the capillaries. This is what some investigators claim. It is more probable, according to the investigations by Asboe and Hansen, that the following mechanism operates. The mast cells that are greatly increased, contain granules that are supposed to consist of theolone acid. These granules are transferred to the interstitial tissues. The mast cells show up in the lipid tissues as well as in the muscles and there follows, at the same time, an increase of acid mucopolysaccharides. This was shown by tests with radioactive sulfur. The accumulation of hydrophilic substances results in the edema of these tissues, the secondary lipid degeneration of the muscles, and the more generalized fibrosis in the orbital tissues. Haddad reports about an increase of cylic acid. Let us see what changes occur in the retrobulbar space of fish. The fish received exophthalmos-producing substance injections. After 2 days, measurements showed approximately 12% enlargement of the intercorneal distance. Histologic sections reveal that infiltrates are responsible for an increase in the retro-orbital space. We found two types of cells in the infiltrate—cells 7.2 μm. in size and cells of about 4.8 μm. Since the large cells had granules, we believed that they were mast cells and the smaller ones were cells from the leukocyte chain. These are mucopolysaccharide-producing mast cells like those in human beings. We, as well as Uemura and co-workers, consider them as mast cells because they contain metachromatic and astra blue–positive granules. In summary, the histologic results of the experimental exophthalmos in the small fish correspond in the main features to the histopathologic changes of the endocrine orbitopathy in human beings, and I believe that one may use the fish test to arrive at a diagnosis of this illness.

EXPERIMENTS TO TRY TO GET A MORE QUANTITATIVE DETERMINATION OF EPS

Since determination of the exophthalmos-producing substance in fish is a biologic test, there is a large margin of error. In the literature one can show that the fish test was negative in patients with endocrine orbitopathy and positive in patients without endocrine orbitopathy. Strangely enough one cannot find in the literature sufficient reports about basic investigations concerning the possibilities of error in the present fish test. In the methodology and experimental technique that have been in use recently, we found the following possibilities of error.

First, the goldfish that have often been used recently were too large. Smaller fish showed a stronger and more uniform reaction. Fish should therefore weigh only 4 to 5 grams. Second, the injection of the serum of patients should proceed through the cloaca into the coelom. By adding a dye to the injection, one can show that there is a considerable loss of fluid when the injection is given subcutaneously. Also the scales become damaged, so that the fish soon sicken and die. Third, only by giving these small fish anesthesia can one perform the injection with sufficient care to avoid injury to the fish. An unanesthetized fish thrashes about in self-defense, and so one is never quite certain how much of the material has been injected; this is particularly true for the smaller fish. Fourth, one must not only put the fish in a moist chamber and hold it with the fingers to measure the intercorneal distance, but also it is very important to avoid pressure to the site since a large vein flows directly beneath the skin in the fish. We fit the narcotized fish loosely and sideways with a dynamometer. It is necessary to observe both corneas of the fish at the same time while measuring. The fish can move their eyes separately, and because of this, the intercorneal distance may change. We used a so-called profile projector such as is used in making the most delicate mechanism for wristwatches. It is important to measure the intercorneal distance not earlier than 36 and no later than 48 hours after the first serum injection. The reason for this is that we found in the serial measurements that we performed on our control subjects that 20% of these cases, especially in males, showed a pseudoexophthalmos that disappeared after 12 hours. The endocrine exophthalmos appears, however, not only to depend on the amount of secreted exophthalmos-producing substance but also to depend on other hormones as well. For instance, ACTH is in a position to increase the effect of exophthalmos-producing substance.

EXPERIMENTS TO SEPARATE THE EXOPHTHALMOS-PRODUCING SUBSTANCE FROM TSH

Up to now there has been a great deal of discussion about the identity of exophthalmos-producing substances. Are the exophthalmos-producing substance and thyrosomatotropic hormones the same substance, or is the exophthalmos-producing substance a precursor of TSH, or is it a metabolite of TSH? We tried to pursue this question. We used a commercial TSH preparation and separated this into 10 different protein fractions with the aid of column chromatography on carboxymethylcellulose according to the method used by Brunisch and co-workers. In each of these protein fractions we determined the exophthalmic activity and also the thyrotropic activity. We measured the exophthalmic activity in our fish test and the thyrotropic activity in the mouse test with radioactive iodine according to

Mackenzie's methods. I cannot go into the details of the TSH determination test in mice because it is rather complicated. However, our results were the following. We noted exophthalmic activity only in three fractions. In the first fraction, although 88% of the total amount of protein remained, we could not find any exophthalmos-producing effect. On the other hand it was not possible to separate any fraction that had no thyrotropic effect without the two last fractions, which also had no exophthalmogenic activity and probably were impurities. In the fractions that had exophthalmic activity, the thyrotropic activity was minor but nonetheless clearly in evidence. One explanation might be that TSH is separated from exophthalmos-producing substance, and since the molecular weight of EPS is 40,500 whereas the molecular weight of TSH is 28,000, the large molecule contains both active substances. To further clarify this problem, we compared the amino acids in a protein fraction having the highest EPS activity with that of the fraction that only contained TSH activity. The differences we found concerned especially the concentration of cysteine, glycine, prolene, and glutamic acid, and the difference in concentration of cysteine and glutamic acid was particularly striking. In the protein, which I should like to consider as TSH, we found 4.5 times more glutamic acid molecules than cysteine molecules whereas the EPS protein contained the same amount of glutamic acid and cysteine. Consequently I believe that both hormones differ not only in their respective molecular size but also in their amino acid composition. I dare not claim more than this.

In reviewing the literature, as Dr. Solomon said, one finds a large number of contradictory reports about therapeutic successes and failures. One reason may be the therapeutic treatment itself; for instance, D-thyroxin or steroids are administered in cases when no improvement can be expected with these drugs. In the treatment of endocrine orbitopathy it seems, in my opinion, to be especially important that the steroids be started early. This follows from the histologic findings of this disease. One cannot expect that a fibrosis or a severe degeneration of the muscle tissue can show improvement with these drugs or x-ray treatment. Scar tissue cannot be repaired any longer. We use D-thyroxin not only in our acute cases but also in our chronic cases if they were in an acute phase of the disease. We often give a very high dosage, up to the limit of electrocardiographic monitoring, since in cases of coronary insufficiency there is some danger involved. In some cases with malignant exophthalmos, it was sufficient to put sutures in the eyelids, and with D-thyroxin therapy, the acute phase disappeared slowly over a period of 3 to 4 weeks. We combined this D-thyroxin with high doses of corticosteroids in very serious cases, which, however, occur seldom with us. We can bring about a sufficient decompression by performing a simple orbitotomy and by using, after this and combined with this, D-thyroxin and corticosteroids. Operations using the Naffziger or Kronlein procedure have not been performed by us for 20 years. The operative procedure for decompression according to Ogura is now usually recommended. In the case of women we found that in mild acute cases but not in severe cases dosages of estrogen were of some therapeutic benefit. We are observing at present a patient who is receiving estrogens for other causes. When her estrogen therapy is stopped, she develops an orbitopathy. It was possible to observe this effect repeatedly. We have not seen any definite success with x-ray treatment of the hypophysis in older chronic cases, but we do not have a great deal of experience with this. We watch over each case by determining the EPS content. We have found a good correlation between the lessening of the EPS content in the blood with an improvement of the symptoms.

If it is true that the hypophysis secretes a hormone that produces an exophthalmos, then only if the secretion is too large should one call this substance an exophthalmos-producing substance. One could, with the same argument, also call insulin a hypoglycemia-producing substance. I believe that exophathalmos-producing substance may have another function, perhaps that of maintaining the normal tissue pressure. For it is well known that exophthalmos-producing substance demonstrates its function not only in the orbit but also, for instance, in the peritesticular and perirenal tissues, as well as in the armpits and even in the normal skeletal muscles.

Ocular involvement in endocrine disease

CHAIRMAN: **H. Stanley Thompson***

Dr. Thompson: The first question I have here is for Dr. Solomon and I will paraphrase it. If the ophthalmologist is faced with a patient with proptosis and lid retraction and the patient is euthyroid by routine screening tests (two-part question), is it true that there is no one laboratory test in common use that identifies a patient with Graves' disease, and if so, what should be the function of the internist in the handling of this patient?

Dr. Solomon: Most patients with Graves' ophthalmopathy also have an abnormality of the thyroid gland revealed by autonomy, that is, nonsuppressibility when triiodothyronine, for example, is given. Not all have this abnormality. Somewhere between 15% and 35% of such patients have normal suppressibility. In those there is no unequivocal way to establish the diagnosis of Graves' disease, except by the usually pathognomonic clinical features. And I believe that almost always one can make the diagnosis by careful physical examination and I believe you would agree with that statement although perhaps the figure is a little high and a little optimistic. But the differential with orbital tumor is ordinarily a very easy one to accomplish.

The other part of that question that usually comes up is whether LATS assay in serum is a useful way to make the diagnosis. Unfortunately in euthyroid ophthalmopathy the incidence of positive LATS assays is down around 20%. It is a very expensive assay procedure and usually costs about $100 in most laboratories. Not many laboratories run it. So after due consideration it isn't really a very valuable test.

Dr. Thompson: In the case of a patient with a monocular elevator palsy and no history of trauma and a positive forced-duction test, which thyroid studies should be done, if any? Again, this is a problem of diagnosis, and how do you make sure of what you're dealing with?

Dr. Kearns: Well, the positive forced-duction test, in my experience, has been a difficult thing for me to do. It's often quite painful. This is easy if you've got the patient asleep, but you don't want to allow this in doing a forced-duction test. But there is more than one way to skin a cat, and so I found it quite

*Department of Ophthalmology, University of Iowa College of Medicine, Iowa City, Iowa.

valuable to check the intraocular pressure with the eye in a slightly up position. Now you can't do this with applanation, but by Schiøtz check the patient with the head level and then check the patient with the head slightly down and then slightly up. In other words, check in the various positions straight ahead with the eye down and then with the eye up, and you will find that if this is a tight depressor causing the defective elevation, the intraocular pressure will be higher with the eye in the up position and I believe this is a pretty infallible test and works for me about as well as doing a forced-duction test with forceps. There is the other question of what test to do. I would send them to a good internist, someone I know and respect and who knows something about thyroid disease. I leave this to the internist. But I do agree though that most of the internists I work with certainly agree with Dr. Solomon's statement that you don't have to have all three. You can have a goiter; you can have hyperthyroidism; you can have ophthalmopathy. You can have two of those or one of them, and even with the ophthalmopathy it is still Graves' disease.

Dr. Thompson: Dr. Podos, is there a published series of normals in how much the intraocular pressure goes up when you look in various directions?

Dr. Podos: No, not really. There are some controls, and I think the paper that Dr. Kearns was referring to was originally by Gay and co-workers and the data can be found there. It is true that in their series, in the normals that they did this on, there was virtually no elevation of intraocular pressure whereas in patients with thyroid there was.

Dr. Newell: Here we are at the University of Iowa, I think we ought to note that Alson Braley noted this change on upward gaze quite some years ago.

Dr. Podos: My apologies.

Dr. Solomon: In adding a comment to what Dr. Kearns said, I think it is important to have an internist or some appropriate individual look at the whole patient situation and get involved because not only are these patients frequently euthyroid despite the presence of Graves' disease, but they may be hypothyroid. Some of these bizarre cases where the hyperthyroid side of Graves' disease is not expressed are such because of the coincidence of chronic thyroiditis with Graves' disease and the chronic thyroditis limits the ability of the gland to sustain the hyperthyroid state. Well, that combination can then proceed to the point where the Hashimoto thyroiditis has essentially destroyed thyroid function and may become hypothyroid. It is extremely important both for the eyes and the rest of the body that the doctor make that diagnosis and treat it. The other side of the matter is that some of them have undetected hyperthyroidism, and sometimes this is so-called T_3 thyrotoxicosis; that is, the serum thyroxin is still within normal range, but serum triiodothyronine, which is a more sensitive indicator, is elevated. So it gets fairly complicated. There are many possibilities and it's worth looking into in detail.

Dr. Thompson: Dr. Bean, reference was made yesterday to the apparently decreasing instance of severe iritis in gout. Do you believe that progressive dysthyroid malignant exophthalmos is less common now than it was say 30 years ago, and if so, why? Does it have something to do with the way Graves' disease is being managed nowadays or does it have to do with the use of steroids?

Dr. Bean: It's very difficult to give you anything more than a brief impression.

I certainly think it's less common to see those conditions than it used to be. Whether that is an artificial selection to the people that you happen to run into or see, or whether this is a secular trend, that is, in fact, a true reflection of a state that prevails generally, I am not prepared to say. There is no question in my mind, though, that there are really radical and important changes that do occur in the natural evolution and history of certain diseases as we see them and there is also a change that occurs in the frequency of certain disorders and complications. Whether you would say this occurs because for so many diseases long-term steroid therapy is being given and this may in some way smother the appearance of the malignant form of exophthalmos that has been discussed this morning, I don't really know. In a disease for which you do not really understand the pathogenesis it's very difficult to tell when the frequency or incidence of severity changes. I cannot give you an answer to the question you asked because I do not know, but I do know that I have seen far fewer of such patients in a general consultation practice than was true formerly.

Dr. Thompson: Thank you. Is there anyone else on the panel who has a strong opinion on that?

Dr. Newell: I think these cases go back to the 1920s and 1930s when thyroidectomy was carried out for a wide variety of disorders. But not necessarily hyperthyroidism. The most severe instances of this, I think, occurred in those patients who had lid retraction and exophthalmos of euthyroidism and then were treated with a removal of the thyroid, and not uncommonly they developed what we call malignant exophthalmos.

Dr. Thompson: Is there a place for sympatholytic drugs, such as guanethidine, in the management of corneal exposure in thyroid ophthalmopathy?

Dr. Podos: I have very little experience with this, but I saw a number of patients. Dr. Gay treats patients with guanethidine in order to bring down the lids. It was toxic by causing miosis and a good deal of irritation. Guanethidine is not available, nor will it be granted FDA approval as far as I understand; so the question is academic. There is another agent that may become available in the United States called thymoximine that we have heard a little bit about in terms of breaking acute angle-closure attacks. I do not know of anybody who has tried thymoximine in lid retraction of thyroid disease, but I think it would be worth a try.

Dr. Thompson: Thymoximine is a very potent drug, and although in low enough concentrations it might not bother the cornea, it still might do something to the Müller's fibers and it burns. Let's pick up that last item and ask Dr. Kearns. I know that some surgical decompressions are being done at the Mayo Clinic. What are your indications for surgical decompressions in malignant exophthalmos?

Dr. Kearns: I am glad you asked that because I was just thinking about it. There are two indications in my mind for the ophthalmologist to recommend surgical decompression to be considered. First, is the problem of corneal ulceration that cannot be controlled and looks progressive, and the second is optic neuropathy. Now sometimes we get into patients that have cosmetic problems, and none of us like to admit this but sometimes we do think, "Well maybe they will be getting optic neuropathy," but this is on touchy grounds and, we have to be careful that we do not do this for cosmetic purposes although I believe sometimes we get talked into this. The interesting thing here is that, as some of you may know, I have been a great advocate of transcranial or transfrontal decompression because Dr. McCarty, head of our neurosurgery department, does a little different technique than the usual Naffziger operation. He unroofs the orbit and then takes down as much of the lateral wall as he can get; so he is really doing a combination Kronlein and Naffziger operation, and there is no question in my mind, since we wrote these up 3 or 4 years ago, that this procedure works.

Dr. Ogura is professor of otolaryngology in St. Louis. Several had mentioned that the Ogura technique is their procedure of choice. Well, we have a young otolaryngologist who has been doing this technique, and I have to admit I am coming around to it. I believe this probably is a superior technique to the transfrontal one. As I understand, there are more diplopia problems and complaints about numbness of the upper lip than with the transfrontal technique.

Dr. Thompson: Dr. Solomon, perhaps you can take this question from an ophthalmologist. Three parts. What are the criteria for giving oral thyroid medication, what is the maximal dose of oral thyroid for patients 60 or over, and can thyroid extract be taken without harm for years?

Dr. Solomon: The indications for oral thyroid medication are hypothyroidism, or chronic thyroiditis with the desire to decrease the size of a goiter, or certain thyroid nodules with the desire to try to suppress TSH output, etc. There are other indications. In the disease we are talking about today there is no indication except hypothyroidism. The dose of thyroid hormone that most of us use today is averaging two tenths of a milligram of thyroxin per day. And the answer to the third part is that there is no harm from prolonged administration.

Dr. Dardenne: Dr. Solomon, if you give x-ray treatment in the retrobulbar space, is there danger of an increase in fibrosis if you give it in *chronic* cases? Normally x-ray treatment increases fibrosis.

Dr. Solomon: I think that's a very good question, Dr. Dardenne. The only thing we really know is what Donaldson, Bagshaw, and Kriss have reported recently in the *Journal of Clinical Endocrinology and Metabolism*. That's the only paper on orbital irradiation in the past 15 years that I know of. And they do not report any worsening of the diplopia or of the extraocular muscle function, but they may not have followed some long enough.

Dr. Herron: I wonder if someone would comment on high-dose steroids, indications for beginning, and experience with getting people off these steroids.

Dr. Solomon: The indications are essentially the same as Dr. Kearns gave for orbital decompression, and if there are no contraindications such as an active peptic ulcer or any of the usual things, then we would generally first try a short course of high-dose prednisone in the range of 60 to 80 mg. a day in the patient with the critical indications that he mentioned. If there is no beneficial response within 1 week in a patient who was having evidence of optic neuropathy, then we would turn to orbital decompression. In the patient with less serious indications, we go 2 weeks, but if there isn't any benefit by 2 weeks, there is no point in continuing it because there won't really be much benefit anyway. So we rapidly taper in that situation. In the patient who does well and shows improvement, we very slowly taper off over a period of months, playing by the Rundall's curve for the natural tendency of this condition to remit once it is past the plateau.

10

Problem of tissue oxygenation in diabetes as related to development of diabetic retinopathy

Jørn Ditzel

Diabetes mellitus is a chronic systemic disease characterized by disorders in (1) the metabolism of carbohydrate, fat, and protein because of a relative or an absolute insulin deficiency and (2) the function and structure of blood vessels.

The principle early symptoms and signs are usually related to the metabolic defect; findings late in the disease are linked with complications resulting from vascular defects. The treatment of the disease diabetes is concerned with the control of the blood glucose by diet and various forms of antidiabetic therapy, and this is a vital aspect in the care of diabetics. Equally important is the management of the various chronic complications to which the diabetic is subject. These complications account for most diabetic morbidity and mortality.

The vascular disease in diabetes involves all types of vessels, of which those of the small blood vessels are of particular importance. The disease of this portion of the vasculature is one of the focal points of current research in diabetes and is referred to as "diabetic microangiopathy." The histologic changes of these lesions share certain similarities in various organs, mainly endothelial proliferation with hyalinization and thickening of basement membranes, which show periodic acid–Schiff positivity.

Of all the late complications of the small blood vessels in diabetes, none are more important than those affecting the retina; important not only because they cause blindness, but also because they help us to recognize the vascular component of diabetes at a stage when we should try to arrest their progress. The specific diabetic retinopathy is characterized by morphologic changes, primarily in the venules and capillaries, with subsequent neovascularization. These changes developing in young diabetic patients seem directly attributable to some disturbance that is a result of diabetes, or associated with it. The disturbance is probably in the functional relationship between insulin, other hormones, and enzyme systems. This may explain why the most skillful use of insulin, a good diet, and medical supervision persistently followed, postpone or prevent such diabetic complications in many patients.

The purpose of this review is to draw attention to the fact that retinal tissue hypoxia may be an important factor in the pathogenesis of diabetic retinopathy. Evidence for this statement is provided

1. by comparison of the various diseases in which the characteristic features of diabetic retinopathy, the retinal microaneurysms, venous changes, and proliferating new vessels occur
2. by the in vivo responses of the conjunctival vessels in diabetics
3. by presentation of some new data indicating the erythrocytes as a cause of disordered oxygen transport in diabetes.

RETINAL TISSUE HYPOXIA—A COMMON FACTOR FOR RETINAL CHANGES?

The histologic picture of diabetic retinopathy is characterized by the following microvascular changes: microaneurysms, phlebopathy, proliferating new-formed vessels.

Microaneurysms

The admirable study by Ballantyne and Loewenstein[8] in 1943 clearly disclosed that most of the so-called punctate hemorrhages observed ophthalmoscopically were actually microaneurysms. There was some controversy at first as to whether they were primarily arterial or venous in origin. The general consensus now strongly favors the latter source, particularly capillaries and small venules. Ashton[3] showed that microaneurysms were not found outside the retina (with the possible exception of the conjunctiva[26]). Their confinement to the retina seems related to local factors such as the peculiar structure and function of the retinal capillary network in the inner nuclear layer. The stages in the development of microaneurysms from the normal capillary are not known. Besides the globular microaneurysms, other ectasias may occur on the retinal capillaries. Ashton has depicted the development of microaneurysms as beginning either as a pouching of the capillary wall or as loops formed by elongation and kinking, the inner portion of which may later become obliterated. Part of the mechanism by which the microaneurysm is formed in diabetes may be through degenerative and proliferative changes in the lining endothelium associated with premature pericyte degeneration. Hypoxia is a well-known stimulus for endothelial proliferation. In a comprehensive comparative study of retinopathies in various conditions, Wise[45] presented considerable evidence for the concept that the microaneurysms actually represented an attempt of neovascularization in response to retinal tissue hypoxia.

From a morphologic point of view the retinal microaneurysms are not specific for diabetes. In the cases in which a relatively large number of microaneurysms have been demonstrated, they have been confined to conditions associated with prolonged venous stasis of the retinal circulation. Thus Ballantyne,[9, 10] Loewenstein and Garrow,[36] Becker and Post,[11] and Ashton[4] have all reported on the presence of numerous microaneurysms in cases of central retinal vein thrombosis. The occurrence of retinal microaneurysms has also been demonstrated in sickle-cell anemia, macroglobulinemia, pulseless disease, and malignant hypertension.[4, 6, 25, 43] Diabetes, however, stands out as being the disease in which microaneurysms are seen most frequently, in greatest number, and in most advanced form, giving rise to hemorrhages and exudates. This indicates that the aneurysms may be related to one or several factors common to many diseases that are present in a particular degree in the diabetic state. The most obvious common determinant for the formation of retinal microaneurysms in the conditions mentioned would appear to be retinal tissue hypoxia, either brought about by a failure of blood supply, by stasis of the venous circulation, or by defective oxygen release from the erythrocytes.

Phlebopathy

The earliest alteration observed in the retinal veins is usually an increased fullness and general dilatation without any major configurative irregularities. Some investigators consider this venous feature to precede the formation of microaneurysms.[1, 28] Larsen[34] studied diabetics serially with a modern retina camera and reported that fullness or dilatation of the retinal veins might be observed even from the onset of diabetes. During the first years of the disease the fullness in dilatation of the retinal vein was reversible, but later on venous dilatation became more permanent. The reversibility of the dilatation of the retinal veins appeared to be related to the degree of regulation of the metabolic disturbance. Jütte[33] carefully measured the retinal veins and found that the retinal veins were dilated in 43 of 100 juvenile diabetics. The dilatation increased with the duration of diabetes during the first 10 years. An increase in vein diameter occurred during periods of poor regulation but was reversible with correction of the diabetic metabolic disturbance. Because of the reversibility of the changes in cases of short-term diabetes, Jütte considered the dilatation as a functional change. He suggested that the capillary venous dilatation was produced by some alteration in the metabolism of the retinal tissue. However, since dilatation of the venules of the microcirculation is a response change of hypoxia, this change in diabetes might similarly indicate a state of retinal tissue hypoxia. Their reversibility with the control of diabetes indicates a relationship between the hypoxic state and poor regulation of the disease.

Proliferating new-formed vessels

As for the retinal microaneurysms new-formed vessels are also seen in various nondiabetic conditions such as in retinal vein occlusion, sickle-cell anemia, macroglobulinemia, and so on. According to Ashton[5] new vessel formation can be stimulated when three basic requirements are present: (1) the presence of living cells to ensure an active metabolism, (2) a low oxygen tension to promote anaerobic metabolism, and (3) a poor venous drainage to permit the accumulation of anaerobic metabolites, wherein the vasoformative factor probably lies. Recall that the retina has the highest metabolism and respiration of any tissue and that the various layers of the retina possess their own peculiar metabolism, with some of the cells being responsible for the high glycolytic activity whereas the others are almost completely oxidative in character. The inner nuclear layer seems to be particularly concerned with anaerobic glycolysis.[42]

These clinicopathologic and other evidences suggest a relationship between retinal tissue hypoxia and the development of diabetic retinopathy.

IN VIVO RESPONSES OF CONJUNCTIVAL VESSELS IN DIABETES

Since a study of another vascular bed could be a further step to a better understanding of the pathogenesis of the microangiopathy in diabetes, we as well as other groups of investigators have studied the cutaneous vessels of the bulbar conjunctiva. It was supposed that the functional disease diabetes might reflect functional changes in the smaller blood vessels, which ultimately could lead to degenerative lesions. These studies have shown that the significanct vascular changes in the diabetics consist of irreversible degenerative changes that are distinctly accelerated as compared to those of normal aging and reversible caliber changes of arterioles and venules.[18, 19] The reversible response changes consisted of various degrees of arteriolar and venular dilatation. Table 10-1 presents measurements of the calibers of the vessels from the negative film of flash photographs of the conjunctival vessels in diabetic and healthy individuals. These measurements were done without the investigators' knowing beforehand whether a photographic negative belonged to a diabetic or to a control subject. Table 10-1 shows that the diameters of the arterioles were significantly larger in the diabetics than in the nondiabetics ($p < 0.05$) and that the venules in the diabetics had diameters significantly larger than those of the nondiabetics ($p < 0.001$). When the diabetics were divided into two groups depending on the duration of diabetes, the diameters of the arterioles were significantly larger in short-term diabetics than in those diabetics with more than 10 years' duration of their disease ($p < 0.01$) (Table 10-2). Table 10-3 shows that both the arterioles and venules were less dilated in the late afternoon ($p < 0.01$), when the insulin effect might be expected to produce the optimal daily metabolic pattern (Fig. 10-1). The conjunctival blood flow is representative of the cutaneous blood flow as a whole. The function of the cutaneous blood flow is to satisfy metabolic needs of the tissue, but additionally it ensures that thermal waste reaches the surface. It is well-known that diabetes mellitus is a unique disease with instability in oxygen consumption. The basal oxygen consumption of adult diabetics is increased by approximately 10% to 15%.[29, 32, 44] However, subsequent to insulin administration there is a transient decrease of the oxygen uptake to normal values, but the effect lasts only

Table 10-1. Average diameters of conjunctival arterioles, venules, and arteriovenous ratio in diabetic and healthy subjects (measured from photonegatives in the morning prior to receiving insulin)

Groups	Number	Number of measurements	Average age (years)	Average duration of diabetes (years)	Diameter (0.01 mm.)		Arteriovenous ratio
					Arterioles	Venules	
Diabetics	47	136	27.6 ± 9.2	12.0 ± 10.4	18.7 ± 6.7	46.9 ± 16.0	0.43 ± 0.16
Healthy controls	48	126	25.9 ± 6.4		16.8 ± 4.6	35.0 ± 12.5	0.52 ± 0.15
Significance					$p < 0.05$	$p < 0.001$	$p < 0.001$

some hours, depending on the type of insulin given.[30, 31] The microvascular dilatation observed during the day with a gradual improvement in the late afternoon might parallel a concomitant normalization of the oxygen consumption of the body, when insulin has its maximum effect. It was also found that the degree of caliber changes in the form of venous dilation was favorably influenced

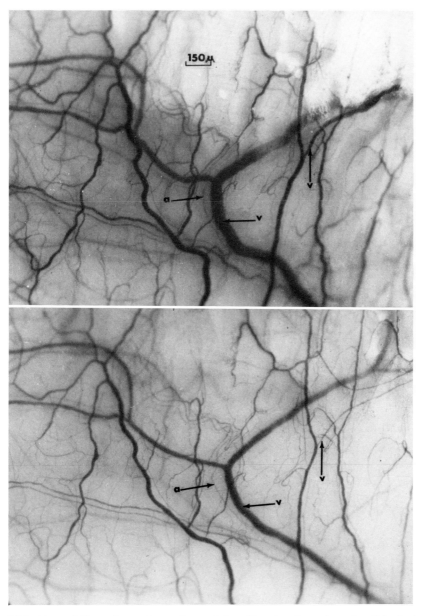

Fig. 10-1. Reversibility of venular and arteriolar dilatation in a juvenile diabetic in the morning prior to NPH-insulin administration *(top)* until in the afternoon of the same day *(bottom)*. **a,** Arteriole. **v,** Venule. (Approximately × 60).

Table 10-2. Average diameters of conjunctival arterioles, venules, and arteriovenous ratio in diabetic subjects with duration of less than 10 years and more than 10 years

Groups	Number	Number of mea-surements	Average age (years)	Average duration of diabetes (years)	Diameter (0.01 mm.) Arterioles	Venules	Arterio-venous ratio
Diabetics of less than 10 years' duration	21	63	25.2 ± 8.6	2.7 ± 2.3	20.6 ± 8.1	46.6 ± 17.3	0.48 ± 0.17
Diabetics of more than 10 years' duration	26	73	29.5 ± 9.5	19.6 ± 7.8	17.1 ± 4.1	47.1 ± 14.9	0.42 ± 0.14
Signifi-cance					$p < 0.01$	Not significant	$p < 0.01$

Table 10-3. Diameters of conjunctival arterioles, venules, and arteriovenous ratio in the morning and in the afternoon of diabetic and healthy subjects

Groups	Number of individ-uals	Number of measure-ments	Average age (years)	Average duration of diabetes (years)	Time of photo-graphing	Diameter (0.01 mm.) Arterioles	Venules	Arterio-venous ratio
Diabetics	47	136	27.6 ± 9.2	12.0 ± 10.4	Morning	18.7 ± 6.7	46.9 ± 16.0	0.43 ± 0.16
					After-noon	17.5 ± 5.7	41.6 ± 14.5	0.45 ± 0.15
Significance						$p < 0.001$	$p < 0.001$	$p < 0.05$
Healthy controls	48	126	25.9 ± 6.4		Morning	16.8 ± 4.6	35.0 ± 12.5	0.52 ± 0.15
					After-noon	16.7 ± 4.5	33.4 ± 11.4	0.53 ± 0.16
Significance						Not sig-nificant	$p < 0.001$	Not sig-nificant

by optimal dietary and insulin prescription.[20] This parallels the fact that the basal oxygen consumption in poorly regulated diabetics is elevated as compared to their oxygen consumption when in optimal metabolic control.

In order to evaluate whether these microvascular responses were related to the development of retinopathy and nephropathy a study of the vascular response patterns observed microscopically in the bulbar conjunctiva was made in 60 young diabetics with varying degrees of complication. A significant relationship between the degree of retinopathy and the conjunctival pattern abnormality was found.[21] This study suggests that the reversible vasomotor changes may play an important role in the development of diabetic retinopathy. Since arteriolar and venular dilatation is a response that parallel changes in the oxygen demand, these studies of the bulbar conjunctival vessels also suggest that there might be some specific disorder in the oxygen delivery to the tissues in diabetes.

ERYTHROCYTES AS A CAUSE OF DISORDERED OXYGEN TRANSPORT IN DIABETES

In the past, the major focus of clinical interest in oxygen transport has centered on factors governing oxygen uptake, and little attention has been paid to the factors governing oxygen release—the unloading of oxygen in the tissue capillaries. It has been assumed that the affinity of hemoglobin for oxygen, as reflected by the position of the oxyhemoglobin dissociation curve, was a fixed parameter that was mainly influenced by changes in pH and temperature. In 1967, Benesch and Benesch[13] and Chanutin and Curnish[15] demonstrated that the affinity of a hemoglobin solution for oxygen could be decreased by its interaction with a number of organic phosphates. Of the organic phosphates tested, 2,3-diphosphoglycerate (2,3-DPG) was most effective in lowering oxygen affinity. The amount of this organic phosphate in the red cell is equivalent to the hemoglobin concentration. Many experimental and clinical data show the great importance of 2,3-DPG in regulating oxygen delivery to the tissues.

During the last 3 years we have conducted a study of the various factors involved in tissue oxygenation in health and in diabetes mellitus. These studies demonstrate the erythrocyte in diabetes as a cause of disordered oxygen transport, a condition that is present from the onset of diabetes and that is partly related to the degree of metabolic control.

The oxygen-transport system in man is based on the erythrocyte and its primary function is to bring oxygen to the tissues at a sufficient pressure to permit rapid diffusion from blood in adequate quantities. Previously it was believed that the release of hemoglobin-dependent oxygen to tissues was satisfactory when the arterial oxygen saturation was close to 100%. However, this measurement pro-

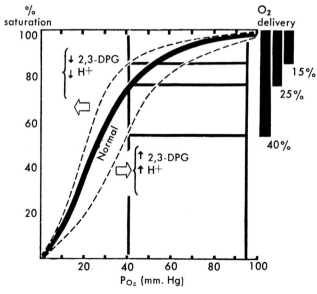

Fig. 10-2. Effect of 2,3-DPG and pH on position of oxyhemoglobin dissociation curve and on oxygen delivery.

vides no information about the potential for oxyhemoglobin to actually unload this oxygen to tissues.

The oxyhemoglobin dissociation curve (ODC) reflects the affinity of hemoglobin for oxygen. As the blood circulates in the normal lung, the arterial oxygen tension rises from 40 mm. of mercury and reaches approximately 100 mm. of mercury, sufficient to ensure at least 95% saturation of the arterial blood (Fig. 10-2). The shape of the ODC is such that a further increase of the oxygen tension in the lung results in only a very small increase in the degree of saturation of the blood. The oxygen tension falls as blood travels from the lungs, and oxygen is released from the hemoglobin. In the normal adult when the oxygen tension has fallen to approximately 26 mm. of mercury at a pH of 7.4 and a temperature of 37° C., 50% of the oxygen bound to hemoglobin has been released. The P_{50} value, the whole blood oxygen tension at 50% oxygen saturation, will thus be stated to be 26 mm. of mercury. When the affinity of hemoglobin is reduced, more oxygen is released to the tissues at a given oxygen tension. In such situations the ODC is shifted to the right of normal. Alternatively, if the affinity of hemoglobin is increased, the blood gives off less oxygen; thus the dissociation curve is shifted to the left.

The hemoglobin molecule is composed of two pairs of polypeptides that in adult hemoglobin are known as α- and β-chains (hemoglobin A is $\alpha_2\beta_2$). Each

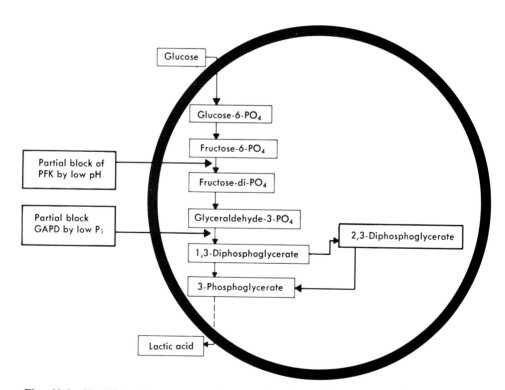

Fig. 10-3. Simplified diagram of erythrocyte glycolysis. Cell membrane is permeable to hydrogen ion, inorganic phosphate (P_i), lactate, and pyruvate, but it is impermeable to the organic phosphate.

chain has a little more than 140 amino acids bound together in a specific sequence. The study by Bunn and Briehl[14] indicates that 2,3-DPG is bound both at the β-143-histidin and to the N-terminal amino groups of the β-chains.

The 2,3-DPG in the red cell is generated by the glycolysis (Fig. 10-3). The erythrocytes are said to be insensitive to insulin. Normally about 90% of glucose is broken down anaerobically to lactic acid. This is the sole pathway for net ATP synthesis, and the rate of glycolysis determines the passage of the intermediate, 1,3-DPG, through the glycolytic Rapoport-Luebering pathway to 2,3-DPG. A decrease in total concentration of 2,3-DPG of about 1 mmol. per liter of erythrocytes induces a shift to the left of 1.5 to 4 mm. of mercury at half saturation.[41] In diabetes at least two factors have major importance for determining the content of red cell 2,3-DPG, that is, the hydrogen-ion concentration (pH) of blood and the concentration of plasma inorganic phosphate. At a blood pH below normal such as during diabetic acidosis the intraerythrocytic glycolysis becomes impaired. Lactate production decreases, the synthesis of 2,3-DPG ceases, while glucose-6-phosphate concentration remains high. These changes are partly attributable to the inhibitory effect of the lower pH on the activities of enzymes involved in 2,3-DPG production, such as DPG-mutase and phosphofructokinase. Inorganic phosphate in the erythrocytes reflecting the concentration of inorganic phosphate in the plasma acts as a cofactor for both phosphofructokinase (PFK) and glyceraldehyde-3-phosphate dehydrogenase (GAPD). Insulin administration induces a sudden carbohydrate utilization by muscle and fat tissues all over the body. As glucose is entering the cell, there is a concomitant cellular uptake of inorganic phosphate in the formation of glucose-6-phosphate. Therefore, insulin administration may lead to a lowering of the concentration of plasma inorganic phosphate (P_i), which again may lead to an inhibition in the formation of 2,3-DPG of the red blood cell.

Decrease in red cell 2,3-DPG in and during recovery from diabetic acidosis with concomitant abnormalities in oxygen release

Diabetic coma or severe diabetic ketoacidosis is the result of the disease when it is uncontrolled. The clinical picture related to the sequelae of insulin deficiency is characterized by mobilization of fatty acids, accumulation of ketone bodies, hyperglycemia, impaired cellular uptake of glucose, and deficits in electrolytes and in body water. Diabetic ketoacidosis is associated with a significant depletion of the phosphorus stores in the body as shown by the immediate response of plasma and urinary phosphorus to insulin. With insulin treatment there occurs a precipitous fall in both plasma phosphate and urinary phosphorus levels and the plasma phosphate level may remain subnormal for as long as a week. Since both low blood pH and low plasma inorganic phosphate are known to act as inhibitors in the glycolysis of the red cells and thereby the formation of 2,3-DPG, the low pH and P_i may be determining factors for the rate of resynthesis of red cell 2,3-DPG and the normalization of the affinity of hemoglobin for oxygen. We have evaluated this supposition by studying the interrelationship between these blood parameters and red cell 2,3-DPG and the position of the oxyhemoglobin dissociation curve in patients in and during recovery from severe diabetic ketoacidosis.[22, 23] Fig. 10-4 shows a typical pattern of changes occurring in plasma

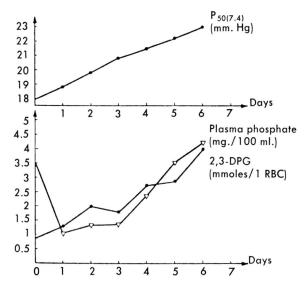

Fig. 10-4. Pattern of changes in 2,3-DPG, plasma inorganic phosphate, and $P_{50(7.4)}$ in a case of severe diabetic ketoacidosis.

phosphate, red cell 2,3-DPG content, and the $P_{50(7.4)}$ of the oxyhemoglobin dissociation curve (ODC) on admission and after treatment with insulin and neutral fluid replacement in diabetic ketoacidosis. P_i on admission was normal or slightly increased, but immediately after insulin administration there occurred a pronounced drop in the P_i to values not infrequently below 1 mg. per 100 ml. The plasma phosphate may remain at such low levels for several days, depending on the condition of the patient, and thereafter the plasma level slowly increased. The red cell 2,3-DPG content was decreased in all ketoacidotic patients, averaging approximately 2 mmol. per 1 RBC on admission. The concentration slowly increased during the following 6 to 8 days to reach concentrations above the normal values. $P_{50(in\ vivo)}$ was usually normal on admission. This was attributable to the low concentration of 2,3-DPG counteracting the Bohr effect on the position of the ODC. $P_{50(7.4)}$ of the ODC was considerably below normal, approximately 18 to 19 mm. of mercury. With insulin treatment the pH usually became normalized approximately 24 hours after initiation of the treatment, and the $P_{50(in\ vivo)}$ became lowered. The values of $P_{50(in\ vivo)}$ and $P_{50(7.4)}$ slowly increased toward normal during the following 6 to 8 days.

Fig. 10-5 shows that there is a close correlation between the concentration of 2.3-DPG of the red cell and the position of $P_{50(7.4)}$ of the ODC ($r = 0.94$, $p < 0.001$). Fig. 10-6 indicates that there is a close correlation between the concentration of P_i and the $P_{50(7.4)}$ of the ODC ($r = 0.80$, $p < 0.001$). Thus the P_i may be an important factor in determining the release of oxygen from the erythrocytes.

These and other studies[2, 12, 27] have shown that diabetic ketoacidosis is associated with a distinct decrease in the content of red cell 2,3-DPG and that during treatment the concentration of this organic phosphate compound may

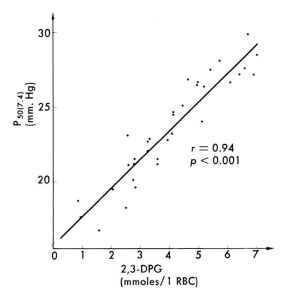

Fig. 10-5. Correlation of red cell 2,3-DPG content and $P_{50(7.4)}$ of the oxyhemoglobin dissociation curve from patients during recovery from severe diabetic ketoacidosis. Regression line: $y = 15.74 + 1.94x$.

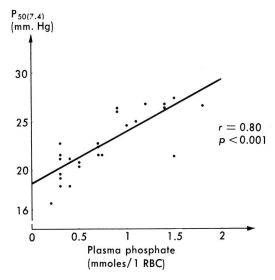

Fig. 10-6. Correlation of plasma inorganic phosphate and $P_{50(7.4)}$ of oxyhemoglobin dissociation curve subsequent to normalization of blood pH with insulin treatment in 10 cases of diabetes recovering from severe ketoacidosis. Regression line: $y = 18.65 + 5.28x$.

only rise slowly. Our study indicates that the decrease of 2,3-DPG is strongly correlated to an increase in red cell affinity of oxygen. Normally, this decrease in oxygen-release capacity would easily be compensated for by an increase in the cardiac output leading to an improved tissue perfusion and a normalization of tissue oxygenation. This compensatory change may take place, but because of dehydration, acidosis, and changes in the microcirculation of many tissues, these compensatory adaptations are not efficient enough. This was observed in our study by a transient rise in the lactate/pyruvate ratio as an indication of absolute tissue hypoxia. Our study also demonstrates the regulatory role of P_i on red cell metabolism and red cell oxygen affinity as shown by a close relationship between P_i and 2,3-DPG content of the red cells and between the P_i and the position of the ODC.

Evidence of a hemoglobin fraction with abnormally high oxygen affinity in nonacidotic juvenile diabetics

In a study of tissue oxygenation in nonacidotic juvenile diabetics we determined red cell 2,3-DPG and the ODC in 32 ambulatory nonacidotic diabetic children and in 49 healthy children.[17, 24] Table 10-4 indicates the result of these and related parameters. It is seen that despite the fact that the diabetic children on an average had an increased hemoglobin concentration, their erythrocytes contained significantly more 2,3-DPG than normal. Both in the diabetics and in the healthy children a negative relationship was found between the content of 2,3-DPG and the hemoglobin concentration.[17] In the diabetics 2,3-DPG was positively correlated to the $P_{50(7.4)}$ and to the $P_{50(in\ vivo)}$ of the ODC. However, despite the significant increase in 2,3-DPG among the diabetic children, the average P_{50} was not increased as compared to the control children (Table 10-4). The combination of changes consisting of an elevated hemoglobin concentration and an increased 2,3-DPG level but a normal position of the ODC in the presence of

Table 10-4. Age of subjects, duration of diabetes, hemoglobin, 2,3-diphosphoglycerate content, P_{50} (at pH 7.4 and at actual pH), pH, and oxyhemoglobin saturation

Group	Age (years)	Duration of diabetes (years)	Hemo-globin (grams per 100 ml.)	DPG (μmoles per gram of hemo-globin)	$P_{50\ (7.4)}$ (mm. of mercury)	$P_{50\ (act.)}$ (mm. of mercury)	pH	O_2 satura-tion (moles per mole)
Children								
Controls (n = 49)								
Mean	9.6	—	13.1	13.9	26.4	25.1	7.44	0.98
± S. D.	—	—	0.44	1.31	0.98	0.94	0.03	0.01
Diabetics (n = 32)								
Mean	11.3	4.6	13.7	15.2	26.3	25.4	7.42	0.98
± S. D.	—	2.5	0.82	1.70	1.40	1.37	0.02	0.01
Significance			$p < 0.001$	$p < 0.002$	Not sig-nificant	Not sig-nificant	$p < 0.01$	Not sig-nificant

a normal arterial oxygen saturation indicates the presence of a hemoglobin fraction with increased oxygen affinity (decreased oxygen availability) in the red cell of diabetic children. Even though the inhibitory factor of a normal 2,3-DPG-hemoglobin-oxygen affinity in diabetic subjects is not known, recent column chromatographic studies of hemoglobin from diabetic subjects suggest this to be the result of an increase in hemoglobin A_{1c}. This hemoglobin fraction is unique in that it is a glycoprotein with a hexose bound by a Schiff-base linkage to the terminal valine of both β-chains of hemoglobin. This glycohemoglobin is increased in patients with diabetes, and the proportion of this hemoglobin appears to be independent of age of the patient and the duration of diabetes.[37, 40]

Bunn and Briehl[14] have shown that the oxygen affinity of hemoglobin A_{1c} is little affected by the addition of 2,3-DPG in contrast to ordinary hemoglobin A because the presence of the carbohydrate on the N-terminal residues of hemoglobin A_{1c} impairs the binding of 2,3-DPG to hemoglobin. It therefore appears that the functional defect in the oxygen-releasing capacity of the red cell in nonacidotic diabetics is caused by the presence of excess amounts of a glycoprotein in an insulin-insensitive cell. In diabetes the formation of glycoprotein appears to be stimulated by the increased concentration of glucose in the extracellular fluid leading to an overutilization of glucose for the synthesis of these abnormal materials.[38] The elevated level of 2,3-DPG in the nonacidotic diabetic children appears to provide a compensatory mechanism whereby the circulating red cells decrease the oxygen affinity of hemoglobin and in the present study the $P_{50(in\ vivo)}$ could be maintained close to a normal level. The question arises, however, whether this adaptation in the diabetic organism is optimal or whether improved metabolic control with respect to the carbohydrate metabolism might further increase the oxygen-releasing capacity of the erythrocytes.

The present study of the oxygen-releasing capacity of the red cells in nonacidotic and in acidotic diabetics indicates that the content of 2,3-DPG fluctuates much more in diabetics than in healthy subjects.

IMPROVEMENT OF TISSUE OXYGEN RELEASE BY DIETARY SUPPLEMENT OF CALCIUM PHOSPHATE IN JUVENILE DIABETICS

During recovery from diabetic ketoacidosis it is evident that P_i is the determining factor for the rate of resynthesis of 2,3-DPG and the position of the ODC. The coefficient of correlation between 2,3-DPG and P_i in 10 patients recovering from severe diabetic ketoacidosis was found to be as high as 0.91 ($p < 0.001$). Also in studies of nonacidotic diabetics we have found an interrelationship between the content of 2,3-DPG of the red cell and P_i. These studies suggest that the red cell metabolism in diabetes is influenced by the concentration of inorganic phosphate in the plasma at levels below, at, and above the normal physiologic plasma level. "Hyperphosphatemia" results in a rise of the level of 2,3-DPG in the red cells and a consequent shift to the right of the ODC, and conversely hypophosphatemia may produce a decrease in red cell 2,3-DPG with increased oxygen affinity. It is likely that the effect of inorganic phosphate is on the enzymes phosphofructokinase and glyceraldehyde-3-phosphate dehydrogenase and that these enzymes in vivo might be in a basically inhibited state. Also in other clinical situations the concentration of plasma inorganic phosphate has

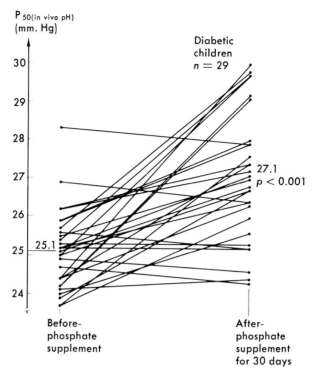

Fig. 10-7. Effect of daily oral dietary supplement of 6 grams of calcium diphosphate to 29 ambulatory diabetic children for 30 days. Oxygen release from erythrocytes measured from $P_{50(in\ vivo\ pH)}$ of oxyhemoglobin dissociation curve is greatly increased ($p < 0.001$).

been shown to influence the metabolism of red cells.[35, 39] Thus, in order to arrive at an optimal oxygen-releasing capacity of the red cells in juvenile diabetics, one needs to maintain a high level of intraerythrocytic 2,3-DPG and P_i. Without a more specific supportive therapeutic approach, this may be difficult to obtain in juvenile diabetics, because several studies have indicated that the metabolism of plasma inorganic phosphate may be disturbed in diabetes, particularly so during poor metabolic control.[7, 16]

We have examined the possible influence of dietary supplement of calcium phosphate on the oxygen-releasing capacity of the red cells in diabetic children by giving 6 grams of calcium diphosphate daily divided into three doses for 30 days. Fig. 10-7 indicates that there occurs a drastic increase in the oxygen-releasing capacity of the erythrocytes with this dietary supplement in diabetic children. We are at present concerned with studies trying to elucidate the underlying mechanism for this interesting finding. It may be hoped that with the use of agents that can specifically support tissue oxygenation, it may be possible to prevent the development of malignant lesions in the retina of the diabetics.

REFERENCES

1. Agatston, S. A.: Clinicopathologic study of diabetic retinitis, Arch. Ophthalmol. **24:**252-257, 1940.

2. Alberti, K. G. M. M., Emerson, P. M., Darley, J. H., and Hockaday, T. D. R.: 2,3-diphosphoglycerate and tissue oxygenation in uncontrolled diabetes mellitus, Lancet **2:** 391-395, 1972.

3. Ashton, N.: Vascular changes in diabetes with particular reference to retinal vessels; preliminary report, Br. J. Ophthalmol. **33:**407-420, 1949.

4. Ashton, N.: Retinal microaneurysms in non-diabetic subjects, Br. J. Ophthalmol. **35:**189-212, 1951.

5. Ashton, N.: Retinal vascularization in health and disease, Am. J. Ophthalmol. **44:**7-15, 1957.

6. Ashton, N.: Diabetic retinopathy. In Pyke, D. A., editor: Disorders of carbohydrate metabolism, London, 1962, Sir Isaac Pitman & Sons Ltd., pp. 195-206.

7. Astrug, A. K.: Studies on the clearance and tubular reabsorption of phosphates in diabetes mellitus and some of its complications, Diabetologia **2:**198-201, 1966.

8. Ballantyne, A. J., and Loewenstein, A.: Pathology of diabetic retinopathy, Trans. Ophthalmol. Soc. U. K. (1943) **63:**95-115, 1944.

9. Ballantyne, A. J.: Observations on pathology of thrombosis of central vein of retina, Trans. Ophthalmol. Soc. U. K. (1943) **63:**137-142, 1944.

10. Ballantyne, A. J., and Loewenstein, A.: Retinal micro-aneurysms and punctate haemorrhages, Br. J. Ophthalmol. **28:**593-598, 1944.

11. Becker, B., and Post, L. T., Jr.: Retinal vein occlusion: Clinical and experimental observations, Am. J. Ophthalmol. **34:**677-686, 1951.

12. Bellingham, A. J., Detter, J. C., and Lenfant, C.: The role of hemoglobin affinity of oxygen and red cell 2,3-diphosphoglycerate in the management of diabetic ketoacidosis, Trans. Assoc. Am. Physicians **83:**113-120, 1970.

13. Benesch, R., and Benesch, R. E.: The effect of organic phosphates from the human erythrocytes on the allosteric properties of hemoglobin, Biochem. Biophys. Res. Commun. **26:**162-167, 1967.

14. Bunn, H. F., and Briehl, R. W.: The interaction of 2,3-diphosphoglycerate with various human hemoglobins, J. Clin. Invest. **49:**1088-1095, 1970.

15. Chanutin, A., and Curnish, R. R.: Effect of organic and inorganic phosphates on the oxygen equilibrium of human erythrocytes, Arch. Biochem. **121:**96-102, 1967.

16. Danowski, T. S.: Clinical endocrinology, Baltimore, 1962, The Williams & Wilkins Co., vol. III, pp. 45-46.

17. Daugaard, N., and Ditzel, J.: Effect of 2,3-diphosphoglycerate and hemoglobin on oxygen affinity of blood in juvenile diabetics. Presented at the Ninth Annual Meeting of the Scandinavian Society for the Study of Diabetes, Aarhus, Denmark, May 24-26, 1973, Acta Endocrinol. (suppl) **181:**4, 1973.

18. Ditzel, J.: Angioscopic changes in the smaller blood vessels in diabetes mellitus and their relationship to aging, Circulation **14:**386-397, 1956.

19. Ditzel, J., and Duckers, J.: The bulbar conjunctival vascular bed in diabetic children, Acta Paediatr. Scand. **46:**535-552, 1957.

20. Ditzel, J., and Moinat, P.: The responses of the smaller blood vessels and the serum proteins in pregnant diabetic subjects, Diabetes **6:**307-323, 1957.

21. Ditzel, J., Sargeant, L., and Hadley, W. B.: The relationship of abnormal vascular responses to retinopathy and nephropathy, Arch. Intern. Med. **101:**912-920, 1958.

22. Ditzel, J.: Importance of plasma inorganic phosphate on tissue oxygenation during recovery from diabetic ketoacidosis, Hormone Metabol. Res. **5:**471-472, 1973.

23. Ditzel, J.: Effect of plasma inorganic phosphate on tissue oxygenation during recovery from diabetic ketoacidosis, Adv. Exp. Med. Biol. **37A:**163-172, 1973.

24. Ditzel, J., Andersen, H., and Daugaard, N. P.: Increased hemoglobin A_{1c} and 2,3-diphosphoglycerate in diabetes and their effects on red-cell oxygen releasing capacity, Lancet **2:**1034, 1973.

25. Edington, G. M., and Sarkies, J. W. R.: Two cases of sickle-cell anemia associated with retinal microaneurysms, Trans. R. Soc. Trop. Med. Hyg. **46:**59-62, 1952.

26. Funahashi, T., and Fink, A. J.: The pathology of the bulbar conjunctiva in diabetes mellitus. Am. J. Ophthalmol. **55:**504-509, 1963.

27. Guest, G. M., and Rapoport, S.: Role of acid-soluble phosphorus compounds in red blood cells, Am. J. Dis. Child. **58:**1072-1089, 1939.

28. Hardin, R. C., Jackson, R. L., Johnston, T. L., and Kelly, H. G.: The development of diabetic retinopathy, Diabetes **5:**397-405, 1956.

29. Holten, C.: The respiratory metabolism in diabetes and the influence of insulin upon it, Copenhagen, 1925, Levin & Munksgaard.

30. Horstmann, P.: The oxygen consumption in diabetes mellitus, Acta Med. Scand. **139:** 326-330, 1951.

31. Horstmann, P.: The effect of adrenaline on the oxygen consumption in diabetes and in hyperthyroidism, Acta Endocrinol. **16:**233-247, 1954.

32. Joslin, E. P.: Diabetic metabolism with high and low diets, Carnegie Institution of Washington, Publ. 323, 1923.

33. Jütte, A.: Über die Erweiterung des Netzhautvenen bei jugendlichen Diabetikern. In Mohnike, G., editor: Diabetische Angiopathie, Berlin, 1964, Akademie-Verlag.

34. Larsen, H. W.: Diabetic retinopathy, Copenhagen, 1960, Munksgaard.

35. Lichtman, M. A., and Miller, D. R.: Erythrocyte glycolysis, 2,3-diphosphoglycerate and adenosine triphosphate concentration in uremic subjects: Relationship to extracellular phosphate concentration, J. Lab. Clin. Med. **76:**267-279, 1970.

36. Loewenstein, A., and Garrow, A.: Thrombosis of retinal choroidal and optic-nerve vessels; pathologic study, Am. J. Ophthalmol. **28:**840-851, Aug. 1945.

37. Paulsen, E. P.: Hemoglobin A_{1c} in childhood diabetes, Metabolism **22:**269-271, 1973.

38. Spiro, R. G.: Glycoproteins and diabetic microangiopathy. In Marble, A., White, A. P., Bradley, R. F., and Krall, L., editors: Joslin's diabetes mellitus, ed. 11, Philadelphia, 1971, Lea & Febiger, pp. 146-156.

39. Travis, S. F., Sugarman, H. J., Ruberg, R. L., Dudrick, S., Delivoria-Papadopoulos, M., Miller, L. D., and Oski, F. A.: Alterations of red-cell glycolytic intermediates and oxygen transport as a consequence of hypophosphatemia in patients receiving intravenous hyperalimentation, New Eng. J. Med. **285:**763-768, 1971.

40. Trivelli, L. A., Ranney, H. M., and Lai, H.-J.: Hemoglobin components in patients with diabetes mellitus, New Eng. J. Med. **284:**353-357, 1971.

41. de Verdier, C.-H., Garby, L., and Hjelm, M.: Intraerythrocytic regulation of tissue oxygen tension, Acta Soc. Med. Ups. **72:**209-216, 1969.

42. Warburg, O., Posener, K., and Negelin, E.: Über den Stoffwechsel der Carcinomzelle, Biochem. Z. **152:**309-343, 1924.

43. Wexler, D., and Branower, G.: Retinal capillary lesions in malignant hypertension, Arch. Ophthalmol. **44:**539-548, 1950.

44. White, P.: Endocrine manifestations in juvenile diabetes, Arch. Intern. Med. **63:**39-53, 1939.

45. Wise, G. N.: Retinal neovascularization, Trans. Am. Ophthalmol. Soc. **54:**729-826, 1956.

11

The eye in diabetes mellitus: signs, symptoms, and their pathogenesis

Paul Henkind*

Few diseases affect the visual apparatus as widely, or as profoundly, as does diabetes mellitus. Thousands of articles, numerous books, and myriads of conferences have been devoted to the ocular effects of diabetes. In this discussion, the variety of ophthalmic lesions related to the diabetic process are presented, and, where possible, the pathogenetic explanation and clinical significance of each entity are considered. First, I will deal with the extraocular manifestations and then with the ocular lesions associated with diabetes.

EXTRAOCULAR MANIFESTATIONS OF DIABETES MELLITUS

Extraocular manifestations of diabetes mellitus are shown as follows:

Tissue	Manifestation	Significance
Lids	Xanthelasma	Cosmetic
Conjunctivae	Microcirculatory alteration	May reflect generalized micro-vascular disorder
Extraocular muscles	Third and sixth nerve palsy	Diplopia; may be mistaken for intracranial neoplasm or aneurysm
Orbit	Mucormycosis	Lethal if untreated

Lids

The lids, conjunctivae, extraocular muscles, and orbits, can all be affected in the diabetic patient. Of limited clinical significance are xanthelasma, which are elevated yellowish plaques, usually occurring at the inner aspects of the lids. They have been reported to occur slightly more frequently in diabetics than in normal individuals.[28] Histologically, xanthelasma is a mass of aggregates of lipid-laden histiocytes, and reflect a disturbance in lipid metabolism, rather than a primary diabetic effect. They constitute a cosmetic blemish and can easily be excised.

*Assisted in part by Grant No. EY00613-04 of the National Institutes of Health.

195

Conjunctivae

Conjunctival microcirculatory alterations have been reported by a number of authors. A paper by Ditzel and his co-workers[11] is of special interest; the subject is reviewed by Caird, Pirie, and Ramsell in their monograph *Diabetes and the eye.*[7] Ditzel noted a diurnal variation in venous dilatation that he believed was characteristic of diabetes; it was independent of blood glucose level or time of insulin therapy. Vasoconstriction of the conjunctival vessels has also been observed, as have conjunctival microaneurysms.[3] Tamura[26] examined by electron microscopy both fenestrated and nonfenestrated capillaries in human conjunctivae. He reported that only the latter type of vessels, which resemble retinal capillaries in morphologic appearance, showed basement membrane thickening in diabetic patients. The significance of this finding is as yet unknown. I have been unimpressed with the significance of conjunctival signs in diabetes as regards diagnosis or prognosis. For example, conjunctival microaneurysms, often near the limbus, occur in many nondiabetics. Conjunctival vascular changes may, however, have value in some instances, and they may reflect the generalized microvascular disturbance that affects diabetics.

Extraocular muscles

Extraocular muscle palsies associated with diabetes are not common, but they can be characteristic. They usually occur suddenly without other central nervous system signs, are often heralded or accompanied by periorbital pain, and generally resolve spontaneously over a period of a few months. The lateral rectus muscle, innervated by the sixth nerve, is more commonly involved than the muscles innervated by the third nerve. Headache is said to be more likely to occur in a diabetic third than a sixth nerve involvement.[7] The pupil is generally spared in a diabetic third nerve palsy, in contradistinction to third nerve involvement from aneurysms or neoplasms.[16] Although many patients developing ocular palsy have had overt diabetes for many years, this may be the presenting sign in some instances. For example, a latent diabetic with a strong familial history of diabetes presented initially with diplopia caused by weakness of the right lateral rectus, which cleared spontaneously within a few months. Several years later he had an episode of painful ophthalmoplegia also involving his right eye, and this, too, subsided in several months. There were no other overt signs of diabetes in this individual.

It has been postulated that the extraocular palsies result from occlusion of the vascular supply to the third or sixth nerves, and thus the condition is primarily an angiopathy with secondary, reversible neural changes. Histologic examination in one case of third nerve palsy revealed focal inflammation within the trunk of the nerve.[12] In another case, involvement of the intraneural vessels of the oculomotor nerve was suggested.[4] Aside from the temporarily disabling diplopia caused by the palsy, the condition is occasionally misdiagnosed, with the patient being subjected to extensive neurologic or neurosurgical evaluation. Caird and co-workers[7] note that carotid angiography can be deferred when the clinical diagnosis of diabetic ophthalmoplegia seems possible.

Orbit

Orbitorhinomucormycosis is a rare, but dreaded complication associated with diabetes. Although not directly related to the diabetic process, it develops most frequently in patients with poor control and severe acidosis. Approximately 50% of individuals developing this complication have diabetes. The condition evolves rapidly, and I have seen a case develop within 24 hours after a dental extraction in a young man. The constellation of findings includes rhinitis, headache, unilateral ptosis, lid edema, ophthalmoplegia, and with or without visual loss. Any diabetic patient with such signs and symptoms should be suspected of having mucormycosis. Untreated, the condition is usually fatal. Amphotericin B therapy, both systemic and local, if initiated early, can be curative.[13]

INTRAOCULAR MANIFESTATIONS OF DIABETES MELLITUS

Intraocular manifestations of diabetes mellitus are shown as follows:

Tissue	Manifestation	Significance
Cornea	Descemet's wrinkles	Unknown, may be an early clinical sign
Iris	Ectropion uveae (without rubeosis)	Unknown, may be an early clinical sign
	Rubeosis iridis	Neovascular glaucoma
	Pigment epithelium vacuolization	Increased pigment of anterior segment
Lens	Refractive changes	Fluctuating vision
	Cataract	Impaired vision
Ciliary body	Basement membrane thickening	Unknown
Vitreous	Asteroid hyalosis	Unknown
Retina	Retinopathy	Visual impairment; may indicate severity of the diabetes
	Lipemia retinalis	Signifies greatly elevated serum lipid
Optic nerve	Optic atrophy	May be part of a syndrome

Our approach to the intraocular manifestations of diabetes mellitus proceeds from cornea to optic nerve.

Cornea

Fine wrinkles in the central portion of Descemet's membrane are a common finding in diabetics[18] (Fig. 11-1). Similar but usually less well-demarcated wrinkles may be observed in elderly nondiabetics. The presence of Descemet's folds in people under the age of 60 should arouse suspicion of a possible diabetic state, and I have personally made the initial diagnosis of diabetes in a number of middle-aged individuals, who had no other stigmas of the disease; laboratory tests later confirmed the presence of diabetes. Obviously, Descemet's wrinkles can only be evaluated by slit-lamp examination and may occasionally be mistaken for corneal nerves. The use of the technique known as specular reflection confirms the deep location of these lesions. There has not been any clinicopathologic correlation of these lesions, and their significance, other than as a signpost of potential disease, is unknown.

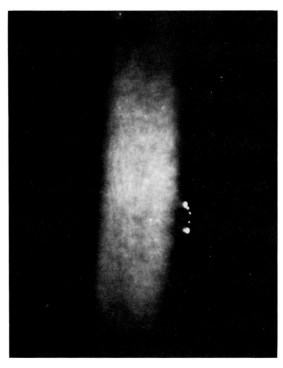

Fig. 11-1. Slit-lamp photograph of corneal endothelium and Descemet's membrane in a diabetic. Fine vertical wrinkles are present in Descemet's membrane. Such folds may also be oblique, but never horizontally arranged.

Iris

The iris shows a number of features indicative of diabetes. Armaly and Baloglou[3] claim to have found ectropion uveae, a migration of the posterior iris pigment epithelium over the pupillary margin, in a large percentage of diabetics. The difference between the diabetic and normal population with regard to this finding was said to be highly significant, particularly in younger individuals. Whether this is a valuable early sign of diabetes has yet to be confirmed by other workers, and I have not noted this in my experience. On the other hand, ectropion uveae is a frequent sequela of rubeosis iridis that occurs in diabetics. In rubeosis, a fibrovascular membrane grows from the iris stroma, eventually covering the anterior surface of the iris and anterior chamber angle, causing an intractable "neovascular" glaucoma. In diabetics, the rubeosis is almost always secondary to retinitis proliferans and is thus an indicator of severe posterior ocular disease. Although the usual outlook for an eye with rubeosis iridis is bleak, I have followed a small number of affected diabetic patients for several years without seeing them develop glaucoma or an anterior chamber hemorrhage; I do not know why these cases appear more benign. Anterior-segment fluorescein angiography is a useful technique for detecting and confirming the presence of early rubeosis, but no therapy has been developed to stay its course. Once glaucoma occurs in these

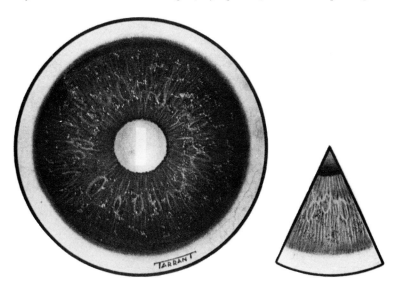

Fig. 11-2. Slit-lamp transillumination of iris in diabetes. Local pigment migration is seen in direct view. (From Abrams, J. D.: Biomicroscopy of the transilluminated iris, Ann. Inst. Barraquer **5:**39, 1964.)

patients, management may be difficult and enucleation must frequently be entertained as a desperate measure to relieve the severe pain that occurs.

Vacuolization of the iris pigment epithelium is a common finding in diabetic eyes. The vacuoles, which contain glycogen,[32] are not specific for diabetes and have also been demonstrated in patients with Hurler's disease, Menke's disease, those on systemic steroids (Samuel Gartner, personal communication), and also in the eyes of infants. The glycogen-laden cells of the pigment epithelium are apparently fragile and may degenerate; they then release pigment into the anterior chamber, from where it gains access to all anterior-chamber structures. This may be particularly striking in cataract surgery, where large amounts of pigment may be liberated during the course of the operation. Although the diagnosis of glycogenous degeneration of the iris pigment epithelium is primarily a histopathologic one, Abrams[1] suggests that transillumination of the iris during slit-lamp examination may reveal a rather characteristic appearance (Fig. 11-2).

Lens

There are two major ways that the lens can be implicated in diabetes: dynamic alterations and cataract formation. The dynamic alterations, which are readily reversible, cause fluctuating refractive errors. It is generally accepted that a tendency towards a more myopic refractive error occurs when the blood glucose is elevated, whereas the opposite trend, toward a hyperopic error, develops when the blood glucose is decreased. According to Caird et al.[7] myopic changes occur as an initial symptom of diabetes in approximately one third of the cases. Although the exact cause of the refractive changes is not known, it has been attributed to the level of blood glucose. Glasses therefore should not be prescribed for uncontrolled diabetics.

The second, and perhaps more important lens change in diabetes is the development of cataract. Cataracts of a type indistinguishable from those found in the aged seem to occur with greater frequency and at an earlier age in diabetics. We have certainly been impressed with the high incidence of diabetes in our cataract population, and vice versa. Another, less common, type of lens opacity has been termed a "true" or "juvenile" diabetic cataract, and this occurs bilaterally in younger diabetic patients.[22] Such cataracts develop rapidly and consist of dense bands of white subcapsular dots, fine needle-shaped opacities of uniform diameter, and posterior subcapsular vacuoles and clefts. The treatment of diabetic cataract is lens extraction when vision is impaired below a useful level. The visual outcome will depend to a large extent on the health of the retina, and it is well to caution diabetic patients about the guarded prognosis for visual improvement after lens extraction. Acute, reversible lens opacities have been described in young diabetics; such cases are rare.

Ciliary body and vitreous

The basement membrane of the ciliary processes tends to be thicker in diabetics than in normal people,[30] but the significance of this finding is unknown.

Asteroid hyalosis, a striking clinical finding that involves the vitreous body, has been reported by some authors to occur with higher frequency in diabetics than in normal individuals; this has been denied by others.[20] In asteroid hyalosis, myriads of small white opacities composed of calcium soaps are noted within the vitreous. Despite their prominent appearance, they rarely cause visual symptoms. There is no obvious relationship between asteroid hyalosis and diabetic retinopathy. Other alterations occurring to the vitreous in diabetics, including neovascularization and hemorrhage, are secondary to retinopathy.

Retina

The most significant ocular alteration in diabetes is retinopathy. "Of those blinded by diabetes, 84% owe their disability to retinopathy."[15] Although none of the clinical features of diabetic retinopathy are absolutely specific, the overall picture is so characteristic as to lead to a correct diagnosis in the majority of cases. Diabetic retinopathy is basically an angiopathy, a disease of the small vessels coursing through the inner retinal layers. There is, at present, considerable question as to whether it is the retinal venule, capillary, or arteriole that is initially involved in the disease process. The usual, initial presenting sign is in the posterior pole and consists of retinal microaneurysms.

Aneurysms of retinal vessels were first noted histologically by Bowman in 1854[6] and were initially associated with diabetes in 1877.[21] It was not until 1943, however, that Ballantyne and Loewenstein[5] firmly established retinal microaneurysms as an undoubted sign of diabetic retinopathy. Indeed, in the early decades of this century there were many who questioned whether there was a specific or characteristic picture to be found in the retina of diabetics. This difficulty is understandable when one considers that prior to the discovery of insulin few diabetics lived long enough to develop the retinopathy. Even the neophyte medical student is now expected to properly label a fundus picture consisting of microaneurysms, hemorrhages, exudates, and neovascularization as probably diabetic. Certain clues point to a retinopathy being diabetic in origin[17]: (1) *Laterality*. The condition is almost always bilateral. If only one eye is involved, one should look for another cause of the "diabetic" retinopathy. (2) *Symmetry*. Diabetic retinopathy is often symmetric, involving similar portions of both fundi and being of approximately equal severity in both eyes.[27] Asymmetry of retinopathy in a diabetic occurs when there is unilateral carotid artery disease,[14] previous chorioretinal or optic nerve disease,[2] and perhaps in some cases of unilateral high myopia or ocular hypertension. (3) *Location*. Diabetic retinopathy is basically a posterior polar disease; the retinal periphery is usually spared. This is the reverse of the situation encountered in sickle-cell disease and the dysproteinemias, disorders that generally involve the anterior retina, either selectively or predominantly. Central retinal vein occlusion in certain stages may occasionally be mistaken for diabetic retinopathy, involving both the anterior and posterior retina in a hemorrhagic process. (4) *Progression*. Diabetic retinopathy may be reversible or may wax and wane; in general it is a progressive disorder.

Since the microaneurysm is the key and perhaps the earliest visible sign of diabetic retinopathy, its pathogenesis should be considered. One popular theory[9] states that the microaneurysm is somehow related to the degeneration of outer cells of the retinal capillary wall, the so-called intramural pericytes, or mural cells. There is abundant evidence that the intramural cells are indeed affected selectively in diabetes,[25, 31] but there is controversy concerning the loss of such cells and their relationship to microaneurysm formation.[10] Many other theories concerning retinal microaneurysm formation have been proposed, but none have been proved correct to date. Retinal microaneurysms, of course, are found in many other conditions, and in these disorders there is no selective loss of intramural pericytes.

Besides microaneurysms, the retinal vascular abnormalities include (1) dilated and hypercellular arterioles, capillaries, and venules, with the hypercellularity being mainly a result of proliferation of endothelial cells; (2) neovascularization both within and anterior to the retina; and (3) "capillary shunts."[8] The last have been shown to be slow-flow channels connecting an adjacent artery and vein, and they traverse a partially or totally obliterated capillary bed. The "shunts" probably develop secondary to capillary-bed obliteration, and rather than being examples of neovascularization, they represent collateral vessel formation from preexisting capillaries. In this regard, they are entirely different from retinal neovascularization or retinitis proliferans. These proliferating vessels develop anew from retinal vessels and cause great difficulty because of their tendency to bleed into the vitreous cavity. A point worth emphasizing is that retinal neovascularization does not arise from vitreous hemorrhage, but rather is a cause of the hemorrhage.[29]

Three relatively new findings concerning diabetic retinopathy are that (1) cotton-wool spots can occur in this condition without concomitant hypertension,[19] (2) macula edema, without evidence of severe retinopathy, may cause severe reduction in vision,[23] and (3) large areas of capillary nonperfusion can be demonstrated by fluorescein angiography in patients who ophthalmoscopically have only mild or moderate retinopathy. Such nonfilling areas have been demonstrated to have concomitant scotoma, but the patient is usually unaware of the defect in his field of vision.

The rather characteristic retinal hemorrhages and exudates of diabetic retinop-

athy are obviously secondary to the vasculopathy. The "dot and blot" hemorrhages tend to lie deep in the retina, with their appearance being attributable to
sequestration of blood in anatomically compact retina. The yellowish exudates,
often displayed in rings (circinate figures) around clusters of microaneurysms,
probably represent leakage of material from a malfunctioning capillary bed.

A number of major questions concerning diabetic retinopathy still puzzle me:
(1) What causes the retinopathy? Does the initial and basic lesion reside in the
small vessels and their basement members, or are the vascular alterations secondary
to an underlying endocrine or metabolic disturbance? We must not forget that
"diabetic retinopathy has been reported in almost every etiological variety of
diabetes,"[7] including chronic pancreatitis, pancreatectomy, hemochromatosis,
Cushing's syndrome, and acromegaly. (2) What is the site of the initial retinal
vascular insult; is it arterial, venous or capillary? (3) Does control of the diabetic
state really modify the course of the retinopathy? I think we have all seen "well-
controlled" diabetics with severe retinopathy and "poorly controlled" diabetics
with little or no retinopathy. (4) What triggers the retinal vessels to proliferate
and cause retinitis proliferans?

Lipemia retinalis is striking but is simply an alteration in the normal appearance of the retinal vessels, which, instead of having a red color, appear pink,
creamy white, or yellow gray. The appearance is attributable to gross hyperlipemia
and total lipids of 3 to 3.5 gm. per 100 ml. are necessary for the phenomenon to
appear. In diabetics the hyperlipemia develops secondary to ketosis, and when this
is corrected, the lipids return to a normal level and the lipemia retinalis disappears
without a sequela.

Optic nerve

If optic neuritis occurs in relationship to diabetes, it must be rather uncommon
and I cannot personally remember making the diagnosis of optic neuritis related
to diabetes during the past decade. However, Caird et al. review the literature
and provide pertinent references to the subject.[7] Optic atrophy has been rarely
associated with juvenile diabetes, and the two conditions may be part of a recessively inherited disorder in which deafness is also a component.[24] Optic atrophy
can also develop in patients who have Friedreich's ataxia and Refsum's syndrome,
disorders in which diabetes is frequently found.

CONCLUSION

It should be evident that this presentation merely skims the surface of a major
problem. It was intended to provide useful information for practitioners who daily
must assess the visual apparatus of diabetics and who, conversely, may consider
the diagnosis of diabetes on the basis of ocular findings. Controversial areas such
as the relationship of diabetes mellitus to chronic simple glaucoma and the role
of various treatment modalities for diabetic retinopathy have not been considered.

REFERENCES

1. Abrams, J. D.: Biomicroscopy of the transilluminated iris, Ann. Inst. Barraquer. **5:**39,
   1964.
2. Aiello, L. M., Beetham, W. P., Balomidos, M.D., Chazan, B. I., and Bradley, R. F.:
   Ruby laser photocoagulation in treatment of diabetic proliferating retinopathy. In Gold-

berg, M. F., and Fine, S. L., editors: Symposium on the treatment of diabetic retinopathy, Public Health Service Publication No. 1890, 1968, p. 437.

3. Armaly, M. F., and Baloglou, P. J.: Diabetes mellitus and the eye. 1. Changes in the anterior segment, Arch. Ophthalmol. **77:**485, 1967.

4. Asbury, A. K., Aldredge, H., Hershberg, R., and Fisher, C. M.: Oculomotor palsy in diabetes mellitus: A clinico-pathological study, Brain **93:**555, 1970.

5. Ballantyne, A. J., and Loewenstein, A.: Diseases of the retina. 1. The pathology of diabetic retinopathy, Trans. Ophthalmol. Soc. U.K. **63:**95, 1943.

6. Bowman, W.: As noted by Ashton, N.: The blood-retinal barrier and vaso-glial relationships in retinal disease (The Bowman Lecture), Trans. Ophthalmol. Soc. U. K. **85:**199, 1965.

7. Caird, F. I., Pirie, A., and Ramsell, T. G.: Diabetes and the eye, Oxford, 1969, Blackwell Scientific Publications, Ltd.

8. Cogan, D. G., and Kuwabara, T.: Capillary shunts in the pathogenesis of diabetic retinopathy, Diabetes **12:**292, 1963.

9. Cogan, D. G., and Kuwabara, T.: The mural cell in perspective, Arch. Ophthalmol. **78:**1967.

10. De Oliveira, L. F.: Pericytes in diabetic retinopathy, Br. J. Ophthalmol. **50:**134, 1966.

11. Ditzel, J., Beavan, D. W., and Renold, A. E.: Early vascular changes in diabetes mellitus, Metabolism **9:**400, 1960.

12. Dreyfus, P. M., Hakim, S., and Adams, R. D.: Diabetic ophthalmoplegia, Arch. Neurol. Psychiat. **77:**337, 1957.

13. Fleckner, R. A., Goldstein, J. H.: Mucormycosis, Br. J. Ophthalmol. **53:**542, 1969.

14. Gay, A. J., and Rosenbaum, A. L.: Retinal artery pressure in asymmetric diabetic retinopathy, Arch. Ophthalmol. **75:**758, 1966.

15. Goldberg, M. F., and Fine, S. L., editors: Symposium on the treatment of diabetic retinopathy, Public Health Service Publication No. 1890, 1968.

16. Goldstein, J. E., and Cogan, D. G.: Diabetic ophthalmoplegia with special reference to the pupil, Arch. Ophthalmol. **64:**592, 1960.

17. Henkind, P.: Diabetic retinopathy: Pathology. International Diabetes Congress, Brussels, 1973, Amsterdam, 1974, Excerpta Medica, p. 448.

18. Henkind, P., and Wise, G. N.: Descemet's wrinkles in diabetes, Am. J. Ophthalmol. **52:**371, 1961.

19. Kohner, E. M., Dollery, C. T., and Bulpitt, C. J.: Cotton-wool spots in diabetic retinopathy, Diabetes **16:**691, 1969.

20. Luxenberg, M., and Sime, D.: Relation of asteroid hyalosis to diabetes mellitus and plasma lipid levels, Am. J. Ophthalmol. **67:**406, 1969.

21. MacKenzie, W., and Nettleship, E.: A case of glycaemic retinitis with comments: Microscopical examination of the eyes, Royal London Ophthalmol. Hosp. Rep. **9:**134, 1877.

22. O'Brien, C. S., Molsberry, J. M., and Allen, J. H.: Diabetic cataract, J.A.M.A. **103:**892, 1934.

23. Patz, A., Schatz, H., Berkow, J. W., Gittelsohn, A. M., and Ticho, U.: Macula edema—an overlooked complication of diabetic retinopathy, Trans. Am. Acad. Ophthalmol. Otolaryngol. **77:**34, 1973.

24. Rose, F. C., Fraser, C. R., Friedmann, A. I., and Kohner, E. M.: The association of juvenile diabetes mellitus and optic atrophy. Clinical and genetical, Q. J. Med. **35:**385, 1966.

25. Speisor, S., Gittelsohn, A. M., and Patz, A.: Studies on diabetic retinopathy. Influence of diabetes on intramural pericytes, Arch. Ophthalmol. **80:**332, 1968.

26. Tamura, T.: Electron microscopical observations on the capillaries of the bulbar conjunctiva in diabetic and non-diabetic patients, Jap. J. Ophthalmol. **11:**193, 1967.

27. Taylor, E., Adnitt, P. I., and Jennings, A. M. C.: An analysis of diabetic retinopathy, Q. J. Med. **42:**305, 1973.

28. Waite, H. J., and Beetham, W. P.: The visual mechanism in diabetes mellitus, New Eng. J. Med. **212:**367, 1935.

29. Wise, G. N.: Retinal neovascularization, Trans. Am. Ophthalmol. Soc. **54:**729, 1956.

30. Yamashita, T., and Becker, B.: The basement membrane of the human diabetic eye, Diabetes **10:**167, 1961.
31. Yanoff, M.: Diabetic retinopathy, New Eng. J. Med. **274:**1344, 1966.
32. Yanoff, M.: Ocular pathology of diabetes mellitus, Am. J. Ophthalmol. **67:**21, 1969.

ADDITIONAL READINGS

Duke-Elder, W. S.: System of ophthalmology, London, 1974, Henry Kimpton. The various volumes contain a wealth of useful information concerning diabetes and its effects on the eye.

Leopold, I. H., and Lieberman, T. W.: The eye in diabetes mellitus, Chapter 38 in Ellenberg, M., and Rifkin, H., editors: Diabetes mellitus: Theory and practice, New York, 1970, McGraw-Hill Book Co. An excellent overview of the effects of diabetes on the eye and an extensive bibliography.

Toussaint, D.: Contribution à l'étude anatomique et clinique de la rétinopathie diabétique chez l'homme et animaux. Pathologica Europa. Brussels, 1968, Presses, Académiques Européennes. An excellent monograph in French dealing with diabetic retinopathy.

Wise, G. N., Dollery, C. T., and Henkind, P.: The retinal circulation, New York, 1971, Harper & Row, Publishers. Chapter 15 provides a comprehensive view of the retinal lesions of diabetes.

Articles on the subject of diabetic retinopathy by Norman Ashton. He has certainly been one of the most prominent investigators in the field of retinal vascular disease and has written widely on diabetic retinopathy.

The clinical articles by the Hammersmith group of investigators including Eva Kohner and Colin Dollery are valuable for their modern approach to the subject of diabetic retinopathy.

PANEL DISCUSSION

Ocular involvement in diabetes

CHAIRMAN: **Robert C. Watzke***

Dr. Watzke: My main interest in diabetic retinopathy at present is in the way of therapy, I would like to start a discussion among various members of the panel concerning the value of photocoagulation. Photocoagulation therapy, as you know has become very popular recently; initially and hopefully we directed it toward the prevention of hemorrhage by closing off small vessels in proliferative disease. Recently, however, there is a recurrence in the use of photocoagulation to destroy large areas of peripheral retina to have some influence on the prognosis of proliferative disease. I would like to ask first Dr. Ditzel if in his opinion he can at least find a common ground between his approach to the pathogenesis of diabetic retinopathy and that of the therapists who are using ablation therapy to ablate large areas of retina and find some common ground between the two.

Dr. Ditzel: I have had no experience whatsoever with photocoagulation or laser therapy. My guess is that what is actually being done is that an area where there is a state of hypoxia is being changed to an infarct. Ashton, for example, states that neovascularization can only be produced if there is venous stasis and the accumulation of what he calls a vasoproliferative factor, and if you are then obliterating the arterioles and venuoles in a small area, you are changing this ischemic area to a complete necrosis and therefore are not producing this vasoproliferative substance whatever that would be.

Dr. Watzke: Dr. Henkind, what is your opinion about the unproved value of retinal photocoagulation either scatter or focal, and do you have an opinion about its possible value in diabetic retinopathy?

Dr. Henkind: I think it's worth reviewing quickly the history of the treatments of diabetic retinopathy. When I reviewed this subject about 15 years ago for the first time, I was convinced that there was no therapy of any value, be it dietary, chemical, or anything else. On a single observation that a woman who was pregnant and who had diabetes that necrotized a pituitary, there developed a whole school in Scandinavia and many hundreds of pituitaries have been ablated on the basis of a single clinical observation and many patients have

*Department of Ophthalmology, University of Iowa College of Medicine, Iowa City, Iowa.

205

been benefited by pituitary abalation according to those who do it. It is interesting that the groups that did it in this country never came out with a follow-up of their work. Other therapies have been utilized by many other people, and now we have photocoagulation based again on clinical observation that patients who have chorioretinitis or severe disease of the retina don't get proliferative retinopathy or retinopathy per se. One could point to high myopia as protective against diabetic retinopathy. On glaucoma, there is a group in New York who are giving patients steroids topically and provoking steroid-induced glaucoma to prevent diabetic retinopathy. One could argue as to the merits of that sort of therapy. Photocoagulation is ablative and, as Dr. Ditzel says, you never see neovascularization in an area of infarcted retina. We do photocoagulation in our center when we think that the vision is going to be threatened by neovascularization whose natural course generally leads to hemorrhage and a downhill course. One would think that if you don't totally photocoagulate an area, you are really producing just the opposite of what you want; you are producing a hypoxic state, and then you'll get vasoproliferation. We have seen that happen. My fear is that there is only one thing to be done and that is to follow Matthew Davis's advice with the collaborative study. You only know about diabetic retinopathy treatment if patients actually do go to the collaborative study. We have specifically stayed out of the study because we don't think it can be done, but that's not a reason why other groups shouldn't go into it, and your group is certainly into it. I think there is a danger that diabetic retinopathy is becoming "ARR," which is a very bad disease. Does anyone want to know what ARR is? *A*cute *r*emunerative *r*etinopathy! And I think the proliferation of machines to treat the disease is caused by mental hypoxia on certain people. I didn't say I'd be kind by giving you my philosophy. I believe that until we have all the data about how this disease should be treated and, unless you are willing to randomize patients and study them except in certain very circumscribed ways, we're going to have photocoagulators sitting in dustbins in the next few years.

Dr. Watzke: Thank you. Dr. Cogan, what is your opinion on this subject?

Dr. Cogan: Well, that's kind of a broad question. I am not sure if I agree with the point that Dr. Henkind differs from us on, but on other points I would. He stated that he believed these shunts were the consequence of ischemia rather than the cause of the ischemia. Our guess is that it is the cause of the ischemia simply because one finds ischemia in the retinal capillaries very commonly. It is a normal occurrence in middle age and later to have a profound capillary ischemia at the periphery and sometimes in the central area, and one doesn't see the shunts. The arteriole venous shunts are very characteristic of diabetes. A few other points. You gave me a rather open invitation. One point is that reference is commonly made to neovascularization of the retina. I don't believe neovascularization ever occurs in the retina. What we see in the retina are dilatations of preformed capillaries, and when we look at them with the ophthalmoscope, we see little pig-tailed vessels. They may look like neovascularization, but it's a remarkable phenomenon that even with the thought of profound necrosis, which rarely occurs in diabetes, one doesn't see any evidence of neovascularization. You don't see these little endothelial buds that one associates with neovascularization. Another point is thickness of the basement membrane. We don't see that except where the vessels are distended, and I'd like to present a very simplistic point of view that appeals to me to explain this myth of basement membrane thickening, on which so much emphasis has been put, in the nonocular vasculopathy at least. It seems to me that when we have a distension of the vessels in consequence to the loss of the mural cells and loss of tone, the vessels just passably distend. When they distend, they get an endothelial hyperplasia as a sort of defense mechanism with laying down of new basement membrane by these proliferated endothelial cells. The endothelial cells become trapped in their own basement membrane. They die. We can see them and microaneurysms, and also in the diffuse distensions we can see trapped endothelial cells die and leave just a thickened wall as a result. Well, that thickening is in consequence of the distension of the vessels rather than any primary effect on diabetes. Many aspects of this are extremely interesting and I thought the presentations were excellent.

Dr. Watzke: Before we leave this question of therapy and get to more specific questions from the audience, I would like to ask Dr. Newell what his opinion is. Particularly, on ablation or scatter therapy and its value in disk vessels.

Dr. Newell: Dr. Watzke, we've never used scatter therapy. However, in a series of cases that Krill and others reported about 3 years ago there are approximately 12 patients in that group that were treated with photocoagulation in a C-shaped figure surrounding the macula because of chronic macular edema and in 5 or so of those 10 or 12 patients there is no sign of background retinopathy at this time. They started with background retinopathy, but there is no sign of this now. There is a large number of patients with optic atrophy who have had background retinopathy disappear, but I believe at the first sign of neovascularization these patients should be treated with photocoagulation. I don't believe one should wait 5 years for these studies to be completed.

Dr. Watzke: I think we will leave this subject.

Dr. Bietti: Professor Henkind mentioned that one of the characteristics of diabetic retinopathy is bilaterality. We should consider high anisometropia because we know that diabetic retinopathy does not occur so easily in highly myopic eyes. You may have cases where in one eye, emmetropic or hyperopic, there is a well-developed retinopathy whereas in the highly myopic eye there is no sign of retinopathy. I wonder if this is a known fact and if it has also been presented as an explanation of the action of photocoagulation, which should produce a sclerosis, as we encounter in myopic eyes. I wonder if some important members of our panel as Professor Henkind and Professor Cogan have a better explanation for this peculiar attitude of the retina of the highly myopic eye.

Dr. Henkind: Well, the observation has been reported a number of times. I have seen a lot of diabetics. I have not seen that many with a pronounced anisometropia where there has been this difference, but it has certainly been reported, and I am willing to accept that. I do not have any reason for knowing unless one assumes that the highly myopic eye is really a totally degenerated eye where the retina is incapable of any sort of vascular alteration.

Dr. Podos: Another relationship here, of course, is the fact that highly myopic eyes are particularly prone to glaucoma and it's conceivable that in a number of these eyes where there is an asymmetry of diabetic retinopathy we are dealing with high myopia, and glaucoma also, or high myopia and elevation of intraocular pressure, and this may be another relationship to bear in mind. Dr. Henkind has mentioned to you that there are some disagreements in terms of the relationships of diabetes and glaucoma. Without going into great detail, I would suggest, for those of you who haven't seen the evidence, that it is well described in Bernard Becker's Jackson Memorial Lecture in the *American Journal of Ophthalmology.*

Dr. Hayreh: Paul Henkind dismissed the subject of ischemic optic neuropathy in diabetes as nonexistent. It might be of interest to hear that within the last 3 weeks I have had two patients with ischemic optic neuropathy caused by diabetes. In fact they were sent as patients with diabetic retinopathy, and since the residents were not really satisfied with the degree of diabetic retinopathy and the amount of visual loss, they brought the patients to me. One patient had a bilateral ischemic optic neuropathy and in both eyes a central scotoma. The other patient had in one eye complete loss of one half of his vision and in the other a quadrantic hemianopia. So these are the types of patients who really suffer a lot, and I do not want to go into a subject of ischemic optic neuropathy and its management, but it might be relevant for me to point out at this stage that in my previous studies of ischemic optic neuropathy by having a controlled study I found out that systemic corticosteroids definitely benefit them and significantly; so with that in mind I put this patient with diabetes on corticosteroids with caution because he is a severe diabetic. His diabetes is being controlled and within 10 days he has progressed from almost counting fingers to where he can see quite a lot. The field defects to bigger targets completely disappeared, and he is left with a tiny central scotoma. His visual acuity is about 20/100 or 20/200. This is the type of person who if you leave untreated lands back to counting fingers because of partial optic atrophy. So the fact that a person has diabetic retinopathy should not mislead you. If he had more pronounced loss of vision that you cannot explain on the basis of diabetic retinopathy, it is valuable looking at the disk.

Dr. Henkind: I did not want to dismiss the subject. All I said is that I have not seen it for 15 years, and furthermore I wonder whether Dr. Hayreh tested for Uhthoff's sign. The fact that a patient has bilateral optic ischemia, or what he calls that, is very peculiar to me and would seem to me that the bilaterality of it would argue against its being diabetic and more likely to be multiple sclerosis or something like that. I would be more convinced if it were unilateral.

Dr. Watzke: I have another question from the audience. This is directed to Dr. Henkind. Does nonproliferative retinopathy progress to the proliferative type? Do you think that these are two stages of a single entity or do you think that they are two different entities?

Dr. Henkind: The answer to that is yes and no. Most cases of diabetic retinopathy do not progress to proliferative retinopathy. There are rare cases, particularly in the young, where there is not a so-called preceding background retinopathy and these are well documented in the Scandinavian literature. I would point out that perhaps only 5% of patients with diabetic retinopathy will get a severe proliferative retinopathy. Most of them will have had at one time or another a lot of background retinopathy and David Cogan brings up a very good and interesting point. Most of what is called "retinal neovascularization" is pre-formed vessels that are just dilating. I would just ask Dr. Cogan the theoretical question, If you can get diabetic preretinal neovascularization, where does it come from? It must come from the retinal vessels, and I presume there must be some stage, be it ever so insignificant, that there must be intraretinal neo-vascularization breaking through that basement membrane. It's really probably a question of semantics, and I don't know how you can prove one point to another, but the retinal neovascularization in my view must precede pre-retinal neovascularization, but I don't know how I can tell the two apart till it has become preretinal.

Dr. Cogan: Preretinal vascularization comes from the large vessels in two places, one is over the disk, as we commonly see it, and also in the periphery of the retina—but always from the point of a large retinal vessel—and because the large retinal vessels are in contact with the basement membrane, they disrupt the basement membrane and grow out a little bit, but they don't grow into the retina. They grow into the vitreous and it's interesting that these are the two places where the internal limiting membrane is most tenuous. Dr. Henkind knows that over the optic disk the internal limiting membrane is practically absent. One sees fractures or disruptions at the thin point where the internal limiting membrane and the large vessels are in contact. I believe that the proliferative retinopathy must be some abnormality or some diabetic susceptibility of the internal limiting membrane rather than any primary change in the vessels themselves.

Dr. Watzke: Thank you. This is one of the disturbing things to me about treatment by photocoagulation of capillaries—ablation of large areas of capillaries—when you hope by doing so to affect new vessels that are probably from a different source. Now, we have neglected the internists on the panel, and I have a question I would like to direct to all of them. Specifically, I will ask Dr. Kirkendall about this. Question from the audience is, what is his opinion about the value of strict control of diabetes in its prevention of diabetic retinopathy? And specifically I would like to add to that; there is some statement in a retrospective study that early control of diabetes, if strict, in the early stages of the disease bears some relation to the later development of diabetic retinopathy. What is your opinion about that Dr. Kirkendall?

Dr. Kirkendall: I don't think the evidence is clear that strict control of the diabetic actually changes the course of diabetic retinopathy. Obviously, there are differences of opinion on this matter. I don't believe the hard evidence is available to support the view that the better the control the better the course of the retinopathy. One of the things that must be equated in all this is how severe the diabetic is in the first place, and if he is controllable, he may be less of a candidate for diabetic retinopathy than if he is difficult to control for any reason. So I am of the opinion that the diabetic ought to be controlled, but not necessarily because he is going to have less trouble from his diabetic retinopathy.

Dr. Ditzel: Well, looking through the literature there is no doubt about it; you cannot say that if you are treating your diabetic patient optimally you will have no retinopathy. Now, of course, what we call control and even what we call optimal control is from a physiologic point of view very poor control. But on the other hand, if you look through the literature and see the number of proliferative retinopathy cases in groups of patients being treated in what the clinician at that particular clinic will call poor and good control, there is a strong feeling that the very malignant lesion is seen more rarely in the well-controlled cases, but we certainly cannot prevent these lesions from appearing.

Dr. Watzke: Also, another question directed to the internists on our panel. Do you feel that there is a significant difference in the effect of not only diabetic retinopathy but other microvascular diabetic disease, whether one uses oral antidiabetic agents or insulin?

Dr. Kirkendall: I don't believe there is, but I'd like to hear Dr. Solomon develop his ideas on both of these issues.

Dr. Solomon: My answer is no. There certainly is no evidence on the point of this last question; that is, a controlled study would provide the only clear evidence and there has been no such study that directed its attention to the ophthalmopathy comparing oral treatment with insulin therapy. In regard to Dr. Kirkendall's statement about tight control, I can add nothing. Here again, the proper study has not been done. Until it has been done, all it is is talk.

Dr. Watzke: Dr. Ditzel, can you reconcile the thickening of the basement membrane so commonly seen in diabetic microangiopathy and your presentation and theory regarding the shift of the oxygen tension curve, and so forth?

Dr. Ditzel: Yes, I can. It is well recognized that each individual tissue in the organism is only optimally functioning at the particular tissue P_{O_2}. The delivery of the oxygen, $\dot{v}_{O_2}$ to the tissue can be described by the balance equation $\dot{v}_{O_2} = \dot{Q} \cdot C_{O_2} \cdot (Sat_A - Sat_V)$, where $\dot{Q}$ is the blood flow, C_{O_2} is the capacity of the blood to bind oxygen (physically dissolved oxygen is not considered here), and $Sat_A - Sat_V$ is the arteriovenous hemoglobin saturation difference. If one of these factors is being changed, there occurs a compensatory change in the others. In diabetes there may be a relative or absolute shift of the oxyhemoglobin dissociation curve to the left; therefore in short-term diabetics, $\dot{Q}$ through the tissue may tend to increase in order to keep the tissue P_{O_2} constant. However, since the autoregulatory dilatation is produced by a lowering of tissue P_{O_2} and since in many tissues a vasodilatation is actually a loss of vascular tone, the dilatation may be accompanied by an increase in plasma permeation. In diabetes, being a chronic fluctuating disease, the episodes of plasma permeation therefore become very frequent. Exudation into the vascular walls leads to an infiltration of the basement membranes with fibrinogen and lipoproteins and, after some years, to the thickening and hyalinization of the basement membranes. Thus the functional changes in the microvessels may lead to the degenerative vascular changes. (For further details see Ditzel, J.: Functional microangiopathy in diabetes, Diabetes **17:**388-397, 1968.)

Dr. Watzke: Would you discuss your concept of the relationship of whole blood viscosities and diabetic retinopathy?

Dr. Ditzel: The investigations of Ashton and others have established that although the clinical picture of diabetic retinopathy is typical and easily recognizable none of its features are specific for diabetes. Microaneurysms with similar hyaline thickening and lipoid and polysaccharide staining, though fewer in number but indistinguishable from those seen in diabetes, have also been found in other conditions such as central retinal vein thrombosis, macroglobulinemia, and myelomatosis. This indicates that the microaneurysms may be related to factors common to many diseases that are present in the diabetic state. The finding of retinal microaneurysms in the nondiabetic conditions mentioned above suggests that their formation may result from prolonged tissue hypoxia, either produced from actual thrombosis or from an increased whole blood viscosity attributable to dysproteinemia. In diabetes there is no indication that the presence of microaneurysms is preceded by actual venous thrombosis, and the problem naturally arises of whether in these cases the blood viscosity is increased.

We compared 40 young juvenile diabetics with 26 healthy individuals of similar ages and found that the whole blood viscosity differed in the two groups. Since hematocrit is an important factor in determining whole blood viscosity, the data have been corrected for this factor (Skovborg, F., et al.: Proceedings of the Fourth European Conference on Microcirculation, Cambridge, 1966, Basel, 1967, Karger, AG, p. 508). When the diabetes is out of control, the increase in whole blood viscosity of the diabetic becomes even more pronounced. The blood viscosity was significantly correlated to the concentration of α_1-, α_2-, and β-hemoglobulin and to fibrinogen. In large groups of diabetics the increase in whole blood viscosity is only on the order of 8%, and from Poiseuille's law, in which the viscosity is one of the factors involved, such a relatively small increase in blood viscosity could be corrected by a very small increase in the diameter of the blood vessels. We have furthermore found that in juvenile diabetics without evidence of long-term vascular manifestations the mean whole blood plasma viscosities were only slightly higher in the diabetic subjects than in their controls. If one accepts the development of diabetic retinopathy as being a slow chain of events starting from the earliest evidence of diabetes, our findings do not support the view that blood viscosity is a major factor in the development of the very early retinal lesions. However, since in diabetics the whole blood viscosity apparently shows fluctuations greater than normal, such a relationship cannot be completely ruled out, nor can the possibility of the increased blood viscosity present in long-term cases of diabetes with evidence of microangiopathy be excluded as a contributing factor in the progression of an already established retinopathy (see Ditzel, J.: Whole blood viscosity and related components in diabetes, Dan. Med. Bull. **15:**49-53, 1968).

12

Retinal changes of hypertension

Walter M. Kirkendall

The vessels of the optic fundi are readily visible with the ophthalmoscope. This represents the sole opportunity for the clinician to see smaller arteries and veins and make observations concerning them. It is important to remember, however, that the changes observed in the vessels of the optic fundi are, in almost every case, nonspecific ones. These vessels have only a limited number of ways to react to a variety of stimuli so that it is not surprising that an exudate may derive from hematologic disorders, diabetes mellitus, arthritis, microembolization, metastatic malignancy, primary renal disorders, or hypertension.

It is also important to remember that narrowing tortuosity, right-angle branching, increased light reflex, irregularity of caliber, localized narrowing, copper-wire reflex, silver-wire arteries, perivascularitis, sheathing, spasm, and crossing phenomena, and other terms describing changes in the appearance of the arterioles are inexact. Recognition and estimation of degree of change depend entirely on the judgment of the examiner. There are no accurate indices for quantitating any of these changes in clinical circumstances although extreme degrees of narrowing and vascular obliteration are readily apparent.

These limitations do not detract from the importance of fundus findings in patients with vascular disease since observation of this bed may suggest new or alternate diagnoses, give clues to the severity of the vascular disease, and provide information about the efficacy of treatment.

ANATOMIC CONSIDERATIONS

Histologically, it has been shown that the central retinal artery within the optic nerve is similar to medium-sized arteries elsewhere in the body.[8] Intima, media, and adventitia layers in the vascular coat with well-developed elastic and muscular components are easily recognized. After passing through the lamina cribrosa of the sclera, the central artery begins to lose the characteristics of a true artery. The internal elastic lamina becomes thinner and usually disappears at the first or second bifurcation. The muscular coat thins, and the muscle fibers lose continuity. Thus, the majority of vessels one sees have the characteristics of arterioles and range in size from 63 to 134 μ in diameter. With fluorescence angiography one can see capillaries, particularly in the region of the macula.

Two distinct processes go on simultaneously in the vessels of the hypertensive patient. These are vasoconstriction and structural changes in the muscle and intima of the arterioles. Additionally nodular arteriosclerosis may occur in the retinal artery and its first branches and provide characteristic findings.

HYPERTENSIVE CHANGES IN RETINAL VESSELS

General and local vasoconstriction, striate hemorrhages, cotton-wool exudates, retinal edema, and papilledema are processes that become more easily recognized and more numerous as blood pressure rises. There is not a strict relationship, however, between the height of the systemic blood pressure and the presence or absence of these signs. For instance, patients with very severe sustained hypertension may have no evidence of cotton-wool spots or striate hemorrhages, whereas, rarely, the full-blown picture of the retinal change of malignant hypertension may appear in a patient with relatively minimal elevated pressure. Of importance is the observation that as blood pressure is reduced by treatment, all signs of hypertensive disease subside quickly.

Generalized and local vasoconstriction

These changes in retinal vessels are extremely difficult to quantify in clinical situations. Few observers question the phenomenon of generalized reversible narrowing of retinal arterioles in patients with severe hypertension, but some believe that localized vasoconstriction rarely occurs, if at all.[19]

Evidence for the presence of vasoconstriction comes from a number of sources. In experimental models of hypertensive disease, general and local vasoconstriction are prominent features of the process in retinal arterioles.[2] Retinal arterioles have the capacity to narrow in response to environmental changes such as increases in the oxygen saturation of the blood.[25] It is agreed that general and local constriction occur in retinal arteries of patients with acute forms of hypertension such as acute glomerulonephritis or toxemia of pregnancy.[6] There have been a number of studies utilizing optic fundus photographs and grid measurements that demonstrate that both the number of visible vessels at stated distances from the disk are fewer and their caliber is less in hypertensive than in normotensive individuals.[13] These vessels increase in size after therapy.[21] A number of competent observers, chief among them Wagener,[28] have reported dilatation of constricted arterioles in the eyegrounds. The evidence supports the view that the majority of localized narrowings of retinal vessels reflect organic changes in these structures. Typical of the comments are those of Dollery, Ramalho, and Paterson[5]: "Scrutiny of sequential color photographs of about 100 major or minor areas of narrowing in retinal arterioles show that the great majority of these areas remained unchanged even if hypertension was apparently cured by renal surgery." Nevertheless the difficulty of defining and recording vessel caliber leaves an important question as to the significance of observed local narrowing of vessels. Should one accept as fact that virtually all narrowed areas are the result of structural changes and hence relatively permanent? Or should one recognize that arterioles of the retinal circulation respond to many stimuli as do arterioles elsewhere and frequently demonstrate local constriction (and local dilatation) as either a consequence or a cause of severe blood pressure elevation? Because of my experiences and the difficulty of documenting ephemeral events in the retinal circulation, I believe local retinal constriction occurs commonly.

A major defect in all currently used methods of classifying eyeground changes in the hypertensive patient is the difficulty in differentiating between normal, mildly narrowed, and severely narrowed retinal arterioles. Even among experienced observers, there is much inter- and intra-observer difference in regard to caliber and variation of primary and distal vessel narrowing. Using conventional methods of assessment of milder forms of hypertension, one group found them virtually useless for quantitation.[12] These experienced observers were able, however, to note signs of generalized and local vascular changes more frequently in hypertensive than in nonhypertensive individuals. The use of the arteriole-venule ratio as a measure of arteriolar caliber also has many pitfalls and is not particularly useful.[26]

Cotton-wool patches

Fluffy, soft-appearing exudates called cotton-wool patches represent thickening and swelling of the terminal nerve fibers of the retina.[3] Although they have no special diagnostic implication, they are common in hypertensive people and in patients with lupus erythematosus, dermatomyositis, occlusion of the central retinal vein, and papilledema. In hypertensives, such exudates appear and grow rapidly and may continue to appear for several days after the blood pressure has been lowered. They usually lie close to the main vessel groups, within three diameters of the disk, and displace large blood vessels as they enlarge. The exudates first appear as a grayish white area in the retina and grow to full size within a few days. During resolution in the hypertensive, they become a dull white color and later develop a coarse granular appearance. At this stage hemorrhages quite frequently appear in the bed of the exudates and fine red dots are visible that correspond with microaneurysms identified in fluorescent angiography. The striate hemorrhages may arise from ruptured microaneurysms. Based on experimental studies, Harry and Ashton[10] believe that soft exudates in hypertensive patients probably are ischemic infarcts. Dollery[3] points out that the cotton-wool spot formed as a result of experimental arteriolar obstruction is shorter lived than that found in the hypertensive patient. Experimental animals do not develop the surrounding rings of aneurysms or fluorescent leakage as is seen in man. Renal hypertension produced in monkeys caused the development of retinopathy with cotton-wool spots, which had the same characteristics of those of man. Arteriole obstruction, central to the development of the cotton-wool spot, may be caused by microangiopathic hemolytic anemia (MHA) and the coagulopathy associated with malignant hypertension. In experimental animals with malignant hypertension at least 50% have major manifestations of microangiopathic hemolytic anemia.[9] Similarly, in man, many patients with malignant hypertension have reduction in platelets, development of schistocytes, increases in fibrin-degradation products, and alteration of coagulation factors characteristic of MHA.[9]

The appearance of even a single cotton-wool spot in the hypertensive is a cause for alarm. Although other processes may cause the exudate, if it is from necrotizing arteriolitis or microangiopathic hemolytic anemia, the patient's prognosis without treatment is poor. Appropriate diagnosis and immediate blood

Table 12-1. Primary malignant hypertension: changes in a 24-year-old woman after malignant hypertension and subsequent therapy

Date	Blood pressure (mm. Hg)	Blood urea nitrogen (mg. %)	Serum creatinine (mg. %)	Creatinine clearance (ml. per min.)	Serum potassium (mEq. per liter)	Hematocrit (vol. %)	Plasma renin activity (ng. per ml.)
5/7	240/140	17	1.1	—	2.3	39	—
5/21	220/140	126	6.2	—	2.8	23	7.2
Treatment							
5/23	140/90	147	7.6	5	2.7	19	—
5/29	120-140/90-100	103	7.5	—	4.8	—	—
9/3	120-140/90-100	28	3	20	3.9	31	3.2

pressure reduction are indicated, since continuation of the process may result in irreversible renal damage within days.

Illustration of how rapidly malignant hypertension may progress is provided by the following case. Four years ago, a 24-year-old woman was seen by a physican because of occipital headache. Her blood pressure was elevated to the level of 240/140 mm. of mercury, but she was said to have had neither retinopathy nor proteinuria. Blood urea nitrogen and creatinine were normal, but her serum potassium was low (Table 12-1). For some reason she was not treated. When seen 2 weeks later, she had severe hypertensive retinopathy with papilledema, striate hemorrhages, and cotton-wool spots. At this time she had azotemia and increased fibrin degradation and schistocytes in the circulating blood. When blood pressure was lowered with furosemide and methyldopa, the malignant stage regressed and the anemia and azotemia improved. She now is doing well on maintenance therapy. In addition to malignant hypertension, this patient had evidence of microangiopathic hemolytic anemia. The rapid deterioration of kidney function before proper treatment emphasizes the critical need for prompt medical attention in such patients.

Hard exudates

In contrast to the cotton-wool patches, hard exudates that lie deep to the retinal vessels and have a sharp margin do not signify the same grave prognosis. These exudates are smaller and disappear much more slowly than do the superficial ones. They frequently appear at a stage in the patient's course when the soft exudates are beginning to dissolve. Hogan and Zimmerman[11] believe the hard lesions originate with fluid, which collects in pools in the various layers of the retina, and they represent degeneration of nervous tissue. The fluid undergoes changes and accumulates as lipid, fibrin, and cellular debris at the junction of the inner nuclear and outer plexiform layers of the retina. Studies by Shakib and Ashton[24] support the concept of primary nervous tissue damage as the cause of hard exudates. In a study of experimental retinal arteriolar embolization, they observed outer plexiform layer changes with cytoid bodies development in the nerve fiber layer. Ultimately there was a complete loss of architecture in the outer plexiform layer. It was the view of Shakib and Ashton that retinal arteriolar occlusion was the common denominator for the production of outer plexiform lesions as well as those in the nerve fiber layer. It should be noted, however, that outer layers of the retina receive nourishment from the choroidal capillaries by diffusion through Bruch's membrane rather than by the central retinal artery and its branches. This raises the question of whether choroidal vascular disease is responsible for the formation of hard exudates.

Drusen, the domed excrescences that project anteriorly from Bruch's membrane, are difficult to distinguish from hard exudates in patients with retinal vascular disease. In most instances, however, drusen can be differentiated from hard exudates after the use of fluorescent angiography. The drusen lie deep to the hard exudates and fluoresce very early because fluorescence shines through from the choroidal circulation while hard exudates do not fluoresce.[1]

Because the macular star figure represents hard exudates that develop in the Henle's layer of the macula, they are arranged in a radial fashion from the central fovea. Macular star figures follow the same course as other hard exudates and usually take months to years to disappear. The macular star figure usually develops in conjunction with other retinal changes of the malignant hypertensive state. Prior to the advent of widespread antihypertensive drug treatment, patients with macular star figures seldom survived for long periods and the star figure was considered to be a fixed lesion. Since the advent of effective antihypertensive therapy, it is the rule for macular star figures to disintegrate and disappear after successful lowering of blood pressure.

Retinal hemorrhages

Hemorrhages associated with severe hypertensive disease characteristically occur near the disk in the nerve fiber layer and extend along the nerve fibers parallel to the retinal surface. As fibers pass peripherally they separate and form a loose network with round bases. Thus, in the peripheral portions of the nerve fiber hemorrhage the lesion may be round or patchy. The hemorrhages overlie the retinal vessels. Hemorrhages from other causes may occur in this nerve fiber layer and resemble the hemorrhages common to hypertension. Other hemorrhages of the hypertensive person occur either secondary to severe arteriolosclerosis with venous occlusion or in the periphery of areas made ischemic by retinal or arteriolar occlusion. These hemorrhages are almost always localized, round or oval, and usually confined to the periphery of the fundus, and when they occur in the macular region, they assume a star-like arrangement. Deep hemorrhages lie below the retinal vessels. In general, peripheral, solitary, or localized round retinal hemorrhages are signs of severe arteriolosclerosis rather than of severe hypertension although the two often coexist.

Patients with retinopathy of diabetes mellitus have hemorrhages associated with vascular obstruction and cause confusion in evaluating vascular damage from hypertension. Hemorrhages associated with anemia and leukemia may have a white center. They occur in the nerve fiber layer and hence may be confused with hypertensive ones in patients with elevated blood pressure. Subhyaloid hemorrhages may appear as extrusions bleeding from the deeper layers of the retina in diabetes, in those with leukemia, after intracranial hemorrhage or trauma or occasionally without demonstrative cause. They are usually sharp bordered, bright red, and raised and may be very large.

Hemorrhages in the nerve fiber layer may regress rapidly in patients with successfully treated accelerated hypertension. In a matter of 2 to 3 weeks one may find no clinical residue. On the other hand, microscopic foci of lipid may persist. Since many of the striate hemorrhages occur in proximity to cotton-wool patches, it is quite likely that some or all may represent leaks of blood from microaneurysms surrounding the cotton-wool patch.

PAPILLEDEMA

This is an ominous sign when caused by malignant or accelerated hypertension. Together with soft exudates, striate hemorrhages, and retinal edema, it implies that renal function has failed or soon will fail to the point of uremia if treatment is not applied. Because of the serious prognosis it is imperative to rule out other causes of papilledema such as brain tumor, pseudotumor cerebri, head trauma, lead poisoning, rupture of an intracranial aneurysm, or other cerebral catastrophies.

Papilledema may develop slowly first, causing loss of the physiologic cup, then distension of the veins and blurring of the nasal margin, and finally obliteration of the temporal margins of the disk. It may resolve in days but may not be completely resolved in 2 or more months after effective therapy. A peripapillary halo, possibly a cuff of unreabsorbed edema fluid, may persist for a year after papilledema has disappeared. In fluorescence studies of the optic fundi[4] and occasionally in conventional photographs, one may see dilated or new vessels at the margin of the disks indefinitely after papilledema has subsided.

Two major postulates have been used to explain the pathogenesis of papilledema. Papilledema is most often observed in patients with elevated intracranial pressure, and there has been a suggestion that it is a manifestation of edema of the brain.[27] Since increased intracranial pressure is not always present, a second hypothesis has been developed that suggests that elevated pressure in the central retinal vein impedes return flow from the capillaries of the nerve head that arise from the circle of Zinn-Haller.[17] The congestion and stasis of the capillaries of that circle then provide mechanisms for the development of edema of the optic nerve and for its location in the fibers anterior to the lamina cribrosa.

ARTERIOLOSCLEROTIC RETINOPATHY

The second major process that goes on in the vessels of the fundus is a diffuse thickening of small vessels. This has been termed by Fishberg and Oppenheimer[7] "arteriosclerotic retinopathy," but since the process occurs primarily in arterioles, "arteriolosclerosis" is a more appropriate term.

The first development of this process is deposition of hyaline material often with considerable lipid just beneath the endothelium. The disease progresses to involvement of the muscularis and eventual invasion of the entire vessel wall. The process should be distinguished from nodular arteriosclerosis, which often appears in the small arteries near the disk.[1]

Characteristic changes of arteriolosclerosis are tortuosity, development of right-angle crossing at the arteriolar-venular junction, widening of the light reflex, development of copper and silver wire arterioles, and changes in the arteriolar-venular crossing. At the arteriolar-venular crossing there is initial mild depression of the vein, later obliteration of the vein for short distances on either side of the arteriole, damming of the blood distally, and finally occlusion of the vein as the process worsens.[23]

Local areas of narrowing from arteriolosclerosis are common. These are associated with widening of the arteriole beyond and are easily recognized. The areas of local sclerosis and the changes at the arteriolar-venular crossing are easiest of the arteriolosclerotic changes to judge. Extreme degrees of narrowing and vascular obliteration are readily apparent, regularly recognized, and fairly accurately graded; lesser degrees tend to be variously interpreted by competent observers.[13]

Arteriolosclerosis is a generalized disorder that appears in small blood vessels of all organs. A question of great importance is whether the sclerosis seen in the eyeground accurately reflects that in other vital tissues. Studies designed to answer this question by comparison of the sclerosis of retinal vessels with nephrosclerosis have tended to support the view that the two processes are parallel in most instances.[29] Nevertheless the observations are not conclusive because in most examples histologic verification of the retinal-artery arteriolar lesion was not documented and the renal biopsy material represented only a small portion of one kidney. The hypothesis that renal and retinal arteriolosclerosis proceed together is an attractive one but needs better support before it can be accepted completely.

NODULAR ARTERIOSCLEROSIS

A third process that goes on in the eyeground of the hypertensive person is nodular arteriosclerosis. This appears in the small arteries near the disk, and occasionally small atheromas are visible. The process may involve surrounding retinal tissues, and because of the common adventitial coat of the artery and vein, the atheromas may invade the wall of the vein, causing occlusion. The absence of nodular arteriosclerosis in this circulation is no assurance that it is not present elsewhere. Its appearance in the fundus makes it likely that the process is in other large vessels.

CHOROIDAL VASCULAR CHANGES

Choroidal vessels are difficult to demonstrate clinically. Histologic sections and serial retinal photographs indicate that the choroidal circulation participates in the arteriolosclerosis and probably in other vascular changes seen in the retinal circulation.[10]

Figs. 12-1, *A* and *B,* reveal the development of a thickened choroidal vessel over a period of 3 years of observation in a hypertensive patient under treatment. Some investigators believe that deep hemorrhages and exudates occur as a result of disease in the choroidal circulation since these areas are nourished by these vessels.

CHANGES IN FUNDUS VESSELS WITH AND WITHOUT TREATMENT IN THE HYPERTENSIVE PATIENT

Several years ago Dr. Mark Armstrong and I studied this problem in a group of patients treated for hypertension and a similar group treated with placebo.[14, 15, 16] We observed increases in the caliber of retinal vessels by crude measurements of patients successfully treated for 1 to 2 years. When blood pressure had not declined, we rarely saw what appeared to be an increase in arteriolar caliber. We occasionally observed areas of local narrowing to clear after therapy. The florid features of hypertensive retinopathy regularly receded when the patient was treated successfully.

After 2 or more years of observation, whether blood pressure stayed the same or was reduced, we were unable to demonstrate significant change in arterio-

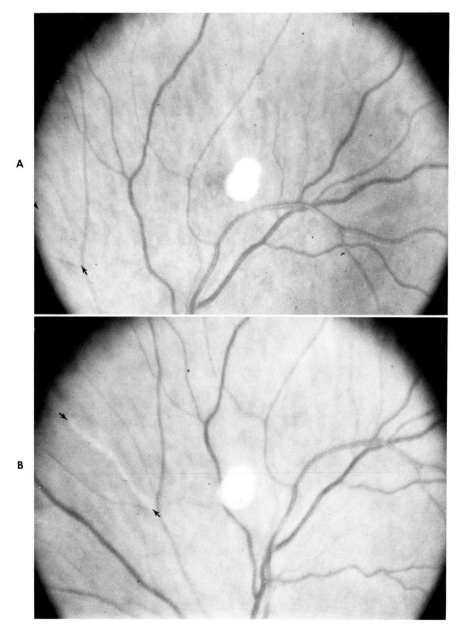

Fig. 12-1. Choroidal sclerosis developed in area between arrows in fundus of 57-year-old hypertensive man. **A** was taken 3 years before **B.**

sclerotic processes in most patients. In some, however, there was a very active repair process observed. We saw obstructed arterioles with lumina severely compromised by sclerosis around which widespread collateral circulation developed so that the obstructed area was effectively bypassed. In some cases, after effective treatment the obstructed arterioles appeared to be recanalized so that collaterals around the obstructed area disappeared. Venous channels that became obstructed at the arteriolar-venular junction by arteriolosclerotic processes likewise were bypassed effectively by the development of collaterals.

These observations are consistent with the thesis that there is reversible general and local narrowing in the hypertensive, that at times arteriolosclerosis may progress while hypertensive changes in the eye ground regress and that, generally, the arteriolosclerotic process is not visibly worsened or improved by blood pressure lowering. The recognition that recanalization of small blood vessels can occur in the presence of lower blood pressure is of importance in justifying long-term treatment. It provides support for vigorous and sustained control of the blood pressure in most clinical situations.

Most long-term evaluations of retinal changes in the hypertensive patient have not had the benefit of adequate retinal photography, and these studies have shown little change in the appearance of arteriolosclerosis after treatment. There is need for information concerning retinal blood flow and the state of retinal vessels after long-term treatment by modern techniques available including fluorescent angiograms, stereoptic photography, and better methods to quantitate blood flow and the size of small vessels.

CLASSIFICATION

Central to an understanding of retinopathy of the hypertensive patient is a classification that meets educational and clinical needs. The Keith-Wagener-Barker classification of hypertensive retinopathy is inadequate since it lumps arteriolosclerotic and hypertensive changes into four groups and gives equal weight to hard exudates and cotton-wool patches and to striate and round hemorrhages. Pickering[20] has pointed out that another reason for this classification to be abandoned "is the invitation to self-deception presented by group one." Mild changes in the retinal artery are notoriously subjective, and the patient with mild elevation of arteriole pressure and doubtful changes in the retinal arteries is inevitably put into this group. Pickering promoted the classification suggested by Foster-Moore.[18] Foster-Moore reorganized arteriosclerotic retinitis and distinguished it from the albuminaric or renal retinitis. Fishberg and Oppenheimer coined the terms "arteriosclerotic retinopathy" and "hypertensive neuroretinopathy" for these.[7]

I am attracted to the classification suggested by Scheie[22] because it separates arteriolosclerotic and hypertensive changes. I have modified this, as depicted in Table 12-2, to emphasize several things. First, I have no confidence in my ability to consistently distinguish between minimal narrowing of the retinal arteries and none at all. Hence, I have left out grade-one changes. Second, I have emphasized the striate hemorrhages and cotton-wool spots of the accelerated or malignant hypertensive patient, which are the important signals for the clinician to recognize. The patient with these hypertensive retinal changes is in great jeopardy and in need of immediate treatment. Third, I have emphasized that arteriolosclerotic

Table 12-2. Classification of retinal vascular changes

Arteriolosclerotic defect	*Changes*	*Hypertensive defect*
Definite arteriolar-venular crossing changes and moderate local sclerosis	II	Severe general narrowing
Invisibility of vein beneath arteriole and severe local sclerosis with segmentation	III	Plus striate hemorrhages and soft exudates
Plus venous obstruction and silver-wire arterioles	IV	Plus papilledema

changes may lead to hemorrhages of an entirely different nature, namely, those secondary to arteriolar-venous compression.

More elaborate classifications than this run the risk of confusing observers by the use of changes that under current circumstances cannot be accurately measured or consistently recognized in clinical situations. Better classifications await better knowledge of the genesis of retinal vascular abnormalities and of their significance.

SUMMARY

The optic fundus provides the physician with the opportunity to gain important information about his hypertensive patient. There, one can readily see the most florid signs of accelerated hypertension and, by correctly identifying them, provide the patient with needed treatment. Identification and classification of the retinopathy for the hypertensive patient can aid the physician in avoiding inappropriate therapeutic measures. Better understanding and better methods of quantitating changes in the eye will improve the value of the fundoscopic examination as an instrument to measure progression of the disease and adequacy of therapy. Recent work has done much to clarify the genesis and significance of cotton-wool exudates and microaneurysms in the hypertensive. Additional information is needed regarding the arteriolosclerotic process, its evolution after successful hypertensive therapy, and the effect of vascular disease on retinal blood flow and distribution. New techniques now available make it possible to provide this information.

REFERENCES

1. Allen, L., Kirkendall, W. M., Synder, W. B., and Frazier, O.: Instant positive photographs and stereograms of ocular fundus fluorescence, Arch. Ophthalmol. **75:**192, 1966.
2. Byrom, F. B.: The caliber of the retinal arteries in hypertension, Am. Heart J. **66:**727-730, 1963.
3. Dollery, C. T.: Circulatory clinical and pathological aspects of the cotton-wool spots, Proc. R. Soc. Med. **62:**1267-1271, 1969.
4. Dollery, C. T., and Hodge, J. V.: Hypertensive retinopathy studied with fluorescein, Trans. Ophthalmol. Soc. U. K. **83:**115, 1963.
5. Dollery, C. T., Ramalho, P. S., and Paterson, J. W.: Retinal vascular alterations in hypertension. In Gross, F., editor: Antihypertensive therapy: Principles and practice. An international symposium, Berlin, 1966, Springer Verlag, p. 152.
6. Epstein, F. H.: Vascular disease of the kidney. Toxemia of pregnancy. In Wintrobe et al., editors: Harrison's principles of internal medicine, ed. 6, New York, 1970, McGraw-Hill Book Co., p. 1422.
7. Fishberg, A. M., and Oppenheimer, B. S.: Differentiation and significance of certain ophthalmoscopic pictures in hypertensive diseases, Arch. Intern. Med. **46:**901, 1930.

8. Friedenwald, J. S.: Retinal and choroidal arteriosclerosis. In Ridley, F., and Sorsby, A., editors: Modern trends in ophthalmology, New York, 1940, Paul B. Hoeber, Inc., p. 77.

9. Gavras, H., Brown, W. C. B., Brown, J. J., Lever, A. F., Linton, A. L., MacAdem, R. F., McNicol, G. P., Robertson, J., Ian, S., and Wardros, C.: Microangiopathic hemolytic anemia and the development of the malignant phase of hypertension, Circ. Res. **28**(Suppl. II):127-141, 1971.

10. Harry, J., and Ashton, N.: The pathology of hypertensive retinopathy, Trans. Ophthalmol. Soc. U. K. **83**:71, 1963.

11. Hogan, M. J., Zimmerman, L. E., editors: Ophthalmic pathology. An atlas and textbook, ed. 2, Philadelphia, 1962, W. B. Saunders Co.

12. Kagan, A., Aurell, E., Dobree, J., Hara, K., McKendrick, C., Michaelson, I., Shaper, G., Sundaresan, T., and Tibblin, G.: A note on signs in the fundus oculi and arterial hypertension: Conventional assessment and significance, Bull. W.H.O. **34**:955-960, 1966.

13. Kagan, A., Aurell, E., and Tibblin, G.: Signs in the fundus oculi and arterial hypertension. Unconventional assessment and significance, Bull. W.H.O. **36**:231-241, 1967.

14. Kirkendall, W. M., and Armstrong, M. L.: Effect of blood pressure reduction on vascular changes in the eye. In Moyer, J. H., editor: The first Hahnemann symposium on hypertensive disease, Philadelphia, 1959, W. B. Saunders, Co., p. 472.

15. Kirkendall, W. M., and Armstrong, M. L.: Effect of blood pressure reduction on vascular changes in the eye. II. Results after two years. In Brest, A. N., and Moyer, J. H., editors: The second Hahnemann symposium on hypertensive disease, Philadelphia, 1961, Lea & Febiger, p. 624.

16. Kirkendall, W. M., and Armstrong, M. L.: Vascular changes in the eye of the treated and untreated patient with essential hypertension, Am. J. Cardiol. **9**:663-668, 1962.

17. Leinfelder, P. J.: Pathogenesis of papilledema, Am. J. Ophthalmol. **48**:107, 1959.

18. Moore, R. Foster-: Retinitis of arteriosclerosis, Q. J. Med. **10**:29, 1917.

19. Pickering, G. W.: High blood pressure, London, 1955, J. & A. Churchill, p. 273.

20. Pickering, G. W.: The Bowman lecture. The eyes as an index of generalized vascular disease, Trans. Ophthalmol. Soc. U. K. **89**:83-124, 1970.

21. Ramalho, P. S., and Dollery, C. T.: Hypertensive retinopathy. Caliber changes in retinal blood vessels following blood pressure reduction and inhalation of oxygen, Circulation **37**:580-588, 1968.

22. Scheie, H. G.: Evaluation of ophthalmoscopic changes of hypertension and arteriolar sclerosis, Arch. Ophthalmol. **49**:117, 1953.

23. Seitz, R.: Die Genese und Ätiologie des Kreuzungsphänomens und seine Bedeutung für die Diagnostik von Netzhautgefässerkrankungen, Klin. Monatsbl. Augenheilk. **139**:491, 1961.

24. Shakib, M., and Ashton, N.: Part II. Ultrasonic changes in focal retinal ischemia, Br. J. Ophthalmol. **50**:325, 1966.

25. Sieker, H. O., and Hickam, J. B.: Normal and impaired retinal vascular reactivity, Circulation **7**:79, 1953.

26. Stokoe, N. L., and Turner, R. W. D.: Normal retinal vascular patterns, Br. J. Ophthalmol. **50**:21-40, 1966.

27. Taylor, R. D., Corcoran, A. C., and Page, I. H.: Increased cerebrospinal fluid pressure and papilledema in malignant hypertension, Arch. Intern. Med. **93**:818-824, 1954.

28. Wagener, H. P.: Retinal arterial and arteriolar lesions associated with systemic hypertension, Am. J. Med. Sci. **241**:240, 1961.

29. Wendland, J. P.: The relationship of retinal and renal arteriolosclerosis in living patients with essential hypertension, Am. J. Ophthalmol. **35**:1748, 1952.

13

Retinal vascular accidents

David G. Cogan

The retina offers a unique opportunity to study vascular accidents. Nowhere else in the body can we witness so readily the evolution of these ministrokes during life, plot their course at successive stages of development, and select areas for subsequent pathologic study. The aim of the present report will be to correlate some of their clinical and pathologic features.

A consideration of occlusive vasculopathy in the retina must include vessels as far posterior as the nerve head since most vascular accidents have their origin at the level of the lamina cribrosa. The scope of the present observations will include, therefore, the vessels in the optic nerve, in addition to those in the retina proper, insofar as they directly involve the retinal vessels. For convenience I have divided the subject under the headings of arteries, veins, and capillaries but with full recognition of the overlap between them and awareness that occlusion of one system may cause secondary changes in the other systems.

ARTERIES

The retinal artery enters the eye by way of the optic nerve. Traversing the center of the nerve, it passes through a membrane called the lamina cribrosa, which is, in effect, a fenestrated continuum of the sclera. This fibrous membrane apparently offers local resistance to expansion of the artery (and vein) and is a common site for lodgment of calcific emboli.

After passing through the lamina, the retinal artery extends to the innermost portion of the nerve head where it, or its branches, abut against the internal limiting membrane that separates the neural compartment from the vitreous or connective tissue compartment. In its intramural and papillary course the retinal artery resembles larger arteries elsewhere in the body in containing a substantial muscular coat and internal elastic lamina. It is therefore susceptible to atheromatosis and to giant cell arteritis, which affect vessels of this constituency.

On leaving the nerve head, however, the retinal arteries lose their internal elastica and much of the muscle to become arterioles (although we will continue to call them retinal arteries in accordance with tradition). They have a diameter of approximately 100 μ or less and rarely show changes that could be interpreted

223

as atheromatosis.[1] Instead, occlusive disease of these vessels shows hyalinization and lipidization of their walls without the endothelial proliferation that characterizes atheromatous stenosis of the larger vessels. Similarly the arteries in the retina do not show the giant cell arteritis that affects vessels containing internal elastic membranes.

Hypertension, on the other hand, does affect the retinal arteries directly. This is characterized clinically by the diffuse narrowing and irregularity of the arterial lumina. Pathologically the changes are most significantly evaluated in flat mounts of the retinal vessels prepared by trypsin digestion and stained by the periodic acid–Schiff method. The conspicuous abnormality is then evident in an increased stainability of the precapillary arterioles.[13]

Complete occlusion of the central retinal artery is characterized usually by sudden blindness with the early ophthalmoscopic picture of stagnation in the retinal vessels, especially boxcar segmentation of blood in the veins, and an opacification of the central retina, with a cherry-red spot, coming on after several hours. Variations from this typical picture are common. The blindness may be preceded by episodes of amaurosis fugax over considerable periods of time. The final episode may be an attack similar to the prior episodes but one that failed to clear. Once the amaurosis has lasted more than one-half hour, it is usually permanent although we have all witnessed exceptions on rare occasion. The boxcar segmentation of blood disappears with reestablishment of the circulation and has usually disappeared by the time the patient presents himself for examination. The retinal vessels may then appear normal. The opacity of the retina however persists for more than a week. It eventually disappears completely, leaving a normally transparent retina, with or without evident narrowing of the arteries, but a telltale pallor of the disk, indicating optic atrophy.

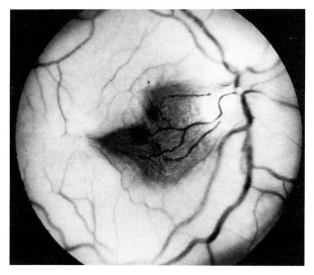

Fig. 13-1. Opacity of retina after embolic occlusion of central retinal artery. Two ciliary arteries emerging from temporal side of disk (and arising in choroid) were uninvolved and consequently spared the retina in centrocecal area. Embolus is evident as a white dot in center of disk where arteries emerge.

A frequent variant is persistence of intact circulation and maintenance of some visual function in an area corresponding to a cilioretinal artery (Fig. 13-1). The cilioretinal artery is derived from the choroidal circulation and is present normally in many persons. Such patients will have sparing of the retina in the area between the macula and the disk. (Of course, the reverse may also be true, wherein the cilioretinal circulation is obstructed, giving rise to a centrocecal scotoma, while most of the retina is preserved.)

The several causes of retinal artery occlusion include chiefly decreased blood flow from carotid stenosis or from increased intraocular pressure, atheroma of the ophthalmic artery or central retinal artery in the optic nerve, emboli, and arteritis. Carotid stenosis is especially likely to be preceded by amaurosis fugax and to be accompanied by contralateral hemiparesthesia or hemiplegia.[7] It cannot always be distinguished from embolic causes of the blindness. Pathologically the retinal arteries may show simply hyalinization of their walls or may show no abnormality despite gross evidence of infarction in the retinal tissue. Atheromatosis of the retinal artery is usually hidden in the nerve head and therefore can be diagnosed only pathologically. The final occlusion has been reported in one case to have been precipitated by hemorrhage into the atheromatous plaque.[3]

Emboli probably account for the majority of retinal artery occlusions. The most commonly identified emboli are the calcific emboli from cardiac vegetations of rheumatic scars or carotid plaques and the lipid emboli from carotid atheromas. Fibrin-platelet emboli also occur and probably account for the migratory emboli that are seen occasionally in transit through the retinal vessels, but they have been less well documented. They occur in hypercoagulable states and after myocardial infarction. Myxomatous emboli from the heart are infrequent but highly significant, since on their recognition may depend the life of the patient.

Calcific and lipid emboli are approximately equal in frequency and together comprise the majority of embolic occlusions. They have somewhat different modes of presentation. Calcific emboli are likely to lodge at the lamina cribrosa (Fig. 13-2) and are evident ophthalmoscopically only when they fragment and enter the circulation within the eye. The fragments do not ordinarily extend far from the disk; they are usually few in number; and they can be recognized as mat-white plugs that appear larger than the lumen of the adjacent vessels. By contrast, lipid emboli are more malleable and gain access to the peripheral vessels where many of them may be identified, especially at bifurcations of the arteries, as yellowish and sometimes scintillating plaques (Fig. 13-3). Occasionally one may see isolated, highly reflectile emboli, consisting of cholesterol plates (Hollenhorst plaques[9]), which are not necessarily obstructive. The histopathologic identification of the emboli has been documented in the case of calcific,[6, 10, 16] lipid,[2, 4, 5, 12] fibrinous,[15, 18] and myxomatous[11, 14] embolism.

The tissue changes with retinal artery occlusion are characterized, as might be expected, by loss of the inner retinal layers but preservation of the outer layers that are supplied by the choroidal circulation. Preserved are the rods and cones, their nuclei, and a portion of the bipolar layer with their connections. Autolysis occurs first in the ganglion cells (Fig. 13-4, *A*). Then follows the remarkably complete disappearance of all the inner layers without appreciable gliosis so that the internal limiting membrane comes to be apposed to the remaining portion of

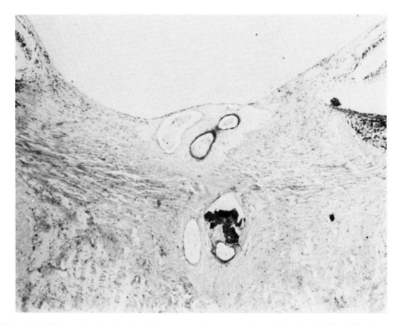

Fig. 13-2. Calcific embolus lodged in central artery immediately behind lamina cribrosa. Occlusion had occurred 6 years previously. (Stain PAS; × 10.)

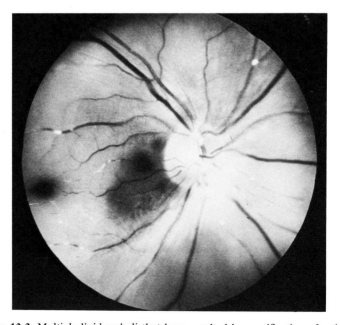

Fig. 13-3. Multiple lipid emboli that have resulted in opacification of retina.

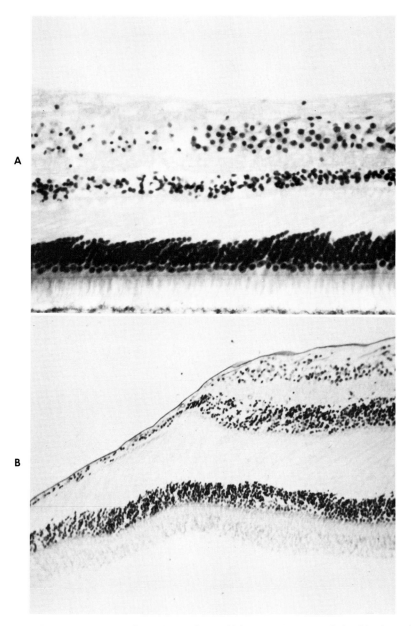

Fig. 13-4. A, Early degeneration of ganglion cell layer and some of the bipolar cell layer at junction of infarcted *(left)* and normal *(right)* portion of retina. The latter, having been supplied by the cilioretinal artery, remained intact. (Stain H & E; × 22.) **B,** Complete disappearance of inner layers of retina in old infarcted portion of retina *(left)* compared with normal portion supplied by a cilioretinal artery. (Stain PAS; ×22.)

the bipolar layer (Fig. 13-4, *B*). This dropout of tissue, pathognomonic for retinal infarction, is most striking in the central area where the inner layers are normally thickest.

VEINS

The retinal veins conjoin at the nerve head to exit from the eye in close association with the central retinal artery to which it is usually bound by a common tunica adventitia. Like the artery its capacity for distension is especially constrained as it traverses the lamina cribrosa, which thereby becomes a preferential site for occlusion (Fig. 13-5). Within the retina proper the retinal veins consist of extremely thin-walled vessels, having a negligible muscular coat but substantial endothelium of the continuous variety, which renders them relatively impermeable. At arteriovenous crossings the arteries and veins are closely apposed to each other, as in the optic nerve, and often bound to each other by a common adventitia. This accounts for the frequent compression and sometimes occlusion of tributary veins by pressure from the arteries.

Occlusion of the retinal veins is characterized by massive hemorrhages (apoplexy) and by dilatation of the veins upstream from the obstruction (Fig.

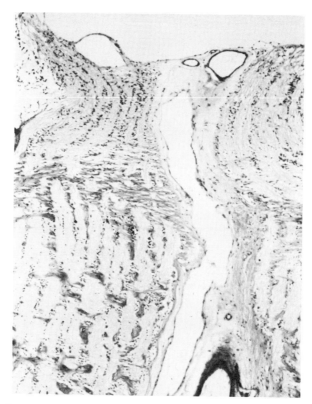

Fig. 13-5. Transit of a normal central vein through optic nerve. Lamina cribrosa, believed to offer a mechanical hindrance to expansion of vein, consists of horizontal fibers in center of photograph. A portion of artery is visible in lower right corner. (Stain **PAS**; × 10.)

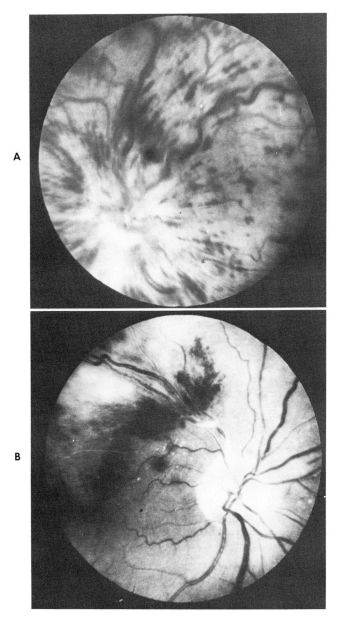

Fig. 13-6. A, Central retinal vein occlusion with extensive hemorrhage and congestion of veins. **B,** Branch retinal vein occlusion with hemorrhages radiating from site of arteriovenous crossing. Elongated white plaques represent opacification ("sclerosis") of arterial wall.

13-6, *A*). With occlusion in the nerve, the entire fundus will be hemorrhagic, with dilated veins intermittently emerging through the hemorrhagic shield. With branch or tributary occlusion, the hemorrhages and venous dilatation are peripheral to the arteriovenous junction that is the site of the obstruction (Fig. 13-6, *B*). The late appearances of venous occlusion are characterized by prominent collateral vessels that bypass the obstruction. In the case of central retinal vein occlusion within the nerve these dilated vessels form at the edge of the disk to drain blood by way of the choroidal circulation. With branch vein occlusion the collateral vessels form dilated, tortuous channels within the retina, sometimes extending into the vitreous, so as to circumvent the site of obstruction.

The causes of venous obstruction are multiple but include especially diabetes, hyperviscosity syndromes, increased intraocular pressure, and arterial disease. This latter consists of an increasing rigidity of the artery, vaguely comprehended under the term "arteriosclerosis," but may, as we have come to learn recently, occur also with arterial emboli or may result from arterial occlusion.[8]

Actually, the pathogenesis of retinal venous occlusion has not been satisfactorily clarified. Is it a thrombotic process as commonly inferred or an endothelial hyperplasia? An answer to this question is not merely of academic interest, since on it depends the rationale of anticoagulant therapy. In his exhaustive study of the subject Dr. Verhoeff did not exactly deny that thrombosis could occur but said that he had never seen it in his pathologic specimens and that by contrast simple endothelial hyperplasia was frequent.[17]

Because of my association with Dr. Verhoeff and my respect for his observations, I have been on the look out for thromboses in retinal veins. Accordingly I would like to cite two cases that were sufficiently fresh to indicate that a thrombotic process is a possible mechanism if the cases are seen sufficiently early. One of these patients who died of polyarteritis nodosa and had had several attacks of amaurosis fugax during the month prior to death showed in the affected eye a fresh thrombus filling the central retinal artery at the level of the lamina cribrosa. The thrombus was considered to be antemortem by reason of the spindle formation of some of the retained cells and because the contained red blood cells showed various stages of disintegration. The other case was a patient whose eye I had an opportunity to study with Paul Sanderson at the National Institutes of Health. The patient, who had myelogenous leukemia with pancytopenia, was a 47-year-old woman who received a transfusion of packed platelets and promptly became blind in her right eye. When seen shortly thereafter she had the typical massive hemorrhages and dilated veins that we associate with central vein occlusion. Two weeks later she died in shock and we had an opportunity to study the eye pathologically. An organizing thrombus filled the length of the vein within the optic nerve. Thus, thrombosis appears to be a possible mechanism for venous occlusion but of course does not preclude endothelial hyperplasia as the cause in the majority of cases.

Pathologic changes in the retina with venous occlusion consist of variable but sometimes massive gliosis and obliterative changes in the veins. These latter may vary from complete replacement of the vessel by acellular basement membrane to a recanalized and functional vessel (Fig. 13-7). Not surprisingly, the adjacent artery may be significantly sclerosed.

An enigmatic but often catastrophic complication of central retinal vein oc-

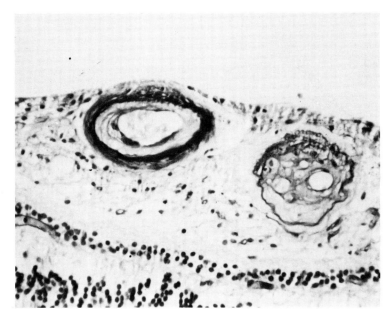

Fig. 13-7. Canalization of occluded vein (vessel on the right) with sclerosed artery nearby (vessel on the left). (Stain PAS; × 80.)

clusion is the development of new vessels on the surface of the iris and angle of the anterior chamber. This occurs several weeks or months after the occlusive episode and results in an intractable and painful form of glaucoma that often requires enucleation. The pathogenesis of this neovascular proliferation is obscure. It does not occur with branch vein occlusion.

CAPILLARIES

Capillary infarcts present a problem essentially indigenous to the eye for only here do they cause significantly functional disturbances.

Retinal capillaries form a glomerulus-like labyrinth of vessels, each approximately 5 μ in diameter, fed by a precapillary arteriole that is not much larger, and conjoining into multiple venules. They are unusual in having, in addition to their lining endothelial cells, another type of cell embedded within the wall variously called "mural cell," or "intramural pericyte." These latter cells appear to be contractile and thereby regulate the flow of blood at the local level through the maze of capillaries.

Obstruction at the capillary or immediately precapillary level causes the cotton-wool spots seen ophthalmoscopically in many vasculopathies (Fig. 13-8, *A*). They are common with hypertension, anemia, collagenoses, and transient embolic occlusion but are relatively inconspicuous with diabetes. The obstructions are best demonstrated by the failure of filling of the capillaries on fluoroangiography. Pathologically cytoid bodies in the nerve fiber layer correspond to the cotton-wool spots seen ophthalmoscopically (Fig. 13-8, *B*). These consist of interrupted

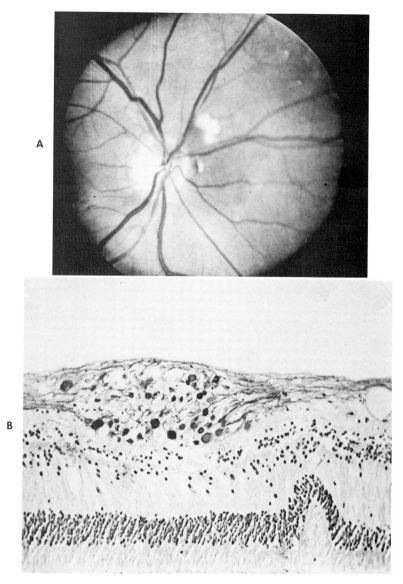

Fig. 13-8. A, Single cotton-wool spot in eye of patient with hypertension. **B,** Cytoid body consisting of nucleoid bodies in nerve fiber layer and resulting from a microinfarct. (Stain Bodian; × 22.)

and swollen nerve fibers with conglomeration of organelles that simulate nuclei by light microscopy.

Aside from the cytoid bodies and local acellularity, the tissue and vascular changes with capillary occlusions are inconspicuous in routine cross sections. Flat mounts of the retinal vessels, however, show a characteristic loss of cellularity from the capillaries, beginning with disappearance of the endothelial cells and later of the mural cells. Ultimately the ischemic capillaries are represented by acellular strands of basement membrane that permanently indicate the site of the former capillary scaffold.

SUMMARY

Vascular accidents in the retina are caused by occlusive disease and present differing clinical and pathologic features depending on whether they are caused by arterial, venous, or capillary obstruction.

Arterial occlusion causes the transient stagnation of blood and opacification of retina with loss of retinal tissue and variable changes in the arteries. Venous occlusion, on the other hand, causes massive hemorrhages with gliosis of the retina and variable obliterative changes in the veins. Capillary occlusions present the familiar cotton-wool spots clinically and cytoid bodies pathologically with nonspecific loss of cellularity from the ischemic capillaries. Together these vascular accidents comprise a well-documented but still open-ended object of study.

REFERENCES

1. Brownstein, S., Font, R. L., and Alper, M. G.: Atheromatous plaques of the retinal blood vessels, Arch. Ophthalmol. **90:**49, 1973.
2. Cogan, D. G., Kuwabara, T., and Moser, H.: Fat emboli in the retina following angiography, Arch. Ophthalmol. **71:**308, 1964.
3. Dahrling, B. E.: The histopathology of early central retinal artery occlusion, Arch. Ophthalmol. **73:**506, 1965.
4. David, N. J., Klintworth, G. K., Friedberg, S. J., and Dillon, M.: Fatal atheromatous cerebral embolism associated with bright plaques in the retinal arterioles, Neurology **13:**708, 1963.
5. DeVoe, A. G.: Ocular fat embolism; a clinical and pathologic report, Arch. Ophthalmol. **43:**857, 1950.
6. Ferry, A.: Unpublished.
7. Fisher, M.: Transient monocular blindness associated with hemiplegia, Arch. Ophthalmol. **47:**167, 1952.
8. Hayreh, S. S.: Pathogenesis of occlusion of the central retinal vessels, Am. J. Ophthalmol. **72:**998, 1971.
9. Hollenhorst, R. W.: Significance of bright plaques in the retinal arterioles, J.A.M.A. **178:**123, 1961.
10. Holley, K. E., Bahn, R. C., and McGoon, D. C.: Calcific embolization associated with valvotomy for calcific aortic stenosis, Circulation **28:**175, 1963.
11. Jampol, L. M., Wong, A. S., and Albert, D. M.: Atrial myxoma and central retinal artery occlusion, Am. J. Ophthalmol. **75:**242, 1973.
12. Kearns, T. P.: Fat embolism of the retina demonstrated by a flat retinal preparation, Am. J. Ophthalmol. **41:**1, 1956.
13. Kuwabara, T., Carroll, J. M., and Cogan, D. G.: Retinal vascular patterns. Part III. Age, hypertension, absolute glaucoma, injury, Arch. Ophthalmol. **65:**708, 1961.
14. Manschot, W. A.: Embolism of the central retinal artery originating from an endocardial myxoma, Am. J. Ophthalmol. **48:**381, 1959.
15. McBrien, D. J., Bradley, R. D., and Ashton, N.: Retinal emboli in stenosis of the internal carotid artery, Lancet **1:**697, 1963.
16. Penner, R., and Font, R. L.: Retinal embolism from calcified vegetations of aortic valve, Arch. Ophthalmol. **81:**565, 1969.
17. Verhoeff, F. H.: Obstruction of the central retinal vein, Arch. Ophthalmol. **36:**1, 1907.
18. Zimmerman, L. E.: Embolism of central retinal artery; secondary to myocardial infarction with mural thrombosis, Arch. Ophthalmol. **73:**822, 1965.

Ocular involvement in vascular disease

CHAIRMAN: **Sohan Singh Hayreh***

Dr. Hayreh: We just had two very interesting papers on two very common problems that interest the ophthalmologist as well as the physician, and I am sure there will be plenty of questions. Since these subjects are of tremendous interest to me personally, I think I will give a chance to other people before I get carried away talking about my own work.

Question: What is the etiology of papilledema in hypertension?

Dr. Cogan: Well, I think all papilledema is attributable to leaky capillaries on the nerve head. I will refer the question to you because of your vast experience.

Dr. Hayreh: There is a first-class paper on this subject by Professor Ashton that he gave at the academy a couple of years ago ("The Eye in Malignant Hypertension," Trans. Am. Acad. Ophthalmol. Otolaryngol. **76:**17, 1972). At that time he discussed the subject with me, and as far as I understand it, he thinks that papilledema in hypertension is part of the ischemic process like hypertensive retinopathy. Ashton and Garner have done a tremendous amount of work on hypertensive retinopathy and have produced it experimentally and based on that, they believe that it is probably caused by swelling of the nerve fibers and leakage from the ischemic vessels. No definite answer on the pathogenesis of papilledema in hypertension is yet known.

Dr. Henkind: I have always assumed that Dr. Singh Hayreh knew the answer.

Dr. Hayreh: There is plenty to learn about that.

Dr. Cogan: I think that Dr. Ashton and many others who have studied papilledema and its cause (Dr. Leinfelder was involved in one of these studies many years ago) have been troubled by the fact that there was no strict correlation between cerebrospinal fluid pressure and optic nerve-head edema. I believe that this was the first thing that made it obvious to others that there had to be another explanation for nerve-head edema, and I believe that Dr. Ashton's explanation is quite a good one. I would like to emphasize the fact that the choroidal circulation is involved in clinical hypertension as well. We don't know very much about it, but certainly from time to time we see choroidal sclerosis develop. In a series of patients we observed over years,

*Department of Ophthalmology, University of Iowa College of Medicine, Iowa City, Iowa.

we saw several instances of severe choroidal vessel sclerosis develop. It was a striking finding in many of them and I think that this is an area that needs exploration.

Dr. Hayreh: It was Pickering and other authors who originally thought that papilledema in hypertension was caused by the raised intracranial pressure. I know of a paper where the authors had two series of patients; one group with papilledema and hypertension and the other one without papilledema and with hypertension. They found that there was a significant rise in the intracranial pressure in patients with papilledema, and there are a few other papers confirming that. But that is not something invariable, as has been shown by other workers. I think one has to look more into the optic disk and the surrounding region rather than the possibility of intracranial hypertension. Incidentally, Dr. Kirkendall, while looking at your angiograms, in one of them I did see that there were filling defects because of the nonfilling of the choroid; so this is a good example of a choroidal pathologic condition in hypertension.

Question: Do the choroidal vessels dilate in retinal artery occlusion?

Dr. Cogan: I don't know whether they do or not.

Dr. Hayreh: I see no reason why there should be choroidal vessel dilatation because the retinal vascular system itself is quite an independent system, unconnected with the choroidal vascular system. I personally would not expect choroidal vessel dilatation; I have done a lot of angiograms in patients with retinal vascular occlusion and have never seen any choroidal abnormality. The only thing that I might mention here, and I think is a worthwhile thing to keep in mind, is that if a patient is over the age of 60 or so (as most of these patients with the central retinal artery occlusion or branch retinal artery occlusion tend to be), there is always the possibility of temporal arteritis being the causative factor. I have just finished analyzing a series of temporal arteritis cases with anterior ischemic optic neuropathy, and I have found that there were some cases who were diagnosed as central retinal artery occlusion, which we in fact associated with anterior ischemic optic neuropathy. According to the latest concept, anterior ischemic optic neuropathy is caused by occlusion of the posterior ciliary arteries; because the whole of the disk is supplied by the posterior ciliary arteries, anything that occludes the posterior ciliary arteries produces anterior ischemic optic neuropathy. In the studies that I did about 12 to 13 years ago I found that up to 40% of cases in human beings had the central retinal artery and one of the major posterior ciliary artery arising by a common trunk from the ophthalmic artery. In patients with central retinal artery occlusion, on doing fluorescein angiography, I could demonstrate the filling defects in the posterior ciliary artery as well as in the central retinal artery, but the ophthalmoscopic appearance was typically that of central retinal artery occlusion, which misled the referring ophthalmologist, and the posterior ciliary artery occlusion and anterior ischemic optic neuropathy were totally missed. Similarly, I had in the same series of cases, what had been diagnosed as branch retinal artery occlusion, which, in fact, was a cilioretinal artery occlusion associated with anterior ischemic optic neuropathy, which was demonstrated on angiography, and was caused by temporal arteritis. So I think as a routine it would be in the interest of the patient to do the erythrocyte sedimentation rate, which doesn't cost very much but can avoid tragedy. Only a month ago I had a patient who went to an ophthalmologist with a loss of vision in one eye, was diagnosed as central retinal artery occlusion, and was told it was hard luck and nothing could be done. Then she had a central retinal artery occlusion in the other eye that ultimately left her totally blind. When we did a temporal artery biopsy, it was positive for temporal arteritis; so this poor lady could have been saved from the tragedy that overtook her, if this had been borne in mind. So, I would very strongly recommend that one should do the erythrocyte sedimentation rate in every patient with central retinal artery occlusion, because even if you catch only a few, it is worth it.

Now, I will give a problem to any member of the panel who would like to attempt it: Outline the treatment for a central or sectoral retinal vein occlusion in the usual patient over 50, seen within 24 hours of the onset and after 2 to 3 weeks from the onset of symptoms. This is a very important problem; after all, to diagnose vascular occlusion is easy, but it is the management that is really still the problem.

Dr. Henkind: You're talking about central retinal or branch vein occlusion, not artery occlusion, right?

Dr. Hayreh: Yes, retinal vein occlusion.

Dr. Henkind: Well, I think that in central retinal vein occlusion the key point is to check if the patient has glaucoma. We have seen more than a few instances where the second eye has obvious evidence of glaucoma and we presume that the first eye also had it. It is interesting, there is a large series out of Scandinavia and a group from Nevada that showed that the eye that sustains a vein occlusion may go into hypotony after the vein occlusion, but these patients started out with a central vein occlusion on the basis of glaucoma. So there are two modes of therapy. One is to protect the second eye, because we have seen vein occlusions develop in the second eye, and then the question is, What do you do in the eye that has had the central retinal vein occlusion? Branch vein occlusion we do not treat unless it is involving of macula. We give it several months with no medical therapy, and then if the occlusion is involving the macula, we may consider photocoagulating it if it has cystic macula edema. From the series presented at the academy this year and some other series I know, there is ample evidence to show that branch vein occlusion can be treated by laser or perhaps gentle light photocoagulation. We have, as you know, George Wise at our institution, and he has written this up with Charlie Campbell. They have had some good results. As far as central retinal vein occlusion is concerned, we are nihilists generally and do not treat these patients. There are reports in the Hungarian literature about all sorts of plasma expanders, and there are reports, basically in the European literature, about anticoagulating these patients. My fear is, from the experience we have had in the past with anticoagulating some of these patients, that some of them come down with kidney bleeds. These are generally older patients who have other systemic disease, and quite frankly I don't feel competent to anticoagulate anybody; if

I do, I send them over to the internists, but in the last 5 years I don't think we have treated one patient medically with any form of anticoagulation. I think we have just followed them. Now, on central retinal vein occlusion there are people who are photocoagulating these patients, but the natural course is so variable that I do not think you can tell which patient is going to do well and which is not. So, maybe someone has a better therapy. We see a lot of vein occlusion, both central and branch. Of course, the great fear in the central retinal vein occlusion is that the patient will go on after 90 days classically to rubeosis. We have had a number of such patients. I have now seen patients with central retinal vein occlusions as young as 16 or 17 years of age. You have to make sure that this is not the entity that Singh Hayreh and others from England have reported, which is not a true central retinal vein occlusion, but an inflammatory process that may or may not respond to steroids, depending on who you believe. The original paper on that by Lyle and Wybar tried to differentiate this different entity. Now I separate the young central retinal vein occlusion from the old one. Do women who take contraceptive pills develop central retinal vein occlusion? The courts say yes; most doctors say no, but I think you had better be responsive to the court opinion on this. It may be that the younger patient does require some therapy, but I don't know whether I would anticoagulate my younger patients, because they have done exceedingly well, I must say, without any therapy.

Participant: We do treatment with streptokinase. It is very important in that case that you work together with a good institute for hematology, but the results seem to be really good if you do not treat patients over 60 years, and only patients who never had brain hemorrhage before, not only brain damage, but also suspected brain vascular occlusion. But I wish to ask this panel if anyone has had experience with this new operating procedure of decompressing the central retinal vein in the optic nerve. We have not yet; we have just begun the use of this technique, but the results of the original investigator himself are really strikingly good. He cut the sclera around the scleral ring of the optic disk, and it seems to me that this is a very logical treatment, so that the blood vessels can dilate, especially in cases when (as Cogan showed) the blood vessels are occluded in the lamina cribrosa.

Dr. Hayreh: Regarding the therapy, from the experience of nearly 100 cases that I have collected, there are now a few things that I feel fairly confident to say. First, regarding surgical treatment, I am aware of that and, in fact, people have talked to me about that since 1965. I cannot believe that it does any good, because what is the size of the vessel? One must take into consideration that, as Dr. Cogan pointed out in the beginning, it is about at a maximum 1 mm. in diameter. Now, if you are going to open a 1 mm. vessel and dilate it and take out the clot, I think that is just about impossible. Secondly, you have to cut through the nerve, and I have manipulated the nerve many times, when opening the sheath of the optic nerve to relieve papilledema or doing orbital manipulation in trying to occlude the various vessels. The optic nerve is very sensitive, even if you strip the pia off it. You

may find you get optic atrophy. So, I think surgery is a fairly theoretical treatment, and you are not likely to get much joy out of it.

Now, coming to the question of central retinal vein occlusion, I personally
believe that one has to consider what the background mechanism is. On
that, I would like to refer to my previous work, where I divided patients
with so-called central retinal vein occlusion into two categories. In fact, I
do not call this condition central retinal vein occlusion, but either venous
stasis retinopathy or hemorrhagic retinopathy, depending on the ophthalmoscopic appearance. In venous stasis retinopathy, the retinal veins are
tremendously engorged, there are a few odd hemorrhages, and these people
usually have very good vision. Some of them are very young patients,
whereas others are old. In the second category, where there is a considerable
loss of vision and lots of hemorrhages, are the cases that I classify as hemorrhagic retinopathy. Hemorrhagic retinopathy, according to my experimental
and clinical evidence, consists of not only the venous block, but also, at the
same time, retinal arterial ischemia. Thus, it is a combination of arterial
ischemia and venous stasis that is responsible for giving that classical picture
the so-called picture of central retinal vein occlusion. Whereas the picture
that represents venous stasis retinopathy, showing good visual acuity, tremendously engorged vessels, and a few hemorrhages, represents pure venous
occlusion without any associated arterial anoxia or ischemia. If one goes to
the literature to estimate the efficacy of anticoagulant treatment, one finds
about 50% of workers saying it gives good results and the other 50% saying
it has bad results. But people have not tried to divide their cases into the
two categories. In fact, I am studying the natural history of the disease. In
the majority of the cases I find that if patients with venous stasis retinopathy
get a small macular hemorrhage right in the center of the macula, this
lowers the visual acuity, but then, as the small hemorrhage clears, the visual
acuity improves again. These patients after a follow-up of 2 to 3 years have
vision of 20/20 or 20/15, and they are the people who would respond
favorably with or without treatment; whereas the patients with hemorrhagic
retinopathy usually do not recover much, and in those cases whatever treatment you give you are going to fail. The only cases whom I have treated,
and still do, are the patients with venous stasis retinopathy who develop
macular edema, because then you find the vision suddenly falls. The peripheral vision is all right, but in the center they have a central scotoma and
poor visual acuity and in my experience they respond dramatically to corticosteroids. In fact, the main thing that is worth keeping in mind in these
cases, and in young patients who come with venous stasis retinopathy, is
that the fundus picture does not show any improvement, but a dramatic
subjective improvement takes place. The patient usually volunteers the information that he is seeing better than he was. You look at the fundus, and
it looks as horrible as it was in the beginning! So the main guiding factor for
me is the subjective improvement and improvement of the visual acuity
and visual fields, rather than the improvement in the ophthalmoscopic appearance. One has to look into the basic pathologic condition to predict
exactly what is going to happen. The central retinal vein and the choroidal

vein anastomose in the prelamina region of the disk, and most of the venous occlusions occur behind the lamina cribrosa. It takes about 2 to 4 months before you really get collateral vessels large enough to shunt the whole retinal blood supply into the choroid. So, if you see these cases, after a few months you find prominent vessels on the disk. These are friendly vessels, and they should never be light coagulated, because this will lead to disaster for the whole eye. Similarly, I have quite a series of young patients with venous occlusion of the venous stasis retinopathy type, and they are the people whom I do not ordinarily treat unless the macula is involved. In that case, I treat them with corticosteroids, and I have a lot of cases who have returned to perfectly normal after treatment with corticosteroids; but this is a treatment that requires being carefully watched, and one should be guided more by the symptomatic relief than by ophthalmoscopy. This, I believe, is where the main fault lies. People look into the fundus, they don't find any improvement from steroids, and they stop the therapy. But if the patient gains a better visual acuity I think that's an important consideration. Mind you, I treat macular edema in these cases and not venous stasis retinopathy, which is a self-limited condition. If macular edema is not treated, the patient will be left with cystic macular degeneration and a central scotoma.

Dr. Ramalho: I want only to add that for 3 years I have done a prospective branch study, not doing anything for central vein thrombosis, and the results are as good as if you treat with anything. Even in the older age group, of course, there are two groups. The young age group may be similar to that reported by Sanders and others in England: they do well. But we find also in the older group, 60 to 70 years of age, that if you do nothing about the central vein thrombosis, after 2½ years the vision is about 18/20 or 16/20. We did this because someone wanted to light coagulate and do other things, but we shall be publishing a full report of the prospective study in about 2 years. One of our patients, in the prospective study, had had central vein thrombosis about 7 years back, and the visual acuity was "hand movements." She is the wife of a doctor, and after several years her vision is now 18/20; so we must be careful what we do. My impression at the present (though we haven't many cases, about 25 cases in nearly 3 years) is that there are cases, perhaps about 80%, that will certainly improve. My other impression is that none of our cases developed glaucoma, and none of them developed rubeosis of the iris.

Dr. Hayreh: I would agree there because I have done a prospective study of central retinal vein occlusion, and the number of people who get glaucoma and rubeosis is very small. I think people tend to be influenced by the distorted fact that most doctors see only those people who get glaucoma. When I took a large series and started analyzing it, I was surprised at the very small number of people who developed rubeosis or its symptoms, as compared to the total number; this is something very surprising.

Let me tell you about another thing that has always bothered me. I ended up in the field of retinal vascular occlusion in a very accidental way. In 1962, I was more interested in producing papilledema in monkeys, and to do that I was blocking the central retinal veins, but I never got any hemorrhages or anything like central retinal vein occlusion. Then one day I accidentally blocked both central retinal artery and vein, and finally I got the hemorrhagic retinopathy—the complete classical picture of so-called central retinal vein occlusion. This excited my interest in the subject. I also found that the side on which I blocked the vessels had a lower intraocular pressure than the normal side, and then I looked back into the literature and found there were a couple of references not mentioning anything but just the intraocular pressure measurement and that the eye in which there was venous occlusion had a lower pressure. Since then Foulds and a lot of other people have come up with a definite proof that the eye with the occlusion near the time of occlusion has a lower intraocular pressure as compared to the other eye. There is a paper, which I think was published in the *British Journal of Ophthalmology* in the mid-1950s, that showed very well that there was a high incidence of glaucoma in these patients, because measuring the intraocular pressure in the normal eye in these patients, they found there was a very high incidence of high intraocular pressure. So perhaps high pressure has some role to play in the pathogenesis, initially by promoting more stasis and thus promoting thrombosis.

Now there is one thing that I would like to know from the internists; I see these patients with retinal vascular occlusion and I send them to the internists for an opinion, and most of them, as you know, have hypertension or arteriosclerosis. How far are they in a position to help us? Are we doing any good to the patient by sending him to the internist, with the cost that is evidently involved? How far are you in a position to help these patients?

Dr. Kirkendall: Well, I am not sure that very much can be done by an internist. From the standpoint of atherosclerosis or nodular arteriosclerosis, which might be the factor behind some of the occlusive processes in the region of the retinal vein and retinal artery, I don't think that much can be done at that point. I think this is really like locking the door after the horse is gone. I do believe that the retinal circulation is a reasonably good place to see nodular arteriosclerosis or atherosclerosis in the area of the disk, and sometimes I think this is a good reflectant of what is going on in the other larger vessels of the individual's body. It may be useful for the ophthalmologist to tell the internist so that, if he has a method to deal with atherosclerosis today, he may apply this information to that patient, or make recommendations, when you see these lesions in his eyes. But after the vein has been occluded, I do not know very much that the internist can do right now.

Dr. Hayreh: A question to Dr. Kearns: Does arteriosclerosis develop in absence of hypertension?

Dr. Kearns: Yes, certainly. There are many situations in man where this has been documented quite well. The question is always whether the individual has had brief periods of hypertension in the past, and we also have the problem of deciding what hypertension is, in terms of actual numbers, but I believe in our society that we must accept the idea that arteriosclerosis in the retinal circulation can occur without overt or obvious hypertension. I believe, on the other hand, that in other societies this is not nearly so often seen, and so one is left with the idea that perhaps in epidemiologic studies we ought to recognize the fact that in the Western world blood pressure tends to rise with age in the population, whereas in most other portions of the world this does not occur. And, perhaps this is simply a reflection of that, and a reflection of the fact that we have more arteriolar disease in our society than in many other areas of the world.

14

Hematologic and reticuloendothelial diseases

Michael C. Brain

Unlike other organ systems the cellular and plasma constituents of the blood subserve distinct and often unrelated physiologic functions. It is not surprising therefore that the ocular manifestations of blood diseases can vary widely depending on the nature of the blood disorder present. In this article the disorders of the blood will be considered in relation to the separate and distinct physiologic functions of the blood rather than in relation to specific hematologic disease entities.

There are three broad physiologic functions performed by the hematologic constituents of the blood:

1. Oxygen delivery by the red cells
2. Cellular and humoral responses to infections by the white cells; granulocytes, monocytes, lymphocytes, and plasma cells
3. Hemostasis provided by the interaction of platelets and the plasma coagulation factors

The disorders of the blood that give rise to diseases of the eye will be considered under the three main physiologic categories listed above. However, one must recognize that because the cellular constituents of the blood, with possible exception of the lymphocytes, arise from a common stem-cell precursor in the bone marrow all the cellular constituents and their related physiologic functions may be affected in disorders of cellular proliferation and differentiation in the bone marrow, such as the leukemias, and by the action of cytotoxic drugs.

OXYGEN DELIVERY BY THE RED CELLS

The transport of oxygen by the red cells to the organs of the body, including the eyes, is determined by factors both influenced and uninfluenced by the blood itself. Indirect factors include adequate oxygenation in the lungs, maintenance of normal cardiac output, and absence of obstruction to blood flow through arteries and arterioles. The factors that influence oxygen transport in the blood itself are changes in hemoglobin concentration, changes in blood viscosity, which influence blood flow through arterioles and capillaries, and changes in the affinity of hemoglobin for oxygen. Only these factors in the blood itself that influence transport of oxygen will be discussed further.

242

Hemoglobin concentration

Severe anemia, irrespective of etiology, has been recognized to cause abnormalities in the optic fundus, superficial retinal edema, cotton-wool spots, Roth spots, capillary microaneurysms, retinal hemorrhages, and, more rarely, papilledema.[27] Although the changes in the retina have been recognized in association with a wide variety of causes of anemia, they correlated most closely with the degree of anemia, are uncommon unless the hemoglobin is less than 7 grams per 100 ml., and are more commonly seen in adults than children.[30] Associated blood disorders such as leukemia or thrombocytopenia predispose to such changes in less anemic patients. It thus seems likely that the principal mechanism for the retinal vascular changes observed is the hypoxia caused by the lowered hemoglobin concentration, because the changes in the optic fundus improve or return to normal when the anemia is corrected either by specific treatment or blood transfusion.

Anemia that may give rise to such retinal changes may be caused by the following:
1. Reduction in red cell formation in the bone marrow because of
   a. Bone marrow aplasia or hypoplasia
   b. Infiltration of the bone marrow by leukemic or other abnormal cells
   c. Failure of erythroid precursor-cell maturation because of the lack of vitamin B_{12} or of folic acid
2. Failure of hemoglobin synthesis because of
   a. Iron deficiency
   b. Inherited defects of globin chain synthesis (thalassemia major)
3. Acute or chronic blood loss
4. Congenital or acquired hemolytic anemia

These causes of anemia can be fairly readily differentiated from the information derived from a complete blood count, examination of the morphology of red cells in the peripheral blood, assessment of the cellularity and morphologic appearances of the bone marrow aspirate biopsy, recognition of leukemia or causes of marrow infiltration, or hypoplasia, and the results of more specific tests of megaloblastic anemia, of hemolytic anemia, or of disturbances of hemoglobin structure or synthesis. It must be recognized that the nutritional anemias that arise from specific vitamin deficiencies may rarely, as in the case of vitamin B_{12}, give rise to optic atrophy, because of the effect of the deficiency on neural function rather than from the consequences of anemia.[18]

Blood viscosity

Oxygen delivery by the red cells will be impaired if, despite a normal hemoglobin concentration, the flow of red cells through the microcirculation is reduced by an increase in the viscosity of the blood. An increase in blood viscosity may come about through changes in either the cellular or plasma constituents of the blood. The viscosity of normal blood is remarkably low despite the high proportion of red cells of which it is constituted. This property is attributable to the behavior of the red cells as "fluid drops" rather than as solid particles.[15] Nevertheless, the viscosity of blood does rise when the total red cell count or hematocrit rises significantly above the normal values, as in polycythemia.[17] The increase in blood viscosity associated with polycythemia in all probability accounts for the retinal vein engorgement long recognized to accompany this disorder. The increase in blood viscosity probably also accounts for the increased incidence of retinal vein thrombosis in this disorder.

The viscosity of whole blood is also influenced by the proportion of white cells present, the white cells having an inherently higher viscosity than do the red cells.[17, 50] The increase in blood viscosity attributable to high white cell counts, particularly when the proportion of immature white cells is increased, may be an important contributory factor in the development of retinal changes in patients with acute or chronic leukemias.

The viscosity of blood is also profoundly influenced by the relative proportions of large molecular weight plasma proteins present and is increased with elevations of IgM immunoglobulins in macroglobulinemia and less commonly IgG in multiple myeloma.

Abnormal red cells and blood viscosity

Loss of deformability of the red cells is accompanied by both an increase in viscosity and impairment of blood flow through microcapillaries. Deformability is reduced as a result of loss of red cell membrane relative to red cell volume in spherocytic hemolytic anemia whether caused by hereditary spherocytosis or appearing in acquired (autoimmune) hemolytic anemia in which partial phagocytosis of the antibody-coated surface leads to membrane loss.[33] However, it is uncertain whether the retinal changes observed in these disorders are caused by the anemia or the alterations in capillary flow.

The loss of red cell deformability and changes in blood viscosity from alterations in the structure or stability of the hemoglobin within the red cell are more clearly related to the optic changes. Increases in blood viscosity and loss of deformability account for the clinical and hematologic features of patients with sickle-cell disease, hemoglobin SS disease, or hemoglobin SC disease and patients with homozygous hemoglobin C.[16, 26, 34] A variety of specific retinal changes have been recognized in patients with sickle-cell disease[25, 51] and SC disease[13, 32, 51] and more rarely in patients with sickle-cell trait and sickle cell–thalassemia disease.[24] These changes include angioid streaks,[23, 37] retinal hemorrhages, peripheral retinal vascular occlusions with new vessel formation, more rarely polar or choroidal arterial or arteriolar occlusions,[1, 14] and glaucoma.[7] Specific changes have been observed in scleral and conjunctival blood vessels[46] and have been correlated with the proportion of irreversibly sickled cells in the peripheral blood in sickle-cell anemia. The severity of the retinal changes in sickle cell–thalassemia disease has been related to the severity of the disorder and the proportion of hemoglobin A present.[24]

The specific hemoglobin disorder encountered can be diagnosed by hemoglobin electrophoresis, after carrying out a screening sickling test. At present no satisfactory treatment is available for the prevention of the vaso-occlusive crises that characterize sickle-cell disease. Treatment with urea has been shown to be ineffective.[6] The modification of deoxygenation of hemoglobin by carbamylation by the use of cyanate compounds, although effective when used in vitro,[11, 45] may be accompanied by undue toxicity in vivo. Currently the best available treatment appears to be the use of intravenous fluids and other measures to lower blood viscosity, and the treatment of associated infections and other general measures.

Blood viscosity and abnormal plasma proteins

Increase in blood viscosity accompanies the rise in IgM macroglobulin in Waldenström's macroglobulinemia and high levels of IgG in patients with multiple myeloma.[8, 22, 49] The retinal vascular changes in these disorders[2, 4, 5, 10, 39] appear to be directly related to the increase in blood viscosity and improve with the reduction in the concentration of plasma proteins by plasmapheresis[44] or by control of the disease with cytotoxic chemotherapy. The extent of the hemorrhagic manifestations observed in the retina and elsewhere may also reflect the influence of the macroglobulins and myeloma proteins on platelet aggregation and on fibrin formation and polymerization.[12, 35, 36, 38, 42] Thus, in certain patients a hyperviscosity syndrome may also be accompanied by a defect of hemostasis.

The abnormal plasma proteins that can give rise to a "hyperviscosity" syndrome may be diagnosed by demonstration of a monoclonal peak in electrophoresis of serum, by the demonstration of a single class of light chains in the abnormal protein, by the finding of free light chains in the serum or urine (Bence Jones protein), and by the presence of abnormal numbers and morphology of plasma cells in the bone marrow. Apart from the retinal changes, infiltration of the bones of the orbit or retro-orbital structures by plasma cell tumors can involve the optic nerve, extraocular muscles, and other structures in the orbit. The impaired immune response in chronic disorders involving the immunoglobins can also result in chronic infections that may affect the eye and orbital contents.

WHITE CELLS AND EYE DISEASE

Granulocytopenia whether from hypoplastic anemia, leukemia, or intensive cytotoxic chemotherapy predisposes patients to bacterial infections that may involve the eye, usually as a sequel to systemic infections. The increase in the white cell count seen in early untreated acute or chronic leukemia, possibly through an influence on blood viscosity,[50] can give rise to retinal manifestations, microaneurysms,[20] exudates and hemorrhage, or leukemic infiltration.[3, 9] Leukemic infiltration may involve the optic nerve,[19] retina, choroid, or periorbital structures. Infiltration of the meninges may give rise to papilledema or extraocular palsies.[28, 47] These late manifestations of leukemia are being encountered more frequently because of the longer survival achieved by intensive chemotherapy and because of the failure of many of the drugs used to induce remission of leukemia to cross the blood-brain barrier. In children with acute lymphocytic leukemia, irradiation of the skull and vertebral column together with intrathecal methotrexate has been successful in preventing the development of meningeal leukemia once a hematologic remission has been induced.[29]

DISORDERS OF HEMOSTASIS AND EYE DISEASE

Normal hemostasis is dependent on both normal numbers of circulating platelets and the presence of normal function of the coagulation factors to produce a stable fibrin clot. Defects of hemostasis can thus arise from reduction in the platelet count or through congenital or acquired disorders of the normal coagulation pathway.

Platelets

Thrombocytopenia leads to spontaneous purpura and prolonged bleeding in response to trauma. Severe thrombocytopenia may be accompanied by retinal hemorrhage,[43] but this is more commonly seen when there is an associated hematologic abnormality, such as anemia, leukemia, or hyperviscosity syndrome. Serious degrees of thrombocytopenia may require treatment with platelet transfusions, but such transfusions are of only temporary benefit, and treatment should be directed at the underlying hematologic disorder giving rise to thrombocytopenia.

The formation of platelet aggregates on atheromatous plaques in the carotid arteries may give rise to platelet emboli that can enter the cerebral circulation,[41] causing transient cerebral ischemic attacks, and can enter the retinal arteries, causing amaurosis fugax.[40] Similar changes have been observed in association with the thrombocytosis accompanying polycythemia rubra vera.[48]

The use of drugs that inhibit platelet aggregation, notably sulfinpyrazone (Anturan) in a dose of 800 mg. daily has been accompanied by a reduction in the incidence of these episodes in a double-blind controlled trial[21]; aspirin has also been used successfully.[31]

Coagulation disorders and the eye

Congenital disorders of coagulation such as hemophilia rarely give rise to spontaneous bleeding into the eye or periorbital structures. Patients with hemophilia and other rarer disorders from congenital deficiencies of coagulation factors and patients on anticoagulants will bleed as the result of accidental trauma or surgical operations involving the eye or orbital structures. Any patient who gives a history of abnormal bleeding tendency should undergo full investigation to identify the nature of the coagulation defect before surgery is undertaken. The availability of factor VIII concentrates to correct the deficiency state and the use of such material, both preoperatively and for a minimum of 8 days postoperatively, should enable surgery to be performed without serious hemorrhagic complications. The investigation and management of patients with both congenital and acquired coagulation disorders undergoing elective surgery or with posttraumatic ocular hemorrhage necessitate close collaboration with a hematology service able to carry out the appropriate investigations and the monitoring of the effectiveness of replacement therapy.

THE EYE AND RETICULOENDOTHELIAL DISEASES

The eye may be involved as a manifestation of the reticuloendothelioses (Hand-Schüller-Christian disease and Letterer-Siwe disease) because of the involvement of periorbital structures by histocytic infiltrations. The lipid-storage diseases—Gaucher's disease and Niemann-Pick disease—although accompanied by typical lipid-loaded reticulum cells in the bone marrow, are perhaps more appropriately considered as inborn errors of metabolism that secondarily affect the reticuloendothelial system, rather than as primarily hematologic disorders.

REFERENCES

1. Acacio, I., and Goldberg, M. F.: Peripapillary and macular vessel occlusions in sickle cell anemia, Am. J. Ophthalmol. **75:**861-866, 1973.
2. Ackerman, A. L.: The ocular manifestations of Waldenström's macroglobulinemia and its treatment, Arch. Ophthalmol. **67:**701-707, 1962.
3. Allen, R. A., and Straatsma, B. R.: Ocular involvement in acute leukemia and allied disorders, Arch. Ophthalmol. **66:**490-508, 1961.
4. Andersson, B., and Samuelson, A.: A case of hyperglobulinemia with pronounced eye changes and acrocyanosis, Acta Med. Scand. **117:**248-260, 1944.
5. Ashton, N.: Ocular changes in multiple myelomatosis, Arch. Ophthalmol. **73:**487-494, 1965.
6. Bensinger, T. A., Mahmood, L., Conrad, M. E., and McCurdy, P. R.: The effect of oral urea administration on red cell survival in sickle cell disease, Am. J. Med. Sci. **264:** 283-287, 1972.
7. Boniuk, M., and Burton, G. L.: Unilateral glaucoma associated with sickle cell retinopathy, Trans. Am. Acad. Ophthalmol. Otolaryngol. **68:**316-328, 1964.
8. Bloch, K. J., and Maki, D. G.: Hyperviscosity syndromes associated with immunogloblin abnormalities, Semin. Hematol. **10:**113-124, 1973.
9. Borgeson, E. J., and Wagener, H.P.: Changes in the eye in leukemia, Am. J. Med. Sci. **177:**663-676, 1929.
10. Carr, R. E., and Henkind, P.: Retinal findings associated with serum viscosity, Am. J. Ophthalmol. **56:**22-31, 1963.
11. Cerami, A.: Cyanate as an inhibitor of red cell sickling, New Eng. J. Med. **287:**807-812, 1972.
12. Cohen, I., Amir, J., Ben-Shaul, Y., Pick, A., and de Vries, A.: Plasma cell myeloma associated with an unusual myeloma protein causing impairment of fibrin aggregation and platelet function in a patient with multiple malignancy, Am. J. Med. **48:**766-776, 1970.
13. Condon, P. I., and Serjeant, G. R.: Ocular findings in hemoglobin SC disease in Jamaica, Am. J. Ophthalmol. **74:**921-931, 1972.
14. Condon, P. I., Serjeant, G. R., and Ikeda, H.: Unusual choroidal retinal degeneration in sickle cell disease. Possible sequele of posterior ciliary vessel occlusion, Br. J. Ophthalmol. **57:**81-88,1973.
15. Dintenfass, L.: Molecular and rheological considerations of the red cell membrane in view of the internal fluidity of the red cell, Acta Haematol. **32:**299-313, 1964.
16. Dintenfass, L.: Rheology of packed red blood cells containing hemoglobin A-A, S-A and S-S, J. Lab. Clin. Med. **64:**594-600, 1964.
17. Dintenfass, L.: Viscosity of packed red and white blood cells, Exp. Mol. Pathol. **4:**597-605, 1965.
18. Ellis, P. P., and Hamilton, H.: Retrobulbar neuritis in pernicious anemia, Am. J. Ophthalmol. **48:**95-97, 1959.
19. Ellis, W., and Little, H. L.: Leukemic infiltration of the optic nerve head, Am. J. Ophthalmol. **75:**868-871, 1973.
20. Duke, J. R., Wilkinson, C. P., and Sigelman, S.: Retinal microaneurysms in leukemia, Br. J. Ophthalmol. **52:**368-374, 1965.
21. Evans, G.: Effect of drugs that suppress platelet surface interaction on incidence of amaurosis fugax and transient cerebral ischemia, Surg. Forum **23:**239-241, 1972.
22. Fahey, J. L., Barth, W. F., and Solomon, A.: Serum hyperviscosity syndromes, J.A.M.A. **192:** 464-467, 1965.
23. Geeraets, W. J., and Guerry, D., III.: Angioid streaks and sickle cell disease, Am. J. Ophthalmol. **49:**450-467, 1960.
24. Goldberg, M. F., Charache, S., and Acacio, I.: Ophthalmic manifestations of sickle cell thalassemia, Arch. Intern. Med. **128:**33-39, 1971.
25. Goodman, G., Von Sallmann, L., and Holland, M. G.: Ocular manifestations of sickle cell disease, Arch. Ophthalmol. **58:**655-682, 1957.

26. Ham, T. H., Dunn, R. F., Sayre, R. W. and Murphy, J. R.: Physical properties of red cells as related to effects in vivo. I. Increased rigidity of red cells as measured by viscosity of cells altered by chemical fixation, sickling and hypertonicity, Blood **32**:847-861, 1968.

27. Holt, J. M., and Gordon-Smith, E. C.: Retinal abnormalities in diseases of the blood, Br. J. Ophthalmol. **203**:145-160, 1969.

28. Hyman, C. B., Bogle, J. M., Brubaker, C. A., Williams, K., and Hammond, D.: Central nervous system involvement of leukemia in children. I. Relation to systemic leukemia, Blood **25**:1-12, 1965.

29. Medical Research Council: Treatment of acute lymphoblastic leukemia: Effect of "prophylactic" therapy against central nervous system leukemia, Br. Med. J. **2**:381-384, 1973.

30. Merin, S., and Freund, M.: Retinopathy in severe anemia, Am. J. Ophthalmol. **66**:1102-1106, 1968.

31. Mundall, J., Quintero, P., Von Kaulla, K. N., Harmon, R., and Austin, J.: Transient monocular blindness and increased platelet aggregability treated with aspirin, Neurology **22**:280-285, 1972.

32. Munro, S., and Walker, C.: Ocular manifestations of sickle cell hemoglobin C disease, Br. J. Ophthalmol. **44**:1-24, 1960.

33. Murphy, J. R.: The influence of pH and temperature on some physical properties of normal erythrocytes and erythrocytes from patients with hereditary spherocytosis, J. Lab. Clin. Med. **69**:758-775, 1967.

34. Murphy, J. R.: Hemoglobin CC disease: Rheological properties of erythrocytes and abnormalities in cell water, J. Clin. Invest. **47**:1483-1495, 1968.

35. Nilsson, I. M., and Wenckert, A.: Hyperglobulinemia as a cause of hemophilia-like disease, Blood **8**:1067-1077, 1953.

36. Pachter, M. R., Johnson, S. A., and Basinski, D. H.: The effect of macroglobulins and their dissociation units on release of platelet factor 3, Thromb. Diath. Haemorrh. **3**:501-509, 1959.

37. Paton, D.: Angioid streaks and sickle cell anemia, Arch. Ophthalmol. **62**:852-858, 1959.

38. Perkins, H. A., MacKenzie, M. R., and Fudenberg, H. H.: Hemostatic defects in dysproteinemias, Blood **35**:695-707, 1970.

39. Rosen, E. S., Simmons, A. V., and Warnes, T. W.: Retinopathy of Waldenström's macroglobulinemia. Photographic assessment, Am. J. Ophthalmol. **65**:696-706, 1968.

40. Ross Russell, R. W.: Observations on the retinal blood vessels in monocular blindness, Lancet **2**:1422-1428, 1961.

41. Ross Russell, R. W.: The source of retinal emboli, Lancet **2**:789-792, 1968.

42. Rozenberg, M. C., and Dintenfass, L.: Platelet aggregation in Waldenström's macroglobulinemia, Thromb. Diath. Haemorrh. **14**:202-208, 1965.

43. Rubenstein, R. A., Yanoff, M., and Albert, D. M.: Thrombocytopenia, anemia and retinal hemorrhage, Am. J. Ophthalmol. **65**:435-438, 1968.

44. Schwab, P. J., Okun, E., and Fahey, J. L.: Reversal of retinopathy in Waldenström's macroglobulinemia by plasmapheresis, Arch. Ophthalmol. **64**:515-521, 1960.

45. Segel, G. B., Feig, S. A., Mentzer, W. C., McCaffrey, R. P., Wells, R., Bunn, H. F., Shohet S. B., and Nathan, D. G.: Effects of urea and cyanate on sickling in vitro, New Eng. J. Med. **287**:59-64, 1972.

46. Serjeant, G. R., Serjeant, B. E., and Condon, P. I.: The conjunctival sign in sickle cell anemia: A relationship with irreversibly sickled cells, J.A.M.A. **219**:1428-1431, 1972.

47. Shaw, R. K., Moore, E. W., Friereich, E. J., and Thomas, L. B.: Meningeal leukemia, Neurology **10**:823-833, 1960.

48. Singer, G.: Migrating emboli of retinal arteries in polycythemia, Br. J. Ophthalmol. **53**:279-283, 1969.

49. Somer, T.: The viscosity of blood, plasma and serum in dys- and paraproteinemia, Acta Med. Scand. (Suppl.) **456**:1-97, 1966.

50. Stephens, D. J.: Relation of viscosity of blood to leucocyte count with particular reference to chronic myelogenous leukemia, Proc. Soc. Exp. Biol. Med. **35**:251-256, 1936-1937.

51. Welch, R. B., and Goldberg, M. F.: Sickle cell hemoglobin and its relation to fundus abnormality, Arch. Ophthalmol. **75**:353-362, 1966.

ADDITIONAL READINGS

Chester, E. M.: The ocular fundus in systemic disease; a clinical pathological correlation, Chicago, 1973, Year Book Medical Publishers, Inc.

Williams, W. J., Beutler, E., Erslev, A. J., and Rundles, R. W., editors: Hematology, New York, 1972, McGraw-Hill Book Co.

Wise, G. N., Dollery, C. T., and Henkind, P.: The retinal circulation, New York, 1971, Harper & Row, Publishers.

15

Hematologic and reticuloendothelial diseases and their relation to the eye

Malcolm N. Luxenberg

The eye offers a unique opportunity for examination of various normal and abnormal processes as they are occurring in the living individual. No where else can one directly observe portions of the vascular and nervous systems so well. This symposium is a testimonial to the important relationship between the eye and systemic disease. As one might suspect, it is impossible to address oneself to all hematologic and reticuloendothelial diseases and their ocular manifestations. Therefore, only the entities where the eye findings may play an important role in diagnosis and treatment will be emphasized. Ocular manifestations are sometimes the first evidence of an underlying hematologic or other systemic disease, and with a careful history and examination a tentative diagnosis can sometimes be made.[54] Early recognition of these problems is becoming more important as many previously untreatable or fatal diseases can now be successfully treated and sometimes cured.

HYPERVISCOSITY SYNDROME

Dilated, tortuous retinal vessels can occur as the result of ocular disease but are probably more frequently seen in association with systemic abnormalities. Hematologic diseases, especially those that produce hyperviscosity, are a common etiology.[11, 60] The differential diagnosis should include diseases causing serum hyperviscosity. Among these are macroglobulinemia,[104] multiple myeloma,[55] and occasionally Hodgkin's disease and other lymphomas when associated with dysproteinemias.

The serum hyperviscosity syndrome is most frequently seen with macroglobulinemia. The increased frequency of elevated serum viscosity with macroglobulinemia as compared to other hyperglobulinemias may be related to the IgM molecule, which has a molecular weight of about 1 million and other characteristics that provide a disposition towards a higher intrinsic viscosity. The viscosity elevation is aided by the fact that about 80% of the IgM molecules are located within the intravascular compartment as compared to about 40% for IgG and

250

albumin. In multiple myeloma hyperviscosity is most often caused by high molecular weight polymers of IgG or IgA paraprotein. Hyperviscosity occurs much less commonly with the other entities mentioned above.

Ocular changes seen with the hyperviscosity syndrome are essentially the same regardless of the underlying cause. The initial abnormality is dilation of the retinal veins, and as distension progresses, they may become tortuous. Dilation of retinal arteries also occurs but is less severe and often hard to visualize. The next stage is constriction at arteriovenous crossings, which produce a beading or sausage-like effect; and occlusion of veins, especially smaller ones, can occur. Retinal hemorrhages of varying size, both superficial and deep, are often seen scattered throughout the fundus. Capillary microaneurysms, exudates, and cotton-wool spots are occasionally found. In advanced stages it may be difficult to differentiate this from papilledema or central retinal vein occlusion. Dilation and increased tortuosity of the conjunctival vessels may also be present.

Concurrent with the eye changes there may be systemic signs and symptoms such as bleeding, vertigo, ataxia, headaches, and cardiac failure associated with the hyperviscosity. Normal serum viscosity relative to water is 1.4 to 1.8. Symptoms have not been reported with a viscosity of less than 4, whereas some patients may have no symptoms even with a viscosity of 8 or 10. Each patient appears to have his own symptomatic threshold. In addition the organ systems affected and their order of involvement varies from patient to patient.[31]

The etiology of the vascular changes, such as dilation, is not fully understood but is probably related to sludging and slowing of the blood flow with increased lateral pressure on the vessels, especially thin-walled veins. Anoxia, expanded plasma volume and other factors such as the high metabolic rate and oxygen demand of the retina and resistance to venous outflow at the lamina cribrosa may also play a role.

It is important to diagnose these diseases early since the symptoms can often be relieved and complications prevented by plasmapheresis, chemotherapy, or other treatment (Fig. 15-1). Plasmapheresis can be carried out indefinitely with minimal risk. Treatment can be given on a symptomatic basis or by following serum protein and viscosity levels.

Experimental hyperviscosity retinopathy has been produced in monkeys by use of high molecular weight dextran.[65] Most of the typical fundus abnormalities, including dilated vessels, hemorrhage, and microaneurysms seen clinically were observed experimentally. The latter have also been demonstrated on trypsin digest mounts of the retinas from these animals (Fig. 15-2).

Multiple myeloma can affect the eye in various ways, both intraocularly and extraocularly. It can directly invade the orbit,[87] surrounding bones, eyelids, lacrimal sac and gland, conjunctiva, and optic nerve[46] with varying symptoms. Ocular involvement[99] includes crystalline deposits in the cornea,[4, 34, 80, 82] infiltration of tumor into iris, choroid, retina[28] and sclera, retinal detachment, pars plana cysts,[5, 33, 51, 52, 98, 109] dilation and tortuosity of the retinal vessels, retinal hemorrhage, and microaneurysms.

Similar findings may occur with blood hyperviscosity that is caused by an increase in the formed elements of the blood as is seen in polycythemia (common) and leukemia (rare). Other fairly common entities to consider as causes of retinal

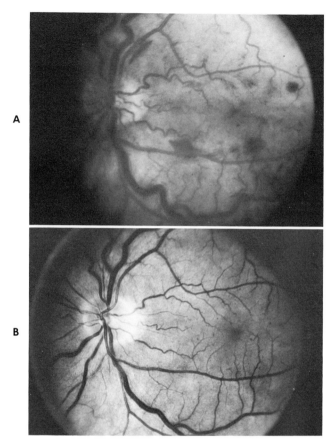

Fig. 15-1. Hyperviscosity syndrome with dilation and tortuosity of retinal vessels, hemorrhages, and microaneurysms. **A,** Before plasmapheresis. **B,** After plasmapheresis.

vessel tortuosity are sickle-cell disease, diabetes mellitus, central retinal vein occlusion, and papilledema.

DISEASES OF LYMPHOID TISSUE

Diseases of lymphoid tissue vary widely in their histologic and clinical manifestations. They range from benign lesions such as lymphoid hyperplasia and pseudotumor of the orbit to malignant lesions such as lymphosarcoma, reticulum cell sarcoma, Hodgkin's disease, and others.* They may be localized to ocular structures or can be widespread throughout the body, with the eye findings being the initial or primary abnormality. Almost any ocular or orbital tissue can be involved. One of the most frequent presentations, especially for lymphomas, is the observation of a firm pink mass in the inferior cul-de-sac or perilimbal region. Pseudotumor of the orbit is also one of the more common forms and may present as a localized or diffuse mass, with or without swelling, tenderness, or exophthalmos[8] and may respond to systemic steroid treatment. Posterior uveitis with or with-

*See references 8, 22, 27, 62, 72, 73, 77, 94, 101, 106, and 108.

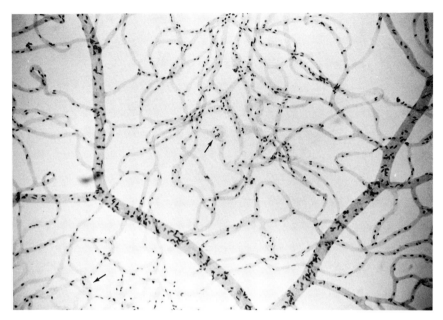

Fig. 15-2. Experimental hyperviscosity syndrome in rhesus monkey. Microaneurysms *(arrows)* seen on trypsin digest mount of retina. (Courtesy Dr. Frederick A. Mausolf, Iowa City, Iowa.)

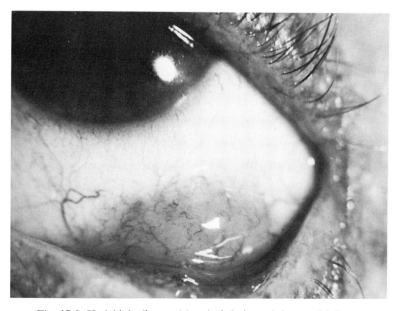

Fig. 15-3. Hodgkin's disease. Mass in inferior cul-de-sac of left eye.

out clinical evidence of direct involvement of the retina or choroid has been reported in association with reticulum cell sarcoma of the brain and may be the initial manifestation of the disease.[76] Benign lymphoid hyperplasia may present as diffuse involvement of the uveal tract, which can be misdiagnosed as a malignant intraocular tumor.[26, 96]

Other forms of lymphoma can invade the lids or orbit producing swelling and exophthalmos. I have treated an elderly female patient in whom the first manifestation of recurrence of a malignant lymphoma, treated 5 years previously, was tearing, with associated swelling of the medial canthal region caused by lymphomatous involvement of the lacrimal sac.

Hodgkin's disease causes most of the same ocular abnormalities as the other lymphomas (Fig. 15-3). In addition there have been reports of retinal vasculitis and severe destruction of the retina in association with Hodgkin's disease.[56] The mechanism is not known, but the possibility of a leukoencephalopathy or toxic reaction has been suggested.

LEUKEMIA

Leukemia can involve all ocular structures either focally or diffusely but is uncommon in nonvascular tissue such as the cornea, lens, and vitreous.* The vascular choroid is most frequently involved with infiltrates, especially in its posterior portion, and hemorrhage is a frequent and probably the most serious complication. The hemorrhages vary in shape and size, can be deep or superficial, and occur anywhere throughout the fundus but are more frequent in the posterior pole (Fig. 15-4, *A*). White centers in the hemorrhages are often seen and are usually caused by accumulations of white cells (Fig. 15-4, *B*). These resemble so called Roth spots. Retinal infarcts manifested as cotton-wool spots may also occur. Dilated tortuous veins probably caused by hyperviscosity are often present and can be an early manifestation of the disease. Pale, broad, fuzzy, whitish lines distributed along vessels may be seen and, when present, strongly suggest the diagnosis of leukemia (Fig. 15-4, *C*). Perivascular infiltration and nodule formation in the retina can occur.[57] Diffuse mottling and clumping of the retinal pigment epithelium, primarily in the posterior fundus, of undetermined etiology has been reported.[13, 50] It is possible that the pigment changes are a nonspecific response from vascular insufficiency of the posterior pole of the eye.[19, 48]

Peripheral retinal neovascularization resembling that seen in the hemoglobinopathies has been observed in chronic myelogenous leukemia with very high white cell counts.[35, 71] These cases had hyperviscosity, which was believed to play an etiologic role possibly through the production of chronic anoxia. Disk edema, either unilateral or bilateral, has been reported and can be the result of direct invasion of the nerve or surrounding tissues or secondary to increased intracranial pressure.[30, 84, 114] Central serous retinopathy and detachment of the retina have also been observed.[9, 114]

Ocular changes are most commonly seen in the acute leukemias. However, there is still controversy regarding the incidence of fundus changes as related to the number of white blood cells, platelets, and red blood cells.

*See references 3, 6, 10, 61, 83, and 112.

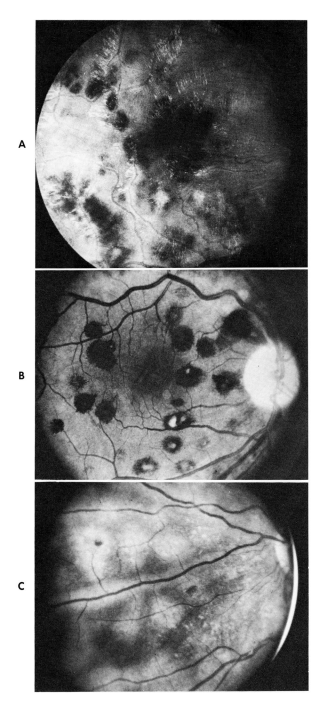

Fig. 15-4. A, Leukemia. Hemorrhages in posterior fundus. **B,** Leukemia. Hemorrhages with white centers resembling "Roth spots." **C,** Leukemia. Perivascular white lines. (**B** Courtesy Mr. Johnny Justice, Houston, Texas.)

POLYCYTHEMIA

Ocular abnormalities occur frequently with polycythemia, especially the primary form. It has been estimated that as many as 80% of these patients may have visual disturbances. The conjunctival vessels may be diffusely engorged resembling conjunctivitis, and the state of engorgement usually varies as a function of the red blood cell count. The fundus appears deeply red or cyanotic in all areas, and there is often associated tortuosity and dilation of the veins, with lesser involvement of the arteries (Fig. 15-5). Deep and superficial hemorrhages often occur, papilledema may be present, and central retinal vein thrombosis is a well-known complication.[89] The fundus changes are not usually seen until the red blood cell level reaches at least 6 million.

SICKLE-CELL DISEASE

Sickle-cell anemia, with its attendant complications throughout the body including the eyes, is a major health problem. Abnormal hemoglobins are present in about 10% of American Negroes. Approximately 8% have the sickle-cell trait (AS), 0.4% have sickle-cell anemia (SS), and 0.2% have sickle cell–hemoglobin C disease (SC). The initial symptoms and signs may be ocular, and it is therefore important for one to be aware of the abnormalities that take place.*

Conjunctival findings in this disorder have been described for many years.†They consist of numerous, short, comma-shaped segments of capillaries that seem to be isolated from the rest of the vascular network. These changes are found on the bulbar conjunctiva particularly in areas where it is covered by the lids and are most common in the inferior fornix. They are seen most frequently with SS disease (96%), less often with SC disease (80%), and rarely with the other

*See references 16, 17, 18, 42, 44, 45, and 75.
†See references 15, 32, 36, 69, and 81.

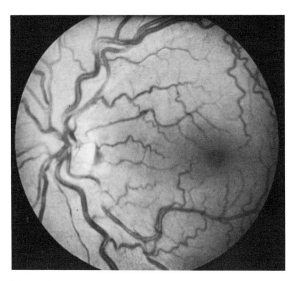

Fig. 15-5. Polycythemia. Dilation and tortuosity of retinal vessels.

hemoglobinopathies. Recent information suggests a relationship between the number of irreversibly sickled cells and the severity of conjunctival vessel abnormality.[101] The mechanism by which sickling may be associated with changes in the conjunctival vessels is uncertain.

Fundus abnormalities occur primarily with SS and SC disease and the manifestations of each vary somewhat.[58, 88, 110] Most of the changes are seen in the middle to peripheral retina. Ocular abnormalities occur much less frequently in the other hemoglobinopathies. Significant venous tortuosity is said to occur in 47% of patients with SS disease. In addition, this group has frequent black disk-shaped scars referred to as "black sunbursts," vascular occlusions (especially arterial), and scattered deposits of refractile material that probably represent

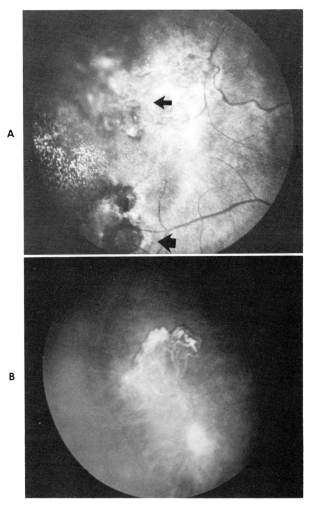

Fig. 15-6. A, Sickle cell disease. "Black sunburst" *(lower arrow)*, "refractile deposits" in retina, "sea fan" with hemorrhages *(upper arrow),* and chorioretinal scarring. **B,** Sickle cell disease. "Sea fan."

old, resorbed hemorrhage in the retina (Fig. 15-6, *A*). Retinitis proliferans is uncommon in SS disease, but occurs in the majority of patients with SC disease. The most typical manifestation of this is the so-called sea fan (Fig. 15-6, *B*). Vascular occlusions and refractile retinal deposits are common, but black sunburst scars occur infrequently. In 1971 Goldberg[10] classified the sequence of events taking place in the fundus of patients with SC disease. In stage 1 peripheral anteriolar occlusions occur, whereas in stage 2 peripheral arteriolar-venular anastomoses are seen. Neovascular and fibrous proliferations take place in stage 3, and in stage 4 vitreous hemorrhage occurs. Lastly, in stage 5 there is detachment of the retina.

With increasing awareness of the hemoglobinopathies and better diagnostic techniques, such as stereoscopic examination of the retina with high magnification and fluorescein angiography, it is becoming apparent that fine-vessel occlusions are occurring in other areas of the eye, especially at the posterior pole around the disk and macula and also in the iris.* Symptoms related to these occlusions vary, and they can be overlooked without careful study. Occlusions of this type with little or no visible change on routine examination may account for some of the cases of unexplained visual loss associated with this disease.

It has recently been recognized that patients with various forms of sickle-cell disease may develop ischemia of the eye during ocular surgery.[29, 95] This is seen most frequently after retinal detachment surgery and may present as anterior segment necrosis with a soft eye, a thickened edematous cornea with folds in Descemet's membrane, iris necrosis, anterior uveitis, and cataract. It is important that the surgeon be aware of this potential complication.

Many of these lesions, especially the areas of abnormal vessels, can be successfully treated and the course of events halted before severe vitreous hemorrhage or detachment of the retina takes place. The most common modes of local ocular treatment are photocoagulation with either the xenon arc or argon laser and cryotherapy.[39, 41] There is currently no proved method of systemic treatment. However, exchange transfusions may be beneficial especially in preventing fine vascular occlusions.[102] Urea and potassium cyanate are of questionable clinical value.[23-25] Patients undergoing ocular surgery, especially retinal detachment procedures, should be kept well oxygenated, and in some cases preoperative exchange transfusions may be indicated to prevent ocular ischemia and anterior segment necrosis. Patients should be warned of the potential hazards of living at high altitudes, flying in nonpressurized aircraft, and ocular trauma.[20, 68]

ANEMIA

Retinal hemorrhage attributable to anemia is frequent, though ophthalmologists do not see many of these cases because of the lack of severe ocular symptoms or decreased vision.[63, 67, 91] The hemorrhages of various shapes, sizes, and numbers can occur anywhere in the fundus but tend to spare the macula with preservation of vision. The level of anemia at which ocular hemorrhage occurs is quite variable between individuals. The incidence of retinal hemorrhage increases when the hemoglobin is less than 5 gm.%, and above 8 gm.% it seems to be infrequent.

*See references 1, 37, 43, 53, 93, and 103.

The incidence and number of hemorrhages significantly increases when there is a concomitant decrease in the platelets, especially below 50,000. The platelet abnormality may be qualitative as well as quantitative. In addition to hemorrhages, one can see exudates and edema of the optic nerve head. The hemorrhages may be caused by anoxia, platelet dysfunction, or possibly viscosity changes, and in many cases they are probably the result of a combination of these factors.

The etiology of anemia is variable and ocular hemorrhages can probably be seen with anemia of any type although the frequency of its occurrence may vary depending on the etiology. The most common cause of anemic ocular hemorrhage is probably leukemia since it decreases both the hemoglobin and platelets and may also affect the viscosity.

COAGULATION DISORDERS

Abnormal platelet aggregation, although not well known to the ophthalmologist, can produce ocular disease, usually as a result of emboli to the retinal vessels.

Platelet emboli are less frequently observed than those composed of calcium or cholesterol.[49, 93] They are white and nonreflective, appear to be the same size as the blood column, and are highly mobile, which probably accounts for their infrequent visualization. They produce the same signs and symptoms as do other types of emboli and frequently cause monocular ischemic attacks, which are manifested as brief episodes of decreased vision or blindness in one eye. These episodes often come and go like the lowering and raising of a windowshade. During an attack one may see ocular changes such as vascular spasm, emboli, hemorrhages, or retinal ischemia, whereas in between attacks the eye examination is usually normal. It is obviously important for one to carefully question patients with apparent monocular ischemic attacks, and if they are believed to be of embolic origin, platelet-survival studies and other appropriate tests should be performed. Careful examination of the heart and large vessels such as the carotids should be done to rule out possible sources of emboli. If shortened platelet survival is present, treatment with either aspirin or dipyridamole (Persantin) can be tried, as both of these agents decrease platelet aggregation.

In the mid-1960s ophthalmologists became concerned about the possible relationship between oral contraceptives and certain neuro-ophthalmic disorders.[12, 64, 98, 108] Two of the main problems are migrane or vascular heaches and vertebrobasilar insufficiency, which may occur in a younger age group than that ordinarily seen. These agents apparently cause hypercoagulability and predispose some patients to intravascular thromboses attributable to very low grade intravascular clotting. These changes occur in 15% to 20% of women on oral contraceptives but do not begin until the drug has been used for at least 2 to 3 months. This abnormality cannot be picked up with routine tests but only by fibrinogen chromatography, which unfortunately, is performed in only a few laboratories. Other simpler tests are under evaluation, but their usefulness has not been determined.

BLEEDING DISORDERS

Occult hemorrhagic disorders, particularly hemophilia, the so-called mild hemophilias and von Willebrand's disease (angiohemophilia), can cause serious eye problems especially during and after surgery.[2, 85, 90, 106, 112] Under ordinary circumstances the eyes are infrequently affected, but hemorrhage, particularly subconjunctival or in the orbit[114] as well as intraocular, can occur even after mild trauma. In the postoperative period bleeding and mild oozing are frequently observed. It is therefore important to take a careful preoperative history with regard to previous bleeding tendencies. The most common sites of hemorrhage are the nose, the gastrointestinal and urinary tracts, and the joints. There is often a history of bruising and prolonged bleeding after cuts or minor surgical procedures such as extraction of teeth or circumcision. These episodes usually begin in childhood but may not occur until later in life, especially if the patient has acquired, rather than congenital, hemophilia. The specific disorder must be identified so that appropriate treatment can be given when needed. Treatment consists of replacement of factor VIII in classic hemophilia, which can be done by transfusions of fresh whole blood, fresh plasma, or concentrates of these.[21, 38, 47, 66] Cryoprecipitates containing factor VIII in a concentrated form can now be produced at reasonable cost and can be used during and after surgery to keep factor VIII at a high enough level to prevent bleeding. It is important to plan for this ahead of time when elective surgery is scheduled so that enough material will be available.[86] There are simple means for calculating the appropriate amount of concentrate or cryoprecipitate that will be needed for a given patient, and with their use the risk of significant bleeding can be greatly reduced.

It is now known that certain drugs may alter coagulation, and these effects take place through various mechanisms that may occur with differing degrees and frequency.[74] For example, aspirin blocks platelet agglutination, and the effect of even a small dose may last for 1 to 2 weeks. Therefore, as commented by Newell,[78] it would seem advisable to discontinue the use of aspirin for a reasonable time before and after eye surgery to prevent possible bleeding problems. Other drugs such as furosemide (Lasix), nitrofurantoin (Furadantin), and cyproheptadine (Periactin) can also affect platelet function. A careful preoperative drug history will help to prevent this type of occult bleeding.

RETICULOENDOTHELIOSES

Comments will be limited to a brief discussion of histiocytosis X, which is the name given to a group of three interrelated syndromes consisting of eosinophilic granuloma of bone, Hand-Schüller-Christian disease, and Letterer-Siwe disease.[7, 14, 59, 70, 79, 92] Eosinophilic granuloma tends to be a benign, localized bony disease seen primarily in children and young adults. It can affect the eye, especially if the orbit or skull is involved. On x-ray examination the lesions appear sharply outlined with a radiolucent, punched-out appearance. Various methods of treatment including local excision, radiation, and steroids are available. Hand-Schüller-Christian disease usually has a chronic course, tends to be more widespread, and occurs primarily in children although adult cases have been reported. It consists of a classic triad of bony lesions, exophthalmos, and diabetes insipidus. Involvement of the skull is very common, and when exophthalmos is present, orbital lesions are often seen. Cranial nerve palsies, papilledema, optic atrophy, and swelling of the eyelids and orbit are among other abnormalities that may be found. Treatment is similar to that for eosinophilic granuloma, that is, radiation, steroids, and excision of the lesion. Letterer-Siwe disease is both the rarest and severest entity in the group. It occurs mainly in infants and young children and is a widespread systemic disorder with a rapidly progressive, often fatal course. Clinically one sees a skin rash (consisting of crops of brown, scaling papules on the head, neck, and trunk), fever, anemia, lymphadenopathy, and enlargement of the spleen and liver. It can involve the eye, with the choroid being the most frequent site. Lesions have also been reported in the retina, sclera, and anterior uveal tract; hyphema can occur when the last one is involved. Steroid therapy may be beneficial.

REFERENCES

1. Acacio, I., and Goldberg, M. F.: Peripapillary and macular vessel occlusions in sickle cell anemia, Am. J. Ophthalmol. **75:**861-866, 1973.
2. Aggeler, P. M., et al.: The mild hemophilias, occult deficiencies of AHF, PTC, and PTA frequently responsible for unexpected surgical bleeding, Am. J. Med. **24:**84-94, 1961.
3. Allen, R. A., and Straatsma, B. R.: Ocular involvement in leukemia and allied disorders, Arch. Ophthalmol. **66:**490-508, 1961.
4. Aronson, S. B., and Shaw, R.: Corneal crystals in multiple myeloma, Arch. Ophthalmol. **61:**541-546, 1959.
5. Ashton, N.: Ocular changes in multiple myelomatosis, Arch. Ophthalmol. **73:**487-494, 1965.
6. Blodi, F. C.: The difficult diagnosis of choroidal melanoma, Arch. Ophthalmol. **69:** 253-256, 1963.
7. Blodi, F. C.: Histiocytosis X in an adult, Trans. Am. Acad. Ophthalmol. Otolaryngol. **64:**1012-1017, 1964.
8. Blodi, F. C., and Gass, J. D. M.: Inflammatory pseudotumor of the orbit, Trans. Am. Acad. Ophthalmol. Otolaryngol. **67:**303-323, 1967.
9. Burns, C. A., Blodi, F. C., and Williamson, B. K.: Acute lymphocytic leukemia and central serous retinopathy, Trans. Am. Acad. Ophthalmol. **69:**307-309, 1969.
10. Cant, J. S.: Dacryocystitis in acute leukaemia, Br. J. Ophthalmol. **47:**57-59, 1963.
11. Carr, R. E., and Henkind, P.: Retinal findings associated with serum hyperviscosity, Am. J. Ophthalmol. **56:**23-31, 1963.
12. Chizek, D. J., and Franceschetti, A. T.: Oral contraceptives: Their side effects and ophthalmological manifestations, Survey of Ophthalmol. **14:**90-105, 1969.
13. Clayman, H. C., Flynn, J. T., Koch, K., et al.: Retinal pigment epithelial abnormalities in leukemic disease, Am. J. Ophthalmol. **74:**416-419, 1972.
14. Codling, B. W., Soni, K. C., Barry, D. R., et al.: Histiocytosis presenting as swelling of orbit and eyelid, Br. J. Ophthalmol. **56:**517-530, 1972.
15. Comer, P. B., and Fred, H. L.: Diagnosis of sickle-cell disease by ophthalmoscopic inspection of the conjunctiva, New Eng. J. Med. **271:**544-546, 1964.
16. Condon, P. I., and Serjeant, G. R.: Ocular findings in hemoglobin sickle cell anemia in Jamaica, Am. J. Ophthalmol. **73:**533-543, 1972.
17. Condon, P. I., and Serjeant, G. R.: Ocular findings in hemoglobin sickle cell disease in Jamaica, Am. J. Ophthalmol. **74:**921-931, 1972.
18. Condon, P. I., and Serjeant, G. R.: Ocular findings in sickle cell thalassemia in Jamaica, Am. J. Ophthalmol. **74:**1105-1109, 1972.
19. Condon, P. I., Serjeant, G. R., and Ikeda, H.: Unusual chorioretinal degeneration in sickle cell disease, Br. J. Ophthalmol. **57:**81-88, 1973.
20. Conrad, W. C., and Penner, R.: Sickle-cell trait and central retinal-artery occlusion, Am. J. Ophthalmol. **63:**465-468, 1967.
21. Cooke, J. V., Holland, P. V., and Shulman, N. R.: Cryoprecipitate concentrates of factor VIII for surgery in hemophiliacs, Ann. Intern. Med. **68:**39-47, 1968.
22. Cooper, E. L., and Riker, J. L.: Malignant lymphoma of the uveal tract, Am. J. Ophthalmol. **34:**1153-1158, 1951.

23. Cooperative Urea Trials Group: Clinical trials of therapy for sickle cell vaso-occlusive crises, J.A.M.A. **288:**1120-1124, 1974.
24. Cooperative Urea Trials Group: Treatment of sickle cell crisis with urea in invert sugar, J.A.M.A. **228:**1125-1128, 1974.
25. Cooperative Urea Trials Group: Therapy for sickle cell vaso-occlusive crises, J.A.M.A. **228:**1129-1131, 1974.
26. Crookes, G. P., and Mullaney, J.: Lymphoid hyperplasia of the uveal tract, Am. J. Ophthalmol. **63:**962-967, 1967.
27. Currey, T. A., and Deutsch, A. R.: Reticulum cell sarcoma of the uvea, Southern Med. J. **58:**919-922, 1965.
28. Delaney, W. V., and Liaricos, S. V.: Chorioretinal destruction in multiple myeloma, Am. J. Ophthalmol. **66:**52-55, 1968.
29. Eagle, R. C., Yanoff, M., and Morse, P. H.: Anterior segment necrosis following scleral buckling in hemoglobin SC disease, Am. J. Ophthalmol. **75:**426-433, 1973.
30. Ellis, W., and Little, H. L.: Leukemic infiltration of the optic nerve head, Am. J. Ophthalmol. **75:**867-871, 1973.
31. Fahey, J. L., Barth, W. F., and Soloman, A.: Serum hyperviscosity syndrome, J.A.M.A. **192:**464-467, 1965.
32. Fink, A. I.: Vascular fine structure changes in the bulbar conjunctiva associated with sickle cell disease, Am. J. Ophthalmol. **69:**563-572, 1970.
33. Foos, R. Y., and Allen, R. A.: Opaque cysts of the ciliary body, Arch. Ophthalmol. **77:**559-568, 1967.
34. François, J., and Rabaey, M.: Corneal dystrophy and paraproteinemia, Am. J. Ophthalmol. **52:**895-901, 1961.
35. Frank, R. N., and Ryan, S. J.: Peripheral retinal neovascularization with chronic myelogenous leukemia, Arch. Ophthalmol. **87:**585-589, 1972.
36. Funahashi, T., Fink, A., Robinson, M., et al.: Pathology of conjunctival vessels in sickle-cell disease, Am. J. Ophthalmol. **57:**713-718, 1964.
37. Galinos, S., Rabb, M. F., Goldberg, M. G., et al.: Hemoglobin SC disease and iris atrophy, Am. J. Ophthalmol. **75:**421-425, 1973.
38. George, J. N., and Breckenridge, R. T.: The use of factor VIII and factor IX concentrates during surgery, J.A.M.A. **214:**1673-1676, 1970.
39. Goldberg, M. F.: Treatment of proliferative sickle retinopathy, Trans. Am. Acad. Ophthalmol. Otolaryngol. **75:**532-665, 1971.
40. Goldberg, M. F.: Classification and pathogenesis of proliferative sickle cell retinopathy, Am. J. Ophthalmol. **71:**649-665, 1971.
41. Goldberg, M. F., and Acacio, I.: Argon laser photocoagulation of proliferative sickle retinopathy, Arch. Ophthalmol. **90:**35-44, 1973.
42. Goldberg, M. F., Charache, S., and Acacio, I.: Ophthalmologic manifestations of sickle cell thalassemia, Arch. Intern. Med. **128:**33-39, 1971.
43. Goldberg, M. F., Galinos, S., Lee, C., et al.: Macular ischemia and infarction in sickling, Invest. Ophthalmol. **12:**633-635, 1973.
44. Goodman, G.: Sickle cell ocular disease. Symposium on surgical and medical management of congenital anomalies of the eye, Transactions of the New Orleans Academy of Ophthalmology, St. Louis, 1968, The C. V. Mosby Co.
45. Goodman, G., von Sallmann, L., and Holland, M. G.: Ocular manifestations of sickle-cell disease, Arch. Ophthalmol. **58:**655-682, 1957.
46. Gudas, P. P.: Optic nerve myeloma, Am. J. Ophthalmol. **71:**1085-1089, 1971.
47. Hattersley, P. G.: The treatment of classical hemophilia with cryoprecipitates, J.A.M.A. **198:**153-157, 1966.
48. Hayreh, S. J., and Baines, J. A. B.: Occlusion of the posterior ciliary artery. II. Chorioretinal lesions, Br. J. Ophthalmol. **56:**736-753, 1972.
49. Hoyt, W. F.: Retinal ischemic symptoms in cardiovascular diagnosis, Postgrad. Med. **52:**85-90, 1972.
50. Jakobiec, F., and Behrens, M. M.: Leukemic retinal pigment epitheliopathy. (In press.)
51. Johnson, B. L.: Proteinaceous cysts of the ciliary epithelium II, Arch. Ophthalmol. **84:**171-175, 1970.

52. Johnson, B. L., and Storey, J. D.: Proteinaceous cysts of the ciliary epithelium I, Arch. Ophthalmol. **84:**166-170, 1970.
53. Knapp, J. W.: Isolated macular infarction in sickle cell (SS) disease, Am. J. Ophthalmol. **73:**857-859, 1972.
54. Kolker, A. E.: Ocular manifestations of hematologic disease. In Brown, E. B., and Moore, C. V., editors: Progress in hematology, vol. 5, London, 1966, William Heinemann, Ltd.
55. Kopp, W. L., Beirne, G. J., and Burns, R. O.: Hyperviscosity syndrome in multiple myeloma, Am. J. Med. **43:**141-146, 1967.
56. Kurz, G. H.: Retinopathy of obscure (toxic?) origin in Hodgkin's disease, Am. J. Ophthalmol. **57:**205-213, 1964.
57. Kuwabara, T., and Aiello, L.: Leukemic miliary nodules in the retina, Arch. Ophthalmol. **72:**494-497, 1964.
58. Levine, R. A., and Kaplan, A. M.: The ophthalmoscopic findings in C + S disease, Am. J. Ophthalmol. **59:**37-42, 1965.
59. Lieberman, P. H., Jones, C. R., Dargeon, H. W. K., et al.: A reappraisal of eosinophilic granuloma of bone, Hand-Schüller-Christian syndrome and Letterer-Siwe syndrome, Medicine **48:**375-400, 1969.
60. Luxenberg, M. N., and Mausolf, F. A.: Retinal circulation in the hyperviscosity syndrome, Am. J. Ophthalmol. **70:**588-598, 1970.
61. Mahneke, A., and Videbaek, A.: On changes in the optic fundus in leukaemia, Acta Ophthalmol. **42:**201-210, 1964.
62. Marcus, H. C.: Malignant lymphoma of the uveal tract, Arch. Ophthalmol. **69:**251-253, 1963.
63. Marker, M. A. M., Peiris, J. B., DeSilva, G. U., et al.: Retinopathy in megaloblastic anaemias, Trans. R. Soc. Trop. Med. Hyg. **63:**398-406, 1969.
64. Masi, A. T., and Dugdale, M.: Cerebrovascular diseases associated with the use of oral contraceptives, Ann. Intern. Med. **72:**111-121, 1970.
65. Mausolf, F. A., and Mensher, J. H.: Experimental hyperviscosity retinopathy, Ann. Ophthalmol. **5:**205-209, 1973.
66. Mazza, J. J., Bowie, E. J. W., Hagedorn, A. B., et al.: Antihemophilic factor VIII in hemophilia, J.A.M.A. **211:**1818-1823, 1970.
67. Merin, S., and Freund, M.: Retinopathy in severe anemia, Am. J. Ophthalmol. **66:**1102-1106, 1968.
68. Michelson, P. E., and Pfaffenbach, D.: Retinal arterial occlusion following ocular trauma in youths with sickle-trait hemoglobinopathy, Am. J. Ophthalmol. **74:**494-497, 1972.
69. Minatoya, H., Acacio, I., and Goldberg, M.: Fluorescein angiography of the bulbar conjunctiva in sickle cell disease, Ann. Ophthalmol. **5:**980-992, 1973.
70. Mittelman, D., Apple, D. J., Goldberg, M. F.: Ocular involvement in Letterer-Siwe disease, Am. J. Ophthalmol. **75:**261-265, 1973.
71. Morse, P. H., and McCready, J. L.: Peripheral retinal neovascularization in chronic myelocytic leukemia, Am. J. Ophthalmol. **72:**975-978, 1971.
72. Mortada, A.: Nature of lymphoid tumors, Am. J. Ophthalmol. **57:**820-826, 1964.
73. Mortada, A.: Reactive reticulum cell hyperplasia of orbit, lacrimal gland, eyelids and conjunctiva, Am. J. Ophthalmol. **74:**307-310, 1972.
74. Mortada, A., and Abboud, I.: Retinal haemorrhages after prolonged use of salicylates, Br. J. Ophthalmol. **57:**119-120, 1973.
75. Munro, S., and Walker, C.: Ocular complications in sickle-cell haemoglobin C disease, Br. J. Ophthalmol. **44:**1-24, 1960.
76. Neault, R. W., Scoy, R. E. V., Okazaki, H., et al.: Uveitis associated with isolated reticulum cell sarcoma of the brain, Am. J. Ophthalmol. **73:**431-436, 1972.
77. Nevins, R. C., Frey, W. W., and Elliott, J. H.: Primary, solitary, intraocular reticulum cell sarcoma (microgliomatosis), Trans. Am. Acad. Ophthalmol. Otolaryngol. **72:**867-876, 1968.
78. Newell, F. W.: Aspirin, bleeding, and ophthalmic surgery, Am. J. Ophthalmol. **74:**559-560, 1972.

79. Niordson, A., and Danø, P.: Letterer-Siwe's disease, Acta Derm. Venereol. **48:**612-617, 1968.
80. Palm, E.: A case of crystal deposits in the cornea, Acta Ophthalmol. **25:**165-174, 1947.
81. Paton, D.: The conjunctival sign of sickle-cell disease, Arch. Ophthalmol. **68:**627-632, 1962.
82. Pinkerton, R. M. H., and Robertson, D. M.: Corneal and conjunctival changes in dysproteinemia, Invest. Ophthalmol. **8:**357-364, 1969.
83. Podos, S. M., and Canellos, G. P.: Lens changes in chronic granulocytic leukemia, Am. J. Ophthalmol. **68:**500-504, 1969.
84. Porter, E. A.: Acute leukaemia presenting with papilloedema: Case report, N. Z. Med. J. **71:**138-140, 1970.
85. Poweleit, A. C.: A procedure for cataract extraction in the hemophiliac, Am. J. Ophthalmol. **59:**315-317, 1965.
86. Richards, R. D., and Spurling, C. L.: Elective ocular surgery in hemophilia, Arch. Ophthalmol. **89:**167-168, 1973.
87. Rodman, H. I., and Font, R. L.: Orbital involvement in multiple myeloma, Arch. Ophthalmol. **87:**30-35, 1972.
88. Romayananda, N., Goldberg, M. F., and Green, W. R.: Histopathology of sickle cell retinopathy, Trans. Am. Acad. Ophthalmol. Otolaryngol. **77:**652-676, 1973.
89. Rothstein, T.: Bilateral, central retinal vein closure as the initial manifestation of polycythemia, Am. J. Ophthalmol. **74:**256-260, 1972.
90. Rubenstein, R. A., Albert, D. M., and Scheie, H. G.: Ocular complications of hemophilia, Arch. Ophthalmol. **76:**230-232, 1966.
91. Rubenstein, R. A., Yanoff, M., and Albert, D. M.: Thrombocytopenia, anemia, and retinal hemorrhage, Am. J. Ophthalmol. **65:**435-439, 1968.
92. Rupp, R. H., and Holloman, K. R.: Histiocytosis X affecting the uveal tract, Arch. Ophthalmol. **84:**468-470, 1970.
93. Russel, R. W. R., and Cantab, M. D.: The source of retinal emboli, Lancet **2:**789-792, 1968.
94. Ryan, S. J.: Occlusion of the macular capillaries in sickle cell hemoglobin C disease, Am. J. Ophthalmol. **77:**459-461, 1974.
95. Ryan, S. J., Frank, R. N., and Green, W. R.: Bilateral inflammatory pseudotumors of the ciliary body, Am. J. Ophthalmol. **72:**586-591, 1971.
96. Ryan, S. J., and Goldberg, M. F.: Anterior segment ischemia following scleral buckling in sickle cell hemoglobinopathy, Am. J. Ophthalmol. **72:**35-50, 1971.
97. Ryan, S. J., Zimmerman, L. E., and King, F. M.: Reactive lymphoid hyperplasia, Trans. Am. Acad. Ophthalmol. Otolaryngol. **76:**652-671, 1972.
98. Salmon, M. L., Winkelman, J. Z., and Gay, A. J.: Neuro-ophthalmic sequelae in users of oral contraceptives, J.A.M.A. **206:**85-91, 1968.
99. Sanders, T. E., and Podos, S. M.: Pars plana cysts in multiple myeloma, Trans. Am. Acad. Ophthalmol. Otolaryngol. **70:**951-958, 1966.
100. Sanders, T. E., Podos, S. M., and Rosenbaum, L. J.: Intraocular manifestations of multiple myeloma, Arch. Ophthalmol. **77:**789-794, 1967.
101. Serjeant, G. R., Serjeant, B. E., and Condon, P. I.: The conjunctival sign in sickle cell anemia, J.A.M.A. **219:**1428-1431, 1972.
102. Smith, V. H.: Malignant lymphatic tumours of the orbit, Br. J. Ophthalmol. **43:**247-251, 1959.
103. Sommer, A., Kontras, S. B., and Craenen, J. M.: Partial exchange transfusion in sickle cell anemia complicated by heart disease, J.A.M.A. **215:**483-484, 1971.
104. Stein, M. R., and Gay, A. J.: Acute chorioretinal infarction in sickle cell trait, Arch. Ophthalmol. **84:**485-490, 1970.
105. Spalter, H. F.: Abnormal serum proteins and retinal vein thrombosis, Arch. Ophthalmol. **62:**868-881, 1959.
106. Strauss, L., and Ramsell, T. G.: Successful cataract extraction in a severe haemophiliac, Br. J. Ophthalmol. **52:**242-244, 1968.
107. Vogel, M. H., Font, R. L., Zimmerman, L. E., et al.: Reticulum cell sarcoma of the retina and uvea, Am. J. Ophthalmol. **66:**205-215, 1968.

108. Walsh, F. B., Clark, D. B., Thompson, R. S., et al.: Oral contraceptives and neuro-ophthalmologic interest, Arch. Ophthalmol. **74:**628-640, 1965.
109. Walsh, F. B., and Hoyt, W. F.: Clinical neuroophthalmology, ed. 3, Baltimore, 1969, The Williams & Wilkins Co., vol. 3, pp. 2321-2322.
110. Walsh, F. B., and Shewmake, B. J.: An unusual case of reticulum cell sarcoma, Am. J. Ophthalmol. **74:**741-743, 1972.
111. Welch, R. B., and Goldberg, M. F.: Sickle-cell hemoglobin and its relation to fundus abnormality, Arch. Ophthalmol. **75:**353-362, 1966.
112. Wong, G. Y., Fisher, L. M., and Geeraets, W. J.: Ocular complications of factor XIII deficiency, Am. J. Ophthalmol. **67:**346-351, 1969.
113. Wood, W. J., and Nicholson, D. H.: Corneal ring ulcer as the presenting manifestation of acute monocytic leukemia, Am. J. Ophthalmol. **76:**69-72, 1973.
114. Zimmerman, A., and Merigan, T. C.: Retrobulbar hemorrhage in a hemophiliac with irreversible loss of vision, Arch. Ophthalmol. **64:**949-950, 1960.
115. Zimmerman, L. E., and Thoresen, H. T.: Sudden loss of vision in acute leukemia, Survey Ophthalmol. **9:**467-473, 1964.

Ocular involvement in hematologic and reticuloendothelial disease

CHAIRMAN: **John Mensher***

Dr. Mensher: Dr. Brain, is there a known reason for the characteristic rebleed in 3 to 5 days after an anterior chamber hyphema? The individual asking the question wonders about local thrombolitic factors.

Dr. Brain: I don't know why there should be a rebleed. One would really need a considerable amount of information on individual patients. There is no doubt that quite a significant number of patients coming to surgery do have problems often for very good reasons not identified ahead of time. Unless one can work them out, they present major therapeutic problems. The practical thing is that the patients may have a mild bleeding tendency, which is not of much significance until you undergo surgery when the whole thing blows up, usually in the face of the surgeon.

Dr. Mensher: Dr. Kearns, can you comment on reticulum cell sarcoma and uveitis with respect to whether you have seen uveitis in other malignancies of the reticuloendothelial system?

Dr. Kearns: Well, that question refers to (in case some of you don't know about it) a time 4 to 5 years ago when we had a run of patients with uveitis who were found to have reticulum cell sarcoma. One of our young ophthalmologists had me see a patient with severe bilateral uveitis. There wasn't anything that could be done about the uveitis. The patient had cataracts, synechias (the whole works), and secondary glaucoma. But I just happened to ask, "Have you had any other trouble?" and he said, "Well, none, but my foot gets to jerking every once in awhile, and my wife has to sit on it to keep it from moving." So we wrote down that this could be reticulum cell sarcoma of the brain, and it turned out it was. So, this is being recognized more and more frequently, and it really isn't uveitis. We presented this at a meeting in Baltimore. Dave Knox sitting here will remember it. And, Dr. Zimmerman pointed out this really isn't uveitis. This is probably actual reticulum cell sarcoma involving the eye. I have seen this occasionally when other areas besides the brain are involved, but for some reason when one sees this, usually a bilateral, uveitis-like process (and it is

*Department of Ophthalmology, University of Iowa College of Medicine, Iowa City, Iowa.

uveitis as far as I can tell, though I find it difficult to differentiate) with neurologic involvement, one should think of reticulum cell sarcoma of the brain.

Dr. Mensher: One of the members of the audience wanted to have some comments on the retinopathy of sickle-cell trait.

Dr. Luxenberg: It's really no different from SS or SC. It can be a combination but occurs much less frequently than do either one of those. You can see peripheral neovascularization, the black sunbursts, and the arteriovenous anastomoses, but the most important thing is that it's much less frequent but should be looked for, and if present, the patient certainly should have a hemoglobin electrophoresis test done.

Dr. Mensher: What is plasmapheresis? Would you like to describe what that is?

Dr. Luxenberg: Well, I think probably Dr. Brain could do that better than myself.

Dr. Brain: It's essentially venisecting a patient, spinning the blood down, removing the plasma, adding some normal saline to the red cells, and reinjecting the red cells. Might I add just one point about the sickle cell and sickle trait. It is interesting that the degree of sickling in terms of clinical crises differs quite remarkably from patient to patient, and sometimes this is certainly modified by the presence of hemaglobin F in the cells, so that it's by no means all or none. We don't really completely understand why some patients with SS apparently go through life with remarkably few episodes yet other patients are very crippled by it. This may account for the variable incidence of retinal disorders in this group.

Dr. Cogan: I have a comment on circulating platelet emboli. This is a patient who I believe had platelet-circulating emboli. The patient had metastatic carcinoma, although I believe that had nothing to do with etiology of the platelets other than inducing maybe a hypercoagulability state. These platelet emboli do not get stuck in the retinal vessels. You would think that they would. They pass through the retinal vessels. Curiously, where they get stuck is in the choriocapillaris. There they produce typical pigmentary epithelial changes and detachment of the retina. The retinal vessels are so small you would think that is where they would get stuck, but they seem to pass through. And in this patient they went through like so many white mice. Platelet emboli in other words, I believe, are the circulating emboli although that is much less well documented than are the lipid or calcific emboli. We recently observed another patient with platelet emboli. The emboli have a rate of about 4 mm. per second. She also had a few little hemorhages in her fundi. We watched these emboli go through repeatedly, and then we heparinized her and they disappeared. Then we stopped the heparin and they recurred. I am not sure what the significance of that is. Occasionally, one can see them in the choroid as well. In postmortem examinations we can see an occasional platelet in the flat mounts of the retinal vessels, but it is in the choriocapillaris where they accumulate and pile up.

Dr. Brain: I believe that one has to recognize that these platelet aggregates are really quite unstable and they will tend to deaggregate. I suspect this is the reason that they don't totally obstruct. But if they do sit there, they are quite capable of presumably producing a local thrombosis. I wondered in the previous talk whether they had any tendency to rest in the venous end rather than in the arteriole end?

Dr. Mensher: Dr. Sanders, did you have a case of lymphoma that you wanted to present?

Dr. Sanders: Ocular changes in lymphomatous meningitis may be extremely important for the ophthalmologist to recognize, as these conditions are rarely diagnosed in life unless specific cerebrospinal fluid studies are undertaken.

The patient I would like to describe had a progressive neurologic disorder with normal CSF pressure and normal cerbral arteriography and pneumo-encephalography. The visual acuity in the right eye was reduced to 20/60, there were vitreous opacities, and fundus examination showed chronic disk edema. Examination of the peripheral retina showed focal areas of perivenous sheathing, and the left eye was entirely normal.

Fluorescein angiography showed considerable dilatation of the retinal papillary and peripapillary capillaries (Fig. 1, *A*) and in the late pictures taken after 10 minutes there is gross perivenous leakage of dye (Fig. 1, *B*).

Further CSF studies with centrifuge and millipore techniques showed large mononuclear cells in the CSF that were diagnostic of a lymphomatous meningitis, and the condition resolved after the use of radiotherapy.

I would also like to show the retinal vascular changes in a young patient with chronic myeloid leukemia with a white blood count of 500,000 cells. Vision in the left eye was reduced to 20/200 because of a preretinal hemorrhage in the macular region. The retinal arteries and veins were dilated with numerous deep retinal hemorrhages. One week after therapy the retinal vessels were restored to their normal size (see fluorescein, Fig. 2).

Examination of the periphery showed white leukemic infiltrates, pale centered hemorrhages and fluorescein angiography showed dilatation of the arteries and veins with numerous microaneurysms situated mainly at the venous end of the capillary bed, similar to those reported by Duke et al. in pathological specimens. One week after treatment retinal vessels had reverted to their normal size and microaneurysms had disappeared (Fig. 3).

I would value the opinions of members of the panel, particularly Drs. Cogan and Henkind, on the pathophysiology of the retinal vascular changes and what part autoregulation may play. The complete resolution of aneurysms within a short period has not been stressed in the past.

Dr. Cogan: I refer this to Dr. Henkind.

Dr. Henkind: Is Dr. Hayreh here? Mike Sanders showed me these pictures before. They are rather dramatic. There are several things about them. I have seen venous dilatation disappear very rapidly after plasmapheresis. I believe one has to recognize that if one gets venous dilatation, then one must get venous tortuosity. They go hand in hand. It's quite obvious. A vessel, at least a vein, has an almost elastic wall. You just can't expand the vein in anteroposterior diameter without expanding its longitudinal direction so there is no condition I am aware of where you get venous dilatation without tortuosity. I think that's quite true in the arteries, too, though perhaps not as profoundly. The muscle wall may be a little different. The fact that those microaneurysms appeared and disappeared within a week . . . ah, I don't know how to explain that. Dave Cogan can probably explain it. It just suggests to me that there is a lot of plasticity in the retinal vascular system and I don't know what autoregulation

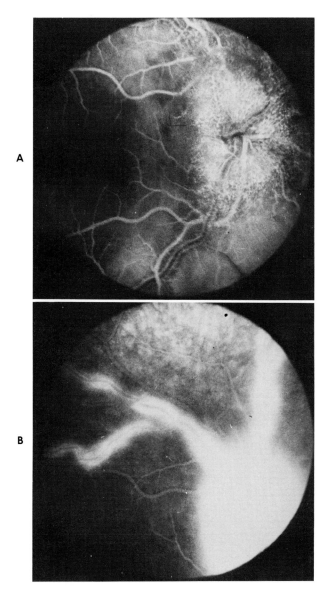

Fig. 1. Lymphomatous infiltration of optic disk. **A,** Arteriovenous phase of fluorescein angiogram of left eye showing pronounced dilatation of disk capillaries. **B,** Late fluorescein angiogram showing extensive perivenous leakage of dye.

is. It's a wonderful term. It's like idiopathic. It means we don't know because we can't identify the site of the autoregulation, but Dave Cogan has worked on this extensively. He hasn't had the answer for a lot of things, but he can probably give us the answer for this one.

Dr. Cogan: I think it's a very interesting case. It might even make the *Archives of Ophthalmology,* but I cannot answer why the microaneurysms resolved so rapidly.

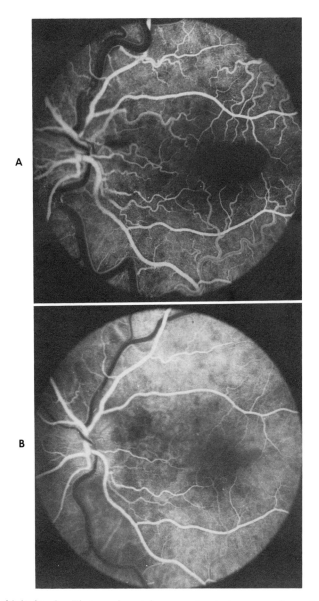

Fig. 2. Myeloid leukemia. Fluorescein angiogram of arteriovenous phase showing dilatation of arterioles, capillaries, and venules, **A,** and resolution to normal after 1 week of therapy, **B.** Macular hemorrhage has also partially resolved.

Dr. Sanders: I'm afraid its booked for the *British Journal of Ophthalmology.*

Dr. Mensher: Would anyone else on the panel like to comment on the bleeding vasculopathy.

Dr. Podos: I think that the case Dr. Sanders showed of meningeal infiltration is different from the reticulum cell sarcoma with focal neurologic signs that Dr. Kearns was talking about. I don't know of any patient with that reticulum cell sarcoma syndrome who has had meningeal infiltrates. It seems to be a disease

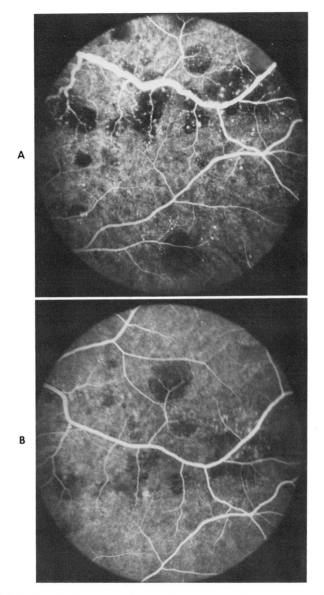

Fig. 3. Myeloid leukemia. Peripheral pictures taken at same time as those of Fig. 2, *A,* showing dilated vessels with numerous microaneurysms, **A,** with pronounced resolution after therapy for 1 week, **B.**

of a focal process in neural tissue of both white matter and gray matter. I am curious, Dr. Sanders, about your patient with multifocal leukoencephalopathy. Was this a thickening of the sensory retina or was this a white patch in the pigment epithelium choroidal layer?

Dr. Sanders: The fluorescein angiogram showed leakage from capillaries and from some of the veins in the macular region. So this is a retinal disturbance.

Dr. Podos: Did this come to histology?

Dr. Sanders: No, I'm afraid it did not.

Dr. Podos: Dr. Kearns, have any of your patients had any meningeal infiltrates?

Dr. Kearns: No, it's a focal neurologic process. They present as a brain tumor.

Dr. Podos: Obviously, this disease can in a sense do anything.

Dr. Kearns: Yes, I've seen a few, one or two, that had reticulum cell sarcoma on the outside of the brain.

Dr. Podos: Yes, there was one case at our hospital that was diagnosed by skin biopsy of the lid.

Dr. Hayreh: Regarding the disappearance of the microaneurysms and the disappearance of the tortuosity. I have quite a few patients with venous stasis retinopathy in whom over the years the whole thing has settled; so it is surprising to see how these kinked veins just go straight and the microaneurysms disappear. There were quite a few instances in which the same thing happened on angiography during the active phase with tortuosity and microaneurysms. Then when the whole thing is settled, everything is clear and not a sign of microaneurysms can be seen. I don't know the mechanism.

Dr. Kearns: One sign that's a bit old I think should be mentioned; that is the sludging of the blood in the retinal veins with light pressure. This was described many years ago and it was really believed to be specific for multiple myeloma. Of course, now we know this isn't true. It happens in any of these diseases that we've talked about with increased viscosity. If you haven't seen it, I recommend that you try it; it's really an amazing thing. The way you do it is to lay your finger across the eye, increase the intraocular pressure above diastolic, and after about 4 seconds, depending on the height of the sedimentation rate and the degree of hyperviscosity, you observe the vessels. First, you watch the artery and get a diastolic pulse and hold it there and get about maybe 8 to 10 beats, and then switch your attention to the vein on the disk or slightly off the disk and you will see these aggregates of red cells running down through. It looks like marbles running down a plastic pipe, and it really is quite amazing. Well, you say, "So what?" Well, it can be very important in diagnosis especially in temporal arteritis. I've used it to advantage a number of times to do a quick sedimentation rate test. I don't think it would ever replace the sedimentation rate test. But, at least, when the patient comes in at 5:30 o'clock on Friday afternoon, and you figure it's temporal arteritis, if you get this positive sludging sign, you know that the sedimentation rate is way up. How many know what I'm talking about? Show of hands. Half a dozen. So it's still remaining a very little or not well-known sign. The next time you have a patient with a high sedimentation rate, try it. It's kind of frightening when you see it. I don't think you could hold it for 10 minutes, but as soon as you see this sludging, let it go, of course. Try it the next time you have a patient with a hyperviscosity syndrome of any type.

Dr. Mensher: Dr. Luxenberg, have you ever seen corneal clouding in macroglobulinemias, and, if so, in which types?

Dr. Luxenberg: No, I haven't.

Dr. Mensher: Has anybody else?

Dr. Podos: I have seen this in multiple myeloma, in macroglobulinemia, and in cryoglobulinemia, and it's well reported in Duke-Elder.

Dr. Henkind: It strikes me very strange that in macroglobulinemia there are huge numbers of microaneurysms. I've seen patients who have gone for years like this. It goes partially to the question of whether the diabetic state always goes into the proliferative state. Dr. Mausolf did a really beautiful study when he produced microaneurysms with hyperviscosity, but really there is no good example of proliferative retinopathy outside of the experimental model of retrolental fibroplasia. Dave Cogan, have you ever seen proliferative retinopathy in this condition?

Dr. Cogan: No.

Dr. Mensher: Dr. Luxenberg, comment on the possibility in SS disease of the concomitant development of angioid streaks.

Dr. Luxenberg: This is seen in approximately 6% of the patients and certainly it's something that should be considered. If you see something resembling angioid streaks, even though there aren't any peripheral fundus changes that are typically associated with sickle disease, it would be worthwhile to test by hemoglobin electrophoresis, particularly in a younger person.

Dr. Mensher: I believe it would be appropriate to have Dr. Mausolf, the individual who organized this symposium, give us a few minutes of his discussion on the experimental hyperviscosity syndrome.

Dr. Mausolf: The hyperviscosity syndrome was produced in one monkey by injection of 300,000 molecular weight dextran intravenously 5 days a week for about 7 weeks. There was an elevation of serum viscosity and a prolongation of retinal circulation time. This resulted in the hemorrhagic retinopathy as reported in the *Annals of Ophthalmology* (**5**:205, 1973). The slide shown by Dr. Luxenberg (Fig. 15-2) is the previously unreported trypsin-digested retina mount demonstrating microaneurysms. We have recently constructed a controlled study in which we have produced microaneurysms in two more monkeys. We hope that this model will prove useful in further studies of the pathophysiology of hemorrhagic retinopathy and microaneurysm formation.

16

Gastrointestinal and ocular disease

David L. Knox
Theodore M. Bayless*

A significant association between ocular disease and disease in another organ or system can be established by several means.

The pathologist utilizes histologic similarities between disease processes in two tissues as points favoring significant pathogenic relationships. Demonstration of identical microorganisms in the eye and other tissues by culture, histology, or electron microscopy has been used as evidence of a cause-and-effect relationship between the organisms and the disease. In this regard, the presence of commensural or adventitious organisms in tissue may lead to a false assumption of causation of disease. Fulfilling Koch's postulates by producing a laboratory model of the disease is considered the best proof of causal relationship.

Parallel or consecutive temporal association between two disorders occurring in a patient population alerts the clinician to the possibility of a significant correlation. A high prevalence of two disorders occurring simultaneously in a patient population may lead to speculation that there is a causal relationship between the two maladies or that they may share the same cause. The science of epidemiology has developed tests and criteria for the significance of such disease-association data.

Single-case reports of the coincident or consecutive development of disease in the eye and some other organ system, although anecdotal, often forms the basis for increased recognition of disease patterns.

Improvement of ocular disease after specific treatment of disease in another organ system leads to the "therapeutic response argument" for disease relationship.

The experience and thoughts of previous workers in an area can be recalled from the literature and used as a historical argument. Differences in general health, geography, epidemics, physiology, and definitions of disease for different populations and eras cannot always be transferred to current studies.

Finally there are times when the biomedical scientist weaves together the facts he has accumulated into a causal web of hypotheses to explain a disorder. Investi-

*Associate Professor, Department of Medicine (Gastroenterology), Johns Hopkins University School of Medicine, Baltimore, Maryland.

gators have the responsibility to fill with solid data the gaps in such webs. No matter how logical by current thinking, hypotheses must be tested and supported before they can be accepted.

It is the purpose of this report to describe four areas where the authors believe there is a significant association between gastrointestinal and ocular disease. These ocular diseases have usually been inflammatory. The methods of association vary; some seem quite valid and others only anecdotal; so our arguments may be easily challenged. It does, however, represent a beginning.

CROHN'S GRANULOMATOUS ENTEROCOLITIS

An association between chronic inflammatory bowel disease and eye disease has been previously reported.[3, 7, 19] In the past, ocular inflammations have been reported with both Crohn's disease and ulcerative colitis. Recently it has become apparent that Crohn's disease can affect the colon without any recognizable involvement of the small bowel so that patients previously classified as having ulcerative colitis should have been identified as having Crohn's disease. In Crohn's disease the ulcers penetrate deep into the wall of the bowel and often perforate, producing fistulas to skin, another loop of bowel, or peritoneum, or retroperitoneally. Granulomas often develop in the walls of inflamed tissue. In contrast, ulcerative colitis is characterized by superficial, extensive areas of ulceration, and giant cells are not seen at the edges or bases of these ulcers. Unfortunately these distinctions were not being made when most of the reports of ocular complications of ulcerative colitis were written.

Extraintestinal manifestations of Crohn's disease include arthralgias, arthritis, fever, erythema nodosum, aphthous stomatitis, and ocular inflammations such as iritis, iridocyclitis, and episcleritis. Granuloma formation with giant cells has been found in mesenteric lymph nodes, in liver, and in a few patients in synovial membranes.

A review of 73 patients with Crohn's disease, primarily of the small bowel, seen from 1958 to 1966 at the Johns Hopkins Hospital listed 7 patients (9.6%) with some ocular complication. These included recurrent conjunctivitis, 2; keratoconjunctivitis, 1; recurrent iridocyclitis, 1; allergic optic neuritis, 1; exudative retinal detachment, 1; and chronic retinitis, 1.

Our personal experience with ocular disease occuring in patients with Crohn's disease has been expanded and now includes 13 different problems in 12 patients, some of whom were included on the previous list.

Chronic iridocyclitis was seen in two patients. Surgical resection of the involved gut was followed by subsidence of the ocular inflammation in one of these.

Macular edema syndromes occurred in three patients. One patient developed classic central serous retinopathy within hours of the onset of intestinal obstruction; another developed a disciform macular edema process; and the third had mild macular edema that subsided only with oral corticosteroids.

An optic neuritis occurred in one male. It was peculiar, with pale edema affecting only the temporal nerve head, suggesting the presence of scleritis adjacent to the nerve head. Episcleritis occurred in two (Fig. 16-1). One patient definitely associated flare-ups of the scleritis with recurrences of diarrhea.

Bilateral multifocal exudative choroiditis with nonrhegmatogeous retinal de-

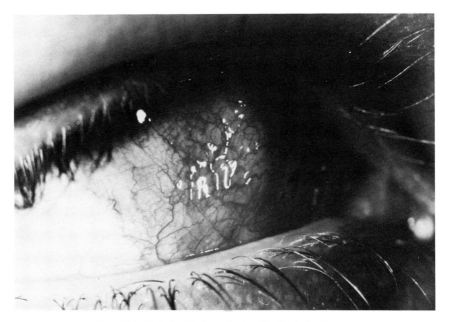

Fig. 16-1. Episcleritis in patient with Crohn's disease.

tachment occurred in one patient with ileal Crohn's disease who was taking large doses of oral corticosteroids (40 mg. of prednisone per day). Increasing the steroids did not cause a decrease in the choroiditis. Six weeks later it became apparent that he had a psoas abscess associated with a fistula from either appendix or terminal ileum. Drainage of the abscess without resection of the affected gut was followed by subsidence of the areas of choroiditis and resorption of subretinal fluid. A peculiar keratopathy has been seen in two patients. This is a subepithelial thickening and white opacification located 1 to 2 mm. inside the limbus. It has not affected central cornea or visual acuity. Management of their Crohn's disease has not relieved the keratopathy. One of the patients also had a deficiency of tear production that was reversed by oral vitamin A therapy. Vitamin A deficiency in these patients can be explained in part by reduced intake of vegetables as part of a low-roughage diet or from affection of the terminal ileum with malabsorption of bile salts and subsequent decreased absorption of fat and fat-soluble vitamins, such as the three carotenes and vitamin A.

A recent patient with peritoneal fistula and abscesses from Crohn's disease developed intraocular candidiasis possibly as a complication of heavy antibiotic and intravenous therapy.

At this time we have seen only one patient with ocular complications of ulcerative colitis. This was a 24-year-old white male whose mother had ulcerative colitis. He also had mild hepatitis that preceded his bilateral smoldering iritis. For some 8 years we have been deeply interested in the association of eye and gut disease so that one of us (D.L.K.) sees most of our hospital's patients with ocular complications of gastrointestinal disease. During this 8-year period there have been approximately 160 patients with ulcerative colitis admitted to the hospital, giving an estimated incidence of ocular complications of 0.63%.

Korelitz and Coles reported 1.9% prevalence of ocular inflammations in a group of 470 patients with ulcerative colitis or granulomatous enterocolitis.[19] Recent review of their patients has led to the clarification that many disorders called "ulcerative colitis" are now defined by current criteria as being Crohn's disease. Evidence was presented in the original paper that surgical excision of the affected gut gave relief of the ocular inflammation in some cases.

Daffner and Brown in a series of 100 patients with Crohn's disease reported two patients with iritis and iridocyclitis, one patient with episcleritis, and one with choroiditis. This gave a prevalence of 4% ocular complications.[7]

WHIPPLE'S DISEASE

Ocular complications or involvement from Whipple's disease have now occurred in at least 18 patients. Intraocular inflammations have occurred in five and ophthalmoplegia in 14. Twelve of these patients have been reported formally in the literature[2, 9, 18, 24, 25] and the remaining six are known to us by way of personal communications from colleagues who know of our interest in this disorder.

Whipple's disease (intestinal lipodystrophy)[28] is a disorder, usually of men over 35, who may have arthritis, fever, serous effusions, cough, lymphadenopathy, and malaise for several years before a final phase in which intestinal malabsorption, steatorrhea, and cachexia lead to death.[10] Most cases, reported before 1955, were diagnosed at autopsy where mucopolysaccharide deposits were found in macrophages in the intestine and intestinal lymphatics. Increasing awareness by physicians and pathologists of the multisystem nature and histopathologic characteristics of Whipple's disease, has led to antemortem diagnoses in recent years. Jejunal mucosal biopsies by way of the mouth, peripheral lymph node biopsy, or abdominal exploration have established or confirmed the diagnosis in many patients who were being studied for diarrhea or malabsorption.

Current criteria for histologic diagnosis require the presence of foamy "Whipple" macrophages[12] PAS (periodic acid–Schiff)–positive granules in jejunal lamina propria. The foamy macrophages and PAS material can also be found in rectal mucosa, mesenteric and extraabdominal lymphoid tissue, heart, lungs, liver, adrenals, spleen, and serous membranes deposits of PAS material, but not foamy macrophages, have been seen in various areas of the brain, arachnoid, retinal, and peripheral and optic nerves.[2, 20, 24-26]

An infectious cause for this disease was considered by Whipple himself, who stated in his original report that he suspected the presence of bacteria in histologic sections stained by the Levaditi's silver technique. This observation attracted little interest until Paulley realized that antibiotic therapy controlled symptoms and reversed the disease process.[21] Electron microscopic studies have supported Whipple's observation by demonstrating "bacillary bodies" extracellularly and in the foamy, "Whipple" macrophages.[6, 15, 30] Bacillary bodies have been seen in the brain of one patient. Bacterial cultures of jejunal aspirates and mucosal biopsies have not demonstrated a single or predominant agent. These studies have not been considered definitive because of the source and possibility of contamination. Whipple's disease is currently considered to be a systemic bacterial infection with the ultimate principal focus being in the intestine. These patients can be shown to have an altered immunologic state with impaired delayed hypersensitivity even while in prolonged remission.[13]

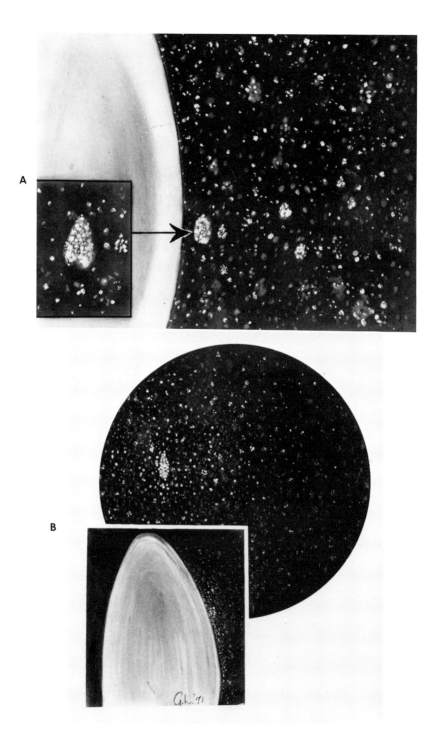

Fig. 16-2. Vitreous opacities seen in eyes of two different patients, **A** and **B,** with Whipple's disease.

A supranuclear type of ophthalmoplegia has been seen in 14 patients. This may involve verticle gaze more than horizontal gaze or may be total but sparing the levators of the lids. Papilledema has been seen in one case.[26] Myoclonic eye, facial, and skeletal muscle action is another feature. Dementia is common, with memory loss and inappropriate behavior. These abnormalities have been seen in patients before they develop characteristic diarrhea, steatorrhea, and weight loss, which might have led to the diagnosis. Some patients have developed their neurologic symptoms after varying periods of antibiotic therapy.

Ocular inflammations have been seen in four patients. One of these has been reported.[18] The second patient had a sudden blurring of vision and was found to have bacteria on Gram staining of the aqueous humor. Two other patients have been seen with intraocular inflammation.[23] Heavy vitreous opacities seem to be a prominent part of the clinical picture of the two patients seen by us[18] (Fig. 16-2). Opacities in the vitreous have been described by other clinicians who did not define that the eyes were inflamed.

The importance of diagnosing Wipple's disease is that it is a medically treatable disorder that if not treated leads to death. Recurrent multisystem inflammatory disease that seems infectious because of elevated white blood cell count and response to antibiotics should alert the clinician to this possibility even before the deterioration phase with diarrhea and weight loss.

INTESTINAL PARASITES

For the past 50 years articles have appeared in the ophthalmic literature implicating intestinal parasites as a cause of ocular disease. The tone of many of these articles is one of caution as evidence by the title of one: "L'Amibiase oculaire existe-t-elle?"[27] Many reports have focused upon *Entamoeba histolytica,* whose pathogenicity for the gut and liver is well established. Most cases have a chorioretinal exudative process,[4, 14, 17] and some have anterior segment inflammation. The similarity of the fundus disease as well as the responses to antiamebic therapy are the evidences that are cited for a cause-and-effect relationship between the parasitic infestation and the eye disease. Challenging arguments are based on the frequency of inactive amebiasis in a general population and whether or not the patient has cysts or motile trophozoites.

Giardia lamblia is also implicated in various case reports and reviews.[5, 8] This is an extremely common intestinal parasite, so that in some geographic areas the frequency of its presence in the stools of "normal" individuals leads clinicians to consider it a nonpathogenic parasite. Reports serve to establish that it is a significant pathogen producing diarrhea, steatorrhea, urticaria, malaise, epigastric distress, and evening belching.[1, 11, 22, 29] The mechanism of these effects is not known. Ocular involvement is usually a central chorioretinal serous exudative process. This has been found in our experience with *Giardia.* In 12 patients found to have *Giardia* as part of a uveitis evaluation; three had central macular processes, three had active retinitis adjacent to an old chorioretinal scar and serologic evidence to support a diagnosis of *Toxoplasma* retinitis, three had chronic iridocyclitis, two had retinal vasculitis, and one, a "pars planitis syndrome."

Other intestinal parasites have been found by our studies of patients with ocular inflammation. *Endolimax nana,* ordinarily a nonpathogen, was found in the stools of two patients, one of whom also had *E. nana* cysts in his urine. Both patients had exudative chorioretinopathies morphologically similar to that labeled as amebic choroidosis (Fig. 16-3). The patient with cysts in both urine and stool had lost one eye because of phthisis after 1 year of inflammation. Vision was reduced to 20/100 in the second eye. Chloroquine therapy reversed the exudative process and vision recovered to 20/20. *Entamoeba coli* has been found in the stools of two patients with exudative chorioretinopathy similar to amebic

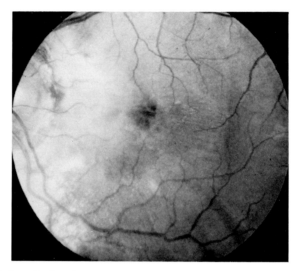

Fig. 16-3. Exudative chorioretinopathy in 30-year-old Negro male who had recurrence of *Endolimax nana* in his stools at same time as this recurrence of ocular disease.

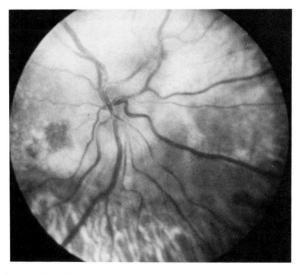

Fig. 16-4. Exudative chorioretinopathy that persisted for 1 year until treatment for *Entamoeba coli,* was followed by improvement in the ocular process.

choroidosis (Figs. 16-4 and 16-5) and in one patient who had chronic irido-cyclitis. *Dientamoeba fragilis* was recovered from both stool and abnormal brown thin mucous at proctoscopy of a patient with 3 months of malaise and 2 weeks of an inflammatory glaucoma. Local therapy helped the eye, and the malaise ceased after therapy for *Dientamoeba fragilis*. One other patient with this parasite had a chronic iridocyclitis. Reports in the literature alert to its capacity as a pathogen.[16] *Strongyloides stercoralis* was found in a patient with bilateral chemosis, proptosis, ophthalmoplegia, and eosinophilia. Treatment of the *Strongyloides* was followed by subsidence of the eye signs and the eosinophilia. Hookworm ova were found in the stools of one patient with central chorioretinopathy (Fig. 16-6).

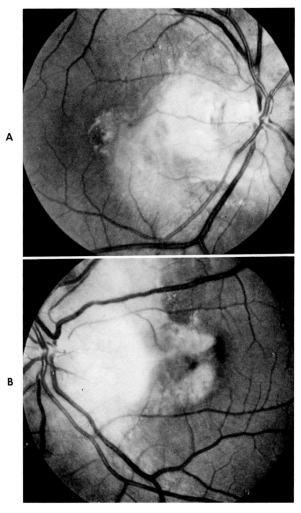

Fig. 16-5. Bilateral exudative chorioretinopathy in woman who was found to have *Entamoeba coli* cysts in her stools. **A,** Right eye. **B,** Left eye.

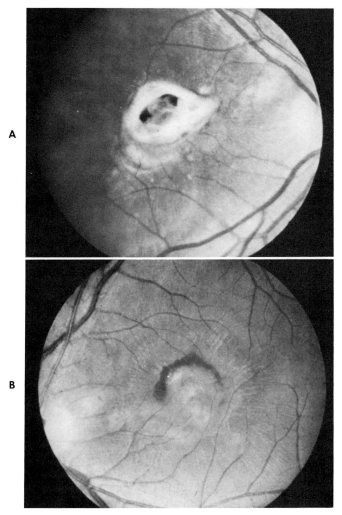

Fig. 16-6. Disciform disease in 16-year-old girl with hookworm infection of gut. **A,** Right eye. **B,** Left eye.

PEPTIC ULCER DISEASE

Peptic ulcer disease is estimated to occur at least once in the adult lives of 10% of American males. It may be subclinical and not cause recognizable symptoms. This was true in 30% of those company executives found to have ulcers when given routine x-ray examinations. Peptic ulcer is so often a "second" disease, and the epidemiologic or statistical tests to implicate it as a cause of other diseases are rarely attempted. Diagnosis and management serve to satisfy a concept of good medicine and patient care.

The clearest association between peptic ulcer disease and an eye disorder occurs when a central optic neuropathy develops from a postgastrectomy vitamin B_{12}–deficiency syndrome. The mechanism of vitamin B_{12} deficiency is the absence of intrinsic factor usually formed in the stomach, which is necessary for absorption of vitamin B_{12} in the small intestine. This eye problem occurs practically always in males and has been well documented by both vitamin B_{12} assays and improvement in central vision with intramuscular vitamin B_{12} therapy.

From our clinical experience the following cases have been selected to implicate active peptic ulcer disease as an etiologic factor in eye disease.

A 45-year-old white male had recurrent iritis from 25 to 37 years of age. He was originally seen at the Wilmer Institute in 1957, at age 37, where studies led to the prescribing of a series of desensitization injections with streptococcal antigens. This was followed by relief of his recurrent iritis until the following events took place. He had experienced intermittent mild epigastric distress until one day he experienced sudden severe epigastric pain. He collapsed in a cold sweat and laid on the floor for 15 to 20 minutes. At a hospital emergency room, no abnormalities were found on physical examination and he was sent home where abdominal pain persisted and he required narcotics for relief. The iritis recurred. He then returned to the Johns Hopkins Hospital, where studies revealed that he had a posterior perforation of a duodenal peptic ulcer. Surgical management of the perforation and topical therapy to the eye were followed by cessation of the iritis.

A 46-year-old white female came for evaluation of an iridocyclitis of 18 months' duration in the right eye and 4 months' duration in the left eye. Her mother and sisters had severe peptic ulcer disease. She herself had had peptic ulcers for 10 years and despite good antacid and anticholinergic management was vomiting every other small feeding. X-ray studies revealed active duodenal ulcer crater, pronounced mucosal edema, and limited passage of contrast material through her duodenum. Surgical management of the peptic ulcer was advised. Gastrectomy with gastrojejunostomy was followed by relief of peptic ulcer symptoms. Six weeks later both eyes were free of signs of inflammation, which have not returned.

Active peptic ulcer occurred in, or was a prominent symptom in, 5 patients with the syndrome known as glaucomatocyclitis crises. The most dramatic of these was a 40-year-old white male who had an x-ray diagnosis of ulcer prior to his first bout of inflammatory glaucoma, which lasted 3 months. A second episode of glaucoma lasted 3 weeks. The third event led to hospital studies that found an intestinal parasite *(Endolimax nana)* and a history of epigastric distress and pain. Upper gastrointestinal x-ray contrast studies found an active peptic ulcer. Treatment of both ulcer and parasites was followed by relief of the glaucoma. He then stopped taking antacids. Six months later the patient ate a raw, ground beef sandwich at midnight and awakened the next morning with halos in his vision. Pressure was elevated, and keratic precipitates were seen again. A repeat upper gastrointestinal tract series demonstrated a new duodenal ulcer in a different location. For 7 years he has maintained antacid therapy prophylactically and has had no return of eye symptoms or peptic ulcer. Four other patients with active inflammatory glaucoma have had active peptic ulcers. In one of the early reports on this syndrome Kraupa mentions *Darmstörung* (gut disturbance) as a concurrent difficulty in one of the patients he had encountered.

As stated, the high prevalence of peptic ulcer in the general male population makes an association of peptic ulcer with another disease a tenuous one. The sequence of events in these patients with relapses of eye disease with recurrence of ulcer and remissions after therapy for the ulcer disease seems to be more than coincidental. Mechanisms for this association can be proposed as follows: antigenic material gains access to the systemic circulation through the defect in the mucosa at the ulcer site; antibodies travel to the mucosa; then partially digested food or damaged tissue at the edge of the ulcer, formed by inflammatory cells at the base of the ulcer, passes into the circulation and combines with appropriate receptors in the eye.

REFERENCES

1. Babb, R. R., Peck, O. C., and Vescia, F. G.: Giardiasis, a cause of traveler's diarrhea, J.A.M.A. **217:**1359-1361, Sept. 1971.
2. Badenoch, J., Richards, W. C. D., and Oppenheimer, D. R.: Encephalopathy in a case of Whipple's disease, J. Neurol. Neurosurg. Psychiatry **26:**203, 1963.
3. Billson, F. A., et al.: Ocular complications of ulcerative colitis, Gut **8:**102-106, 1967.
4. Braley, A. E., and Hamilton, H. E.: Central serous choroidosis associated with amebiasis, Arch. Ophthalmol. **58:**1-14, 1957.
5. Carroll, M. E., Anast, B. P., and Birch, C. L.: Giardiasis and uveitis, Arch. Ophthalmol. **65:**775-778, 1961.
6. Cohen, A. S., Schimmel, E. M., Holt, P. R., and Isselbacher, K. J.: Ultrastructural abnormalities in Whipple's disease, Proc. Soc. Exp. Biol. Med. **105:**411, 1960.
7. Daffner, J. E., and Brown, C. H.: Regional enteritis. Clinical aspects and diagnosis in 100 patients, Ann. Intern. Med. **49:**580-594, 1958.
8. Djabri, S. E., and Diallinas, N.: L'Importance de la lambliase comme facteur étiologique dans la choriorétinite centrale séreuse, Ophthalmologica **147:**264-272, 1964.
9. Enzinger, F. M., and Helwig, E. B.: Whipple's disease, a review of the literature and report of fifteen patients, Virchow's Arch. Pathol. Anat. **336:**238-269, 1963.
10. Farnam, P.: Whipple's disease, the clinical aspects, Q. J. Med. **28:**163-182, 1959.
11. Gleason, N. N., et al.: A stool survey for enteric organisms in Aspen, Colorado. Am. J. Trop. Med. Hyg. **19:**480-484, May 1970.
12. Gonzalez-Licea, A., and Yardley, J. H.: Ultrastructural observations on PAS positive granules of Whipple's disease and muciphages in rectal biopsy tissue, Am. J. Pathol. **50.** May 1967.
13. Groll, A., et al.: Immunologic defect in Whipple's disease, Gastroenterology **63:**943, Dec. 1972.
14. Harris, D., and Birch, C. L.: Bilateral uveitis associated with gastrointestinal *Entamoeba histolytica* infection, case report, Am. J. Ophthalmol. **50:**496-500, 1960.
15. Haubrick, W. S., Watson, J. H. L., and Sieracki, J. C.: Unique morphologic features of Whipple's disease—a study of light and electron microscopy, Gastroenterology **39:**454-468, 1960.
16. Kean, B. M., and Malloch, C. L.: The neglected ameba: *Dientamoeba fragilis,* Am. J. Dig. Dis. (New Series) **11:**735-746, 1966.
17. King, R. E., Praeger, D. L., and Hallett, J. W.: Amebic choroidosis, Arch. Ophthalmol. **72:**16-22, 1964.
18. Knox, D. L., Bayless, T. M., Yardley, J. M., and Charache, P.: Whipple's disease presenting with ocular inflammation and minimal intestinal symptoms, Johns Hopkins Med. J. **123:**175-182, 1968.
19. Korelitz, B. I., and Coles, R. S.: Uveitis (iritis) associated with ulcerative and granulomatous colitis, Gastroenterology **52:**78-82, 1967.
20. Krucke, W.: Über Veränderungen im Zentral-nervensystem bei Whipple'scher Krankheit, Verh. Dtsch. Ges. Pathol. **46:**198-202, 1962.
21. Paulley, J. W.: A case of Whipple's disease (intestinal lipodystrophy), Gastroenterology **22:**128-133, 1952.
22. Peterson, H.: Giardiasis (lambliasis), Scand. J. Gastroenterol. **7:**Supplement 14, 1972.

23. Schlaegel, T. F.: Personal communication.
24. Sieracki, J. C., Fine, G., and Horn, R. C.: Central nervous system involvement in Whipple's disease, J. Neuropathol. Exp. Neurol. **19:**70-74, 1960.
25. Smith, W. T., French, J. M., Gottsman, M., Smith, A. J., and Wakes-Miller, J. A.: Cerebral complications of Whipple's disease, Brain **88:**137, 1965.
26. Switz, D. M., Casey, T. R., and Bogaty, G. V.: Whipple's disease and papilledema, Arch. Intern. Med. **123:**74-77, 1969.
27. Toulant, P.: L'Amibiase oculaire existe-t-elle? Bull. Soc. Ophthalmol. Fr., pp. 351-361, April 1936.
28. Whipple, G. H.: A hitherto undescribed disease characterized anatomically by deposits of fat and fatty acids in the intestinal and mesenteric lymphatic tissues, Bull. Johns Hopkins Hosp. **18:**382, 1907.
29. Wilhelm, R. T.: Urticaria associated with giardiasis lamblia, J. Allergy **28:**351-353, 1957.
30. Yardley, J. H., and Hendrix, T. R.: Combined electron and light microscopy in Whipple's disease—demonstration of "bacillary bodies" in the intestine, Bull. Johns Hopkins Hosp. **109:**80-98, 1961.

Ocular involvement in gastrointestinal disease

CHAIRMAN: **Frederick A. Mausolf**

Dr. Mausolf: Thank you for the interesting paper. Dr. Sanders will now make some comments.

Dr. Sanders: I would like to describe a patient under the care of Dr. D. Croft of St. Thomas' Hospital in London with a 20-year history of intermittent pyrexia, fleeting arthropathy, floaters in front of both eyes, and more recently the development of diarrhea and then steatorrhea. Peroral jejunal biopsy confirmed the diagnosis of Whipple's disease.

Ocular signs included slight reduction in visual acuity to 20/30 right and left, and cells were present in the vitreous. Fundus examination since 1967 has shown bilateral disk swelling with abnormal dilated vessels and superficial hemorrhages.

Fluorescein angiography in 1970 showed considerable dilatation of the papillary and superficial peripapillary capillary plexus with involvement of the macular vessels (Fig. 1, *A*). Residual pictures taken after 10 minutes showed pronounced peripapillary cystoid retinopathy extending to the macular region (Fig. 1, *B*).

After the commencement of antibiotic therapy, there was considerable symptomatic improvement with some resolution of the retinal vascular changes (Fig. 1, *C*).

The fundus changes in this patient have not previously been described and suggest retinal vasculitis involving mainly the capillaries of the posterior pole. Autopsy examination has demonstrated cerebral perivascular small round cell infiltration in a patient with other neurologic findings. The importance of this case is the identification of a retinal vasculitis in conjunction with a systemic disease involving the immune mechanism, which is amenable to treatment. This case is being reported fully in the *British Journal of Ophthalmology*.

Dr. Mausolf: Thank you. Are there any comments?

Dr. Bole: Arthropathy has been mentioned in Whipple's disease, and I would merely emphasize the gaps that can occur between the various so-called classic system involvements. We occasionally see people because of the acute and mysterious cycling polyarthritis. I believe that, even though rare, Whipple's

is an important disease to recognize and I would underscore the long chrono-
logic history of years between these isolated episodes. I believe that makes it
very difficult to make the diagnosis.

Dr. Prewitt: I would like to ask Dr. Knox that since a great deal of work on food
allergies has been done and many of the immunologists around the country
are finding that food plays a definite part in a good bit of our retinal pathology,

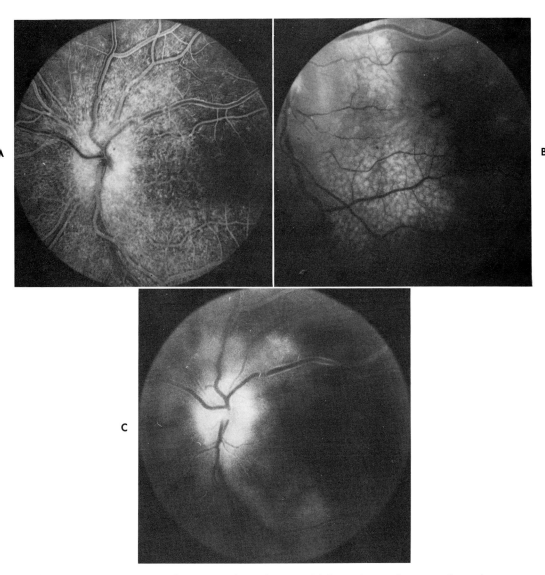

Fig. 1. Whipple's disease. **A,** Fluorescein angiogram of left eye in arteriovenous phase, showing pronounced dilatation of papillary and peripapillary capillaries. **B,** Residual picture (5
minutes) of left eye showing peripapillary cystoid retinopathy. **C,** Residual picture (5 minutes)
showed resolution of cystoid retinopathy 6 months after antibiotic treatment.

might food allergies be an answer to some of the questions asked the other day? I might say that the otolaryngologists now for over 6 years have had a society that has been doing excellent work on different techniques for discovering food sensitivities. We have outstanding men in nearly all the states now giving these courses, and I would suggest that some of the allergists and some of the men interested in finding the answer to some of these retinal lesions would do well to take up a little study on the immunoallergic site to find out the diagnosis in these cases.

Dr. Knox: I appreciate Dr. Prewitt's comments. We know of his long interest in this particular area. The diagnosis and management of food allergies is a tough one, but I think there are definite patients whose histories are so clear that you have to give them some credence. I liked Mike Sanders' pictures concerning his patient because it amplifies what I'm trying to emphasize as the multisystem and multilocular involvement of this particular disease. Why the retinal capillaries and arteries at the nerve head should leak, I don't know, but probably we can explain it as a migration of the organisms, which then become PAS-positive granules in macrophages, setting up some sort of mild inflammation around the blood vessel. The fact that there is some disorder in the way the host manages his bacteria is crucial to the understanding of this particular disease. How much is an allergic component or a vasculitis added on to that, we cannot say. There is a man who had smoldering papilledema for almost 5 years and who was lucky enough not to be so sick that it killed him before the diagnosis was made, but this is often what occurs. The gastrointestinal symptoms are late. Another thing we have learned is that patients with this particular disease are prone to late neurologic complications, and sometimes with their memory defect, they forget they have been treated for Whipple's disease and they come in with ophthalmoplegia and memory problems. Sort of out of the past somebody says, "Oh, he had Whipple's disease 3 years ago." So think about it; it's a disorder for which treatment saves the patient's life.

Dr. Hayreh: Dr. Knox pointed out the association of episcleritis with Crohn's disease, and in one case he said the first patient had episcleritis and then he had scleromalacia. In our experience of more than 400 cases of episcleritis and scleritis we found that a patient with episcleritis never developed scleritis, whereas a patient with scleritis has always associated overlying swelling and involvement of the episclera; so I personally would be inclined to believe that the patient originally had scleritis because the scleritis that goes on to scleromalacia involves episcleritis. At Moorfields we found that referring to patients as episcleritis patients was a very common thing, but then on detailed examination we found they turned out to be scleritis patients. So I get a feeling that that patient was perhaps one with scleritis that went on to scleromalacia because we never had any patient with episcleritis going on to scleromalacia. The second point is that there was one patient with central serous retinopathy and one patient with optic neuritis, and so is it a significant association or is it just a coincidental finding? This is something one has to consider before attributing these associations to Crohn's disease.

Dr. Knox: In all of medicine it is a great difficulty to decide when we have a significant association, when it is a coincidence, and when it is just totally unrelated. At this point I don't believe that there is any common sort of ocular involvement with Crohn's disease. Lillian Boniuk has a patient with a scleritis process that she biopsied and it did show giant cells from a patient with Crohn's disease. At this point I have not been able to get her to give up a slide that I can put into my lecture, but this seems to be at least one association. I think it's difficult to say what causes Crohn's disease and also what causes the eye problem. Is it some sort of effect of Crohn's disease in the inflammatory immunologic events occurring with Crohn's disease that somehow targets in on the eye? These are questions that we may never answer, but I think it's good to make the association.

Dr. Henkind: A point that bothers me a little about the amebiasis story or the parasitic story—in New York City there are literally hundreds of thousands perhaps millions of people who are positive for parasites. As a matter of fact, I remember as a medical student and resident in New York that it was exceptionally common to have people with an eosinophilia and then you'd get a stool sample and they'd have a parasite and yet the fundus picture that is described today and has been described was exceptionally rare. We just don't see this picture very commonly, despite seeing many fundus pathologies, and I just wonder if Dave Cogan or anybody in the audience, perhaps Dr. Braley, can tell us what factor they think it is besides the parasite that's causing it because if it's the parasite itself then the incidence of ocular findings in the parasite disease must be exceptionally uncommon.

Dr. Braley: I saw my first cases of amebiasis when I was in New York. I used to be up at the Eye Institute there, and that's when I saw my first cases. I was unable to be sure what the diagnosis was, and it was kind of by exclusion and waiting around, and I think the best treatment was when we would treat them with chloroquine and emetine. You can see these things clear up with this therapy. Now I believe these are still being missed every once in a while and being called histoplasmosis and treated usually with light coagulation or something like that. I would like to ask one thing and that is in relation to Crohn's disease—of course, its counterpart, which is so well known, is the simple enteritis that occurs. I wonder has anyone ever seen the severe conjunctivitis that sometimes occurs with enteritis?

Dr. Knox: I appreciate Dr. Braley's remarks. It's always fun bringing coals to Newcastle! I agree that being solidly scientific and having the data that will make a skeptic a believer about the chorioretinopathy that occurs in intestinal parasites is very difficult, and I also end up saying, "Well, this is what I am going to do with my patients. If you want to listen to me that is fine, and you do with yours what you want to do, if you do not believe." I think that if we are going to be therapists, it's a therapeutic avenue that ought to be driven down in the effort to help the patient. Of how scientific one should be about it is another matter. In Crohn's disease I do not remember seeing a patient with conjunctivitis. You don't think this is the beginning of a case of Reiter's syndrome?

Dr. Braley: So many people have chronic diarrhea and frequently these people have a recurrent conjunctivitis, and I know this: I see people all the time with recurrent conjunctivitis that have been treated with every kind of medication.

Why all the ophthalmologists in this room get drugs from the pharmaceutical houses, and they do not really study the patient. If the patient complains of something wrong, why they just give them a drop to use. I know it happens all the time. So, if you will study some of these people, you will find that many of them have a diarrhea or an enteritis of one kind or another, and you can cure them by trying to get rid of that enteritis.

Dr. Knox: Are these more often women?

Dr. Braley: Yes, more often women.

Dr. Zahoruk: There is a recent book on Crohn's disease by a man by the name of Truelove, and Dr. Sanders who had talked to the department earlier this week had some comments on the high incidence of iritis that Truelove alludes to in patients with Crohn's disease.

Dr. Sanders: I think Truelove in his book shows an instance of iritis of about 15%, and apparently he got his ophthalmic residents to dilate the pupils and then they looked at the anterior chamber and found one or two cells and so they wrote it down as iritis. So I think the incidence is much lower than in his book and I think there is probably a rather fallacious reading.

Dr. Knox: Obviously, if somebody is going to make the diagnosis of iritis on cells after pupillary dilatation, it will be high. A report out of the Mt. Sinai Hospital gave an incidence of something like 1.9% or 3.6% or something like that, very small, but again they were mixing a case of ulcerative colitis and Crohn's disease.

17

Dermatology and the eye

Harold O. Perry

The close association between various skin diseases and alterations within the structures of the eyes has long been known. By recognizing dermatologic disease in which there may be associated eye findings, the dermatologist can make an important contribution in diagnosis. The ophthalmologist then can examine the eye and provide therapy for the eye involvement. Likewise, the ophthalmologist, on the basis of findings within the eye, can seek the help of the dermatologist in determining whether a specific cutaneous eruption might be the cause of the eye disease. This cooperative spirit has been particularly helpful in studying a disease such as pseudoxanthoma elasticum.

This monograph emphasizes the eye findings in a group of diseases, some in which the findings are purely dermatologic and others in which the skin involvement is only part of the syndrome. The diseases will be discussed on the basis of the following five sections: (1) dermatologic diseases with ocular involvement, (2) hereditary dermatoses with ocular involvement, (3) infectious diseases with ocular involvement, (4) syndromes with skin and ocular involvement, and (5) dermatoses and cutaneous syndromes with cataracts.

DERMATOLOGIC DISEASES WITH OCULAR INVOLVEMENT

Some clinical entities have eye findings not only because the skin lesions are located near the eyes but also because the disease itself is within the eye (see list below). Also some cutaneous lesions that are clinically distinctive in themselves are associated with equally distinctive ocular findings, with neither lesion resembling the other. Most often the ocular findings are not limited to a single change but consist of various changes that may be either mild and only transitory or long-standing and severe, interfering with the comfort of the patient, and eventually leading to loss of vision.

Dermatologic diseases with ocular involvement

Hemangiomas	Psoriasis
Nevus of Ota	Pemphigoid
Dermatitis venenata	Erythema multiforme
Atopic dermatitis	Behçet's syndrome
Seborrheic dermatitis	Juvenile xanthogranuloma
Acne rosacea	Porphyria cutanea tarda
Hidradenitis suppurativa	Nevus sebaceus of Jadassohn

Hemangiomas

Among the commonest of the nevoid disturbances of the skin are those related to the vascular system. Port-wine nevi in the midline of the forehead or the nuchal area are frequently seen at birth or early in life. These nevi often disappear spontaneously during the early years of life. Strawberry and cavernous hemangiomas may be present at birth but also may develop during the first weeks to months of life and may increase in size. Hemangiomas may occur anywhere on the body, but of special concern are those involving the exposed areas of the body. Those involving the eyelids may be so large that closure of the eye occurs. Under these circumstances, the conjunctival surface of the lids may contain the hemangioma.

The strawberry hemangiomas usually disappear spontaneously without treatment during the first 2 years of life. Cavernous hemangiomas, however, may require surgical intervention for their control.

A hemangioma on the eyelid may be of cosmetic importance (Fig. 17-1). Its association with retrolental fibrosis has not yet been proved as being statistically significant. When the hemangioma is excessively large and the child cannot open his eye, amblyopia may occur.

Nevus of Ota

In the nevus of Ota some pigmentary alteration of the eyelids may be so striking as to be cosmetically disfiguring, yet others may be so mild that they can be readily covered by cosmetics so as to be unnoticeable.

The nevus of Ota usually involves the scleras, bulbar and palpebral conjunc-

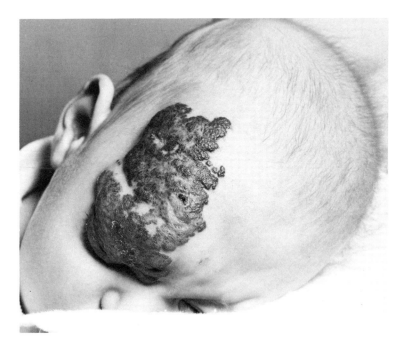

Fig. 17-1. Hemangiomas involving eye not only may be a cosmetic disfigurement to patient but may cause amblyopia.

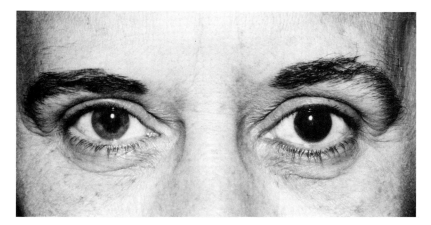

Fig. 17-2. Deeper brown color of one of irides may first direct attention to presence of nevus of Ota.

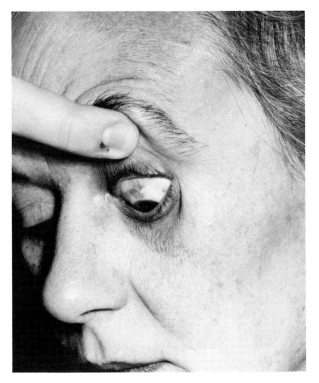

Fig. 17-3. Pigmentary changes of skin in distribution of first two branches of trigeminal nerve with pigmentary changes of cornea are characteristically seen in nevus of Ota.

tivae, and skin areas restricted to the first and second divisions of the trigeminal nerve.[11] The oral mucosa also may be involved. Detailed studies have shown involvement of Tenon's capsule, cornea, iris, fundus, and muscles and fatty connective tissue of the orbit. Increased color of the iris on the involved side may be present (Fig. 17-2).

The pigmentary changes may be punctate or diffuse and present a tan, grayish brown cast to the sclera. When the skin is involved, it is usually gray although it may have shades of red, thus the name "nevus fuscoceruleus ophthalmomaxillaris" (Fig. 17-3).

This disorder is common in Japanese and Oriental people but also is seen in Negroes and Caucasians. The pigmentary changes are present in 50% of the patients at birth but may be noted later in childhood, and the changes usually become increasingly prominent with age. Hidano and associates[11] reported fading of some lesions. Involvement is usually unilateral, but it may be bilateral and is always asymptomatic. Approximately 80% of the patients are females.

Skin involvement is seen with ocular involvement in about 65% of patients. Melanosis oculi, sometimes considered a hereditary disease, has pigmentary changes limited to the ocular tissues. The similarity of pigmentation, differing only in degree, has suggested to some that melanosis oculi is a variant of nevus of Ota.[16]

Malignant melanoma developing in the skin in patients with nevus of Ota is rare. Even more rare is the development of melanoma in the choroid.

The melanosomes found deep in the dermis are similar histologically to some pigmentary disorders of the skin, such as the Mongolian spot, the pigmentation of the sacral area of Indian and Oriental children, East African natives, American Indians, and less frequently Caucasian children. This type of lesion fades with advancing age. The nevus of Ito is a bandlike pigmentary disorder involving the acromiodeltoid area. Neither of these types of lesions, however, has associated eye changes.

Dermatitis venenata

Acute and chronic dermatitis of the eyelids is of mutual interest to the dermatologist and the ophthalmologist. Because of the relatively increased sensitivity of skin of the eyelids to contactants, whether these are primary irritants or allergens, contact dermatitis is seen with great frequency in the eyelid areas. Exposure may occur from direct contact such as the application of cosmetics or from the mists and fumes of aerosols. Contactants may include chemicals encountered in one's occupation, products employed in the home, substances used in a hobby, and various toiletries used by both men and women.

In contrast, the ophthalmologist must be aware of the acute allergic reaction not only to the active ingredients of medications used in the eyes for primarily eye problems but also to the vehicles, preservatives, and stabilizers used in those medications.

The dermatitis may present initially as an erythematous blush to the involved skin. With more prolonged exposure, the skin may become edematous, vesicles may form, and eventually exudation with crust formation occurs (Fig. 17-4). Pruritus is always present. In more chronic exposure, lichenification may be

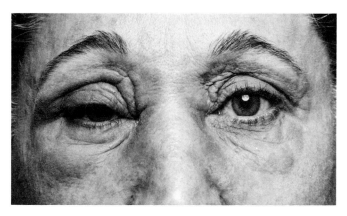

Fig. 17-4. Acute dermatitis of eyelids may represent dermatitis venenata to medicaments instilled into eyes or sensitivities to external contactants.

superimposed on the edema and erythema, and exudation may be minimal. Reproduction of the dermatitis on normal skin by the application of the suspected material in a patch test confirms the role of that substance in the production of the dermatitis.

Atopic dermatitis

Atopic eczema is a part of an inherited diathesis that also includes hayfever and asthma. The disease characteristically begins during the first months of life and may be present for a few years, gradually abating with time. Thus, the name of "infantile eczema" has been applied. There may be a recurrence at puberty, with subsidence of the active disease again during the midteens. Additional flares may occur later during the early adult years when the stresses of college work, occupational pursuit, or marriage seemingly precipitate the disease once again. The flare at puberty may persist into adulthood, with periods of exacerbations and only partial remissions.

During infancy, the skin may be dry, erythematous, and scaling, or with minimal rubbing, it may become exudative, resulting in crusting and at times secondary infection. The face, neck, and upper trunk may be involved early but with time, perhaps 2 to 5 years, a more flexural involvement of the cubital and popliteal areas may occur, with dry, scaling, lichenified plaques in these areas.

Pruritus is a predominant feature of the disease, with the patients almost habitually scratching the same localized areas of the skin, producing pronounced lichenification of the tissues.

The cause of atopic dermatitis remains unknown. The relationship of atopic dermatitis to hayfever and asthma suggests an allergic phenomenon. Patients with atopic dermatitis ordinarily have elevated levels of IgE, but these elevated levels have not been related causally to the disease; some patients with active atopic dermatitis have normal levels of IgE. Local factors of excessive dryness and irritants, as well as psychologic factors, have occasioned the name "disseminated neurodermatitis" to be applied to the clinical complex.

Other factors precipitating the disease are dryness of the skin (particularly

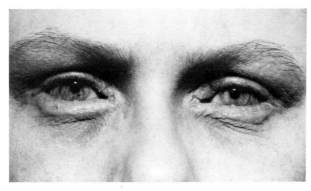

Fig. 17-5. Because of pruritus in atopic dermatitis, patient constantly rubs skin, producing thickening of skin with exudation, crusting, and scaling. Eyelids are commonly involved.

during the winter months), sweating (particularly during the summer months), the wearing of wool clothing, and at times the ingestion of certain foods. Contact dermatitis commonly occurs in the atopic person. The young patient with atopic dermatitis may develop conjunctivitis and lose his eyebrows as a consequence of the acuity of the process and the accompanying pruritus (Fig. 17-5).

Cataracts have been recognized as occurring in approximately 10% of the patients with atopic dermatitis,[6] but these patients ordinarily have long-standing severe disease. The cataracts in atopic dermatitis are usually bilateral, although one side may mature more rapidly than the other. Keratoconus also may be seen with atopic dermatitis. The cataracts that develop in atopic dermatitis must be differentiated from those that develop from the long and continued systemic use of steroids, which are given as treatment for the disease.

Seborrheic dermatitis

Seborrheic dermatitis is among the commonest of the dermatoses and is characterized by erythema and scaling of the scalp and in the facial creases, for example, about the nasolabial folds and the postauricular areas (Fig. 17-6). When the condition is severe, the intertriginous areas of the body, the axilla, the groin, the presternal area, and the upper back also may be affected and even generalized involvement may occur.[8c, 18b]

In its commonest form, the condition affects the scalp, with minimal involvement of adjacent cutaneous surfaces. Pruritus may be present, and itching and scratching, sometimes with excoriations and secondary infection, may occur. When the scaling is dry and flaky, the condition is referred to as "seborrhea sicca," and when the scale is more greasy, it is referred to as "seborrhea oleosa." The cause of the disease remains unknown, but the association of this dermatitis with hyperactive sebaceous glands probably is part of the basic pathologic process. No abnormalities in the sebum itself have been recognized.

Ocular findings may be characterized by involvement of the eyelids themselves, particularly the lateral angles of both eyes. Scaling along the lid margins may become extensive and produce a localized blepharitis. With more scaling, the reac-

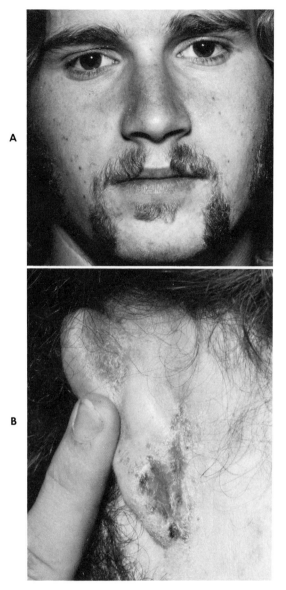

Fig. 17-6. A, Seborrheic dermatitis is characterized by erythema and scaling about central portion of face, including eyebrows, eyelids, and nasolabial folds. **B,** Intertriginous involvement of seborrheic dermatitis may become exudative as in postauricular area. (Same patient as in **A.**)

tion of the lid margins may become so pronounced that epithelial debris is continually shed onto the surface of the eye, producing a blepharoconjunctivitis.

The management of the seborrhea of the scalp requires frequent shampooing, and antiseborrheic substances (sulfur, salicylic acid) and anti-inflammatory agents (topical steroids) should be used for the involved cutaneous areas. The reaction of the ocular tissues will then sympathetically subside.

Acne rosacea

Acne rosacea usually has its onset insidiously in early middle age, although the cutaneous characteristics of persistent erythema and telangiectasias of the center of the face do not become severe until a few years later. The cosmetic problem is of paramount concern to the patient.

The disease is characterized early by pustules, with some diffuse erythema, over the central face, with the forehead and nose being more frequently involved. Crops of pustules recur, with the more chronic inflammatory papules persisting for long periods (Fig. 17-7). The erythema, which initially may be transient, becomes persistent; so the involved tissues become red. Telangiectasia of the skin eventually occurs and is considered a consequence of episodic flushing of the skin. Eventually in long-standing disease, hypertrophy of the involved tissues occurs and, when the nose is especially involved, produces the so-called rhinophyma.

Acne rosacea probably is related to acne vulgaris and sebaceous gland overactivity. Oiliness of the facial skin and seborrheic dermatitis are common accompaniments of the disease. The cause remains unknown although the ingestion of hot and spicy foods, alcohol, and certain medicaments may aggravate the disease.

Blepharoconjunctivitis is not uncommonly seen in acne rosacea. Only in patients with long-standing severe disease do keratitis and ulcers of the cornea develop and lead to loss of vision (Fig. 17-8). Iritis is less common.[20] Although ocular complications in the disease were commonly encountered a few years ago, now

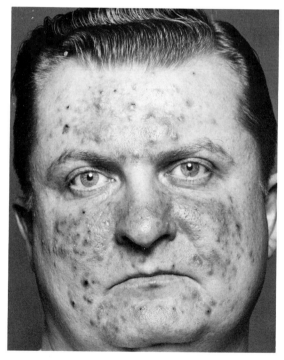

Fig. 17-7. Inflammatory papules and pustules over central portion of face are characteristic of acne rosacea.

because of better control of the rosacea with systemic medications, fewer ocular complications are seen.

Hidradenitis suppurativa

A variant of the problem of acne vulgaris is that of hidradenitis suppurativa, which has, as its major clinical presentation, purulent, draining, and inflammatory cystic lesions of the axillas and anogenital region, particularly in the female, and of these regions as well as the nuchal region in the male (Fig. 17-9). The presence of single, double, and multiple comedones in these regions indicates the relationship of hidradenitis suppurativa to acne vulgaris. The profound degree of inflammatory and purulent reaction, together with considerable pain and discomfort attending these soft-tissue reactions, at times completely disables the patient. In

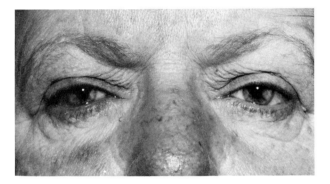

Fig. 17-8. Ocular complications of acne rosacea may even occur in mild cutaneous disease.

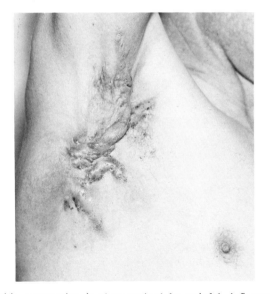

Fig. 17-9. Hidradenitis suppurativa is characterized by painful, inflammatory, and purulent draining lesions of intertriginous areas, commonly the axillas.

our experience, local measures give temporary symptomatic relief only, whereas surgical excision and skin grafting of the involved regions offer the patient more permanent relief.

Bergeron and Stone[2] studied 62 patients who had hidradenitis suppurativa and found that 4 patients had an associated interstitial keratitis. These authors found no relationship of this interstitial keratitis to congenital syphilis.

Psoriasis

The typical erythematous papules of psoriasis, with their micaceous scaling and predominant localization over the bony prominences, make the diagnosis of this common disease relatively easy.[8b] However, because of variations in its presentation, psoriasis may be mistaken for other papulosquamous dermatoses.

The disease occurs in families and is transmitted as an autosomal dominant trait with incomplete penetrance. The primary lesion is an erythematous papule, with scaling on its surface, that enlarges peripherally and eventually forms a plaque (Fig. 17-10). Widespread and eventual generalized involvement of the skin occurs by coalescence of the lesions. Pruritus is a common accompaniment, but excessive shedding of scales may be equally distressing.

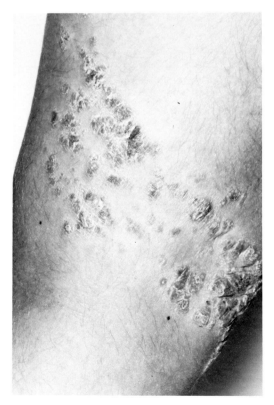

Fig. 17-10. Erythematous papules of psoriasis topped with micaceous scaling are characteristic of disease.

Arthralgias and arthritis, which may be rheumatoid or specifically diagnosed as psoriatic, are seen in 15% of patients. Psoriatic arthritis classically involves the distal interphalangeal joints and is accompanied by dystrophic nail changes of the involved digit. In patients with "true" psoriatic arthritis, the test for rheumatoid factor is negative.

Subtle changes in the nails (consisting of pitting and lateral and distal onycholysis), the Koebner reaction (production of lesions in sites of trauma), and a pink color to the tissues of the intergluteal cleft are findings helpful in making the diagnosis of psoriasis when the cutaneous changes are not clinically characteristic.

The scaling, a predominant feature of the disease, accounts for the conjunctivitis that can be present and results from the deposition of scales in the conjunctival sac. The presence of "true" psoriasis on the conjunctival surface of the lids may be responsible for the ocular irritation. Unless the psoriasis on the skin of the lids transgresses the lid margins and extends onto the mucosal surface, the diagnosis of psoriasis of the conjunctivae cannot be made with certainty. A rare complication of the psoriasis consists of involvement of the cornea with inflammatory infiltration, erosions, vascularization, and eventually opacification.[12]

Benign mucous membrane pemphigoid (cicatricial pemphigoid)

Advances within the past 15 years have permitted better classification of the blistering diseases of the skin. The recognition of acantholysis as a lytic process of epidermal cells differentiates true pemphigus from diseases resembling pemphigus, namely, pemphigoid and dermatitis herpetiformis. However, acantholysis cannot always be observed in biopsy specimens. Later the differences between the two groups were further clarified by the discoveries that circulating serum antibodies against intercellular substance of the epidermis characterized patients with pemphigus and that other circulating serum antibodies against the basement membrane zone characterized patients with pemphigoid.[7]

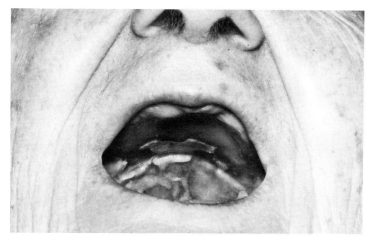

Fig. 17-11. Recurrent crops of blisters, which rupture easily, produce erosive and ulcerative lesions of oral cavity in cicatricial pemphigoid.

Table 17-1. Cutaneous and mucous membrane involvement in 81 patients with cicatricial pemphigoid

Site	Percent
Mouth	84
Eyes	77
Pharynx	43
Nose	38
Larynx	30
Genitalia	30
Female	35
Male	21
Anus	11
Esophagus	7
Skin	23

Pemphigoid can be grouped into major categories: the generalized bullous form in which blisters on urticarial plaques predominate in the intertriginous regions (mucous membrane lesions are uncommon) and the benign mucous membrane form in which blistering of the mucosal surfaces predominates and in which skin blistering is uncommon. Because of the severe scarring of the mucous membranes, the disease may be more appropriately called "cicatricial pemphigoid."

Although antibodies previously were considered to be present only in the serum of patients with generalized bullous pemphigoid and to be absent in patients with cicatricial pemphigoid, more recent studies indicate that antibodies to the basement membrane zone can be detected in both forms. The relationship of these two forms may be closer than had been considered in the past.[1]

In cicatricial pemphigoid, blistering of the mucosal surfaces predominates over that of the skin; the oral tissues are the most frequently involved (Fig. 17-11), and the conjunctivae, the next.[10] Crops of blisters recur and rupture, producing raw and denuded ulcers. The disease stimulates a proliferative reaction of the mucosal tissues: granulation tissue forms, followed after several weeks by fibrosis and scarring. The site of involvement with the blistering determines the clinical presentation of the disease. In a series of 81 patients, the sites of involvement varied (Table 17-1).

Local discomfort with burning and pain at the sites of blister formation characterized the disease. When oral tissues are severely involved, the patient's state of nutrition may suffer, and pharyngeal involvement may produce some respiratory distress. Involvement of the anogenital region may cause stricture of the urethra, vagina, or anus. The eyes are commonly involved, and it is at this location that the disease causes the most trouble.

Initially, the patient may experience burning of the eyes and recognize a mild conjunctival reaction. With progression of the disease, the conjunctival sacs become filled with granulation tissue, and a proliferative reaction progresses onto the sclera (Fig. 17-12). Photophobia may be intense. Adhesions between the lids and bulb may occur; so the lids cannot be closed. Drying and scarring of the cornea ensue. Blindness in one eye or in both eyes is the consequence of long-standing progressive disease. Trichiasis may aggravate the corneal damage, and corneal perforation may occur (Table 17-2).

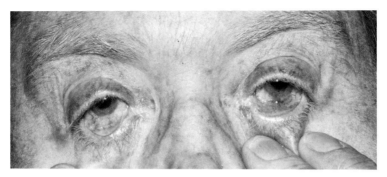

Fig. 17-12. Ocular involvement in cicatricial pemphigoid is characterized by obliteration of conjunctival sac by proliferation of granulation tissue and fibrosis.

Table 17-2. Ocular involvement and complications in 62 patients with cicatricial pemphigoid

Involvement	Percent
Eyes	77
Both eyes	87
Bullae without sequelae	11
Trichiasis	23
Scarring	89
Blindness	34
Both eyes	81
Corneal perforation	8
Bilateral	20

To date there is no effective therapy for cicatricial pemphigoid. Corticosteroids are helpful in some patients, but the therapeutic response to their use is not uniformly good. Immunosuppressive drugs are also employed, but sufficient experience has not accrued to recommend their routine use. Very often the disease is progressive despite therapy.

Pemphigus vulgaris, characterized clinically by large bullae on the skin and a predominance of oral lesions when mucous membranes are involved, can be diagnosed histologically if acantholysis is noted in the epidermal cells above the basal layer and if antibodies to intercellular substance are found by both direct and indirect immunofluorescent techniques. The ocular conjunctivae rarely are involved, but conjunctivitis, proliferation of granulation tissue, symblepharon, and photophobia, indistinguishable from cicatricial pemphigoid, may be seen (Fig. 17-13).

Erythema multiforme

Erythema multiforme[18c] is a disease in which various-sized and -shaped erythematous macules, papules, and plaques, sometimes in association with blistering of the lesions, are present over the body and in which the lesions are precipitated by various infections (bacterial, viral, and fungal) and by reactions to various drugs (Fig. 17-14). The condition may be associated with other systemic

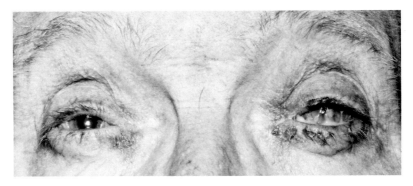

Fig. 17-13. Only rarely are ocular tissues involved with pemphigus vulgaris, but clinical presentation may be indistinguishable from that in cicatricial pemphigoid. (See Fig. 17-12.)

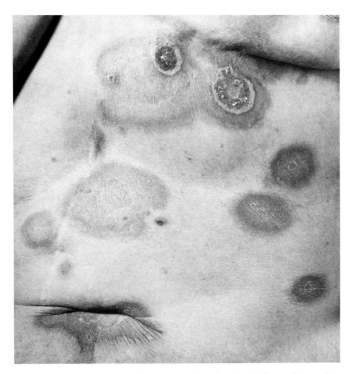

Fig. 17-14. Lesions of erythema multiforme consist of urticarial papules and annular lesions, some of which may present blistering on their surfaces.

diseases such as lupus erythematosus, periarteritis nodosa, Wegener's granulomatosis, and various carcinomas, as well as be a response to physical agents such as x-ray therapy.

The primary lesion begins with an erythematous maculopapular lesion that, as it increases in intensity, tends to form a bulla within the central portion of the lesion, producing a so-called iris configuration. The various forms of the disease have been classified clinically (Table 17-3).

Table 17-3. Clinical forms of erythema multiforme

Form	Comment
Papular or simplex	Maculopapular lesions of extremities
Vesiculobullous	Mucous membranes often involved
Severe bullous (Stevens-Johnson syndrome)	Systemic illness, fever, involvement of multiple organs, extensive involvement of mucous membranes
Atypical	Large erythematous plaques, atypical histologic findings

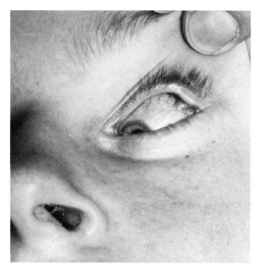

Fig. 17-15. Adhesions with symblepharon may be seen in erythema multiforme and may cause confusion in differentiating them from other blistering diseases.

In the more severe forms of the disease, the systemic complaints of lassitude and fatigue accompany pronounced constitutional symptoms and a high fever. Joint arthralgias are a frequent accompaniment. Ocular findings are common and consist of a catarrhal or purulent conjunctivitis, corneal ulcerations, anterior uveitis, and panophthalmitis. Symblepharon, resembling that in cicatricial pemphigoid, can be seen (Fig. 17-15). Ocular involvement, on rare occasions, produces corneal ulcers, which may perforate the globe and cause blindness.[17]

Behçet's syndrome

Behçet's syndrome[3, 9, 15] is characterized by ulcers of the mouth and genital regions that resemble aphthous ulcers and by a progressive iritis that sometimes causes blindness and is complicated by varied combinations of systemic manifestations consisting of fever, fatigue, arthritis, neurologic problems, and psychologic disturbances. The disease commonly affects young adult males. Unfortunately, there are no specific laboratory tests to confirm the diagnosis; the cause of the syndrome remains unknown.

Because of its many differing presentations, Behçet's syndrome is difficult to

Table 17-4. Criteria for diagnosis of Behçet's syndrome

Criteria	Series (25 patients) Number	Series (25 patients) Percent
Major		
Buccal ulceration	25	100
Genital ulceration	19	76
Eye lesions	19	76
Skin lesions	17	68
Minor		
Gastrointestinal lesions	6	24
Thrombophlebitis	6	24
Cardiovascular lesions	1	4
Arthritis	19	76
Central-nervous-system lesions	1	4
Family history	4	16

Modified from Mason, R. M., and Barnes, C. G.: Behçet's syndrome with arthritis, Ann. Rheum. Dis. **28:**95-103, March 1969.

diagnose. Recently, Mason and Barnes[13] have reviewed the problem and have employed major and minor criteria in the diagnosis, believing that a minimum of two major and two minor criteria are required for the diagnosis to be made (Table 17-4).

The stomal and genital ulcers frequently are the presenting signs and eventually develop in all patients sometime during the course of the disease. The ulcers do not differ from those ordinarily described as aphthae. Other skin lesions consist of erythema nodosum (in approximately one third of the patients), erythema multiforme, other nonspecific erythematous maculopapular eruptions, and pyodermatous lesions (impetigo, superficial and deep folliculitis, furuncles, cellulitis, and ulcers).

Thrombophlebitis, frequently superficial and commonly involving the legs, occurs in 25% of the patients. The central-nervous-system involvement, representing a serious complication, may resemble the changes seen in multiple sclerosis and may include, in addition, cranial nerve palsies, respiratory failure, and long-tract signs.

Ocular involvement, most often beginning as iritis, may be conjunctivitis, uveitis, progressive loss of vision, and retinal hemorrhages. The eye symptoms may lead to severe visual damage and even to total blindness.

Juvenile xanthogranuloma (nevoxanthoendothelioma)

Considerable confusion has existed about the nosologic position of this entity.[8a] In the past, because of its histiocytic histopathologic features and resemblance to xanthoma, juvenile xanthogranuloma was included among the xanthomas. However, results of blood lipid studies are always normal in these patients.

Juvenile xanthogranuloma is the disease of infancy and early childhood in which a few or multiple, yellowish brown to red infiltrated papules or plaques may occur on the skin of a young child, usually during the first months of life (Fig. 17-16). After an initial period of growth, the lesions remain unchanged for months, after which they gradually involute. The child's general health is un-

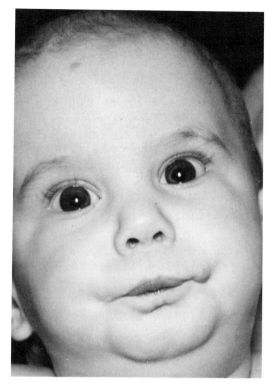

Fig. 17-16. Yellowish papules or plaques of skin in young child should always prompt consideration of xanthogranulomas.

affected. Skin lesions may be generalized over the body, without predilection for any region of the body.

Similar lesions may involve the iris and ciliary body. Previously, the involvement of the ciliary body was confused with a hemangiomatous lesion, but histologic study has now shown that the iris lesions have the same composition as do the lesions on the skin. Ocular involvement is generally unilateral, with glaucoma, spontaneous hyphema, and congenital or acquired heterochromia iridis also being seen.[21] Only rarely will other tissues be infiltrated with histiocytic cells, as seen in the skin. These tissues include bone lesions and pulmonary infiltrate.

Frequent association of xanthogranuloma with café-au-lait spots has been recognized, and numerous reports indicate an association between juvenile xanthogranuloma and neurofibromatosis.[14]

Porphyria cutanea tarda

The diseases of altered porphyrin metabolism are known as porphyria and can be divided into erythropoietic and hepatic types, depending on the major site of origin of the porphyrins. The dermatologist has a major interest in porphyria cutanea tarda because the important clinical characteristics are related to the skin.[5]

The pathologic porphyrin in porphyria cutanea tarda, uroporphyrin, is considered responsible for the photosensitivity seen in these patients and can be found

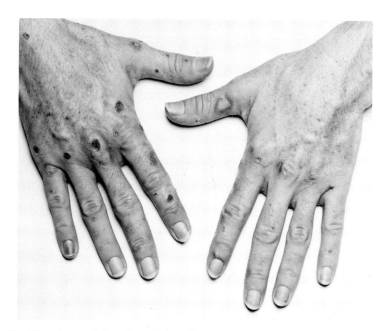

Fig. 17-17. Blistering and fragility of skin in sun-exposed areas characterize patients with porphyria cutanea tarda.

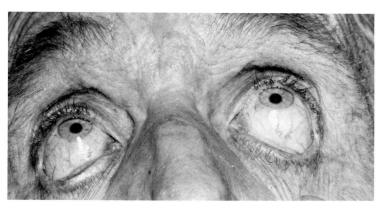

Fig. 17-18. Scleral and conjunctival injections are of major concern to patient with porphyria cutanea tarda and are of diagnostic significance.

in excessive amounts in the urine during the acute stage of the disease. Hepatic insult or impaired liver function seems to be the main cause of the disease.

Blistering and friability of the sun-exposed skin indicate that photosensitivity is a cause of the skin eruption (Fig. 17-17). The blisters rupture and, in the absence of continued insult, gradually heal, with scar formation. Other cutaneous signs include a suffusion to the face, neck, and upper trunk, together with injection of the scleras (Fig. 17-18), hyperpigmentation, sclerodermoid changes to the sun-exposed areas, hirsutism, darkening of the hair, and milia at sites of previous blis-

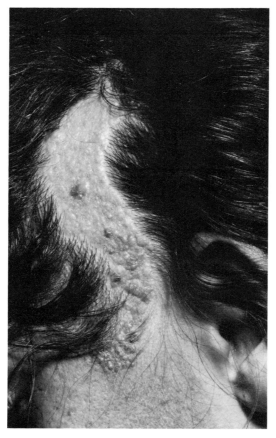

Fig. 17-19. Yellow verrucous plaques devoid of hair and occurring on scalp may eventually show local development of carcinoma or indicate eventual development of neurocutaneous syndrome consisting of seizures, mental deficiency, and ocular abnormalities.

tering. Scleromalacia has developed in porphyria cutanea tarda, and more recently the scleral perforation has been related to photosensitivity secondary to the porphyrins.[19]

Nevus sebaceus of Jadassohn (neurocutaneous syndrome)

Nevus sebaceus of Jadassohn is a discrete, light brown plaque, devoid of hair, and occurring on the scalp; the condition is congenitally present or develops during infancy. The plaques have a pebbled appearance, but there are no discrete papular lesions within the plaque (Fig. 17-19). During childhood, the plaque may become slightly thickened, but at puberty the plaque becomes more elevated and verrucous. Lesions are usually single but may be multiple and may occur in a linear configuration.[18a]

In later life, the plaque may develop various papillary or nodular excrescences, some of which may become secondarily infected with exudation and crusting. Approximately 20% of patients with nevus sebaceus of Jadassohn develop basal cell carcinomas or other hamartomatous growths within the plaques (Fig. 17-19).

The association of nevus sebaceus of Jadassohn with seizures, mental deficiency, and ocular abnormalities recently has been recognized; the ocular abnormalities include colobomas of the irides and choroid, conjunctival lipodermoids, horizontal and rotary nystagmus, and vascularization of the cornea.[1]

HEREDITARY DERMATOSES WITH OCULAR INVOLVEMENT

Many of the entities in this group originally were not recognized as being hereditary dermatoses. With advances in knowledge about the inheritable disorders, more of the so-called idiopathic dermatologic diseases have been found to be genetic in origin. These entities are in the hereditary group because for many years they were considered to be dermatologic, even though their systemic nature is now recognized (see list below). The cutaneous changes in each entity are distinctive; the ocular changes are varied.

> *Hereditary dermatoses with ocular involvement*
> Pseudoxanthoma elasticum
> Incontinentia pigmenti
> Xeroderma pigmentosum
> Anhidrotic ectodermal dysplasia
> Lamellar ichthyosis
> X-linked ichthyosis
> Other ichthyotic disorders
> Epidermolysis bullosa

Pseudoxanthoma elasticum

The cutaneous changes in pseudoxanthoma elasticum may be so subtle that they are overlooked on cursory examination of the skin. But close inspection of the intertriginous areas of the body—particularly the axillas and cubital fossae and the sides of the neck—will reveal the characteristic lesions. The creased areas of the abdominal wall and the buttocks and the popliteal areas also may be involved.

The early primary lesion is a chamois-colored, slightly elevated papule (Fig. 17-20). When the skin in the involved region is slightly tensed, the papular lesions are recognized as being uniform in size and arranged in a linear fashion. Older lesions become more yellow and more prominent because the skin becomes more distended and relaxed and the follicular orifices become readily recognizable over the papules. At this stage, the skin lesions resemble the skin of a plucked chicken.

Pseudoxanthoma elasticum is a disease inherited as an autosomal recessive trait, affecting the elastic tissue throughout the body and resulting in degenerative changes in the structures that possess elastic tissue as a major component.[1] Most noticeable are changes in the skin. Occlusive peripheral arterial disease was present in approximately 15% of 106 patients in one study.[3] Angina pectoris, myocardial infarctions, and cerebrovascular accidents occurred less frequently. Hypertension may be present. Gastrointestinal bleeding from the rupture of elastic tissue may occur in the stomach and the small or large bowel.[1] The histopathologic features of the cutaneous changes are characteristic. The elastic tissue predominantly localized to the middle and upper dermis shows twisting and curling, presenting as tightly wound basophilic masses when stained with hematoxylin and eosin. Special stains show calcium deposited on the altered elastic tissue.

Elastic tissue in the eye is also involved, and degenerative changes result in

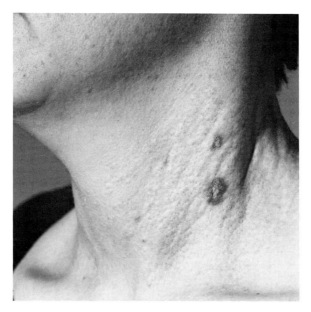

Fig. 17-20. Chamois-colored papules arranged in linear and reticulated pattern are characteristic for pseudoxanthoma elasticum.

cracks in the lamina vitrea (Bruch's membrane), with the production of angioid streaks. Angioid streaks, although most frequently associated with pseudoxanthoma elasticum, are not specific for this entity. The combination of skin and eye findings in pseudoxanthoma elasticum is referred to as the Grönblad-Strandberg syndrome. The streaks may vary from dark brown to red, predominate in the area of the optic lens, and branch, much as blood vessels, toward the periphery. In one third of the patients, hemorrhage accompanies the angioid streaks.

The eye changes are ordinarily bilateral, though asymmetric in the involvement of each eye, and most commonly affect the patient after the age of 30 years. The ocular changes are usually slowly progressive, with trauma to the eye as a factor accelerating the changes. The patient usually is unaware of the ocular changes until sufficient hemorrhage occurs so that the retina is destroyed and vision is lost. In our experience, almost 75% of the patients with angioid streaks had defects in vision. Other ocular findings include hemorrhage into the vitreous, glaucoma, and retinal detachment.

Incontinentia pigmenti

The striking panorama of vesicles, verrucous papules, and whorl-like areas of hyperpigmentation occurring in early childhood makes the diagnosis of incontinentia pigmenti easy. This disease occurs almost exclusively in females; there is a single mutant gene on the X chromosome that has a dominant effect in females and is lethal in males.[10a]

Four stages of the disease are readily discerned.[6] The first, the inflammatory stage, can be present at birth, possibly indicating evolution of the disease in utero. More commonly, however, the disease develops during the first few weeks of life. The inflammatory, papular, and plaque-like lesions, at times with blistering, are the most common on the extremities (Fig. 17-21). The second, the hypertrophic stage, develops within weeks to months, with warty overgrowth of some of the previous bullous lesions. At times, large indurated plaques may form. The third, the pigmented stage, occurs after months. The previous skin lesions disappear and macular or slightly papular whorls, bands, and streaks of hyperpigmentation occur over the trunk (Fig. 17-22). Whereas the verrucous lesion of the second stage may be superimposed on those lesions of the first stage, the pigmentary changes on the trunk during the third stage are unrelated to those on the extremities in the first and second stages. The fourth stage, involution, takes place when the patient is in the late teens or early twenties. The pigmentary changes gradually lessen so that all cutaneous evidence of the disease disappears. Other cutaneous findings may in-

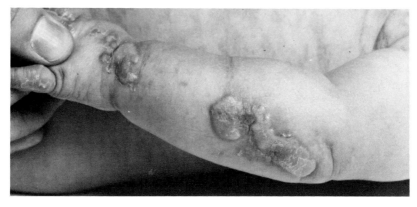

Fig. 17-21. Early lesions of incontinentia pigmenti consist of inflammatory papules and plaques, sometimes with blistering and most often occurring on extremities.

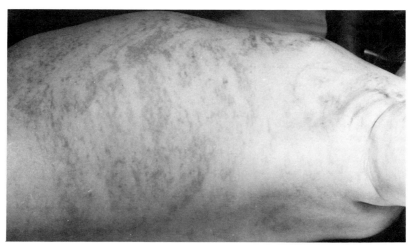

Fig. 17-22. Macular whorls and streaks of pigmentation on trunk are highly suggestive of pigmentary stage of incontinentia pigmenti.

clude thin, flat, or spoon-shaped nails and hair abnormalities including alopecia cicatrisata.

Dental, ocular, musculoskeletal, and central-nervous-system anomalies frequently accompany the disease (alone or in combination). Delayed dentition, pegged teeth, impactions, and abnormalities of crown formation characterize the dental changes. The absence of the lateral upper incisor may be a marker for the presence of the disease after the cutaneous lesions have faded. Neurologic anomalies are present in approximately half the patients and include seizures, mental retardation, and paresis.[8]

Ocular findings, which occur in one third of the patients, include most frequently strabismus, cataracts, and blue scleras and less frequently nystagmus and chorioretinitis. Cole and Cole[2] have emphasized that one third of the patients with ocular findings have a mass in the posterior chamber. They believe that the mass represents a congenital retinal fold or ablatio falciformis and that malignant neoplasm never develops in those patients.[2, 11]

Xeroderma pigmentosum

Xeroderma pigmentosum is a hereditary disease transmitted as an autosomal recessive trait in which the major features are photosensitivity with premature aging of the skin and the subsequent development of various skin malignancies. Defective DNA repair after ultraviolet light exposure probably is responsible for the clinical findings.[5b]

The child is normal at birth, but later erythema develops, which is followed by spotted macular hyperpigmentation of the skin from exposure to the sun. With

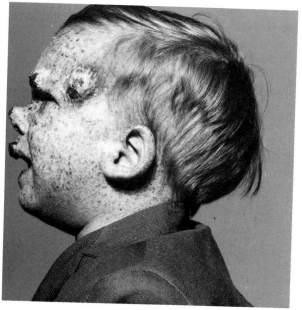

Fig. 17-23. Patient with xeroderma pigmentosum develops prematurely aged skin and various cutaneous malignancies, including basal and squamous cell carcinomas and melanoma.

repeated exposure to the sun, premature aging of the skin occurs, manifested by hyperpigmentation, atrophy, and telangiectasia (Fig. 17-23). Depending on the severity of the reaction, these changes may occur at an early age, and once the changes are established, squamous cell and basal cell carcinomas and kerato-acanthomas may develop. Malignant melanoma often is responsible for the death of the patient. Most patients die before the age of 20 years.

Other findings may include growth and mental retardation, microcephaly, epilepsy, spastic paralysis, deafness, and hypogonadism. A neurologic variant of xeroderma pigmentosum, the De Sanctis–Cacchione syndrome, includes dwarfism, gonadal hypoplasia, and microcephaly in addition to the xeroderma.

Ocular findings are common. Photophobia is an early finding, with blepharo-spasm, excessive lacrimation, and conjunctivitis commonly present. Eyelid involve-ment produces damage to the structures, with loss of lashes, scarring of lids, and the development of ectropion. The ensuing inflammatory reaction may lead to symblepharon and pterygium formation of the conjunctivae, inflammation and vascularization of the cornea, and progressive loss of vision.

Anhidrotic ectodermal dysplasia

Patients with this genetic disorder, which is transmitted as a sex-linked recessive trait, resemble one another to a greater degree than they resemble their siblings.

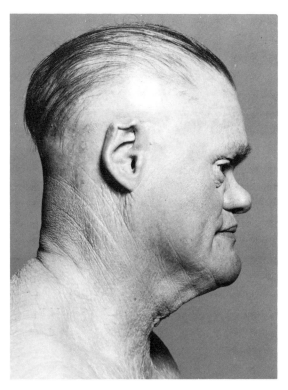

Fig. 17-24. Patient with anhidrotic ectodermal dysplasia can be recognized readily and should be followed because of possibility of cataracts developing.

The syndrome is characterized by absence of eccrine sweating, faulty dentition, and a characteristic facies.[9]

The child seems normal at birth, but by 1 year of age, he already may have developed the features that characterize the disease. Males are involved more frequently than females (ratio of 5:1). Because of the lack of eccrine glands, the child may experience periodic bouts of unexplained fever, especially in hot weather.

The facies is characteristic with a square forehead, prominent frontal bossing and supraorbital ridges, depression of the central face, a pointed and upturned nose, a pointed chin, and sparse hair of the scalp and beard (Fig. 17-24). Dentition is usually delayed. The gonads and skeletal system may be abnormal.

Ocular findings include an unusual increase in periorbital pigmentation (often from birth), a mongoloid slant to the eyelids, absent eyebrows and eyelashes, decreased lacrimation, photophobia, and, less frequently, stenosis of the inferior puncta, corneal opacities, corneal dysplasias, congenital cataracts, absence of the iris, luxation of the lens, and pupillary abnormalities.

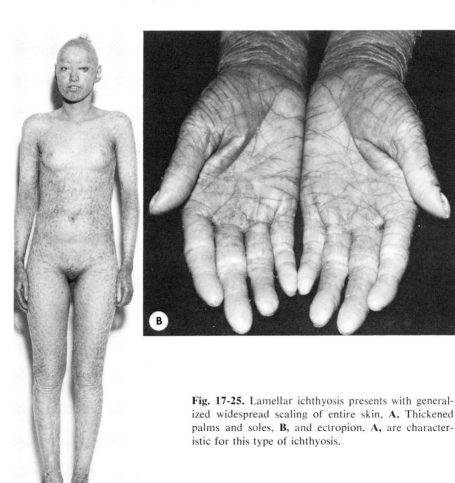

Fig. 17-25. Lamellar ichthyosis presents with generalized widespread scaling of entire skin, **A.** Thickened palms and soles, **B,** and ectropion, **A,** are characteristic for this type of ichthyosis.

Ichthyosis

In the past, all patients who had a dry scaling outer cuticle have been considered as having ichthyosis. With newer staining techniques in histopathology, x-ray diffraction studies, epidermal turnover studies, electron microscopy, and genetic studies, the various forms of the disease can be classified more exactly. All the patients have dry and scaling skin with a discoloration of the skin that varies from green to tan to black. The scales may be small, fine, and flaky, as in ichthyosis vulgaris, or large and coarse, as in lamellar ichthyosis (Fig. 17-25, *A*).

Distribution of the scaling helps in the differentiation, as characteristically the flexural creases, palms, and soles are not involved in ichthyosis vulgaris; in contrast, extensive thickening of the palms and soles occurs in lamellar ichthyosis (Fig. 17-25, *B*). Continual exfoliation of the scales, unrelieved by the usual lubricants, is a cosmetic problem for most patients. The dryness of the skin is accompanied by itching, which causes considerable stress to the patient. Moreover, the dryness of the skin and its lack of suppleness produce a characteristic ectropion that distinguishes lamellar ichthyosis from other forms of the disease.

Fitzpatrick[5a] has outlined the differential considerations in the major types of ichthyosis (Table 17-5).

The ocular findings in the various forms of ichthyosis aid in their differentiation. Ectropion, especially if severe, in association with an ichthyosis characterized by large, coarse scales and thickened palms and soles, means that the patient most likely has lamellar ichthyosis. Comma- and dot-shaped opacities in Descemet's membrane of the cornea identify the males with X-linked ichthyosis and the females as carriers. Corneal scarring and vascularization as a result of exposure, with decrease in vision, also may be present.[12]

Various ichthyotic states that are different from the major types, but which

Table 17-5. Classification of ichthyosis

	Ichthyosis vulgaris	*X-linked ichthyosis*	*Epidermolytic hyperkeratosis**	*Lamellar ichthyosis†*
Heredity	Autosomal dominant	X-linked	Autosomal dominant	Autosomal recessive
Onset	In childhood	At birth	At birth	At birth
Clinical features	Fine scales; spares flexures	Large scales; especially neck and trunk	Large scales; accentuated in flexures	Large scales; thick palms and soles
Associated clinical features	Prominent palmar and plantar markings; atopy	Asymptomatic; corneal opacities	Vesicles and bullae occur	Ectropion
Histopathology	Hyperkeratosis; absent granular layer	Hyperkeratosis; granular layer present	Hyperkeratosis; reticulated degeneration of granular layer	Hyperkeratosis; granular layer present
Epidermal kinetics (cell turnover)	Normal	Normal	Rapid	Rapid

*Bullous congenital ichthyosiform erythroderma.
†Nonbullous congenital ichthyosiform erythroderma.
(Modified from Fitzpatrick, T. B.: Dermatology in general medicine, New York, 1971, McGraw-Hill Book Co., p. 252.)

nevertheless are distinct clinical entities, have been reviewed by Heijer and Reed.[7] The Sjögren-Larsson syndrome, clinically similar to ichthyosiform erythroderma, may have as its ocular accompaniments degeneration of the pigmented epithelium of the macula and its surroundings. Another of the ichthyotic syndromes, described by Refsum, shows retinitis pigmentosa in addition to cerebellar ataxia, chronic polyneuritis, and progressive nerve deafness.

Epidermolysis bullosa

Epidermolysis bullosa is a disease in which blisters, particularly over the bony prominences of the skin, develop either spontaneously or in reponse to trauma. Various modes of inheritance occur in this disease, and the type of inheritance determines the severity of the disease in the individual patients[10b] (Table 17-6). Because the blisters develop commonly in response to trauma, their presence over the hands and feet is common. Yet the lesions may develop anywhere on the body and even on the mucous membrane surfaces.

In the severest form of the disease (polydysplastic type) in which the disease is present at birth and in which mutilation of the skin and digits takes place, the mucosal surfaces are generally involved. Because of scarring secondary to the blistering, interference with function of the tissue is common. The oral cavity and upper gastrointestinal tract may be so severely involved that the child suffers nutritionally. Eye involvement in the polydysplastic form produces scarring of the conjunctiva, with subsequent scarring and dystrophy of the lids.

INFECTIOUS DISEASES WITH OCULAR INVOLVEMENT

Infections often involve the eyelids. Some of these infections may cause minimal discomfort only, with no findings specifically occurring on the eyes. Contrariwise, some relatively uncommon infections frequently cause eye difficulties when they occur on the lids (see list below). Eliminated from consideration are the acute viral exanthemas but included are those few diseases, primarily dermatologic, in which the skin lesions and their specific causes may be the basis for the unusual ocular findings.

Classification of infectious diseases associated with ocular changes

Syphilis	Molluscum contagiosum
Herpes simplex	Pediculosis
Herpes zoster	Vaccinia

Table 17-6. Classification of epidermolysis bullosa

Type	Inheritance	Clinical characteristics
Simplex	Autosomal dominant	Bullae on hands and feet, no scarring; mucous membranes mildly affected
Hyperplastic	Autosomal dominant	Bullae on extremities, resolving with scarring; mucous membranes affected in 20%
Polydysplastic	Recessive	Onset early in life, with bullae resulting in severe scarring; mucous membranes usually involved
Lethalis	Variant of polydysplastic	Present at birth; severe cutaneous and mucous membrane involvement; death by 3 months

Syphilis

Syphilis is seen less frequently today than it was 30 years ago—a decrease related to the introduction of penicillin. Early detection and early penicillin treatment have been important factors in this decreasing incidence of disease. But the development of secondary lesions and heredosyphilis seems less frequent in the overall manifestations of the disease.

The presence of a primary chancre, dark-field positive for spirochetes, remains the most reliable test for the diagnosis of the primary lesion of syphilis. Serologic tests, now employing immunofluorescent techniques with actual spirochetes (fluorescent treponema antibody tests), give specific confirmatory serologic evidence of the disease.

Because of the frequency of skin lesions in the secondary phase of the disease, the dermatologist becomes involved in the diagnosis and management of the disease. Secondary skin lesions, even today, may be the presenting sign that alerts the physician to the presence of the disease. Stokes et al. delineate in exacting fashion the cutaneous presentations of the disease in the secondary stage.[6] They reported that approximately 3% of patients had eye complications in this stage of the disease, the complications consisting of neuroretinitis, iritis, conjunctivitis, and, rarely, interstitial keratitis.

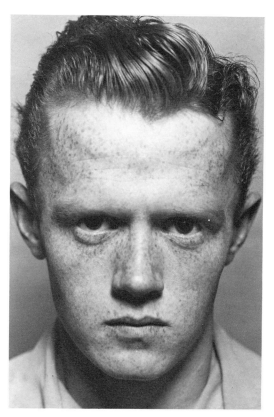

Fig. 17-26. "Pan" facies of congenital syphilis produced by depressed nasal bridge and frontal bossing should suggest possibility of associated interstitial keratitis.

In the late stages of syphilis, tertiary neurosyphilis, involvement of third, fourth, and sixth cranial nerves produces disorders of the function of the ocular muscles.

Early infantile congenital syphilis may present with skin lesions of secondary syphilis and, in addition, bullous lesions, which are characteristic for this stage of the disease. The latter, in a child with snuffles and a marasmus, was always considered presumptive evidence of early hereditary syphilis. Fortunately, this condition is rarely seen today.

Late congenital syphilis is manifested in the child in its classic form of Hutchinson's triad—Hutchinson's incisors, eighth-nerve deafness, and interstitial keratitis (Fig. 17-26). But other stigmas of tardive congenital syphilis consist of mulberry molars, osteitis, saddle deformity of the nose, rhagades, frontal bossing, and scaphoid scapula. The most common of the findings is interstitial keratitis, which occurs in approximately 50% of the patients with congenital syphilis.

Herpes simplex

One of the commonest infections involving the skin about the eye, with secondary complications of the eye, is that caused by the herpes simplex virus.[2a, 3a] Ordinarily, the disease is manifested by grouped vesicles on an erythematous base, localized about the lips and face and rarely elsewhere on the body (Fig. 17-27). Herpes simplex can occur as a primary infection in persons who have no circulating antibodies or in a secondary form known as recurrent herpes simplex in which the patient has circulating antibodies, but repeated episodes of the infection occur at or near the same site of previous involvement.

Infections above the level of the waist (thus those involving the mouth and eyes) are caused by herpes simplex virus, type 1, whereas infections below the waist (genital infections) are caused by herpes virus, type 2.

In many instances, the primary infection may not even by recognized clinically.

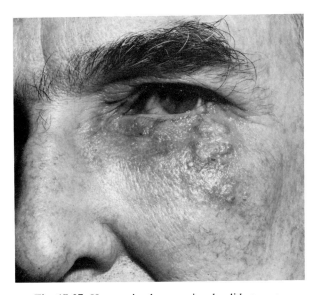

Fig. 17-27. Herpes simplex may involve lids or eye.

In the remainder, severe systemic symptoms consisting of fever, malaise, and toxicity are present for a 7- to 10-day period, with gradual resolution of symptoms and healing of the skin during this period. In contrast, recurrent infections are ordinarily accompanied by fewer constitutional symptoms. However, when the secondary infection is widespread, as in eczema herpeticum, severe constitutional symptoms may be present. The infection is precipitated by physical agents such as fever; exposure to sunlight, wind, or cold; trauma; and such excitants as menstruation and psychic and gastrointestinal upsets.

Primary and secondary herpes simplex infection involving the skin and mucous membranes may take many clinical forms (see outline below). A keratoconjunctivitis may be part of the primary infection, with involvement of the cornea sufficiently severe that scarring results and interferes with vision. Recurrent herpes simplex frequently occurs on the skin and, when the cornea is involved, accounts for the dendritic corneal ulcers that affect the epithelium and corneal stroma and interfere with vision. Recurrent herpes simplex of the eye is associated with pain in the eye, a foreign-body sensation, and initially a corneal epithelial infiltrate that may progress to ulcer formation and eventually scarring. Early, the virus can be isolated from the lesion, but later this is impossible. Iridocyclitis as a part of recurrent herpes simplex infection is not uncommon. The severity of the herpes simplex infection is enhanced by underlying immunologic deficiencies such as in the Wiskott-Aldrich syndrome and in malignant lymphomas.

Classification of clinically recognized varieties of herpes simplex infections*
 I. Subclinical infections (more than 90%)
 II. Clinically evident infections (1% to 10%)
   A. Localized involvement
     1. Genital
       a. Acute vulvovaginitis (balanitis)†
       b. Herpes genitalis (recurrent)
       c. Urethritis
     2. Ocular
       a. Keratoconjunctivitis†
       b. Keratitis, conjunctivitis
     3. Oronasal and gastrointestinal
       a. Acute gingivostomatitis†
       b. Rhinitis†
       c. Herpes labialis; oral, pharyngeal, esophageal, and anal lesions
     4. Cutaneous
       a. Traumatic herpes†
       b. Herpetic whitlow and paronychia†
       c. Zosteriform lesions†
       d. Any skin area; for example, chin, cheek, ear, buttock
   B. Systemic or disseminate involvement
     1. Kaposi's varicelliform eruption†
     2. Meningoencephalitis†
     3. Herpes generalisatus (prematures and neonates)†
     4. Disseminated herpes simplex infections associated with severe malnutrition, malignant neoplasms, and corticosteroid administration†
     5. Infectious mononucleosis–like syndrome†

---

*Modified from Muller, S. A.: Las infecciones clínicas debidas al herpes simple, Medicina Cutánea **3:**1-12, 1968.
†Indicates clinically typical primary infection with herpes simplex.

Herpes zoster

The varicella-zoster virus uncommonly involves both the skin and eye when presenting as a primary eruption in childhood. In contrast, herpes zoster involving the ophthalmic branch of the fifth cranial nerve not uncommonly has eye complications during its course.[1] Herpes zoster may initially present as grouped vesicles along the course of a nerve. The vesicles become pustular, crusting occurs, and, depending on the depth of the ulcers that ensue, a variable degree of scarring occurs. Pain may attend this eruption or may first appear after the eruption has subsided. Pain, without any skin lesions, may be present for days before cutaneous signs of the disease are evident.

The grouped lesions occurring in herpes zoster ophthalmicus are generally unilateral and sharply marginated by the midline. An occasional single lesion may cross the midline. Grouped lesions may be clustered over the eyelids and forehead, with extension into the frontal scalp. Severe erythema and soft-tissue swelling may accompany the vesicles. The maxillary and mandibular branches of the fifth nerve are only rarely involved simultaneously. Involvement of the tip of the nose, representing involvement of the nasociliary branch of the division of the trigeminal nerve (Hutchinson's sign), is presumptive evidence that ocular complications will occur[3b] (Fig. 17-28).

Involvement of the ophthalmic branch of the fifth nerve has always been feared because of the blindness that can occur (rarely). Frequently, patients may complain of photophobia, and evidence of a mild conjunctivitis and keratitis may be present. Excessive lacrimation may occur. More severe involvement may result in corneal ulcers, scarring, and eventual blindness. Perforation of the globe by the corneal ulcers occurs only rarely. Uveitis, accompanied by glaucoma and sometimes by the loss of vision from phthisis bulbi, may occur.

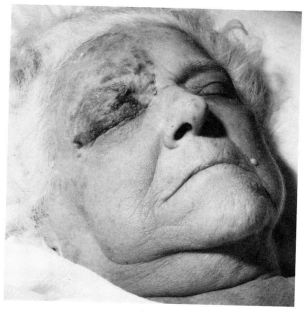

Fig. 17-28. Involvement of tip of nose in herpes zoster suggests possible ocular complications.

Molluscum contagiosum

Molluscum contagiosum is caused by a virus and is characterized by gray to flesh-colored, translucent hemispherical papules that present a verrucous crateri- form umbilication on the surface of the individual lesion as the condition pro- gresses. The lesions may be located anywhere on the skin, but involvement over the trunk and in the anogenital region is common (Fig. 17-29). In older patients, a single lesion is often confused with a basal cell carcinoma. The lesions of molluscum contagiosum are usually asymptomatic.

Individual lesions may persist for a long period, but when they are traumatized and secondary infection supervenes, involution of the lesion promptly occurs. Spon- taneous resolution is also recognized as a regular phenomenon. The histopathologic features of the lesion are specific and are characterized by a pear-shaped lobulated area of degeneration of the epidermis, which represents epidermal cells that have been parasitized by the virus, the so-called molluscum bodies.

The disease spreads by autoinoculation and direct contact. Lesions about the eyes and particularly involving the lid margins produce a follicular or papillary con- junctivitis and occasionally a superficial punctate keratitis. Removal of the indi- vidual lesions from the margin of the lid resolves the eye difficulty.[1]

Pediculosis

Lice may parasitize the hair of the scalp, body, and pubic region, and the re- sulting conditions are clinically designated as pediculosis capitis, pediculosis cor- poris, and pediculosis pubis, respectively.[2b] The lice causing pediculosis capitis and corporis (*Pediculus humanus* var. *capitis* and var. *corporis,* respectively) are not readily distinguished, but the long body parts of these lice are easily distinguished from the "crablike" body form of the louse that causes pediculosis pubis (*Phthirus pubis*).

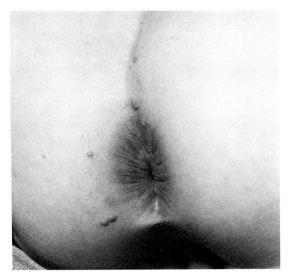

Fig. 17-29. Molluscum contagiosum can be diagnosed clinically because of umbilicated pearly papules of skin.

In pediculosis pubis, the lice cling to the hair at the level of the skin and intermittently feed on the skin and appear as yellowish or gray spots. At the sites of the bites, gray or blue macules, considered to be attributable to the interaction of the saliva of the louse on the blood of the host, develop. The nits of pubic lice attach to the hair approximately 0.5 cm. above the follicular opening.

At times the pubic lice attach themselves to other hairy regions of the body and even to the eyelids. Their presence in the latter location causes irritation of the lids, and when the patient rubs the eye, the louse is crushed, extravasating the louse's tissue juices derived from the host's hemoglobin. Thus, the "bloody-tear syndrome" is produced.

Head lice only rarely attach themselves to the eyelashes, and under these circumstances, they may produce corneal lesions.

Vaccinia

Vaccinia becomes an important dermatologic problem because of its ready transmission to patients with eczema.[2c, 5] Vaccinia in an otherwise normal person results from the secondary inoculation of the vaccinia virus from the patient's recent vaccination or from that of another person, frequently the patient's sibling. Predisposing dermatoses for the development of generalized vaccinia include not only atopic dermatitis but also dermatitis herpetiformis, pemphigus, herpes simplex lesions, and varicella. Extensive burn areas also possess the same potential hazard. Vaccinia developing on otherwise normal skin is relatively innocuous, but when it occurs in an infant, the mortality is 30%.

After the inoculation of the skin, there follows an incubation period of approximately 10 days in which the vesicles abruptly erupt and rapidly become purulent. These are generally grouped and predominantly involve the previously damaged skin, but when on normal skin, the vesicles are widely disseminated over the body. New crops of lesions appear every 5 to 7 days. The constitutional symptoms of fever and regional lymphadenopathy may be present. After the fever subsides in 4 to 5 days, the pustular lesions heal slowly, resulting in punctate scarring at the sites of previous lesions.

The accidental vaccination may involve the tissues of the eyelids and lid margins or conjunctivae. Under these circumstances, involvement of the cornea with keratitis is a hazard. The keratitis from vaccinia may be associated with persistent corneal clouding. It is important to determine whether corneal involvement is present. In its absence, the administration of vaccinia globulins is warranted; in the presence of keratitis, other antiviral agents should preferably be administered, namely, idoxuridine or thiosemicarbazone.

In the nonimmune patients, lid involvement, consisting of severe edema of the lids in association with the pustules along the lid margins, is present. One third of the patients with lid lesions develop corneal complications.

SYNDROMES WITH SKIN AND OCULAR INVOLVEMENT

This group includes many entities, some of which are recognized because of their major involvement of the skin and others of which the cutaneous changes are almost insignificant when compared to the other organ system involvement (see list below). Nevertheless, the cutaneous findings are often a clue to the specific diagnosis.

Syndromes with skin and ocular involvement

Sturge-Weber syndrome	Multiple lentigines syndrome
Tuberous sclerosis	Dyskeratosis congenita
Neurofibromatosis	Marfan's syndrome
Basal cell nevus syndrome	Turner's syndrome
Ataxia-telangiectasia	Rendu-Osler-Weber syndrome
Wiskott-Aldrich syndrome	Disseminate palmoplantar keratoderma
Reiter's syndrome	Cockayne's syndrome
Multiple mucosal neuromas	Klein-Waardenburg's syndrome
Vogt-Koyanagi-Harada syndrome	Progeria (Hutchinson-Gilford syndrome)
Focal dermal hypoplasia	Ehlers-Danlos syndrome

Sturge-Weber syndrome (encephalotrigeminal angiomatosis)

Encephalotrigeminal angiomatosis is characterized by angiomatous formation consisting of a nevus flammeus in one or more distributions of the trigeminal nerve, together with a venous angioma of the cerebral cortex on the same side.[21] Subsequently, calcification of the cerebral angioma occurs. It is then associated early with epilepsy and subsequently with a hemiparesis on the contralateral side from the port-wine stain. Mental retardation is common. Ocular changes consisting of buphthalmos, amblyopia, glaucoma, choroid angioma, homonymous hemianopia, and retinitis pigmentosa may be seen.[2]

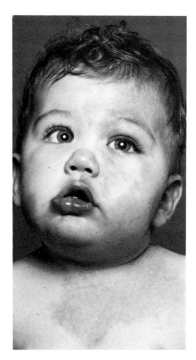

Fig. 17-30. Nevus flammeus in Sturge-Weber syndrome involves skin in one or more distributions of trigeminal nerve.

The striking clinical presentation is that of a port-wine stain over the face (Fig. 17-30). When the nevus flammeus involved the forehead or upper eyelid, Alexander and Norman[1] found that cerebral angiomatosis was present; if the nevus occurred below the level of the palpebral fissure, they could not find cerebral angiomatosis. Close inspection of the oral cavities may show unilateral involvement on the same side as the facial nevus flammeus. The buccal mucosa, maxillary gingiva, and lips may be involved. Less frequently, the tongue, palate, and mandibular gingiva are affected.

The cerebral calcification does not correspond specifically in all cases to the anomalous vessels. The epilepsy, beginning in infancy, consists usually of focal motor seizures rather than generalized convulsions and seems to have no relationship to the extent of the cutaneous vascular lesions or to the cerebral calcification.

Tuberous sclerosis (epiloia, Bourneville's disease)

The striking features of tuberous sclerosis are those of adenoma sebaceum of the face, mental retardation, and epilepsy, but there are also numerous findings in almost every organ of the body.[19] The three classic findings are sufficient to suggest that other of the protean manifestations of the disease should be sought out.

The disease is transmitted as an autosomal dominant trait with variable expressivity. Mental retardation is common although not necessarily present; many patients are confined to various institutions for care.

The skin lesions in the disease are considered under the categories of adenoma sebaceum of the face, ungual fibromas of the digits, shagreen spots, and leaflike areas of depigmentation of the trunk. The facial lesions of tuberous sclerosis, although referred to as adenoma sebaceum, are in reality angiofibromas (Fig. 17-31, *A*). They usually appear during the first few months of life but may have their onset anytime during the first two decades. They may be seen first as small, erythematous maculopapular lesions over the face that increase in number, become more papular and verrucous, and finally concentrate about the central portion of the face and the nasolabial folds. Lesions scattered about the periphery of the face also may be seen. This type of skin lesion is seen in 90% of patients with the disease.

Larger fibromatous lesions, usually single or few in number, may be seen over the forehead or face in an asymmetric distribution (Fig. 17-31, *A*). These are also angiofibromas, but they may be several centimeters in diameter. These lesions are more likely to be seen in those patients who are mentally retarded.

Similar fibromas may be seen about the terminal digits protruding from beneath the nail fold or at times from beneath the nail. The ungual fibromas tend to occur later in life and after the facial lesions have appeared. At times, the size of the fibroma interferes with the growth of the nail and produces a linear groove on its surface (Fig. 17-31, *B*). The toes may be similarly involved. Shagreen patches occur as slightly elevated plaques of the skin in which the follicular orifices are particularly prominent. Their sizes may vary, and they are commonly located in the lumbar region, although they are also present on the upper trunk and about the neck. The plaques are asymptomatic and represent proliferation on the collagen bundles but without the vascular components seen in the other lesions.

Lesions that consist of depigmentation in the form of leaf-shaped macules,

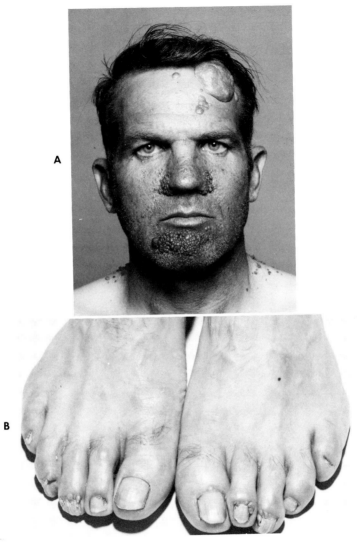

Fig. 17-31. A, Note clusters of small papules (adenoma sebaceum) about nose and chin and larger lesions of forehead (fibromas), both characteristic lesions of tuberous sclerosis. **B,** Fibromas about nails often cause dystrophy of nails. Same patient as in **A.**

which in the light-skinned person may be barely detectable, may be present. Poliosis may accompany areas of leukoderma. Less frequently, café-au-lait spots, fibroepithelial tags, lipomas, and dermatofibromas may be seen.

Nickel and Reed[19] have divided the skin changes into the following categories: *Major (pathognomonic)*—(1) facial angiofibromas (adenoma sebaceum), (2) shagreen patches, (3) ungual fibromas, and (4) large fibromas of forehead and scalp; and *minor (contributory or coincidental)*—(1) leukoderma, (2) poliosis, (3) fibroepithelial tags, (4) café-au-lait spots, and (5) port-wine hemangiomas.

Internal manifestations of tuberous sclerosis are variable and multiple organ systems besides the skin are involved.[25]

Brain. Pearly white nodules consisting of masses of glial tissue produce an undulating configuration on the surface of the brain and may protrude into and occupy the ventricles. Calcification of these nodules occurs in more than half of the patients and produces the classic mottled appearance of the skull on roentgen examination. Calcification deposits may be seen within the brain and are common within the basal ganglia; when they are present only in this latter region, they are indicative of a forme fruste of the disease. The degree of cranial calcification seems to be related to the degree of brain damage and mental deterioration.

Eye. Retinal tumors of gliomatous origin (drusen or hyaline bodies), similar to those seen in neurofibromatosis, are waxy and somewhat translucent and are located on the optic papilla and may interfere with vision. The eye lesion may be the first evidence of tuberous sclerosis. If careful examinations are carried out, eye lesions may be found in 50% of patients and may include, in addition to the gliomas, congenital cataracts, congenital blindness, chorioretinitis, optic atrophy, and areas of depigmentation of the retina.

Kidney. Hamartomas, cysts, and congenital anomalies (ectopic kidney) are found in 50% of patients with tuberous sclerosis. The hamartomas are usually bilateral, multiple, and of variable size, consisting of mixed embryonal tissue but commonly containing muscle and adipose tissue—leiomyosarcoma or liposarcoma. They do not metastasize and are therefore not considered malignant.

Heart. Striated muscle cell tumors that have become large and vacuolated by the intracellular accumulation of glycogen (spider cells) are referred to as rhabdomyomas. These tumors are usually multiple and are seen at autopsy in children who have died early in life—50% during the first year of life and 90% before puberty.

Lung. Cysts containing smooth muscle in their walls occur frequently in the lung and diffusely involve the lung, giving a "honeycomb" appearance on roentgen examination of the chest.

Bones. Roentgenographic changes in bones, consisting of cystic changes of cortical thickening, are found in 80% of patients with tuberous sclerosis who are more than 10 years old.

Others. Hamartomas in the liver, thyroid, and testes and subcutaneous tumors of mesenchymal origin rarely may be present.

Neurofibromatosis (von Recklinghausen's disease)

Neurofibromatosis is considered to be transmitted as an autosomal dominant trait. The high rate of mutation accounts for the development of the disease in patients without a family history.

The clinical diagnosis of the disease is based on the presence of multiple, variously sized, soft, pedunculated, and senile tumors over the body. They may be flesh-colored or vary from pink to red-brown (Fig. 17-32). The neurofibromas usually increase in number with advancing age. The patients are asymptomatic except when the size of the lesion interferes with body function or its location impinges on the space of the vital structure.[9b]

Concomitantly, pigmented macular areas, varying in size up to several centi-

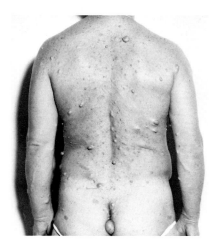

Fig. 17-32. Soft red-brown tumors of back and café-au-lait spots of buttocks easily confirm diagnosis of von Recklinghausen's disease.

Table 17-7. Ocular manifestations of neurofibromatosis

Site	Manifestations
Orbit	Pulsating proptosis
Lids	Plexiform neuromas, café-au-lait spots
Cornea	Buphthalmos (congenital glaucoma, associated with upper lid tumors)
Iris	Neurofibromas
Retina	"Mulberry" tumors
Optic nerve	Optic atrophy (secondary to optic nerve gliomas), papilledema, drusen, myelination of nerve fibers
Neurologic	Corneal reflex decreased (acoustic neuromas), muscle palsies

From Demis, D. J., Crounse, R. G., Dobson, R. L., and McGuire, J.: Clinical dermatology, Hagerstown, Md., 1972, Harper & Row, Publishers, vol. 4, sect. 28, p. 12.

meters, are seen over the body (Fig. 17-32). Their colors vary from light tan to dark brown (café-au-lait spots). Single or few lesions may be seen in otherwise normal persons, but patients with von Recklinghausen's disease usually have more than six such pigmented lesions. Clustering of lesions in the axillas is considered pathognomonic of the disease (Crowe's sign). The cosmetic problem of both the neurofibromas and the macular pigmentation may be considerable.

Mental deficiency may be present in some patients with von Recklinghausen's disease, whereas others may have normal or even superior intelligence. Neurologic disease commonly occurs with symptoms related to the site of the tumors on specific nerves, that is, eighth-nerve involvement (deafness) and trigeminal nerve involvement (with focal pain and numbness).

Osseous involvement because of neurofibromas that are close to or within the bone may include erosive changes or overgrowth of bone and intraosseous lesions that may produce scoliosis, congenital bowing, and pseudoarthritis.

Ocular complications[8] develop because the neurofibroma, which involves all

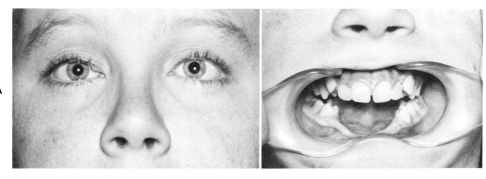

Fig. 17-33. **A,** Small translucent papules of face, including eyelids, are basal cell hamartomas seen in basal cell nevus syndrome. Note widely spaced eyes. **B,** Treatment of dentigerous cysts in basal cell nevus syndrome results in loss of teeth. Same patient as in **A.**

structures of the eye and adnexa except the lens and vitreous, impinges on structures through excessive growth of the tumors. Ocular findings in neurofibromatosis are numerous and varied (Table 17-7).

Basal cell nevus syndrome

The basal cell nevus syndrome is readily recognized when basal cell hamartomas are present predominantly on the face, although they may be present on the trunk as well as in association with cysts of the jaw. The basal cell hamartomas and jaw cysts indicate that these patients also may have multiple defects of ectodermal and mesodermal origin that involve bone, soft tissues, the central nervous system, and the eye.[4, 5]

The basal cell lesions of the skin usually begin after puberty, although the disease may have its onset in childhood as flesh-colored or pigmented papules, with the lesions increasing in number with age. The face is the most striking site of involvement. When the basal cell hamartomas involve the lids, excessive growth of the lesions and their treatment may result in dystrophy (Fig. 17-33, *A*). The patient cannot close the lids completely, ectropion develops, and corneal changes occur. Milia, epithelial and sebaceous cysts, lipomas, and fibromas may be seen on the skin, as well as punctate depressions over the palms and soles, in addition to the basal cell epitheliomas of the skin.

Most common among the osseous lesions are the mandibular cysts (Fig. 17-33, *B*), bifid ribs, and scoliosis; other lesions include synostosis of ribs, spina bifida occulta, and brachymetacarpia. The frontal bossing and a saddle nose in some of the patients produce a facial configuration not unlike that seen in congenital syphilis. Basal cell nevi on the face, together with a jaw cyst, offer ready differentiation, however.

Soft-tissue alterations include calcification of the falx cerebri as well as calcification in some of the pelvic viscera. Ovarian fibromas are frequently seen, as are lymphatic mesentery cysts. Mental retardation, psychiatric problems, abnormal electroencephalographic changes, hydrocephalus, and brain tumors including medulloblastoma are now recognized as occurring with great frequency in the basal cell nevus syndrome.

Hypertelorism, dystopia canthorum, and lateral displacement of the inner canthi are frequent ocular findings readily visualized in the basal cell nevus syndrome. Strabismus, congenital blindness from cataracts, colobomas or glaucoma, and multiple chalazia are also seen.

The syndrome is inherited as an autosomal dominant polymorphic trait with good penetration but with variable expressivity.

Ataxia-telangiectasia (Louis-Bar syndrome)

Ataxia-telangiectasia is an autosomal recessive disease whose earliest manifestations are related to cerebellar ataxia. However, cutaneous and bulbar telangiectasias soon become apparent, and these establish the hereditary nature of the neurologic problem. The severe consequences of the disease in children, because of their altered immunologic status, are chronic sinopulmonary infection and the subsequent development of malignancies, particularly of the lymphoreticular system.[22] The oculocutaneous telangiectasia is accentuated in the sun-exposed areas, with the butterfly area of the face, the bridge of the nose, and the periorbital tissues particularly involved. Subsequently, this vascular reaction may also involve the skin areas on the neck, the popliteal and cubital areas, and the trunk. Telangiectasias of the hard and soft palate also have been reported.[24]

In addition to the telangiectasias in the sun-exposed areas, the skin shows degenerative changes from sun exposure, producing skin that becomes inelastic and somewhat sclerodermatous, with hyperpigmentation and hypopigmentation. Cutaneous malignancies consisting of senile keratosis and basal cell carcinoma have occurred in these areas. Café-au-lait spots, partial albinism, and halo nevi may be seen.

Bullous impetigo is a manifestation of the patient's impaired immunologic status and is a frequent occurrence in patients with ataxia-telangiectasia. Seborrheic dermatitis, follicular keratosis, and dry skin are commonly present. Hirsutism in the female patient older than 10 years of age is common.

The telangiectasia of the bulbar conjunctivae is bilateral, symmetric, and at times resembles conjunctivitis because of the red hue imparted to the scleras. Other ocular findings of ataxia-telangiectasia, in addition to the prominent telangiectasia, consist of peculiar eye movements that simulate ophthalmoplegia—a spasmodic blinking and strasbismus. In addition, Boder and Sedgwick[3] have described a halting that occurs midway on lateral or upper gaze.

Ataxia-telangiectasia is transmitted as an autosomal recessive trait. Decreased levels of immunoglobulins A, E, and G are recognized.

Wiskott-Aldrich syndrome

The Wiskott-Aldrich syndrome is of interest to the dermatologist because of the cutaneous findings of eczema, purpura, and recurring skin infection. The importance of this disease, as representing an immunologically deficient state predisposing the patients to lymphoreticular malignancies, has been appreciated only recently. The disease is transmitted as an X-linked recessive trait and is manifested by decreased levels of immunoglobulin M and increased levels of immunoglobulin A. The condition affects only males.

Its most specific cutaneous finding is petechiae or purpuric eruption on the skin and mucous membranes. The eczema, which usually occurs on the face, the flexural areas, or about the buttocks, is not specific and may be exudative or very dry with fine scales. Secondary infection frequently produces furuncles and abscesses.[17]

A review of the ophthalmologic manifestations of the Wiskott-Aldrich syndrome was undertaken by Podos and investigators,[23] who recognized that 18 of 80 patients described in the literature had ocular complications. These consisted of a blepharoconjunctivitis associated with molluscum contagiosum and herpes simplex keratitis, as an isolated finding or accompanied by disseminated mucocutaneous herpes simplex infection.

Reiter's syndrome

Reiter's syndrome is now recognized as consisting of a tetrad of findings: nonspecific urethritis, asymmetric arthritis of major weight-bearing joints, conjunctivitis, and lesions of the mucous membrane and skin, the last resembling psoriasis to a considerable degree.[9a]

The cause of the syndrome remains unknown, though pleuropneumonia and *Mycoplasma* organisms have been implicated. The nonspecific urethritis, present in patients seen in the United States and western Europe, has never been proved as having a recognized venereal origin, although sexual promiscuity seems to predispose to the development of the disease. A dysenteric form in which gastrointestinal symptoms are predominant occurs in eastern Europe and North Africa.

The skin eruption begins as vesiculopustular lesions that soon dry in situ and become hyperkeratotic, producing the so-called keratosis blennorrhagica. Similar vesiculopustular lesions originate beneath the nails, causing onycholysis, dystrophy, and shedding of the nails (Fig. 17-34, *A*). Erythematous, dry, and scaling plaques

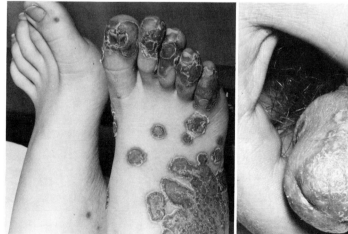 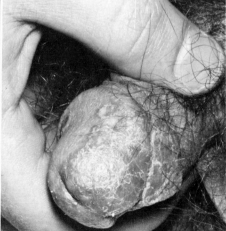

A
B

Fig. 17-34. A, Red, scaling, and crusting lesions (keratosis blennorrhagica) are seen about feet and hands in Reiter's syndrome. Note discoloration and dystrophy of some nails. **B,** Red, scaling lesions encircling urethral meatus on glans penis (balanitis circinata sicca) are common in cutaneous expression of Reiter's syndrome.

about the genitalia and on the glans penis (balanitis circinata sicca) are considered characteristic of the disease (Fig. 17-34, *B*). The more chronic skin lesions resemble psoriasis and emphasize the relationship between psoriasis and Reiter's syndrome (see list below).

Cutaneous and mucosal lesions in Reiter's syndrome
Cutaneous lesions
    Keratosis blennorrhagica
    Hyperkeratotic scaling plaques (psoriasiform lesions)
    Scrotal and penile erosions
    Onycholysis, dystrophy, and shedding of nails
Mucosal lesions
    Balanitis circinata sicca
    Oral and pharyngeal lesions
        Diffuse injection
        Erythematous macules and papules
        Purpuric lesions
        Erosions

Ocular findings in Reiter's syndrome are common. Conjunctivitis is characteristic in the presentation of the disease. Iritis, which may be severe and associated with attacks of prostatitis and sacroiliitis, frequently is seen. Keratitis, corneal ulceration, uveitis, and iridocyclitis are less frequently encountered.

Multiple mucosal neuromas with pheochromocytoma and medullary carcinoma of the thyroid

The syndrome of multiple mucosal neuromas has implication for the presence of either or both pheochromocytoma and medullary carcinoma of the thyroid. The mucosal neuromas are particularly frequent about the eyes and mouth. When they occur on the margins of the lips, the lesions give the borders a serrated appear-

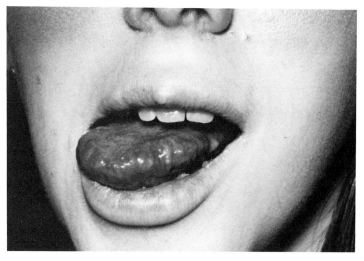

Fig. 17-35. Patient with mucosal neuromas that present as uniform-sized firm nodules along lateral margins on tongue anteriorly, and lips, and along eyelid margins should prompt an investigation for carcinoma of thyroid and pheochromocytoma.

ance and a fullness that has been likened to blubbery lips. When the tongue is extruded, the uniform-sized neuromas can be seen along the lateral margins toward the tip of the tongue[20] (Fig. 17-35).

These same mucosal neuromas are readily apparent on the margins of the eyelids, and the lesions may be so numerous as to cause eversion of the lids, giving the patient a starey appearance. The patients often have a marfanoid habitus. Inspection of the eyes often will be the initial clue to the diagnosis of this significant syndrome.

Vogt-Koyanagi-Harada syndrome

This rare syndrome of unknown cause has, as its cutaneous markers, hypomelanosis that occurs predominantly about the eyes, poliosis of the eyelashes and scalp, and a patchy alopecia.[9c] Associated with these cutaneous findings are ocular changes in the uveal tract, exudative choroiditis, retinal detachment, and sometimes blindness. Deafness may occur. Central-nervous-system involvement is indicated by headaches, vertigo, and vomiting.

Focal dermal hypoplasia

Focal dermal hypoplasia emphasizes the least important of a triad of findings in which the skin is of secondary importance to defects in the bones, cartilage, and eyes.[10] The disease is transmitted as an X-linked dominant trait that is lethal in the male. The skin lesions, which commonly are localized to the upper trunk and extremities, develop at birth and consist of blisters that eventually crust and resolve, with atropic and linear pigmentation of the skin. Brown macules, digitate papules, and fibromas are present in intertriginous areas. Localized superficial fatty deposits are readily seen within the skin because of associated dermal hypoplasia in these areas. Multiple papillomas of lips and oral cavity, defects in enamel formation, and hypoplasia of dentition also are seen.

Severe defects of the bones consist of agenesis of the clavicle, absent digits, syndactylism, oligodactylism, clinodactylism, spina bifida, and scoliosis. Hypoplasia of the nails is common. Ocular findings consist of strabismus, coloboma, epiphora, blue scleras, microphthalmia, nystagmus, and microphthalmus of the iris, retina, or choroid.[12]

Multiple lentigines syndrome

The skin changes in this syndrome consist of numerous lentigines over the body, with only the mucosal surfaces being spared. Ocular changes include hypertelorism and defective oculomotility and strabismus. The cutaneous and ocular findings indicate more severe involvement of other organ systems.[28]

Gorlin and co-workers[11] applied the mnemonic name "leopard syndrome" to the varied findings:

Lentigines multiple
Electrocardiographic conduction defects
Ocular hypertelorism
Pulmonary stenosis
Abnormalities of genitalia
Retardation of growth
Deafness, sensorineural

This syndrome is inherited as an autosomal dominant trait with high penetrance and variable expressivity.

Dyskeratosis congenita

This syndrome is characterized by a triad of findings consisting of nail dystrophy, cutaneous pigmentation, and leukokeratosis progressive to leukoplakia (contrast with pachyonychia congenita). The disease is transmitted as an X-linked recessive trait. The nails become dystrophic when the child is between 5 and 13 years of age and are later shed; a reticulated pigmentation with atrophy and telangiectasia of the trunk, neck, face, and thighs occurs next, followed by leukokeratotic changes of mucosal surfaces, particularly the oral tissues. Keratotic changes involving the tarsal conjunctivae obliterate the lacrimal puncta and account for constant tearing once the syndrome is well developed. Diffuse loss of scalp hair, eyelashes, and eyebrows and premature loss of the teeth may occur.[27b]

Marfan's syndrome

The outstanding features of Marfan's syndrome are those changes associated with the skeletal system in which the body stature draws attention to the possible presence of other features of the disease, namely, defects in the cardiovascular and ocular systems.[15] The tall stature of the patient with Marfan's syndrome presents with Lincolnesque features characterized particularly by arachnodactyly and loose jointedness (Fig. 17-36). Other osseous defects include a high arched palate, dolichocephalic skull, and pectus excavatum or carinatum. These changes should suggest investigation for other major findings of this syndrome. In the cardiovascular system, dissecting aneurysms, mitral valve disease, and atrial septal defects may be seen, and in the ocular system, ectopia lentis, myopia, and retinal detachment commonly occur. Ectopia lentis probably is found in 50% of patients with Marfan's syndrome.[14]

The major defect in Marfan's syndrome is an abnormality in the elastic tissue, which accounts for the loose jointedness and the defects in the cardiovascular system. Absence of elastic tissue accounts for the striae distensae and annular extrusion of elastic tissue through the epidermis for the annular hyperkeratotic lesions (keratosis follicularis serpiginosa) that can occur about the neck and upper trunk[15] (Fig. 17-37).

Turner's syndrome (Bonnevie-Ullrich-Turner syndrome, gonadal dysgenesis)

Cataracts have rarely been found in Turner's syndrome, a syndrome that is partly familial and is perhaps even genetically determined.[18] General dysgenesis involving the connective tissue[9d] and ectodermal structures presents characteristic clinical features that consist of webbing of the neck, axillas, and digits, sexual infantilism, failure to develop secondary sex characteristics at puberty, and osseous defects that include cubitus valgus, pes planus, hallux valgus, a "shield" or stocky chest, clinodactyly, and less frequently thoracic and lumbar scoliosis and pigeon chest. Hypermobility of the joints and hyperelasticity of the skin are commonly present. Cardiovascular defects, vascular anomalies, and anomalies of the genitourinary tract are present in a large proportion of patients. Turner's syndrome occurs predominantly in females who have an XO phenotype.[18]

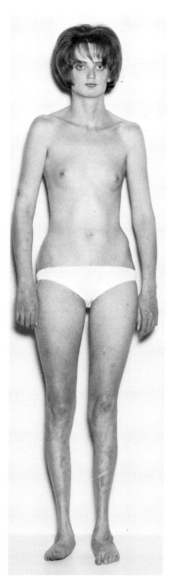

Fig. 17-36. Tall Lincolnesque stature associated with arachnodactylia and loose jointedness permits ready recognition of Marfan's syndrome.

Ocular anomalies, in addition to congenital cataracts, include blue scleras, strabismus, ptosis, idiopathic exophthalmus, colobomas, and retinitis pigmentosa.

Rendu-Osler-Weber syndrome (hereditary hemorrhagic telangiectasia)

The cutaneous manifestations of hereditary hemorrhagic telangiectasia consist of tortuosity and dilatation of vessels, which present as red puncta, tufts, or papules that are most striking on the skin of the face (Fig. 17-38). Additional lesions may be present over the trunk and the mucosal surface of the oral cavity and nose and throughout the mucosal surface of the gastrointestinal tract.

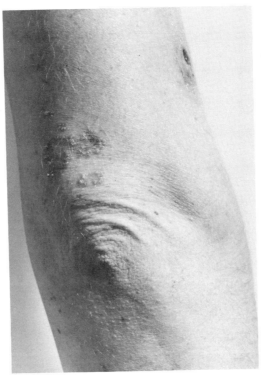

Fig. 17-37. Hyperkeratotic annular lesions (keratosis follicularis serpiginosa) can be seen in Marfan's syndrome as well as in other congenital cutaneous syndromes.

Lesions of the gastrointestinal tract and upper respiratory system can cause bleeding. The association of pulmonary arteriovenous fistulas in members of these families has been delineated.[13] Specific ocular findings of the syndrome consist of tortuosity and segmental dilatation of retinal vessels, neovascularization of the retina and optic papilla, and vitreous and retinal hemorrhages.[6] The disease is transmitted as an autosomal dominant trait.

Disseminate palmoplantar keratoderma

Keratoderma of the palms and soles may present as punctate papules, striate lesions, or plaques, or it may be diffuse and involve the entire palms and soles. The clinical forms have a variable inheritance pattern, being both of recessive and dominant traits. Among the keratodermas is that of a very rare syndrome consisting of punctate and striate keratoderma, inherited as an autosomal dominant trait, which appears in children between the ages of 12 and 15 years and is associated with corneal dystrophy.[27c]

Cockayne's syndrome

Children with this rare syndrome seem to be normal at birth but, at an early age, show an eruption of the butterfly area of the face, which is exacerbated by exposure to sunlight and resembles lupus erythematosus. This is one of

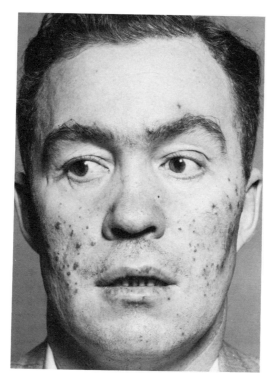

Fig. 17-38. Vascular puncta, tufts, and telangiectasia over face are easily recognized as cutaneous manifestations of Rendu-Osler-Weber syndrome.

the first evidences of this syndrome. In addition to dermatitis on the butterfly area of the face, there is loss of the fatty tissues of the face, producing a senile appearance. Severe mental and physical retardation occurs and microcephaly, large hands and feet, and prominent ears develop, progressive hearing loss occurs, and an unsteady gait, unintelligible speech, birdlike quickness of actions, and emotional instability ensue. The ocular findings that can occur consist of optic atrophy, retinal degeneration, and cataracts.[27a]

Klein-Waardenburg syndrome

Patients with the Klein-Waardenburg syndrome are recognized by their distinctive facies presenting with the inner canthi of the eyes displaced laterally, heavy eyebrows, a prominence of the root of the nose, and partial or complete heterochromia iridis.[26] Deafness is the most common feature. An additional striking finding is that of a white forelock (present in 50% of the patients). The syndrome is inherited as an autosomal dominant trait.

Progeria (Hutchinson-Gilford syndrome)

Children affected with progeria have the onset of their disease early in life. The disease consists of premature aging, such that the child usually dies from coronary thrombosis[7] before he is 20 years old. The disease has been considered transmitted as an autosomal recessive trait with no sex predilection, but recent studies cast doubt on this. These children do not mature normally, with major changes involving the skin and skeletal system. A number of osseous defects including dwarfism, prominent joints, thin bones, small clavicles, coxa valga, and defective ossification of the skull are noted. The skin shows generalized atrophy of the muscles and subcutaneous tissue, with prominence of the veins noted particularly over the scalp, alopecia of the scalp, eyebrows, and lashes, and scleroderma-like plaques and spotted pigmentation over the body. Absence of the earlobes and atrophy of the nails are also observed. The facial appearance is characterized by a recessed chin, prominence of the nose with a glyphic tip, cyanosis of the central face, and craniofacial disproportion (Fig. 17-39). These facial changes, together with alopecia and prominence of veins of the scalp, give the patients with progeria a characteristic appearance. Alopecia of the eyebrows and eyelashes produces a pseudoprominence of the eyes. Intelligence is normal. Sexual maturation does not occur.

Ehlers-Danlos syndrome

The hyperelasticity of the skin and hyperflexion of joints permit ready identification of patients with Ehlers-Danlos syndrome.[16] However, these findings may

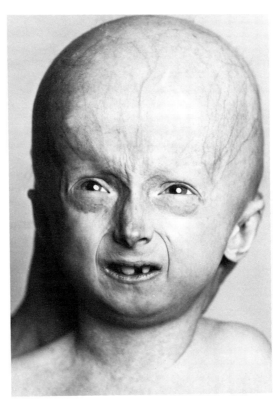

Fig. 17-39. Absence of hair of scalp, eyebrows, and eyelashes, together with craniofacial disproportion, characterizes patients with progeria.

be accepted as "normal" by the patient, and unless the physician carefully queries the family, the subtle presence of these traits in some family members may be missed. An additional striking cutaneous finding is the development of hemorrhagic pseudotumors at sites of trauma. These are areas of ecchymosis, and as they resolve, the skin becomes atrophic with the characteristic cigarette-paper wrinkling on the surface.

The skin of the patient with Ehlers-Danlos syndrome feels soft and supple, and when stretched, it readily returns to the normal contours of the body (Fig. 17-40). Thus, this syndrome can be readily differentiated from cutis laxa, in which the skin hangs in redundant folds and distorts the physical appearance of the patient. Less frequently occurring cutaneous signs of the syndrome are subcutaneous cysts that calcify (the so-called spherules), blisters, elastosis serpiginosum perforans, and neurofibromatosis.

Other multisystem defects are present in this syndrome. The hyperextensibility of the joints (Fig. 17-41), frequent discoloration of joints, kyphoscoliosis, and spondylolisthesis are readily recognized as a part of the commonly present musculo-skeletal defects. The patient with Ehlers-Danlos syndrome has a rather slant-eyed appearance because of the redundance of the tissues of the lids. The patients may have widely spaced eyes, but true hypertelorism is not present. Blue scleras,

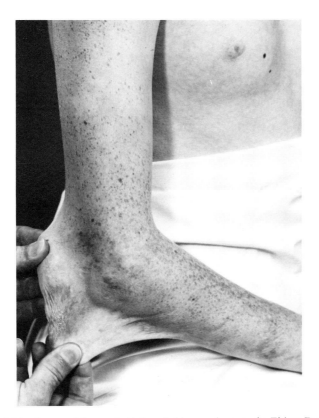

Fig. 17-40. Variable degree of hyperelasticity of skin can be seen in Ehlers-Danlos syndrome.

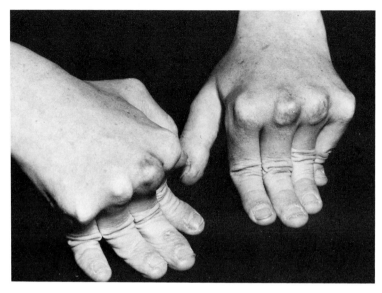

Fig. 17-41. Hyperflexibility of joints may be associated with dislocations of these joints in patients with Ehlers-Danlos syndrome.

microcornea, keratoconus, and defects in the ocular adnexa and the suspensory mechanisms of the lens and in the fundus are common. There may be gastrointestinal manifestations consisting of hiatal hernias and gastrointestinal diverticula; cardiovascular manifestations consisting of dissecting aneurysms of the aorta and other vessels and congenital cardiac defects such as interatrial septal defects; and urologic manifestations.

For many years, the Ehlers-Danlos syndrome has been considered to be transmitted as an autosomal dominant trait, but more recent studies indicate that some forms are transmitted as X-linked and autosomal recessive traits.

DERMATOSES AND CUTANEOUS SYNDROMES WITH CATARACTS

The association of cataracts and dermatologic disease is expected inasmuch as the lens and the skin and its appendages have a common embryonal origin—the surface ectoderm. The finding of cataracts in the various dermatoses has depended on the long-term observation of the patient as well as on the frequency and meticulous nature of the eye examinations.

The term "syndermatotic" cataracts indicates that the lenticular and cutaneous changes are related, and indeed they might have a common origin. The cataracts in the diseases to be described may be congenital or acquired and may develop slowly or rapidly. The exact method by which the cataract develops in the dermatologic disease is not known, but in some instances at least, the dermatologic disease can be controlled, resulting in retardation of cataract development.

In some dermatoses and dermatologic syndromes, cataracts occur with sufficient frequency to suggest a positive association (see outline below). Moreover, cataracts occur as the major ocular pathologic change. The other dermatologic entities

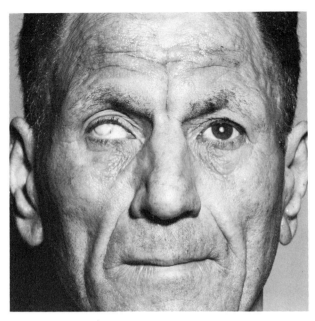

Fig. 17-42. Patient with atopic dermatitis had injury to right eye, with subsequent loss of vision. Cataract developed in left eye, as part of atopic disease.

in which cataracts occur but are a part of numerous other changes already have been discussed (Fig. 17-42; also see Fig. 17-24).

Dermatoses and dermatologic syndromes associated with cataracts

Alopecia universalis	Atopic dermatitis
Pemphigus foliaceus	Incontinentia pigmenti
Pachyonychia congenita	Anhidrotic ectodermal dysplasia
Rothmund-Thomson syndrome	Basal cell nevus syndrome
Werner's syndrome	Cockayne's syndrome
Hallermann-Streiff syndrome	Tuberous sclerosis
Conradi's disease	Turner's syndrome

Alopecia universalis

Alopecia areata designates the patchy loss of scalp and body hair that occurs from an inflammatory reaction of unknown cause. When the reaction involves all the hair of the body, the condition is known as alopecia universalis. These patients have a striking facies because of their lack of scalp and facial hair and their lack of eyebrows and eyelashes, which produces a prominence of their eyes (Fig. 17-43).

Alopecia universalis is a part of the problem of alopecia areata and may be related to an atopic diathesis in the patient or to psychic stress. Histologic study of a biopsy specimen of a hair-bearing area gives the diagnostic, histopathologic picture characterized by a chronic lymphocytic infiltrate about the residual hair follicles. In their studies of persistent, long-standing, generalized alopecia universalis, Muller and Brunsting[5] found that, although rare, cataract formation can occur.

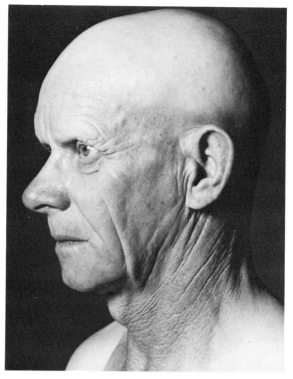

Fig. 17-43. Patient with severe chronically recurrent or persistent universal alopecia is devoid of all body hair and is likely to develop cataracts. No abnormalities of features are otherwise present.

Pemphigus foliaceus

Pemphigus foliaceus is a true pemphigus, with acantholysis of epidermal cells as its major histologic finding. Acantholysis in pemphigus foliaceus occurs high in the epidermis, frequently in the granular cell layer. In pemphigus foliaceus, there are areas of blisters superficially located in the epidermis; the lesions are flaccid bullae that readily rupture and proceed rapidly to scale and crust formation. There are two major types of pemphigus foliaceus: the generalized type in which all cutaneous surfaces are involved in the process, and the localized type in which the blistering is confined predominantly to portions of the scalp, face, neck, and upper trunk. Frequently, the lesions involve the butterfly area of the face and only spotted areas of the rest of the body. Thus the lesions are interspersed in normal-appearing skin. Pruritus and burning pain are common accompaniments of either type of involvement.

The more localized form of the disease, also referred to as pemphigus erythematosus, or Senear-Usher syndrome, has a counterpart in South America known in Portuguese as *fogo selvagem* ('wild fire'). It is clinically, histologically, and immunologically the same disease. Epidemiologically, the disease has been considered to be infectious because of its occurrence in endemic regions in Brazil. Amêndola[1]

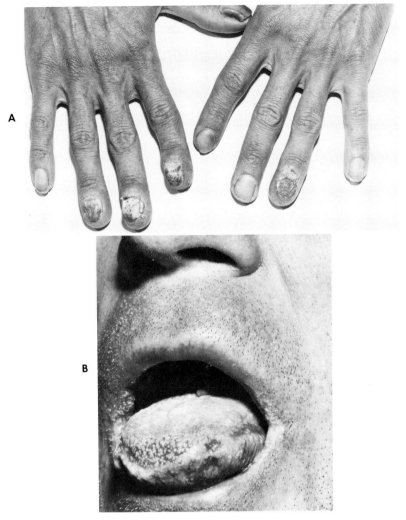

Fig. 17-44. A, One of earliest signs of pachyonychia congenita is occurrence of nail dystrophy. **B,** Leukoplakia of oral mucosa is a later development in pachyonychia congenita. Malignant degeneration of these tissues occurs at an earlier age than anticipated.

reported 12 instances of cataracts in 240 patients with Brazilian pemphigus foliaceus *(fogo selvagem)*. The cataracts resembled those seen in atopic dermatitis.[4]

Pachyonychia congenita

This rare syndrome, transmitted as an autosomal dominant trait, has as its major cutaneous finding hypertrophy of the nails, which is present at birth or shortly thereafter.[3] Keratoderma of the palms and soles begins in early life, when the child is 2 to 4 years old, and bullae sometimes precede or are concomitant with (or both) the thickening of the nails (Fig. 17-44, *A*). Leukokeratosis oris is frequently present, and malignant degeneration of mucosal surfaces involved may oc-

Table 17-8. Frequency of findings in Rothmund-Thomson syndrome

Findings	Percent
Poikiloderma of skin (atrophy, pigmentation, telangiectasia)	100
Cataracts	50
Short stature	50
Skeletal defects (frontal bossing, absent or rudimentary bones, shortening of long bones)	33
Partial or total alopecia (scalp, eyebrows, and eyelashes)	50
Nail defects (small, dystrophic)	25
Dental defects (microdontia, early caries)	14
Hypogonadism	25

Modified from Silver, H. K.: Rothmund-Thomson syndrome: An oculocutaneous disorder, Am. J. Dis. Child. **111**:182-190, 1966.

cur at an early age (Fig. 17-44, *B*). Diffuse alopecia and altered dentition (precocious eruption or delayed) may be present. Ocular findings, including corneal dyskeratoses and cataracts, may be present.

Rothmund-Thomson syndrome (oculocutaneous disorder)

This is a hereditary syndrome transmitted as an autosomal recessive trait, with most of the affected persons being the offspring of consanguineous marriages. Approximately 70% of the patients are females.[6]

The disease begins early in life, frequently between the third and the sixth month, as erythematous patches over the face, and rapidly extends onto the arms, legs, and buttocks. During the ensuing 3 to 5 years, a reticulated pattern of poikiloderma, consisting of atrophy, telangiectasia, hyperpigmentation, and hypopigmentation, replaces the initial dermatosis. Light sensitivity is present in one third of the patients. Silver[7] believes that there are common manifestations of the syndrome (Table 17-8).

Werner's syndrome

The habitus and cutaneous features in Werner's syndrome make the diagnosis of this syndrome easy. Patients frequently are short because growth is arrested at puberty. The arms and legs are thin, and the feet and hands are small. The facial features are distinctive: a beaked nose, a bald scalp, and stiff and inelastic ears. A high-pitched voice is a distinctive finding.[8]

The patient often is sclerodermatous, with the skin being stretched tautly over areas about the face and distal extremities, particularly the feet. Adipose tissue, connective tissues, and musculature are often atrophic. Hyperkeratoses over bony prominences, ulcerations on the feet, generalized hyperpigmentation alternating with depigmentation, and telangiectasias are not uncommon.

Systemic complications are not unusual in this syndrome. Generalized vascular disease consisting of calcification of the peripheral vessels, the aortic valves, and the coronary vessels may occur. Diabetes mellitus is noted in approximately 50% of the patients. Affected persons have poorly developed genitalia and never develop secondary sex characteristics. Some patients may be mentally retarded, and neurologic deficits consisting of loss of deep tendon reflexes, paresthesias, and dizziness may be present.

The eye findings consist of an apparent prominence of the eyes because of the relative loss of supporting circumorbital tissue. Senile cataracts, invariably bilateral, eventually develop. Retinitis pigmentosa, senile macular degeneration, and chorioretinitis are sometimes additional eye findings.

Hallermann-Streiff syndrome (François's syndrome)

These children are characterized by proportionate nanism and a facies with a thin, tapering nose that resembles a parrot's beak, atrophy of the facial skin with a prominence of veins, and dyscephaly (usually microcephaly) with aplasia of the mandible.[4] Hypertrichosis, vitiligo, dental anomalies, and delayed psychomotor development are sometimes present. Total congenital cataracts and microphthalmia are almost always present. No pattern of inheritance of the disease has been determined.

Conradi's disease (congenital stippled epiphyses, chondrodystrophia congenita punctata)

The major diagnostic finding in this syndrome is epiphyseal calcification seen on roentgenograms of the skeleton. This is a rare multisystem disease in which the cutaneous changes, ordinarily present at birth, consist of an erythroderma with micaceous scales that form a whorl pattern over the body. The erythroderma clears during the first year of life and is replaced by follicular atrophoderma, asteatosis, hypotrichiasis, and palmar keratoses.[2]

Skeletal changes, in addition to chondrodystrophy, include rhizomelic micromelia and a high-arched palate (50% of the patients). The cataracts in Conradi's disease usually are congenital, bilateral, and total. Children with Conradi's disease and cataracts usually die before they reach 2 years of age. This syndrome, affecting girls more often than boys, probably is inherited as a recessive trait.

REFERENCES
Dermatologic diseases with ocular involvement

1. Bean, S. F., Waisman, M., Michel, B., Thomas, C. I., Knox, J. M., and Levine, M.: Cicatricial pemphigoid: Immunofluorescent studies, Arch. Dermatol. **106:**195-199, Aug. 1972.
2. Bergeron, J. R., and Stone, O. J.: Interstitial keratitis associated with hidradenitis suppurativa, Arch. Dermatol. **95:**473-475, May 1967.
3. Berlin, C.: Behçet's disease as a multiple symptom complex, Arch. Dermatol. **82:**73-79, July 1960.
4. Bianchine, J. W.: The nevus sebaceous of Jadassohn: A neurocutaneous syndrome and a potentially premalignant lesion, Am. J. Dis. Child. **120:**223-228, Sept. 1970.
5. Brunsting, L. A., and Mason, H. L.: Porphyria with cutaneous manifestations, Arch. Dermatol. Syphilol. **60:**66-79, July 1949.
6. Brunsting, L. A., Reed, W. B., and Bair, H. L.: Occurrence of cataracts and keratoconus with atopic dermatitis, Arch. Dermatol. **72:**237-241, Sept. 1955.
7. Demis, D. J., Crounse, R. G., Dobson, R. L., and McGuire, J.: Clinical dermatology. Vesiculobullous diseases, vol. 2, units, 6-7, 6-12, and 6-13, Hagerstown, Md., 1972, Harper & Row, Publishers.
8. Fitzpatrick, T. B.: Dermatology in general medicine, New York, 1971, McGraw-Hill Book Co.; *a,* p. 208; *b,* pp. 219-236; *c,* pp. 717-721.
9. France, R., Buchanan, R. N., Wilson, M. W., and Sheldon, M. B., Jr.: Relapsing iritis with recurrent ulcers of the mouth and genitalia (Behçet's syndrome), Medicine (Baltimore) **30:**335-355, Dec. 1951.

10. Hardy, K. M., Perry, H. O., Pingree, G. C., and Kirby, T. J., Jr.: Benign mucous membrane pemphigoid, Arch. Dermatol. **104:**467-475, Nov. 1971.

11. Hidano, A., Kajima, H., Ikeda, S., Mizutani, Miyasato, H., and Niimura, M.: Natural history of nevus of Ota, Arch. Dermatol. **95:**187-195, Feb. 1967.

12. Kaldeck, R.: Ocular psoriasis: Clinical review of eleven cases and some comments on treatment, Arch. Dermatol. Syphilol. **68:**44-49, July 1953.

13. Mason, R. M., and Barnes, C. G.: Behçet's syndrome with arthritis, Ann. Rheum. Dis. **28:**95-103, March 1969.

14. Newell, G. B., Stone, O. J., and Mullins, J. F.: Juvenile xanthogranuloma and neurofibromatosis, Arch. Dermatol. **107:**262, Feb. 1973.

15. O'Duffy, J. D., Carney, J. A., and Deodhar, S.: Behçet's disease: Report of 10 cases, 3 with new manifestations, Ann. Intern. Med. **75:**561-570, Oct. 1971.

16. Palmer, D. D., and Perry, H. O.: Melanosis oculi, a variant of nevus of Ota, Arch. Dermatol. **85:**740-742, June 1962.

17. Patz, A.: Ocular involvement in erythema multiforme, Arch. Ophthalmol. **43:**244-256, Feb. 1950.

18. Rook, A., Wilkinson, D. S., and Ebling, F. J. G.: Textbook of dermatology, ed. 2, vol. 1, Oxford, 1972, Blackwell Scientific Publications; *a,* pp. 155-156; *b,* pp. 263-267; *c,* pp. 889-893.

19. Sevel, D., and Burger, D.: Ocular involvement in cutaneous porphyria: A clinical and histological report, Arch. Ophthalmol. **85:**580-585, May 1971.

20. Wise, G.: Ocular rosacea, Am. J. Ophthalmol. **26:**591-609, June 1943.

21. Zimmerman, L. E.: Ocular lesions of juvenile xanthogranuloma: Nevoxanthoendothelioma, Am. J. Ophthalmol. **60:**1011-1035, Dec. 1965.

Hereditary dermatoses with ocular involvement

1. Cocco, A. E., Grayer, D. I., Walker, B. A., and Martyn, L. J.: The stomach in pseudoxanthoma elasticum, J.A.M.A. **210:**2381-2382, Dec. 29, 1969.

2. Cole, J. G., and Cole, H. G.: Incontinentia pigmenti: associated with changes in the posterior chamber of the eye, Am. J. Ophthalmol. **47:**321-328, March 1959.

3. Connor, P. J., Jr., Juergens, J. L., Perry, H. O., Hollenhorst, R. W., and Edwards, J. E.: Pseudoxanthoma elasticum and angioid streaks: A review of 106 cases, Am. J. Med. **30:** 537-543, April 1961.

4. Eddy, D. D., and Farber, E. M.: Pseudoxanthoma elasticum: Internal manifestations; a report of cases and a statistical review of the literature, Arch. Dermatol. **86:**729-740, Dec. 1962.

5. Fitzpatrick, T. B.: Dermatology in general medicine, New York, 1971, McGraw-Hill Book Co.; *a,* pp. 249-265; *b,* pp. 436-439.

6. Gordon, H., and Gordon, W.: Incontinentia pigmenti: Clinical and genetical studies of two familial cases, Dermatologica **140:**150-168, 1970.

7. Heijer, A., and Reed, W. B.: Sjögren-Larsson syndrome: Congenital ichthyosis, spastic paralysis, and oligophrenia, Arch. Dermatol. **92:**545-552, Nov. 1965.

8. McPherson, A., and Auth, T. L.: Bloch-Sulzberger syndrome (incontinentia pigmenti): Report of a case with prominent neurological features, Arch. Neurol. **8:**332-339, March 1963.

9. Reed, W. B., Lopez, D. A., and Landing, B.: Clinical spectrum of anhidrotic ectodermal dysplasia, Arch. Dermatol. **102:**134-143, Aug. 1970.

10. Rook, A., Wilkinson, D. S., and Ebling, F. J. G.: Textbook of dermatology, ed. 2, vol. 2, Oxford, 1972, Blackwell Scientific Publications; *a,* pp. 1255-1258; *b,* pp. 1299-1303.

11. Scott, J. G., Friedmann, A. I., Chitters, M., and Pepler, W. J.: Ocular changes in the Bloch-Sulzberger syndrome (incontinentia pigmenti), Br. J. Ophthalmol. **39:**276-282, May 1955.

12. Sever, R. J., Frost, P., and Weinstein, G.: Eye changes in ichthyosis, J.A.M.A. **206:**2283-2286, Dec. 2, 1968.

Infectious diseases with ocular involvement

1. Becker, F. T.: Herpes zoster ophthalmicus: Results of treatment with transfusions of convalescent blood, Arch. Dermatol. **58:**265-274, Sept. 1948.

2. Demis, D. J., Crounse, R. G., Dobson, R. L., and McGuire, J.: Clinical dermatology, Hagerstown, Md., 1972, Harper & Row, Publishers; *a,* vol. 3, unit 14-3; *b,* vol. 4, unit 18-27, pp. 26-28; *c,* vol. 3, unit 14-9.
3. Fitzpatrick, T. B.: Dermatology in general medicine, New York, 1971, McGraw-Hill Book Co.; *a,* pp. 1878-1892; *b,* pp. 1892-1898.
4. Mathur, S. P.: Ocular complications in molluscum contagiosum, Br. J. Ophthalmol. **44:** 572-573, Sept. 1960.
5. Rook, A., Wilkinson, D. S., and Ebling, F. J. G.: Textbook of dermatology, ed. 2, Oxford, 1972, Blackwell Scientific Publications, vol. 1, pp. 572-575.
6. Stokes, J. H., Beerman, H., and Ingraham, N. R., Jr.: Modern clinical syphilology: Diagnosis, treatment, case study, ed. 3, Philadelphia, 1944, W. B. Saunders Co., pp. 604-649; 967-1169.

Syndromes with skin and ocular involvement

1. Alexander, G. L., and Norman, R. M.: Cited by Berkow, J. W.[2]
2. Berkow, J. W.: Retinitis pigmentosa associated with Sturge-Weber syndrome, Arch. Ophthalmol. **75:**72-76, Jan. 1966.
3. Boder, E., and Sedgwick, R. P.: Ataxia-telangiectasia: A familial syndrome of progressive cerebellar ataxia, oculocutaneous telangiectasia and frequent pulmonary infection, Pediatrics **21:**526-553, April 1958.
4. Clendenning, W. E., Block, J. B., and Radde, I. G.: Basal cell nevus syndrome, Arch. Dermatol. **90:**38-53, July 1964.
5. Clinical Staff Conference (National Institutes of Health): Basal cell nevus syndrome, Ann. Intern. Med. **64:**403-421, Feb. 1966.
6. Davis, D. G., and Smith, J. L.: Retinal involvement in hereditary hemorrhagic telangiectasia, Arch. Ophthalmol. **85:**618-623, May 1971.
7. DeBusk, F. L.: The Hutchinson-Gilford progeria syndrome: Report of 4 cases and review of the literature, J. Pediatr. **80:**697-724, April 1972.
8. Demis, D. J., Crounse, R. G., Dobson, R. L., and McGuire, J.: Clinical dermatology, Hagerstown, Md., 1972, Harper & Row, Publishers, vol. 4, unit 24-2, pp. 1-7.
9. Fitzpatrick, T. B.: Dermatology in general medicine, New York, 1971, McGraw-Hill Book Co.; *a,* pp. 236-243; *b,* pp. 1393-1396; *c,* p. 1419; *d,* pp. 1466-1470.
10. Goltz, R. W., Peterson, W. C., Gorlin, R. J., and Ravits, H. G.: Focal dermal hypoplasia, Arch. Dermatol. **86:**708-717, Dec. 1962.
11. Gorlin, R. J., Anderson, R. C., and Blaw, M.: Multiple lentigines syndrome, Am. J. Dis. Child. **117:**652-662, June 1969.
12. Gorlin, R. J., Meskin, L. H., Peterson, W. C., Jr., and Goltz, R. W.: Focal dermal hypoplasia syndrome, Acta Derm. Venereol. **43:**421-440, 1963.
13. Hodgson, C. H., Burchell, H. B., Good, C. A., and Clagett, O. T.: Hereditary hemorrhagic telangiectasia and pulmonary arteriovenous fistula, New Eng. J. Med. **261:**625-636, Sept. 24, 1959.
14. Kachele, G. E.: The embryogenesis of ectopia lentis: An uncommon dermatological manifestation, Arch. Ophthalmol. **64:**135-139, July 1960.
15. Loveman, A. B., Gordon, A. M., and Fliegelman, M. T.: Marfan's syndrome: Some cutaneous aspects, Arch. Dermatol. **87:**428-435, April 1963.
16. McKusick, V. A.: Heritable disorders of connective tissue, ed. 4, St. Louis, 1972, The C. V. Mosby Co., pp. 292-371.
17. Mills, S. D., and Winkelmann, R. K.: Eczema, thrombocytopenic purpura, and recurring infections, Arch. Dermatol. **79:**466-472, April 1959.
18. Muller, S. A., and Brunsting, L. A.: Cataracts associated with dermatologic disorders, Arch. Dermatol. **88:**330-339, Sept. 1963.
19. Nickel, W. R., and Reed, W. B.: Tuberous sclerosis: Special reference to the microscopic alterations in the cutaneous hamartomas, Arch. Dermatol. **85:**209-224, Feb. 1962.
20. Perry, H. O., Kiely, J. M., and Moertel, C. G.: Cutaneous clues to visceral cancer, Minn. Med. **51:**1719-1726, Dec. 1968.
21. Peterman, A. F., Hayles, A. B., Dockerty, M. B., and Love, J. G.: Encephalotrigeminal angiomatosis (Sturge-Weber disease): Clinical study of thirty-five cases, J.A.M.A. **167:** 2169-2176, Aug. 30, 1958.

22. Peterson, R. D. A., Cooper, M. D., and Good, R. A.: Lymphoid tissue abnormalities associated with ataxia-telangiectasia, Am. J. Med. **41:**342-359, Sept. 1966.
23. Podos, S. M., Einaugler, R. B., Albert, D. M., and Blaese, R. M.: Ophthalmic manifestations of the Wiskott-Aldrich syndrome, Arch. Ophthalmol. **82:**322-329, Sept. 1969.
24. Reed, W. B., Epstein, W. L., Boder, E., and Sedgwick, R.: Cutaneous manifestations of ataxia-telangiectasia, J.A.M.A. **195:**746-753, Feb. 28, 1966.
25. Reed, W. B., Nickel, W. R., and Campion, G.: Internal manifestations of tuberous sclerosis, Arch. Dermatol. **87:**715-728, June 1963.
26. Reed, W. B., Stone, V. M., Boder, E., and Ziprkowski, L.: Pigmentary disorders in association with congenital deafness, Arch. Dermatol. **95:**176-185, Feb. 1967.
27. Rook, A., Wilkinson, D. S., and Ebling, F. J. G.: Textbook of dermatology, ed. 2, Oxford, 1972, Blackwell Scientific Publications; *a,* vol. 1, p. 113; *b,* vol. 1, pp. 117-118; *c,* vol. 2, p. 1181.
28. Selmanowitz, V. J., Orentreich, N., and Felsenstein, J. M.: Lentiginosis profusa syndrome (multiple lentigines syndrome), Arch. Dermatol. **104:**393-401, Oct. 1971.

Dermatoses and cutaneous syndromes with cataracts

1. Amêndola, F.: Cited by Muller, S. A., and Brunsting, L. A.[4]
2. Bodian, E. L.: Skin manifestations of Conradi's disease, Arch. Dermatol. **94:**743-748, Dec. 1966.
3. Fitzpatrick, T. B.: Dermatology in general medicine, New York, 1971, McGraw-Hill Book Co., pp. 346-349.
4. Muller, S. A., and Brunsting, L. A.: Cataracts associated with dermatologic disorders, Arch. Dermatol. **88:**330-339, Sept. 1963.
5. Muller, S. A., and Brunsting, L. A.: Cataracts in alopecia areata, Arch. Dermatol. **88:**202-206, Aug. 1963.
6. Rook, A., Wilkinson, D. S., and Ebling, F. J. G.: Textbook of dermatology, ed. 2, Oxford, 1972, Blackwell Scientific Publications, vol. 1, pp. 109-111.
7. Silver, H. K.: Rothmund-Thomson syndrome: An oculocutaneous disorder, Am. J. Dis. Child. **111:**182-190, Feb. 1966.
8. Smith, R. C., Winer, L. H., and Martel, S.: Werner's syndrome: Report of two cases, Arch. Dermatol. **71:**197-204, 1955.

18

Eye involvement in skin diseases

Giambattista Bietti

The incidence of eye involvement in skin diseases is extremely high. This relationship may well be explained by the embryonic affinity of many components of the ocular apparatus with skin structures, as well as by the continuity of the outer eye tissue toward the surrounding skin area. The conditions reported will be represented by ocular changes related to skin diseases more or less strictly adjacent to the eye, with ocular changes appearing concomitantly with or successively to, morbid localizations in the skin, and in the mucous membranes far from the eye. We have so far recorded more than 200 oculodermatologic conditions, but in agreement with Dr. Perry, I shall illustrate only some of the most frequent and important yet sometimes less known occurrences.

There are important reports on this subject already available, such as those of Groenouw (1930),[2] Sala and Noto (1948),[5] and more recently Thygeson (1951-53),[7, 8] Schreck (1959),[6] Lebas (1966),[4] Casanovas and Villanova (1967),[1] and Korting (1969).[3] The classification criteria followed by various authors in their research are different from ours and thus are not quite adaptable to the present report. We have attempted to follow the most modern trends in our classification, such as those of Lebas, Thygeson, and Korting. Because of the limit of space, I shall briefly mention the ocular manifestations that occur in various degrees in the following groups of diseases in accordance especially with the criteria of Korting and partially with Lebas and Thygeson:

1. Malformations and dystrophies on congenital basis
2. Skin infections
    a. Acute
    b. Chronic
3. Viral, chlamydial, and rickettsial infections
4. Mycoses
5. Zoonoses
6. Erythemas and acute exanthemas
7. Erythrodesquamative dermatoses
8. Eczemas
9. Strophulus; prurigo; and urticaria

10. Pigmentary changes
11. Vascular diseases and circulatory disturbances
12. Bullous dermatoses and pemphigus
13. Diseases of the hair apparatus
14. Diseases of the sebaceous glands
15. Benign and malignant tumors of the lids
16. Phakomatoses
17. Physical, chemical, and drug-provoked changes (including xeroderma pigmentosum)
18. Keratoses and dystrophies (including elastorrhexis)
19. Skin atrophies (including elastosis)
20. Hemorrhagic diatheses
21. Leukosis, reticulosis, etc.
22. Collagenoses
23. Metabolic changes and thesaurismoses

In agreement with the suggestions of Dr. Perry, the following material has been divided into four main groups. For practical purposes in each group several types of diseases are listed but only a few of them will be discussed at length. In the fifth section I have listed in summary the syndermatotic cataracts. Dr. Perry has already illustrated not only the dermatologic but also the etiologic and hereditary aspects of the skin diseases discussed here.

SOME IMPORTANT DERMATOLOGIC DISEASES WITH EYE FINDINGS

In this group the diseases of eczematous type will first be treated. They may present various aspects involving mainly the lid, skin, conjunctiva, and sometimes also the cornea (in addition to the manifestations in the deeper eye structures, such as the lens in some forms of eczema).

Ota's nevus, or oculodermic melanocytosis. Ota's nevus, or oculodermic melanocytosis, consists of usually a unilateral fuscocerulean melanosis of the lid skin, conjunctiva, and sclera. There is sometimes a slight involvement of the cornea and in some cases also of the iris and the eye fundus. This gives place respectively to an iris heterochromia caused by hyperpigmentation of the affected eye and by a grayish ophthalmoscopic reflex. Tenon's capsule and eye muscles may also be pigmented. These manifestations are usually present at birth but may have an evolutive character, and sometimes even a late development has been observed.

A malignant melanoma of the choroid arising from Ota's nevus has been exceptionally found.

In Negroes, Mongolians, and pigmented races there is a frequent occurrence of melanosis oculi. The picture is morphologically close to the one of Ota's nevus.

Hemangiomas. The hemangiomas involving the palpebral skin, conjunctiva, and more rarely the orbit, have been already exhaustively dealt with in the introduction. However, in the topic concerning phakomatoses (p. 378) some particular types of hemangiomas will be fully reconsidered.

The problem that the ophthalmologist has to face in the angiomas (including lymphangiomas) is mainly the therapeutic one, keeping in mind the capacity of evolution, localization, size, and the cosmetic necessities. Also in the ophthalmologic field, the treatment may be based either on classical surgery, physical means (diathermocoagulation, photocoagulation, cryoapplication) or on radiation therapy (Figs. 18-1 to 18-3).

Dermatitis venenata. Dermatitis venenata, or otherwise called contact eczema, involves the lids and the surrounding area. It is important because of the frequency of its occurrence and also as an isolated phenomenon limited to the ophthalmologic field. Dermatitis venenata occurs when particular substances come into contact with the lid skin and conjunctiva.

The substances capable of determining this picture are numerous, such as effects of accidental contact with various stimulating agents of either vegetable, animal, or mineral origin or to various drugs. These substances are used above all topically on the conjunctivae and the lids or may be involved because of the action of cosmetics employed locally or at a distance from the eyes (such

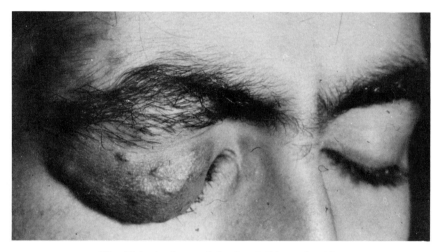

Fig. 18-1. Angioma of forehead, lids, and orbit.

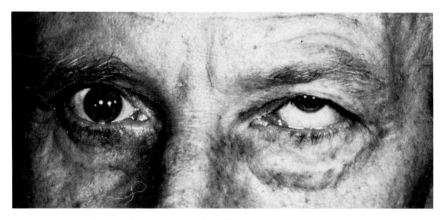

Fig. 18-2. Palpebroconjunctival hemangiopericytoma.

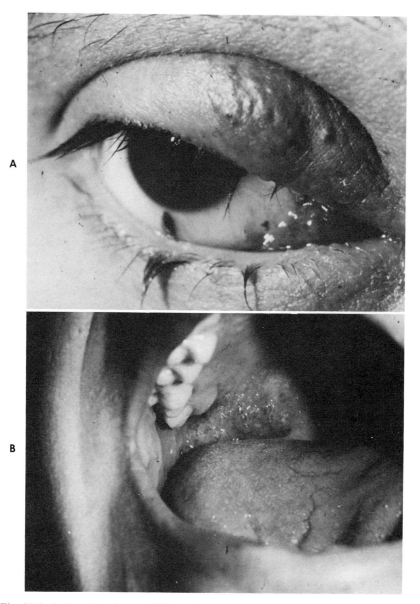

Fig. 18-3. A, Lymphangioma of lids, conjunctiva, and orbit. **B,** Buccal localization in **A.**

as hair dye containing paraphenylenediamine). The reactions to medicaments used topically in ophthalmology are mainly attributable not only to sulfonamides and antibiotics (such as penicillin, chloramphenicol, streptomycin, neomycin, tetracyclines) but also to anesthetics (procaine), pupillokinetics (atropine), and even plastic eyeglass frames (Fig. 18-4).

One should keep in mind that in the course of systemic treatments with chemotherapeutic agents and antibiotics serious eye involvement may be ob-

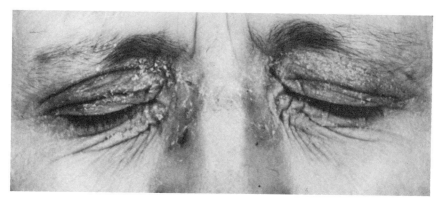

Fig. 18-4. Glass-frame allergy.

served in the presence of severe generalized dermatoses, such as *Lyell syndrome* (or epidermolysis combustiformis) and the *Stevens-Johnson syndrome*. It is known that the patch test may prove useful to determine the substances responsible for the skin reaction when the cause does not appear evident from the clinical history. The excipients or ointments of the eye drops may also be responsible for contact dermatitis. From the therapeutic point of view it is superfluous to recall that antihistaminics and corticosteroids are an excellent way to treat the ocular lesions.

Atopic dermatitis. In the atopic dermatitis (neurodermitis disseminata, prurigo of Besnier, or eczema allergicum) we observe first either seasonal (from hay) or vernal conjunctivitis with both tarsal and limbal localizations and eosinophilia in the secretion. In the second or so-called vulgar type, a keratitis may develop first under the aspect of a keratitis veriscularis disseminata, or keratitis superficialis punctata. In the third phase there are deep opacities with folds of Descemet's membrane preceded by massive serous conjunctivitis. The occurrence of corneal ulcerations is possible. The three stages of eczema correspond to the erythematous, the vesiculated and madidans ('moist'), and the pustulous ones.

Occasionally I have observed a keratoconus accompanied by vernal catarrh (Fig. 18-5). However, the keratoconus and the vernal catarrh are not related in the sense that the keratoconus develops as a consequence of a weakening of the cornea because of the vernal catarrh localization (as it has been pretended recently by Gormaz). In fact atopic dermatitis may be accompanied by either vernal catarrh or keratoconus alone. We have seen moreover the cases of a brother and sister, one affected only by vernal catarrh and the other only by keratoconus, and of two brothers with keratoconus but only one with conjunctivitis. This fact demonstrates that the two diseases arise independently with a common link, such as atopic dermatitis. Keratoconus with vernal catarrh generally occurs earlier in life than keratoconus alone.

The development of a cataract is a relatively frequent occurrence (8.5%). It begins with capsular and subcapsular anterior opacities but may have an evolutive tendency. I should emphasize that the lens changes may appear even

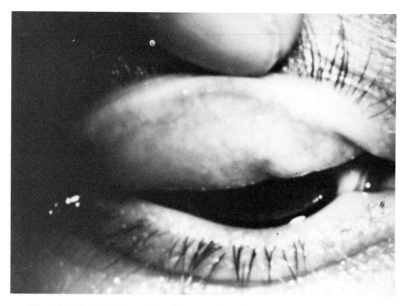

Fig. 18-5. Atopic dermatitis with vernal conjunctivitis and keratoconus.

before the dermatologic alterations. In two thirds of the cases the cataract is bilateral. Also the occurrence of a retinal detachment has been pointed out, and this is interpreted above all as a postoperative complication of a cataract operation.

Seborrhea. Seborrhea is a common occurrence among the various types of *eczema* involving the eye apparatus. There are associations of processes in other areas (mainly scalp) with desquamation of the palpebral skin, which shows a greasy aspect. This can happen in association with chronic conjunctivitis caused not only by bacteria (presence of staphylococcic blepharitis) but also by particles of the skin scales dropped into the conjunctival sac.

The conjunctivitis may be associated with corneal involvement (mostly superficial keratitis), and more infrequently iris reaction is observed. Cataracts and optic neuritis have also been recorded.

Thygeson, Gots, and Waisman found in seborrheic blepharitis the presence of *Pityrosporon ovale,* which is considered responsible for the epithelial keratitis, through an allergic mechanism.

The treatment of the forms not complicated with bacterial infections (which are favorably influenced by antibiotics) is not easy. Every ophthalmologist knows the scarce value of a limited diet (reduction of fats), salicylic products, and resorcinol on the lids.

Acne rosacea. Acne rosacea is characterized by a squamous or ulcerous blepharitis (sometimes accompanied with multiple chalazions). A conjunctival involvement is also frequent. This may develop as a simple hyperemia, or as a meibomian, telangiectatic, or nodular bulbar conjunctivitis. The interpalpebral area is prevailingly affected. The keratitis, appearing in the course of the acne rosacea, may develop not only as marginal ulcers, and subepithelial infiltrates,

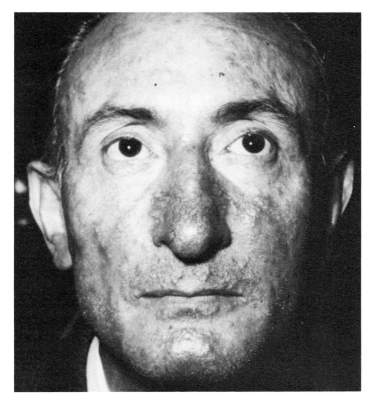

Fig. 18-6. Acne rosacea with lid border involvement and slight corneal involvement.

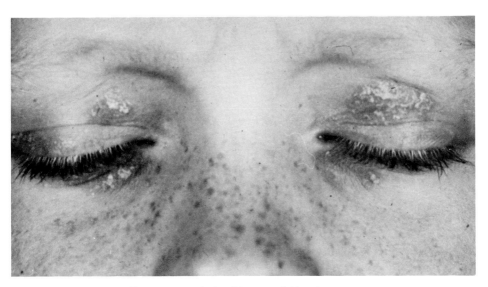

Fig. 18-7. Psoriasis with upper lid involvement.

but also as ulcerations of the progressive "ulcus rodens" type. As a peculiar feature the infiltrates may sometimes present a cretaceous aspect (Fig. 18-6). I should emphasize that the skin lesions sometimes develop independently from the corneal lesions. After the keratitis the occurrence of scleritis (exceptionally perforating) and iris reactions has been observed.

Hidradenitis suppurativa. Hidradenitis suppurativa has been considered as a variant of acne vulgaris. The ophthalmologic interest consists mainly in the appearance of a hidradenitis profunda with interstitial keratitis (Bergeron and Stone). Korting points out the presence of interstitial keratitis also in cases of ecthyma gangrenosum and in infections from *Pseudomonas aeruginosa* (formerly *P. pyocyanea*). This was also observed by Jess, Hitschmann, and Kreibich.

Psoriasis vulgaris. Ocular involvement in psoriasis vulgaris may be characterized first by desquamation foci on the lids, which is sometimes seborrheic in aspect (Korting) and may be followed by madarosis, trichiasis, and ectropion (Fig. 18-7). On the conjunctiva, especially in the tarsal area, small yellowish red granulations covered by sparkling scales may be seen; however, common chronic conjunctivitis is more frequent.

Peculiar features have been attributed to the corneal involvement by Pillat. In this "psoriatic keratitis" there is the presence of either foci originating from the limbus, vascularized, and with a tendency to ulcerations, or minute punctiform opacities located in the layers of the parenchyma far from the limbus. Nodular episcleritis rarely occurs. The presence of iritis in the arthropathic form has been pointed out. There is also to be considered the possible appearance of lens opacities, mainly, subcapsular and cortical anterior, with a tendency to progression. Exceptional is the occurrence of optic neuritis and chorioretinal degenerative changes, which are observed in families with hereditary psoriasis. On the whole, the course of the ocular changes is more or less parallel to that of the skin lesions.

Another erythrosquamous dermatosis is the *pityriasis rubra pilaris.* There is concomitance of supraciliary and palpebral lesions of squamous or crustaceous aspect but less serious than on the surrounding skin. Also observed on the border of the lids and ectropion are ulcerations and efflorescences. On the conjunctiva may be present eruption of the papulas as well as diffuse thickening hyperemia and chemosis. As to the cornea, the aspects are polymorphous. Superficial opacities, keratoses, linear whitish striae, facets, diffuse opacities, ulcerations secondary to the epithelial exfoliation caused by keratosis also occur. More infrequent is the interstitial keratitis having as a main characteristic scarce or no vascularization. In case of severe corneal involvement, secondary iritis may occur.

In *lichen ruber planus* ocular lesions accompanying the papular skin eruptions are infrequent. However palpebral localizations, analogous to the cutaneous ones, are observed. Presence of white, opaline spots with striated or nodular arrangement on the palpebrobulbar conjunctivae is an exceptional occurrence. The concomitant corneal opacities are of limited importance and rather superficial. Isolated cases of iridochoroiditis and of macular pigmentations have been observed.

Pemphigoid changes. The picture of the pemphigoid changes is very complex

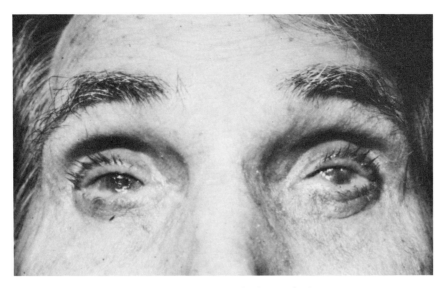

Fig. 18-8. Ocular pemphigoid in terminal stage.

and confused because of the difficulty of separating the various types and the inclusion of the essential retraction of the conjunctivae. The ocular lesions in the advanced stages, however, are substantially analogous in the various types, independently if they are preceded by bullous manifestations of the conjunctival mucous membrane or of other ones. In any case, we are dealing with a serious conjunctivitis, sometimes with the presence of pseudomembranes, followed by cicatricial shrinking of the conjunctiva, trichiasis, ectropion, symblepharon, ankyloblepharon, and blepharophimosis. In the most severe cases this picture is accompanied by sclerotic phenomena. In general, the cornea becomes opacified only later after the appearance of the conjunctival lesions, even if they are already in an advanced stage. The condition may be accompanied by remarkable functional impairment aggravated also by the difficulty of performing ocular movements in the presence of the pronounced symblepharon. This form is in general bilateral, even if with a different degree of gravity in the two eyes. Its course may have a more or less long duration, and an arrest has also been observed (Fig. 18-8). These forms are known also under the names of *cicatricial ocular pemphigoid, bullous dermatitis, or conjunctivitis leading to mucosynechias and atrophy* that may have a familial character with or without skin or mucous involvement. According to François and co-workers, these expressions should replace the term "pemphigus." The differential diagnosis with advanced trachoma is important. I would like to point out that a viral etiology of the pemphigoid changes has been considered. Recently Bettelheim, Zehetbauer, and co-workers (1973) found in the ocular tissues evidence of immunofluorescent antibodies and suggest that the disease might be considered as an autoimmune manifestation. Immunosuppressive drugs have therefore been advised for its treatment.

In *dermatitis herpetiformis* (Duhring) there are some aspects that may re-

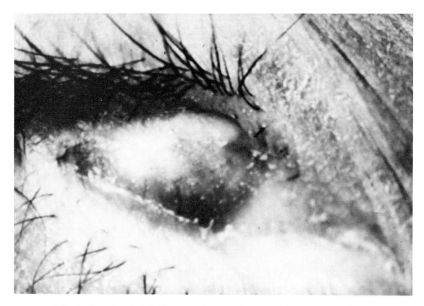

Fig. 18-9. Cicatricial phase of dermatitis herpetiformis (Duhring).

semble those encountered in pemphigus. The lesions of the palpebral skin are rather infrequent. On the conjunctiva, changes from dermatitis herpetiformis are also infrequent and analogous to those observed in the pemphigus forms (Fig. 18-9). Corneal involvement is uncommon too. Bilateral central chorio-retinitis is an exceptional finding.

In the course of *pemphigus foliaceus* (or *fogo salvagem* of Brazil) another occurrence to note is the appearance of a cataract, probably secondary to degenerative iris lesions.

The pemphigoid eye manifestations are favorably influenced, but within a limited degree, by cortisone and fibrinolytic therapies, to which treatment with immunosuppressive drugs has been recently added. It may become necessary to resort to conjunctival and eventually to corneal plastic surgery.

Erythema multiforme. In the severe cases of erythema multiforme not only are there lid lesions with edema, but there may also occur conjunctivitis with catarrh, viscous secretion, subconjunctival hemorrhages, erythematous papulas and large follicles or episcleral noduli, and more rarely, ulcerous keratitis, purulent uveitis, cataracts, and optic neuritis. The complications of the so-called *Stevens-Johnson disease* and of the ectodermosis erosiva pluriorificialis of Fiessinger-Rendu belong to this symptomatology (Fig. 18-10). *Toxic epidermal necrolysis (Lyell's disease,* also *epidermolysis combustiformis),* generally attributed to drugs, also gives place to ocular sequelae, similar to those just described, but often more serious (Fig. 18-11). These sequelae require mainly surgical treatment.

In *erythema nodosum,* small noduli are observed on the lids and frequently on the bulbar conjunctivae, with the aspect of phlyctenae, in the interpalpebral limbic area. Episcleritis and scleritis, as well as keratitis of phlyctenular type, also occur.

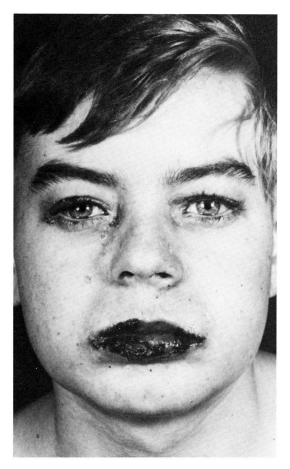

Fig. 18-10. Mild Stevens-Johnson conjunctivitis.

Anterior or posterior uveitis with polymorphous appearances are observed also. Also of ophthalmologic interest are manifestations of *erythema nodosum,* which may be present in other particular dermatologic affections such as in Reiter's and Behçet's disease.

Behçet's disease. In our classification and in the group we are dealing with there is also Behçet's disease. Despite geographic differences in its occurrence, the disease is well known to the ophthalmologists today. We have studied extensively and followed for several years in Italy more than 60 cases. The ocular symptoms generally consist of recurrent hypopyon iritis, but also in posterior uveitis, papilloretinitis, and retinal vasculopathy with vitreous recurrent hemorrhages. The lesions are, in general, bilateral (88% of cases), but they may appear at different times. The visual prognosis is unfavorable, mainly in relation to complicated cataract, secondary glaucoma, and optic atrophy. In about 15% of the cases meningoencephalitic manifestations appear, to which the jargon term of "neuro-Behçet" has been given. Not only is the visual prognosis unfavorable but also

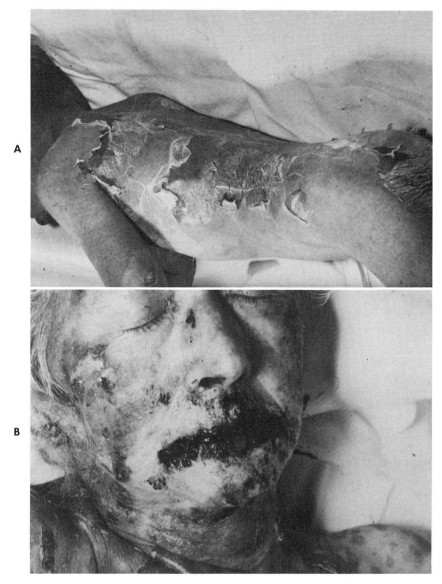

Fig. 18-11. A, Cutaneous exfoliation in epidermolysis combustiformis of Lyell. **B,** Oral, facial, and eye involvement in Lyell syndrome.

the prospect of health and longevity *('quoad vitam')*. The results obtained today with corticosteroids and immunosuppressive drugs are good but not durable. This disease, in which the well-known buccal aphthae, genital, joint, or skin alterations may theoretically even be absent, is ascribed today mostly to the collagenoses.

Collagenoses. The collagenoses merit being mentioned, even if only briefly. Besides the *sclerodermatitides* (Fig. 18-12) in their various aspects (where especially the occurrence of a cataract and also glaucoma should be mentioned), the eye manifestations of the following diseases should not be omitted: *poikiloderma*

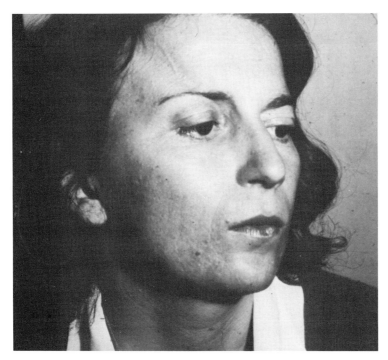

Fig. 18-12. Sclerodermitis *en coup de sabre* with homologous juvenile open-angle glaucoma (right side).

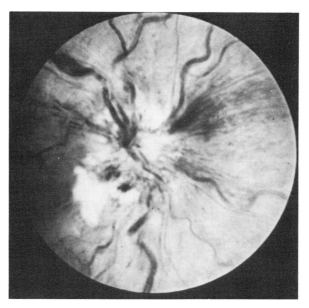

Fig. 18-13. Papillomacular aspect in a case of lupus erythematosus. (Courtesy Jerome T. Pearlman, Los Angeles, Calif.)

(microcornea, high myopia, blepharophimosis caused by cicatricial retraction, lid skin lesions, maculopapular edema, cataract), *dermatomyositis* (lesions of the lids and of the retina, such as cytoid bodies and cotton-wool exudates), *lupus erythematosus* (conjunctival, palpebral, and corneal lesions, iridocyclitis, papilloretinitis, retinal hemorrhages, chorioretinitis, etc.), and (Fig. 18-13) *periarteritis nodosa* (lid skin lesions and conjunctival lesions; parenchymatous, marginal, and sclerosing keratitis; scleritis; uveitis; exudative pseudoalbuminuric hypertensive hemorrhagic retinitis; and oculomotor paralysis). It is known that besides Behçet's disease already mentioned, *Sjögren's disease* (keratoconjunctivitis sicca), pseudopolyarthritis rhizomelica (iridocyclitis), *Horton's disease* (arthritis temporalis with papilloretinal ischemia), *chronic relapsing polychondritis* (scleritis, uveitis), *Takayasu's disease* (retinal vascular changes, especially venous; complicated cataract), *Cogan's disease* (interstitial keratitis with deafness), and *Wegener's granulomatosis* or *lethal midline granuloma* (orbital pseudotumors, keratitis, scleritis) have also been recently included into the group of collagenoses by some authors.

Nevoxanthoendothelioma. Nevoxanthoendothelioma (juvenile xanthogranuloma) may affect the lids and the orbit (Fig. 18-14), as other thesaurismoses (Hand-

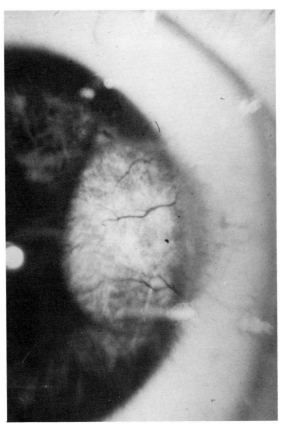

Fig. 18-14. Nevoxanthoendothelioma of the eye. (Courtesy German Ophthalmological Society, Heidelberg.)

Schüller-Christian disease or cutaneous xanthomatoses). Besides palpebral skin lesions, one may observe also conjunctival infiltrates (sometimes involving also the cornea), granulomatous uveitis, hemorrhages in the anterior chamber, and secondary glaucoma.

Porphyria. Porphyria cutanea tarda (a type of mixed porphyria hepatica—the classification systems proposed are still in flux) is one of the most important among many types of idiopathic or symptomatic porphyrias. In this disease, besides hyperpigmentation and the sclerodermoid aspect of the exposed regions on the palpebral skin as well as in the area of the palpebral opening with conjunctival and scleral injections, we note hypertrichosis of the eyebrows, which may lead to synophrys (Fig. 18-15).

Kuhnt, Sevel, and co-workers' observations of scleral perforation secondary to keratomalacia and attributed to the photosensitivity caused by porphyria, appear to be exceptional. Corneal involvement may also be observed with polymorphous aspect, going from the punctiform to the bullous, phlyctenular, or dendritic types.

Iris involvement is essentially secondary to the sclerocorneal lesions. However cases with choroidal and neuroretinal localizations having various morphology, as well as oculomotor paralysis, have also been noted.

The evolution of *porphyria,* with generally seasonal *poussées* ('paroxysms') occurring repeatedly in the course of years, may lead to severe palpebroconjunctival sequelae.

Another important aspect of disordered porphyrin metabolism is the eye changes in *hydroa vacciniforme.* In this disease eye involvement occurs in nearly 20% of the cases with various aspects. There are skin eruptions on the lids with possible cicatricial deformations. Serious inflammation is noted on the conjunc-

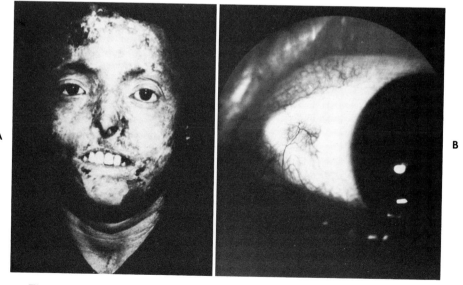

Fig. 18-15. A, Porphyria of the face. **B,** Conjunctival involvement in porphyria.

tiva with chemosis, formation of vesicles, ulcerations followed by necrosis, and cicatricial retractions that may alter the position of the lids, as previously mentioned. Another particularity is the possible appearance of perilimbic infiltrates resembling the bulbar involvement in vernal catarrh and susceptible of giving origin to neovascularizations.

Exfoliations and ulcerations occur on the cornea in the area of the palpebral fissure. There are also sometimes deep parenchymal opacities with neovascularization. Infrequently there is the appearance of scleral necroses and of successive staphylomas. Lens opacities are rare; they are generally of the anterior subcapsular type. One should also note the association of porphyrinuria with chorioretinitis, retinal hemorrhages, retinal edema, optic neuritis, and papilledema. Color vision disturbances have been described. A possible connection of *porphyrinuria* with certain types of vernal conjunctivitis and with anterior subcapsular lens opacities has been considered.

Sebaceous nevus. In sebaceous nevus of Jadassohn, or neurocutaneous syndrome, the frequent appearance of basalomas is well known. The sebaceous nevus may also involve the conjunctiva (with a papillomatous aspect). Regarding the cutaneous manifestations (Blianchine), it has already been pointed out in the dermatologic part that besides epileptic manifestations with spasms and mental deficiency, conjunctival lipodermoids (sometimes with corneal vascularization), rotatory horizontal nystagmus, and uveal coloboma are observed.

Pigmented tumors (melanomas). Various are the types of pigmented tumors (melanomas) affecting the skin (nevi, nevus fuscoceruleus, juvenile melanoma, preblastomatous circumscribed melanosis, malignant melanoma) and being susceptible to single or multiple localization also on the lid skin, the conjunctiva, and

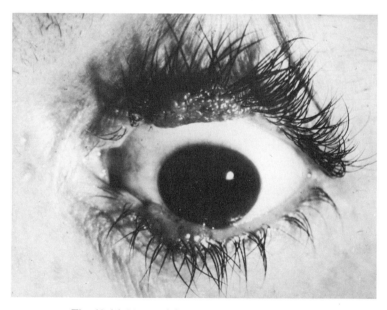

Fig. 18-16. Nevus divisus of upper and lower lids.

exceptionally the cornea. A characteristic finding that shows the precocious development of the nevus is the so-called naevus divisus, which occupies both lids, being separated only by the palpebral fissure at the moment of its formation (Fig. 18-16).

Some neoformations, as the juvenile melanoma (nevus fascicularis) and the malignant melanoma, may notoriously involve also the uvea, giving place to findings that every ophthalmologist knows also from the anatomopathologic point of view. I shall not deal in detail, therefore, with the morphology of the above-mentioned melanomas and their either conservative or radical treatment. I should like to call attention to the difficulty of the clinical diagnosis as far as the malignancy of the conjunctival nevi is concerned, as well as to the prudence in resorting to biopsy, which, according to some authors, may stimulate an atypical proliferation.

HEREDITARY DERMATOSES WITH EYE FINDINGS

Pseudoxanthoma elasticum. In this section on the *hereditary dermatoses* with ocular findings I would like to devote our attention first to the pseudoxanthoma elasticum of Darier caused by elastorexis. As it is well known this cutaneous disease is associated with the so-called angioid streaks of the retina (Knapp, 1892), giving place to the *Grönblad-Strandberg syndrome*.

The "angioid streaks" are caused by lesions of the lamina vitrea of the choroid. The elastic tissue is here furrowed by dehiscence arranged radially to the optic disk. They sometimes originate from an annular circumpapillary formation with an irregular course, which resembles somewhat that of the retinal vessels. They are brownish in color. This characteristic aspect is supposed to be attributable to the stretching phenomena of Bruch's membrane (Fig. 18-17).

After a first functionally silent stage, visual problems follow in relation to

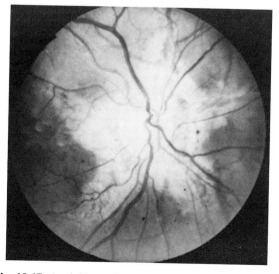

Fig. 18-17. Angioid streaks of retina moderately advanced.

retinal hemorrhages at the posterior pole (expression of elastorexis also vasal). These retinal hemorrhages may become pigmented or scarred, giving place to findings closely similar to the disciform degeneration described by Junius and Kuhnt (Fig. 18-18).

Among the other less outstanding lesions of the eye fundus are hyaline verrucosities, the presence of little whitish-yellowish-brownish retinal foci, and a peculiar "mottled aspect" of the eye fundus. Corneal opacities, keratoconus, Descemet's wrinkles, lens subluxation, cataract, optic atrophy (leading sometimes to amaurosis), and exophthalmos (from recurrent orbital hematomas) are exceptional findings. The oculomotor paralyses, sometimes observed, are caused by vascular lesions of the central nervous system.

The possible occurrence of an elastorexis of Bruch's membrane must be taken always into account in the presence of retinal hemorrhagic phenomena not connected to visible vessel changes or to retinal tears.

Even if infrequently, retinal angioid streaks have been observed also in the course of other systemic diseases such as senile or actinic elastosis, Ehlers-Danlos disease, sickle cell anemia, Paget's deformant osteitis, acromegalia and after injuries.

Incontinentia pigmenti. Also included in the same chapter is the incontinentia pigmenti, or Bloch-Sulzberger disease. Besides pigment changes on the lid skin, malformative or inflammatory eye symptoms appear mostly unilaterally in 30% to 35% of the cases. The most severe lesions are represented by "pseudoglioma" and a peculiar retrolental fibroplasia attributable either to persistence of the primary vitreous or to total retinal detachment, but the lesions may also be a consequence of inflammatory phenomena (metastatic ophthalmitis).

Other eye manifestations consist of disorders of the extrinsic ocular motility, superficial or parenchymal diffuse corneal opacities at the limbus, as well as in

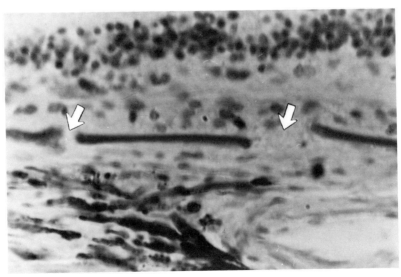

Fig. 18-18. Choroidal changes in angioid streaks. *Arrows*, Defects of Bruch's membrane.

anomalies of the chamber angle. These manifest themselves also by strands of anterior synechias of the iris, which may be atrophic and with pigment irregularities. Complicated cataracts, frequently present at birth, may also be observed. At the fundus examination one may find papillitis, optic atrophy, exudative chorioretinitis with important foci, neovascularization, diffuse hyperpigmentations of the chorioretina, hemorrhages, vessel tortuosities, and retinal edema. Finally, the eyeballs may be microphthalmic or even atrophic. Some ocular findings resemble those observed in the dysgenesis mesodermalis of Rieger.

Xeroderma pigmentosum. In xeroderma pigmentosum the palpebral lesions are thoroughly similar to the cutaneous ones, which tend to become malignant. They are prevailingly localized at the palpebral fissures, especially at the medial canthus and may be accompanied secondarily by ciliary alopecia, madarosis, entropion, symblepharon, and ankyloblepharon (Figs. 8-19 and 18-20).

The conjunctival lesions may present various aspects. They are sometimes simply irritative with pigmentation of various degrees, telangiectatic, or properly neoplastic. Pseudopterygium may also be observed. Secondary neoplastic invasion of the tarsus and the sclera may occur from the palpebral skin and from the conjunctiva. The picture is often accompanied with keratitis, mainly in the interpalpebral limbic zone, with involvement of the adjacent conjunctiva. Edemas and neoplastic infiltrations also occur. Iris atrophy and cataract may be observed. Surgical treatment may become necessary.

Anhidrotic ectodermal dysplasia. In anhidrotic ectodermal dysplasia there may be a hyperkeratosis as a result of retention (retention hyperkeratosis), which may be accompanied with ichthyosis or palmoplantar keratosis. The eye changes are represented sometimes by palpebral opening of mongoloid type, supraciliary and

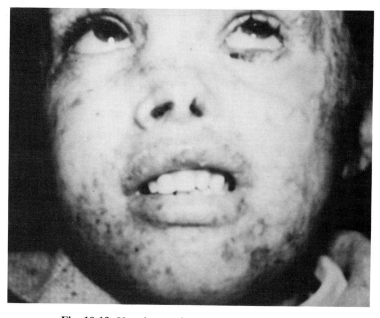

Fig. 18-19. Xeroderma pigmentosum involving eyes.

ciliary alopecia, palpebral pigmentation, absence or reduction of the palpebral glands, hypolacrimia, and also stenosis of the lacrimal puncta. More severe changes consist of corneal involvement in the form of opacities or of dysplastic phenomena, aniridia, pupillary anomalies, subluxation and luxation of the lens, and congenital or juvenile cataract with various morphology (cortical, polar, and nuclear). Phenomena of chorioretinal atrophy at the posterior pole are infrequent, but have sometimes been described.

Ichthyoses. Ichthyoses also belong to this group of diseases and, as previously seen, the disease may appear with different characteristics. Ocular lesions are more frequent in congenital forms. The lesions mainly consist of ichthyotic changes of the lid skin accompanied with conjunctivitis. They may lead to entropion

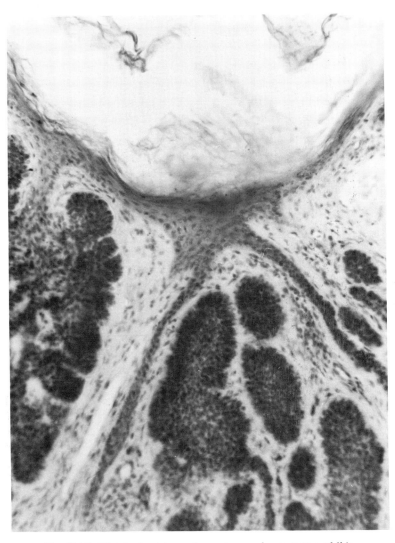

Fig. 18-20. Histologic picture of xeroderma pigmentosum of lids.

caused by retraction and symblepharon or ectropion. The ophthalmologists speak of "corneal ichthyoses" in regard to the various forms of the opacities. Deep punctiform opacities have been observed among them.

There are especially in some syndromes representing a variety of ichthyoses (Rud's syndrome, Sjögren-Larssen syndrome, Refsum's syndrome) the probability of finding a cataract, syntropia with hydrophthalmos, retinal phlebitis, pigmentary retinitis, and macular degenerations. There was also recorded the presence of microphthalmos, oculomotor paralyses and strabismus (Fig. 18-21).

Epidermolysis bullosa. In the course of an epidermolysis bullosa, conjunctivitis leading to symblepharon, lagophthalmos, and cicatricial lacrimal stenoses may be observed. The corneal involvement consists above all of bullae and erosions that are mostly superficial; rarely were there found maculated corneal dystrophies. Retinal detachment is exceptional.

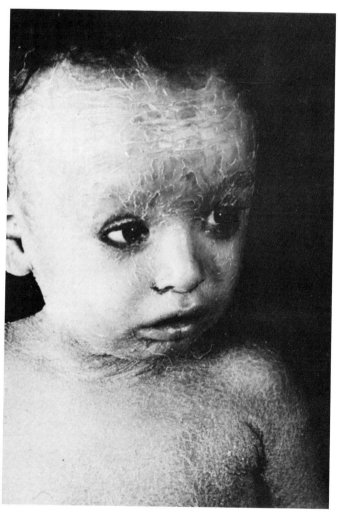

Fig. 18-21. Diffuse congenital ichthyosis.

INFECTIONS

Numerous are the alterations of infectious origin of dermo-ophthalmologic interest, and several of them have been extensively treated by Dr. Perry. I felt it advisable however to rearrange the material, following more closely a classification familiar to ophthalmologists.

Pyogenics. We have previously discussed infection of the palpebral skin attributable to pyogenics, which may affect also the cornea and the conjunctiva with both an acute and a chronic course (Fig. 18-22). The fact that *leprosy* is responsible for typical development of palpebral, conjunctival, and corneal lepromas, uveitis, fundus changes, and disorders of both intrinsic and extrinsic ocular motility (Fig. 18-23) should also be noted. Cutaneous *tuberculosis* may also cause lupus forms of the lids, conjunctiva, sclera and cornea. The so-called scrofulous or eczematous affections do not belong in this category. They are in fact mostly considered, as it is well known, not attributable to Koch's bacillus, but to a tuberculous allergic origin. These affections involve not only the conjunctiva and the cornea, with the appearance of phlyctenae, but also the palpebral skin and the adjacent facial skin (Fig. 18-24). Many other bacterial manifestations are also known but are less frequent or less important.

Viruses. A particular emphasis should be made about the ocular changes caused by viruses. Many viruses are responsible for dermatologic lesions, and they have already been extensively discussed by Dr. Perry. The lesions may occur as a concomitant reaction of the lid skin, conjunctiva, cornea, and more rarely uvea in generalized forms of exanthema (such as in measles, chickenpox, etc.). They may also occur as simultaneous localizations in the eye and in the surrounding skin area as in *herpes zoster of the first branch of the trigeminus* (Fig. 18-25) (blepharitis, conjunctivitis, keratitis, scleritis, uveitis, optic neuritis, glaucoma,

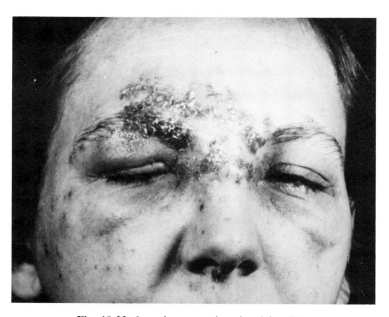

Fig. 18-22. Impetigo contagiosa involving lids.

changes in the pupillary reactivity and intraocular pressure, exophthalmos, ocular paralyses, and localizations in the intracranial pathways) and in *herpes simplex,* which is responsible for infrequent blepharitis and conjunctivitis, but above all for keratitis and uveitis and rarely for optic neuritis and glaucoma. These manifestations of herpes simplex occur, however, in the majority of cases without simultaneous skin involvement (Fig. 18-26).

The lesions of the lid skin and border, involving the conjunctiva and some-

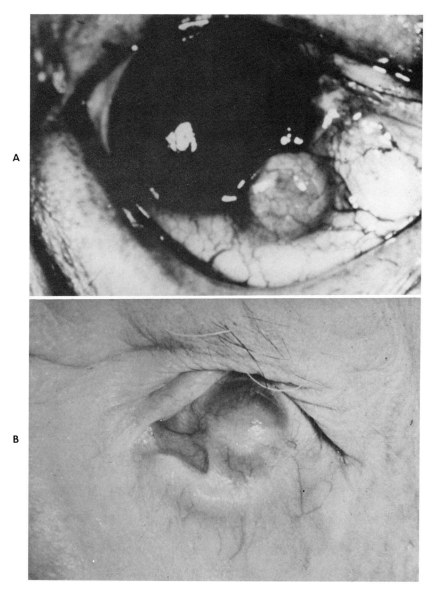

Fig. 18-23. A, Limbal leproma. **B,** Leukoma and symblepharon after corneoconjunctival leproma.

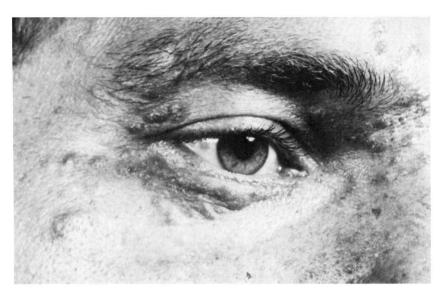

Fig. 18-24. Lupus miliaris facies with lid involvement.

times the cornea in the infection from *vaccinia* are extremely serious. Also in *smallpox* a generally less violent involvement of the outer eye may be observed.

Molluscum contagiosum. I would like to report here also on the toxic follicular conjunctivitis caused by molluscum contagiosum sometimes complicated with keratitis (punctate, more rarely pannous).

Verruca vulgaris. A somewhat analogous picture, generally without follicles, may be determined by implantation of the verruca vulgaris on the lid border.

Rickettsiosis. In the different forms of rickettsiosis (exanthematic typhus, tsutsugamushi, Mediterranean button fever, Q fever, murine typhus) there may be seen, besides more severe eye involvement, also conjunctival phenomena (mostly moderate hyperemia with slight secretion). In Mediterranean button fever, the conjunctiva may be the site of entrance of the disease.

Chlamydioses. There are, moreover, diseases caused by *Chlamydia* (called also *Bedsonia,* or agents of the PLT groups—"psittacosis-lymphogranuloma-trachoma"). This group has to be separated from the true viruses. These agents consist of elementary bodies with a limiting membrane of muramic acid, containing both RNA and DNA, and are sensitive towards antibiotics and sulfonamides. Among the chlamydial diseases, first of dermo-ocular interest is *lymphogranuloma venereum.* This condition may be localized on the palpebral skin, conjunctiva, and cornea. These aspects are similar to the ones encountered in Parinaud's conjunctivitis.

In *Reiter's disease* (oculourethrosynovial syndrome, or Fiessinger-Leroy-Reiter syndrome), considered today as a chlamydiosis by some authors (Ostler et al., Jones et al.), there is the occurrence of conjunctivitis, with various characteristics, in 80% to 90% of the cases. They may consist of simple diffuse or sectorial hyperemia as well as of catarrhal, hemorrhagic or follicular hypertrophic

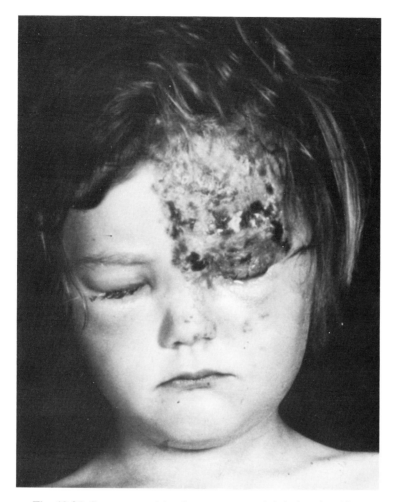

Fig. 18-25. Severe necrotizing herpes zoster ophthalmicus in child.

forms. The ocular localization (bilateral in general, sometimes unilateral) is in most cases successive to manifestations at the level of the urethra, the joints, and sometimes also the intestine. In the latter case there is a late onset.

The cornea is sometimes involved secondarily to the conjunctival lesions with epithelial, at times transitory, edema, epithelial keratitis, roundish subepithelial infiltrations, and also true ulcerations. The interstitial infiltration is an exceptional occurrence. The sequelae are of scarce importance. In some cases episcleritis and scleritis also occur.

The most serious eye manifestations is the iridocyclitis occurring in 5% to 10% of the cases. In general, it appears later (mostly bilaterally), not necessarily in connection with other ocular manifestations. Its course may be acute (with fibrinous exudate and hypopyon or hyphema), but may have also chronic characteristics. Relapses are possible; however, in general, the tendency of the formation of posterior synechias is small.

Secondary glaucoma, optic neuritis, and cataract have been exceptionally observed.

Syphilis. Syphilis is among the infectious process of interest in dermatology and ophthalmology. It may notoriously affect every section of the ocular apparatus with typical aspects, which cannot be recalled here in short (Fig. 18-27). Several data,

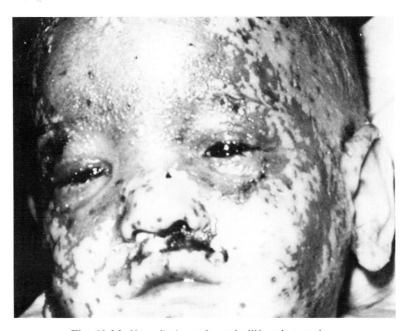

Fig. 18-26. Kaposi's herpetic varicelliformis eruption.

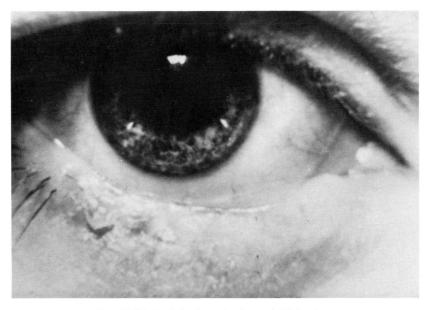

Fig. 18-27. Noduloulcerative lues of lid border.

some of ophthalmologic interest have been reported in Dr. Perry's paper (Chapter 17).

Mycoses. Mycoses are also capable of many ocular localizations. They may involve especially the lids, lacrimal canaliculi in form of concretions, cornea, conjunctiva, and orbit. More rarely intraocular localizations occur.

Zoonoses. Among the *zoonoses,* pediculosis pubis and pediculosis capitis are of ophthalmologic interest. As already mentioned, one may observe localization on the border of the lids and in the area of the eyelashes by the lice *Phthirus pubis* or by *Pediculus capitis.*

SYNDROMES WITH SKIN AND EYE FINDINGS

In this section some peculiar syndromes with *simultaneous lesions of the skin and eye* are considered. They are mainly the so-called phakomatoses, which deserve particular attention. In the *phakomatoses* we shall deal only with those having a dermatologic concomitance: neurofibromatosis, tuberous sclerosis, and various vascular forms of phakomatoses.

Neurofibromatosis. In neurofibromatosis there are congenital plexiform neuromas, especially of the upper lid, and ptosis (Fig. 18-28). The palpebral and

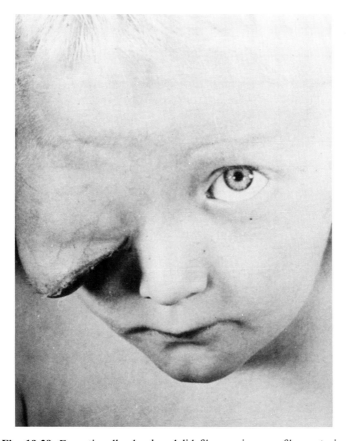

Fig. 18-28. Exceptionally developed lid fibroma in neurofibromatosis.

skin lesions (café-au-lait spots) are similar to those of other areas. There are also pigmented anomalies of the eyelashes and eyebrows. A thickening of the outer edge with atrophy of the temporal muscle has been observed. The presence of small lid tumors is uncommon. A peculiar finding is the thickening of the corneal nerves with possible myelinization, sometimes with the appearance of neurinomas, mainly on the limbus area. The types of corneal opacities are various: those that are diffuse, those with or without vascularization, and those that are degenerative according to Sehr. A secondary phenomenon is the ulcer caused by lagophthalmos.

To Schwannoma's ciliary nerves are attributed the hydrophthalmos and the choroidal thickening of connective aspect. The sclera and episclera may be melanotic. An episcleral choristoma has been seen. Pigmentation, small tumors, and telangiectasias may be observed on the iris. This sometimes appears to be atrophic with heterochromia. Pupillary anomalies are present. The rare occurrence of cataract is a secondary one.

Besides choroidal pigmentations and new growths, the fundus reveals the classic tumors of the retina (single and multiple, grayish white gliomas, originating in the fibrillary layer) as well as of the optic disk, optic nerve, and chiasm (Fig. 18-29). There exist also other more uncommon eye manifestations, such as true choroidal melanomas, retinal angiomas, optic atrophy, exophthalmos (sometimes pulsating), oculomotor paralysis, etc.

It is important to know that the eye manifestations may be the monosymptomatic expression of neurofibromatosis.

Multiple mucosal neuromas. Worthy of mention is the occurrence of multiple mucosal neuromas observed also on the lid margins, originating from the conjunctiva and which provoke a characteristic ectropion of the lids. This finding

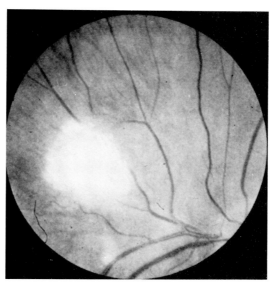

Fig. 18-29. Retinal tumor in sclerosis tuberosa. (From Korting, G. W.: Haut und Auge, Stuttgart, 1969, Georg Thieme Verlag.)

has been considered to be related to neurofibromatosis and from certain aspects also to Sipple's syndrome (medullary thyroid cancer, pheochromocytoma, etc.).

Sclerosis tuberosa. In *sclerosis tuberosa,* apart from sebaceous adenomas, which may involve also the palpebral skin, the outstanding lesions occur at the level of the retina. They are represented by white-yellow-grayish, oval or round spots, with unsharp edges located in the internal layers. Changes of the optic disk (more or less prominent, sometimes mulberry-like papillary or papilloretinal

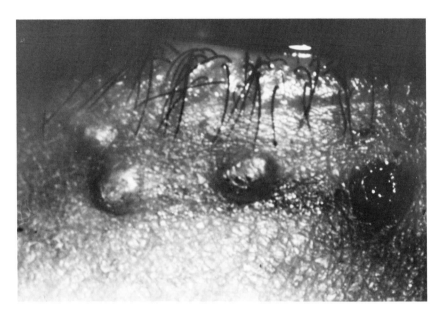

Fig. 18-30. Sebaceous adenoma in sclerosis tuberosa.

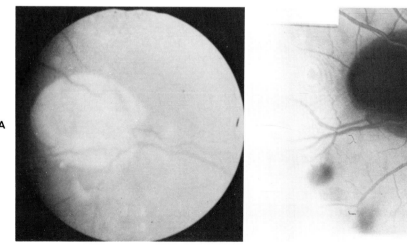

A

B

Fig. 18-31. A, Retinal phakomatoses in tuberous sclerosis. **B,** Fluorescein angiogram of retinal phakomatoses in tuberous sclerosis demonstrating leaking points.

tumors) are also important and typical (Figs. 18-30 and 18-31). Less frequent ocular changes are thickening or noduli of the conjunctiva, central or band-shaped corneal opacities, heterochromia of the iris, ciliary body proliferations, nodular lens opacities, cysts of the vitreous (which is sometimes troubled by retinal material), and chorioretinitis, sometimes with hemorrhages. Cases of total blindness have been recorded.

Vascular phakomatoses. Among the vascular phakomatoses, first there is *meningo-oculofacial angiomatosis,* or Sturge-Weber-Krabbe syndrome. The main characteristic is the palpebral angiomatosis (especially superior, flat, or uneven) with conjunctival and episcleral involvement. One may also observe angiomas of the uvea, which, if located posteriorly, give to the eye fundus a dark aspect (Fig. 18-32).

An important ocular sign is the occurrence of glaucoma. This may develop early with hydrophthalmus, or late without enlargement of the eyeball (Lawford's syndrome), with an incidence of 70% and 30%, respectively. The angiomatosis, accompanied with or without glaucoma, is bilateral in nearly 10% of the cases.

According to François also monosymptomatic and bisymptomatic forms may be considered in the group of angiomatosis. He proposed the following classification of the encephalofacial angiomatosis (dates of discovery are in parentheses):

1. Complete trisymptomatic forms: neurooculocutaneous angiomatosis
    a. Sturge (1879)–Weber (1922) syndrome: early and late congenital glaucoma
    b. Jahnke's syndrome (1930): choroidal angioma without glaucoma
2. Bisymptomatic form
    a. Oculocutaneous angiomatosis

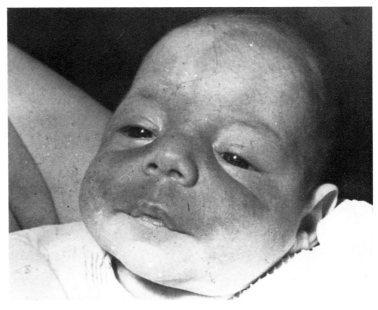

Fig. 18-32. Bilateral nevus flammeus with congenital glaucoma.

(1) Schirmer's syndrome (1860): early congenital glaucoma with an increase in the growth of the globe

(2) Lawford's syndrome (1884): late glaucoma without increase in the growth of the globe

(3) Milles's syndrome (1884): choroidal angioma

    b. Trigeminoencephaloangiomatosis (Krabbe syndrome) (1932)

    c. Oculoencephaloangiomatosis: theoretically possible but not yet described

3. Monosymptomatic form

    a. Facial angioma

    b. Meningeal angioma

    c. Choroidal angioma—certain early and late congenital glaucoma

The pathogenesis of ocular hypertension is to be referred to as malformation of the chamber angle and depends on the effect of uveal and scleroconjunctival angiomas. These angiomas may be responsible for a difficult aqueous outflow because of venous obstruction (Bucci). Tensional oscillations from vascular congestion may be found. In regard to the treatment of the angiomatotic glaucoma, goniotomy has proved particularly effective in our hands (over two thirds of cures in 15 cases); a tendency to recurrence has been seen by us in some cured eyes after several years.

Another vascular phakomatosis is *von Hippel–Lindau disease,* or *angiomatosis of the retina and cerebellum.* From the ophthalmologic joint of view it is characterized by pronounced dilation and tortuosity of both arterial and venous retinal vessels (bilateral in one third of the cases, generally single in two thirds of the cases) and sometimes multiple, especially in the lower fundus. Other features are arteriovenous capillary anastomoses, glial proliferation, and exudative infiltration of the retina. Inflammatory uveal complications and retinal detachment may occur. The treatment consists of photocoagulations, diathermy, and cryocoagulations, as well as electrolysis.

Telangiectatic ataxia, or *Louis-Bar syndrome,* also belongs to the vascular phakomatoses. In this syndrome one can observe multiple telangiectases of the bulbar conjunctiva, developing after the ataxia. They are generally bilateral and especially present in the bulbar conjunctiva not covered by the lids. There is also occasionally the presence of cataract and of peculiar oculomotor disorders (nystagmus, convergence insufficiency, strabismus, and difficulty or paresis of the conjugate movement of gaze (Cogan et al., Boeder and Sedgwich, Gimenes et al.). Among the other *minor vasculocutaneo-ocular phakomatoses* (less known and less important) is first the *Klippel-Trénaunay-Weber syndrome* (osteohypertrophic nevi) in which conjunctival hemangiectasias with limbic hypertrophy are observed. A congenital cataract has been seen. In the *Rendu-Osler-Weber syndrome* (telangiectasia hereditaria hemorrhagica), besides palpebral and conjunctival telangiectases, there is also tortuosity and dilation of the retinal veins, fundus neovascularization, sometimes with hemorrhages, and retinal detachment. In *Bonnet-Dechaume-Blanc syndrome* (mesencephalic cirsoid aneurysm with involvement of the face and of the eye fundus), cirsoid aneurysms of the retina and of the optic pathways are observed. Also worthy to be mentioned is *Weskamp-Cotlier-Gass nevo-oculocutaneous syndrome* where, in association with skin angiomas, cavernous angioma of the retina and sometimes of the optic nerve

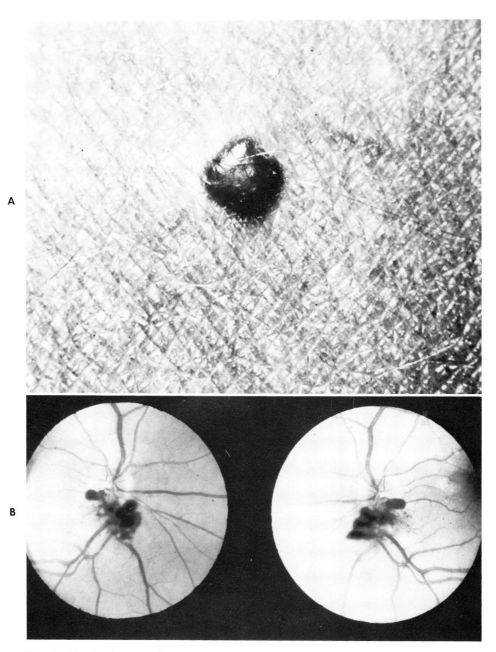

Fig. 18-33. Weskamp-Cotlier-Gass nevo-oculocutaneous syndrome. **A,** Angioma cutis. **B,** Optic nerve. **C,** Retinal angioma. **D,** Histologic examination showing cavernous hemangioma of retina. (**A** from Gass, J. D. M.: Differential diagnosis of intraocular tumors, St. Louis, 1974, The C. V. Mosby Co.; **B** and **C** from Gass, J. D. M.: Cavernous hemangiomas of the retina, Am. J. Ophthalmol. **71:**799-814, 1971; **D** from Hogan, J. M., and Zimmerman, L. E., editors: Ophthalmic pathology, ed. 2, Philadelphia, 1962, W. B. Saunders.)

occurs (Fig. 18-33). In Milner's case there was a retinal capillary angioma.

There are other more or less systemic angiomatous conditions in which angiomas of the lids, conjunctiva, and orbit are present (Brégeat, Riley-Smith, Maffucci, Ullmann, van Bogaert, Bloom).

Basal cell nevus syndrome. The basal cell nevus syndrome (or Ward's syndrome) is an epithelial phakomatosis (the fifth according to some authors) and strictly related to basal cell epithelioma and epithelioma adenoides cysticum, with very similar pathologic conditions. It is, however, 250 times more frequent than

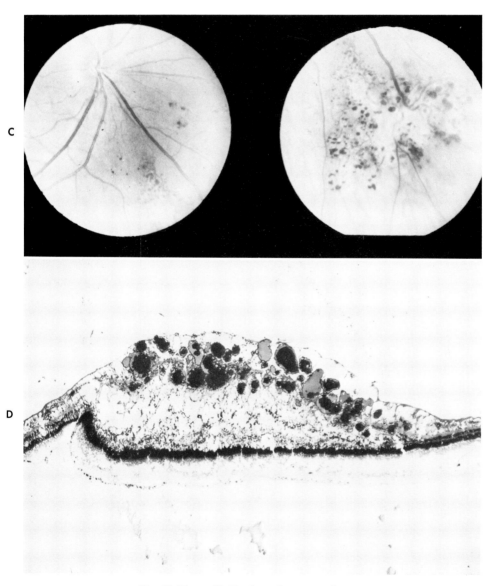

Fig. 18-33, cont'd. For legend see opposite page.

the well-known ordinary basaloma and occurs with autosomal dominant heredity. The early appearance of the basal cell nevus including the lids and conjunctiva, and of general manifestations (osseous and dental anomalies) is accompanied by hypertelorism, lid-angle dystopia, congenital cataract, colobomas, and even blindness and bulbar atrophy.

Multiple lentigines syndrome. Multiple lentigines syndrome, or leopard syndrome of Gorlin, has been fully discussed by Dr. Perry in Chapter 17. Besides the lentigines on the lid skin, there has also been observed hypertelorism, strabismus, and anomalies of ocular motility (Fig. 18-34).

Wiskott-Aldrich syndrome. In the *Wiskott-Aldrich syndrome,* characterized by thrombocytopenia purpura, eczema and relapsing infections caused by immunologic deficiency, changes of the lids, swelling with edema, and difficulty in opening the palpebral fissure may accompany the skin lesions. A purulent conjunctivitis may be simultaneously observed, with presence of hemorrhages, which are a peculiar feature of this disease and also as far as other areas affected are concerned. Various germs, mainly the pyogenic ones, are responsible for the conjunctivitis. Of course, secondary corneal involvement is possible. The association with mulluscum contagiosum of the lids and herpes corneae also occurs. The existence of affinities with the atopic eczema has been pointed out but, as far as we know, they are not established in the ocular symptomatology.

Alopecia. Among the different aspects of *alopecia,* there are the eye changes in *universal alopecia.* Besides the lack of hair in areas of the eyebrows and eyelashes there may occur a strabismus, nystagmus, pupillary changes, pronounced astigmatism, tortuosity of the retinal vessels, congenital but also acquired cataract, and tapetoretinal degenerations.

Vogt-Koyanagi-Harada syndrome. In the Vogt-Koyanagi-Harada syndrome, there occurs an acute, subacute, or chronic inflammation of the anterior uvea (Vogt-Koyanagi syndrome) or the posterior one (Harada). The uveitis is accompanied by dysacousis, meningeal reaction, skin vitiligo, and poliosis of the eyelashes, eyebrows, and hair (Fig. 18-35). Optic neuritis has also been described. The posterior exudative retinal detachment of Harada's forms is accompanied by circumscribed or diffuse fundus depigmentation (Fig. 18-36). The etiology remains uncertain on whether the condition is caused by virus or, more likely by an autoimmune allergic reaction. Some manifestations resemble those encountered in sympathetic ophthalmia.

Focal dermal hypoplasia. In focal dermal hypoplasia the ocular manifestations are represented by epiphora, blue scleras, nystagmus, strabismus, coloboma of iris and choroid, and microphthalmus.

Dyskeratosis congenita. In dyskeratosis congenita (Zinsser-Engman-Cole syndrome) the most striking is the congenital obliteration of the lacrimal puncta of Engman and Cole. Also one may see a vesicular conjunctivitis with tarsal conjunctival keratosis and irregularities in the fundus pigmentation. The keratosis may provoke early loss of eyebrows and eyelashes. A cataract has been seen.

Marfan's syndrome. The clinical findings of Marfan's syndrome are well known not only to the pediatricians but also to the ophthalmologists. Every ophthalmologist knows the ectopia of the lens in patients suffering from this disease, which may be followed by a true lens luxation. This condition is present in nearly

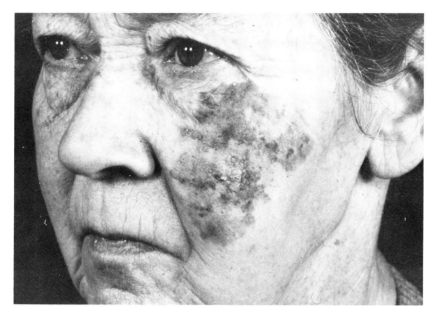

Fig. 18-34. Malignant lentigo involving partially the lids.

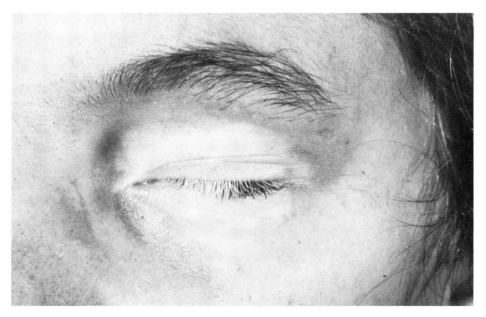

Fig. 18-35. Vitiligo and poliosis of lids in Vogt-Kojanagy-Harada syndrome.

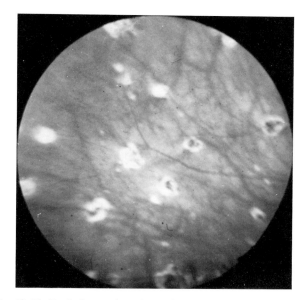

Fig. 18-36. Typical sequelae of eye fundus in Harada's syndrome.

half the cases. Myopia is frequently found. A possible complication occurring mainly from surgical interventions on the lens, consisting either of discission (in young patients) or of lens extraction (often followed by loss of vitreous), is the retinal detachment. This may occur, however, also spontaneously, and I could observe a familial appearance of it. Often there are the anomalies of ocular motility such as strabismus, especially divergent and accommodative paralysis. Other occurrences of ophthalmologic interest are glaucoma (secondary to the lens dislocation), cataract, pigmentary retinitis, and colobomas of the uvea, of the lens (also personal observation), and of the optic nerve.

Bonnevie-Ullrich-Turner syndrome. In this syndrome exophthalmos, ptosis, strabismus, epicanthus, corneal dysplasias, and thinning of the sclera (blue sclera) have been repeatedly observed. Also congenital cataracts, uveal colobomas, and atypical retinitis pigmentosa are sometimes encountered.

Dyskeratosis palmoplantaris. In this disease hyperkeratosis of the lid skin with supraciliary and ciliary alopecia and sometimes ectropion may be present. The tarsal conjunctiva may show a follicular hypertrophy and scars. The most important ophthalmologic changes, however, consist of corneal hyperkeratosis with recurrent exfoliation of the epithelium, grayish white superficial opacities, and ulcerations resembling the dendritic herpetic form (Fig. 18-37). Bilaterality and symmetry are frequent. A pronounced photophobia is usually present. The skin lesions may be associated also with hereditary optic atrophy.

The similarity between the above described findings and that of Hanhart's syndrome should be stressed.

Cockayne's syndrome. In Cockayne's syndrome, besides a defective tear secretion and a sensitivity to sunlight, which may involve also the lid skin and conjunctiva, there may be present also a superficial corneal atrophy, a possible congenital, but also early acquired, cataract, pigmentary atypical retinal degenera-

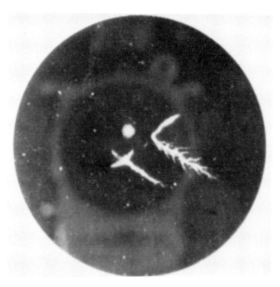

Fig. 18-37. Dendritiformis corneal dystrophy in keratosis palmoplantaris.

tion with vessel constriction, atrophy of the optic nerve and the orbital fat, and nystagmus.

Waardenburg-Klein syndrome. From the ophthalmologic point of view in Waardenberg-Klein syndrome (hereditary, congenital anomaly dominant autosomal with variable penetrance and expression), one of the first observations is a hyperplasia of both bony and soft intraocular tissues. These determine hypertelorism (euryopia), lateral displacement of the internal canthus, as well as of the lacrimal puncta, with consequent lengthening of the canaliculi, and blepharophimosis. These changes are usually present in 95% of the cases. Partial circumscribed or total albinism of the iris leading to heterochromia may be present in nearly 25% of the cases (Lebas). The eyebrows tend to become medially united (synophrys). Association of palpebral ptosis, palpebral vitiligo, ciliary poliosis, strabismus, and anisocoria is not a frequent occurrence.

Dermochondrocorneal dystrophy. In this disorder described by François, changes of bones and cartilages may be accompanied by subepithelial corneal opacities and by keratoconus.

Crouzon's disease. In Crouzon's disease, one of the points noted is the increased interpupillary distance (euriopya, hypertelorism), exophthalmos as a result of reduced depth of the orbits after cranial platybasia, and esotropia are also present. Frequently there is atrophy of the optic nerves, secondary to the precocious synostosis of cranial sutures and to the deformations of the optic foramina caused by the alterations of the basis of the skull, but also as a possible consequence of secondary papillary edema. Cataract has been seen.

Hallermann-Streiff-François syndrome (oculomandibulofacial dysmorphia). In this syndrome, besides dyscephalic bony lesions, one of the important features is the presence of microphthalmos and of congenital cataract.

Treacher-Collins syndrome. Typical in Treacher-Collins syndrome (mandibulofacial dysostosis) is the antimongoloid feature of the palpebral fissure. Hypo-trichosis of the eyelashes and eyebrows may also be present. A particularly im-portant finding is the presence of a congenital cataract. This syndrome also goes under the names of Franceschetti and Zwahlen.

Progeria. In progeria the alopecia of the scalp may be accompanied by loss of the eyebrows and eyelashes. Moreover pseudoexophthalmos, exophthalmos, and microphthalmos, as well as strabismus, uveal colobomas, and cataract, have been observed.

Ehlers-Danlos syndrome. In this syndrome various signs of eye involvement are seen such as epicanthus, laxity of the lid skin (which permits one to evert the upper lid very easily), palpebral ptosis, strabismus, and sometimes exophthalmos.

Other changes involving the eyeball are microcornea, keratoconus, and mainly the blue scleras. The thinning of the scleras facilitates scleral ruptures caused even by slight injuries and implies moreover serious surgical difficulties in the course of intervention on the eyeball (such as strabismus and retinal detachment).

Other ocular findings are tapetoretinal degenerations, choroidal, and vitreal hemorrhages with proliferating retinopathies sometimes with disciform aspect, retinal detachments secondary to tractions, and subluxation of the lens, which may become opaque. Erosions of the lamina vitrea of the choroid (angioid streaks) also occur, with pigment migration of the pigment epithelium of the retina. Possible affinities and sometimes true association of elastorexis with Ehlers-Danlos syndrome as well as with Marfan's syndrome are to be taken into con-sideration.

Mucopolysaccharidoses. Among the mucopolysaccharidoses, I shall mention here only Hurler-Pfaundler syndrome (gargoylism, dysostosis multiplex) and scleredema adultorum (Buschke's syndrome). In the former disease in nearly 75% of the cases, besides the presence of euryopia, there is diffuse parenchymal opacification of the cornea, grayish in color and composed of numerous densely distributed small points. As to the pathologic condition, there are round or fusiform cells filled with mucopoly-saccharides, while the corneal stroma con-tains basophilic granulations. Bowman's membrane may be eroded in many points.

In the forms described by Scheie, hypertrichosis of the ocular region, besides the corneal lesions and the pigmentary retinal degeneration, was observed.

Also other types of mucopolysaccharidosis are mostly accompanied with ocular lesions, however, I shall not deal with them here because of the moderate degree of skin involvement.

SYNDERMATOTIC CATARACTS

Some forms of cataract accompanied by dermatologic lesions, the so-called dermatogenic (Andogsky) or syndermatotic (von Kugelberg) cataracts, have been extensively dealt with by Dr. Perry in Chapter 17. The cataract, associated with skin diseases, finds its fundamental explanation in the embryologic affinities of the skin and the lens. One should note, however, that the strictly syndermatotic forms should be distinguished from those that may develop as complications of uveitis or retinal detachment. In the course of this report I have already men-tioned various dermatologic conditions accompanied by cataract with different incidence, besides those illustrated by Dr. Perry. The syndermatotic cataracts may be of either congenital or acquired type, with characteristic features for the different diseases. Both congenital and acquired cataracts may, however, be observed in the same disease.

Although I believe it is superfluous to repeat in detail each condition and the related cataracts, I felt it useful to enumerate the different diseases accompanied by cataracts in the lists below. I followed mainly the list of Lebas but slightly enlarged it.

SYNDERMATOTIC CATARACTS
Congenital forms

1. Rothmund-Thomson syndrome (congenital forms, however, generally acquired)
2. Hutchinson's progeria
3. Zinsser (congenital dyskeratosis)
4. Siemens' idiopathic cutaneous atrophy
5. Bloch-Sulzberger pigmentary dermatosis (incontinentia pigmenti)
6. Ullrich-Fremerey-Dohna-François syndrome (dyscephaly with hypertrichosis)
7. Sjögren's syndrome (cataracta oligophrenica, trophic changes of nails)
8. Congenital ichthyosis
9. Anhidrotic ectodermal dysplasia (also acquired juvenile)
10. Bonnevie-Ullrich-Turner syndrome (gonadal dysgenesis) or pterygium syndrome (also acquired)
11. Alopecia universalis (also acquired)
12. Embryopathia rubeolaris
13. Anetodermia erythematosa
14. Klippel-Trénaunay-Weber phakomatosis (osteohypertrophic nevi)
15. Basal cell nevus, or Ward's, syndrome (also acquired)
16. Hallermann-Streiff syndrome
17. Conradi's syndrome (chondrodystrophia congenita punctata) (also rarely acquired)
18. Cockayne's syndrome
19. Treacher-Collins syndrome (Franceschetti-Zwahlen syndrome)
20. Pachyonychia congenita (Jadassohn-Lewandowsky syndrome; Siemens-Schäfer, or Riehl syndrome)
21. Fabry's disease (possibly also acquired)

Acquired forms

1. Rothmund's syndrome with infantile poikiloderma—type Zinsser
2. Werner's syndrome with progressive poikiloderma—type Arndt-Jaffe (senile)
3. Atopic dermatosis with chronic eczema; neurodermitis or prurigo
4. Telangiectasias
5. Alopecia (also congenital)
6. Scleroderma
7. Poikiloderma
8. Mongolism
9. Anhidrotic ectodermal dysplasia (also congenital)
10. Psoriasis
11. Pemphigus foliaceus (especially Brazilian type)
12. Pellagra
13. Xeroderma pigmentosum
14. Darier's follicular dyskeratosis
15. Hyperkeratotic nevus (basal cell nevus syndrome)
16. Vitiligo
17. Pachyonychia congenita
18. Ichthyosis

19. Keratodermia dermoplantaris with alopecia
20. Erythema exudativum multiforme
21. Osteogenesis imperfecta (possibly also congenital)
22. Grönblad-Strandberg syndrome
23. Hydroa vacciniforme (polymorphous light eruption)
24. Sclerosis tuberosa
25. Nevus comedonicus
26. Reiter's disease (oculourethrosynovial syndrome of Fiessinger-Leroy-Reiter)
27. Seborrheic dermatitis
28. Porphyrinuria
29. Ehlers-Danlos syndrome
30. Neurofibromatosis
31. Lichen follicularis keratosicus atrophicans (Piccardi, Little, Lawsser)
32. Dupuytren's disease
33. Crouzon's disease (also congenital)

Our tables give a full view of the skin diseases in which a cataract may occur, separating the prevailing congenital from the prevailingly acquired forms.

The most important and frequent of these cataracts are those occurring in the course of Rothmund's syndrome, Werner's syndrome, atopic dermatosis (besides pemphigus foliaceus) (Fig. 18-38). I believe it would therefore be useful to present Table 18-1, which is a synoptic table published by Maeder in 1949. It not only illustrates the clinical features of the most important types of cataracts, but also reports other extraocular and systemic data, facilitating the diagnosis of the type of eye manifestation.

As far as the dermatologic and ocular symptomatology, the etiology, and the mode of appearance are concerned, only some of the various dermatologic diseases possibly accompanied by cataracts listed in our tables have not yet been dealt with already.

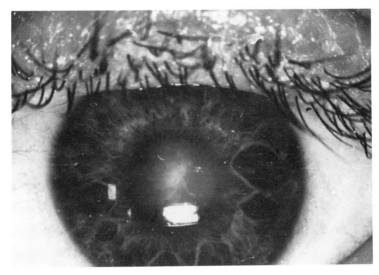

Fig. 18-38. Syndermatotic cataract in Besnier prurigo. (Courtesy Jules François, Ghent, Belgium.)

Among the diseases that have not been mentioned by Dr. Perry and myself are *Zinsser congenital dyskeratosis* and some other forms of congenital skin dysplasia, some of which are accompanied by cataract. There is also the *Siemens-Schäfer* or *Riehl syndrome,* a special form of pachyonychia congenita of Jadassohn and Lewandowsky, where a polykeratosis, thickening of the fingernails, and acneiform follicular, palmoplantar keratosis have been encountered.

Table 18-1. Syndermatotic cataracts*

Symptoms	Rothmund (1868)	Werner (1904)	Neurodermatitis
Cataract	Infantile (2 to 5 years), sometimes congenital subcapsular, anterior and posterior, cortical onset; equal in both eyes; maturation from 4 days to 14 months	Juvenile (15 to 35 years), cortical, posterior onset; equal in both eyes; maturation from 2 to 6 years	Third decade; mainly subcapsular, anterior or posterior onset; unequal in the two eyes; maturation from a few months to 3 years
Skin lesions	Vascular atrophizing poikiloderma (Zinsser's infantile form, Thompson's congenital form)	Progressive diffuse sclerodermia, scleropoikiloderma (Arndt, Jaffe)	Eczema, neurodermatitis, prurigo
Onset	0 to 3 to 6 months	After puberty, 15 to 30 years	0 to 60 years
Evolution	Stationary; face, ears, upper limbs (trunk, lower limbs)	Progressive; lower limbs to knee (face, upper limbs to elbow)	Chronic; face, neck, flexory face of limbs
Telangiectasias	Constant	Inconstant	
Particular features	Hyperpigmentation, depigmentation	Leg ulcers, hyperkeratosis	
Manifestations on fingers and hair	Changes in nails and in hair system	Changes in nails and in hair system, early graying	
Endocrine disorders	Hypogenitalism	Hypogenitalism, diabetes	Various
General anomalies	Mean size; saddle nose, acromicria	Small size, thin extremities, progeria, precocious senility, muscular atrophy, laryngeal difficulty (hoarse "falsetto" voice), acromicria (sclerodactylia), psychic problems, vascular calcifications.	
Sex	In women more than men (16:5)	In men more than women (27:20)	Equal in men and women
Heredity	Recessive	Regular recessive or dominant with anticipation and aggravation	Recessive (?)
Familial characters	Constant (frequent consanguinity) (Alps)	Frequent	Rare
Cause	Pluriglandular endocrine disorders	Pluriglandular endocrine disorders	Allergic and metabolic disorders
Facies	Marbled	"Hard" mask	Lion's face

*Derived from Maeder, G.: Ann. Ocul. **182:**809-854, 1949. Adapted and completed by Lebas, P.: Bull. Soc. Belge Ophtalmol. **124:**140, 1960.

A cataract described as a congenital or acquired form has been found in skin *anetodermia erythematosa* (Jadassohn) belonging also to skin atrophies. A zonular cataract associated with blue scleras, keratoconus, hypoplasia of the iris, and glaucoma has been sometimes described.

Congenital *rubella* cataract is an occurrence familiar to any ophthalmologist. This is after Gregg's first observations in 1944 of a skin rash affecting the expectant mother during the first weeks of pregnancy. One important fact, recently discovered, is the presence of the rubella virus in the opaque lens for many months after birth. It is well known that many other ocular manifestations (strabismus, nystagmus, uveal coloboma etc.) also occur, besides the general ones.

Fabry's disease (angiokeratoma corporis diffusum) is a dermatologic manifestation with a family history and usually with sex-linked transmission. Besides the lid involvement there are many and various ocular lesions, as vascular anomalies of the conjunctiva, tortuosity and dilation of retinal veins, optic disk edema and atrophy, neuro-ophthalmologic disorders, and especially the well-known peculiar whorl-like opacities of the cornea. Recently (after the observation of Spaeth and Frost of postcapsular cataract), A. T. Franceschetti has called attention also to minute anterior wedge-shaped opacities of the lens as well as on branching opacities along the sutures.

In the well-known picture of *mongolism,* which may be accompanied by cutaneous manifestations (akrocyanosis, cutis marmorata, cutis laxa, ichthyotic disorders, pterygium colli, etc.) as well as ocular anomalies (such as epicanthus, hypertelorism, mongoloid direction of the lid opening, and Wölfling or Brushfield's spots, which are nodules on the iris, and keratoconus), a cataract is found in about 50% of the cases.

Pellagra (from nicotinic acid deficiency), along with the well-known cutaneous changes that gave the name to the disease, shows ocular manifestations (mainly of the lids, conjunctiva, cornea, and optic nerve). A cataract in pellagra is a rare occurrence. I have however obtained an experimental pellagra cataract in swine.

Darier's follicular dyskeratosis is a genodermatosis occurring in children or or young people with follicular or parafollicular, squamous, crustaceous, greasy eruptions, especially in the areas of seborrheic secretion or intertrigo. Ophthalmologically, the development of a cataract has been rarely seen in connection with lid-skin lesions, nodular corneal opacities, and nystagmus.

Vitiligo may have different origins. It is hard to assess how far the lens opacities are related to the skin depigmentation or to the cause of it.

Osteogenesis imperfecta represents one of the oculocutaneous manifestations where anomalies of the skeleton occurs. Here a zonular cataract has been described (see anetodermia).

In the unilateral nevus comedonicus, a cataract is an exceptional finding (see Whyte, 2 cases out of 100).

Lichen follicularis keratosicus atrophicans is a variety of lichen planus. It is characterized by a rapidly involving alopecia, cicatricial atrophy of the scalp and of some hairy areas of the body, lichenoid eruptions in other parts of the body, and sometimes small punctate or reticulate hyperchromic eruptions.

Dupuytren's disease (where recently a cataract has been described in association) is represented by a progressive thickening and retraction of the palmar aponeurosis of the hand. It provokes a bending of the fingers, and it is generally observed in males over 50 years of age. Its etiology is controversial.

ACKNOWLEDGMENTS

I am particularly indebted to P. Thygeson, P. Lebas, J. Casanovas, and H. Reich for the many illustrations they have allowed me to publish and to Dr. C. Stadelmann for the bibliographic assistance and Dr. P. Pivetti-Pezzi for the choice of illustrations.

REFERENCES

Extensive bibliographies may be found in the following books and articles.

1. Casanovas, J., and Vilanova, X.: Dermato-oftalmología, Barcelona, 1967, Editorial Almacen.
2. Groenouw, A.: Beziehungen des Auges in den Hautkrankheiten. In Handbuch der Haut- und Geschlechts-Krankheiten. Bd. XIV/I, Berlin 1930, Springer-Verlag.
3. Korting, G. W.: The skin and eye, Philadelphia, 1973, W. B. Saunders Co.
4. Lebas, P.: Les syndromes oculo-cutanés, Bull. Soc. Belge Ophtalmol. **124:**5-537, 1960.
5. Sala, G., and Noto, P.: Malattie cutanee e veneree ed alterazioni oculari, Palermo, 1948, S. F. Flaccovio Editore.
6. Schreck, E.: Veränderungen des Sehorgans bei Haut- und Geschlechtskrankheiten. In Dermatologie und Venereologie, Handbuch Gottron-Schönfeld, Stuttgart, 1960, Georg Thieme Verlag.
7. Thygeson, P.: Dermatoses with ocular manifestations. In Sorsby, A.: Systemic ophthalmology, London, 1951, Butterworth & Co., p. 581.
8. Thygeson, P.: Mucocutaneous ocular syndromes. In Sorsby, A.: Modern trends in ophthalmology. Third series London, 1955, Butterworth & Co., p. 146.

The additional references reported in the bibliography represent a choice among the most recent and sometimes most important publications.

BIBLIOGRAPHY
Some important dermatologic diseases with eye findings

OTA'S NEVUS, OR OCULODERMIC MELANOCYTOSIS
1. Albert, D. M., and Scheie, H. G.: Nevus of Ota with malignant melanoma of the choroid, Arch. Ophthalmol. **69:**774-777, 1963.
2. Bertoni, G.: Oculo-dermal melanocytosis, Ann. Ottalmol. Clin. Ocul. **94:**217-227, 1968.
3. Bozzoni, F., and Bozzoni, G.: Su due casi di sindrome di Ota o melanocitosi oculo-dermica, Boll. Oculist. **36:**652-657, 1957.
4. Coriglione, G., Bellomio, S., and Greco, S.: Sulla melanosi oculare congenita o "faco-melanosi"; contributo clinico, Minerva Oftalmol. **9:**59-62, 1967.
5. Cullman, B.: Ein Fall von Naevus Ota, Ber. Dtsch. Ophthalmol. Ges. **70:**80-82, 1970.
6. Fishman, G. R. A., and Anderson, R.: Naevus of Ota. Report of two cases, one with open-angle glaucoma, Amer. J. Ophthalmol. **54:**453-457, 1962.
7. Font, R. L., Reynolds, Jr., A. M., and Zimmerman, L. E.: Diffuse malignant melanoma of the iris in the nevus of Ota, Arch. Ophthalmol. **77:**513-518, 1967.
8. Frezzotti, R., Guerra, R., Dragoni, G. P., and Bonanni, P.: Malignant melanoma of the choroid in a case of naevus of Ota, Br. J. Ophthalmol. **52:**922-924, 1968.
9. Gold, D. H., Henkind, P., Sturner, W. Q., and Baden, M.: Oculo-dermal melanocytosis and retinitis pigmentosa, Amer. J. Ophthalmol. **63:**271-279, 1967.
10. Jay, B.: Malignant melanoma of the orbit in a case of oculodermal melanosis (naevus of Ota), Br. J. Ophthalmol. **49:**359-363, 1965.
11. Kraus, E., and Jung, E.: Pigmentierungen der Hornhoutrückfläche bei Naevus fusco-coeruleus ophthalmo-maxillaris Ota, Ber. Dtsch. Ophthalmol. Ges. **68:**442-444, 1967.
12. Lumbroso, B. D., and Melchionda, C.: Melanocitosi oculo-dermica, Arch. Ottalmol. **69:**175-180, 1965.

13. Sabates, F. N., and Yamashita, T.: Congenital melanosis oculi complicated by two independent malignant melanomas of the choroid, Arch. Ophthalmol. **77:**801-803, 1967.
14. Tosti, E., and Renna, V.: Insorgenza di melanoblastoma nella coroide in sindrome di Ota, Boll. Oculist. **45:**862-870, 1966.
15. Volpi, U.: Melanoblastoma della coroide in sindrome di Ota, Ann. Ottalmoi. Clin. Ocul. **92:**219-227, 1966.

HEMANGIOMAS

1. Badran, I. G., and Shoukry, I. I.: Hemangiomata of face and eye lids (a preliminary report), Bull. Ophthal. Soc. Egypt **55:**181-188, 1962.
2. Farina, R., Magalhaes, P. B., De Castro, O., Attadia, E. R., and Goleman, B.: Hemangioma cavernoso palpebral e orbito-palpebral, Arch. Brasil. Oftalmol. **27:**61-70, 1964.
3. Flores Y Sanchez, G.: Hemangiomas conjunctivo-palpebrales, Boll. Hosp. Oftalmol. Nuestra Señora de la Luz (Mex.) **17:**64-71, 1964.
4. Gass, J. D. M.: Cavernous hemangioma of the retina. A neuro-oculo-cutaneous syndrome. Am. J. Ophthalmol. **71:**799-814, 1971.
5. Yancey, W. A.: Spontaneous regression of orbital and facial hemangioma, Calif. Med. **108:** 300, 1968.
6. Weskamp, C., and Cotlier, I.: Angioma del cerebro y de la retina con malformaciones capillares de la piel, Arch. Oftalmol. Buenos Aires **15:**1, 1940.

DERMATITIS VENENATA

1. Bandmann, H. J.: Das periorbitale Ekzem (Klinik, Pathogenesis, Therapie), Klin. Monatsbl. Augenheilk. **138:**585-586, 1961.
2. Bandmann, H. J., and Hardieck, L.: Periorbitales "Gummi"-Kontaktekzem durch Augentropfpipette, Hautarzt **11:**468, 1960.
3. Boelcke, U.: Kosmetik-Farbstoffe an Schleimhauten mit besonderer Berücksichtigung der Anwendungstechnik und des Milieus (Lippen, Augenlider, Wimpern), Aesthet. Med. (Berlin) **13:**287-292, 1964.
4. Coles, R. S., and Laval. J.: Retinal detachments occurring in cataract associated with neurodermatitis, Arch. Ophthalmol. **48:**30-39, 1952.
5. Kirton, V., and Munro-Ashman, D.: Contact dermatitis from neomycin and Framycetin, Lancet **1:**138-139, 1965.
6. March, C., and Greenwood, M. A.: Allergic contact dermatitis to proparacaine, Arch. Ophthalmol. **79:**159-160, 1968.
7. Sander, S. H., and Taub, S. J.: Allergic manifestations of the eye and adjacent structures, Eye Ear Nose Throat Monthly **44:**71, 1965.
8. Saraux, H.: L'Allergie des tuniques externes de l'appareil oculaire, Clin. Ophtalmol. **1:**103-107, 1968.
9. Schubert, H.: Kontaktekzeme in Augenumgebung, Klin. Monatsbl. Augenheilk. **151:**457-465, 1967.

ATOPIC DERMATITIS

1. Copeman, P. W. M.: Eczema and keratoconus, Br. Med. J. **2:**977-979, 1965.
2. François, M. J.: Dermatite atopique, cataracte et kératocone, Bull. Soc. Belg. Ophtalmol. **124:**890-897, 1960.
3. Gormaz, A.: Keratoconus secondary to vernal conjunctivitis. In Polack, F. M.: Corneal and external disease of the eye, Springfield, Ill., 1970, Charles C Thomas, Publisher.
4. Hurlbut, W. B., and Domonkos, A. N.: Cataract and retinal detachment associated with atopic dermatitis, Arch. Ophthalmol. **52:**852-857, 1954.
5. Ingram, R. M.: Retinal detachment associated with atopic dermatitis and cataract, Br. J. Ophthalmol. **49:**96, 1965.
6. Lemke, L., and Jütte, A.: Augenbefall bei Neurodermatitis disseminata, Dermatol. Wochenschr. **152:**921-927, 1966.
7. Pillat, A.: Über atypisches beim Frühjahrs Katarrh, Wien. Klin. Wochenschr. **65:**381-384, 1953.
8. Sabiston, D. W.: The associations of keratoconus, dermatitis and asthma, Trans. Ophthalmol. Soc. N. Z. **18:**66-72, 1966.

9. Singh, G., and Mathur, J. S.: Atopic erythroderma with bilateral cataract, unilateral keratoconus and iridocyclitis, and undescended testes, Br. J. Ophthalmol. **52:**61-63, 1968.
10. Spencer, W. H., and Fisher, J. J.: The association of keratoconus with atopic dermatitis, Am. J. Ophthalmol. **47:**332-334, 1959.

SEBORRHEA

1. Korting, G. W.: Formenkreis der Ekzemkrankheiten. In von Riecke, E., editor; Bode, G., and Korting, G. W., revisers: Lehrbuch der Haut- und Geschlechtskrankheiten, ed. 9, Stuttgart, 1962, Gustav Fischer Verlag.
2. Wright, J. C., and Meger, G. E.: Allergic keratoconjunctivitis, secondary to seborrheic dermatitis, Am. J. Ophthalmol. **53:**686-687, 1962.

ACNE ROSACEA

1. Ayres, Jr., S., and Mihan, R.: Rosacea-like demodicidosis involving eyelids, Arch. Dermatol. **95:**63-66, 1967.
2. Cowan, M. A.: Rosacea and its treatment, Trans. Ophthalmol. Soc. U. K. **86:**719-725, 1967.
3. Richter, S.: Skleraperforation bei Rosaceakeratitis, Klin. Monatsbl. Augenheilk. **146:**422-424, 1965.
4. Roper-Hall, M. J.: The ocular aspects of rosacea, Trans. Ophthalmol. Soc. U. K. **86:**727-732, 1967.

HIDRADENITIS SUPPURATIVA

1. Bergeron, J. R., and Stone, O. J.: Interstitial keratitis associated with hidradenitis suppurativa, Arch. Dermatol. Syph. **95:**473-475, 1967.

PSORIASIS VULGARIS

1. Christophers, E.: Pathogenetische Aspekte der Psoriasis, Med. Klin. **67:**317-319, 1972.
2. Eustace, P., and Pierse, D.: Ocular psoriasis, Br. J. Ophthalmol. **54:**810-813, 1970.
3. Lavergne, G.: Psoriasis associé au syndrome de Behçet. Bull. Soc. Belge Ophtalmol. **124:**909-912, 1960.
4. Manna, F., and Jankowski, W.: Badania biomikroskopowe soczewki w przypadkach łuszczycy [Biomicroscopic examination of the lens in psoriasis], Klin. Oczna **36:**371-374, 1966.
5. Marghescu, S.: Immunologische Aspekte der Psoriasis vulgaris, Med. Klin. **67:**320-322, 1972.
6. Maxwell, J. D., Greig, W. R., Boyle, J. A., Pasieczy, T., and Schofield, C. B. S.: Reiter's syndrome and psoriasis, Scott. Med. J. **11:**14-18, 1966.
7. Meenan, F. O. C., and Fitzpatrick, C. M.: Psoriasis and strabismus, J. Irish Med. Assoc. **65:**42-43, 1972.
8. Rassner, G.: Therapie der Psoriasis, Med. Klin. **67:**323-326, 1972.
9. Stuart, J. A.: Ocular psoriasis, Am. J. Ophthalmol. **55:**615-617, 1963.

Pytiriasis rubra

1. Friede, R.: Über einen Fall von Pityriasis lichenoides chronica der Lider und der Conjunctivae, Z. Augenheilk. **44:**253, 1920.

Lichen ruber planus

1. Goldsmith, J.: Keratosis associated with lichen planus, Am. J. Ophthalmol. **31:**224-225, 1948.
2. Michelson, H. E., and Laymon, C. W.: Lichen planus of the eyelids, Arch. Dermatol. Syph. **37:**27-29, 1938.

PEMPHIGOID CHANGES

1. Amêndola, F.: Pênfigo ocular e pênfigoide ocular, Arch. Brasil. Oftalmol. **26:**29-93, 1963.
2. Bettelheim, M. G., Zehetbauer, G. et al.: Direkte immunofluoreszenzoptische Untersuchungen beim Pemphigus ocularis (narbenbildendes Pemphigoid), Klin. Monatsbl. Augenheik. **163:**361, 1973.
3. David, M., Pascu, M., Chiriceanu, M., and Stoicanu, N.: Aspects cliniques du pemphigus oculaire, Ann. Oculist. **195:**38-47, 1963.
4. François, J., Pierard, J., et al.: Pemphigoïde cicatricielle oculaire. Dermatite bulleuse muco-synéchiante et atrophiante, Ophthalmologica **166:**401, 1973.

5. Kleine-Natrop, H., and Haustein, U. F.: Benignes Schleimhautpemphigoid mit rascher Erblindung und generalisierten vernarbenden Hautveränderungen, Hautarzt **19:**6-12, 1968.
6. Nelson, C. T.: Die Behandlung des Pemphigus mit Cortisonpräparaten, Hautarzt **15:**486-487, 1964.
7. Postić, S.: Pemphigoide Augenveränderungen, Ber. Dtsch. Ophthalmol. Ges. **67:**246-252, 1965.
8. Rycroft, B.: The surgery of ocular pemphigus, Proc. Roy. Soc. Med. **54:**111-112, 1961.
9. Tripodi, G.: Osservazioni sopra un caso di pemfigoide associato a vitiligine, Boll. Oculist. **50:**26-33, 1971.
10. Van der Werf, P. J. P.: Ocular pemphigus, Ophthalmologica **152:**547-552, 1966.

Dermatitis herpetiformis

1. Bonavolontà, A.: Dermatite di Dühring-Brocq con manifestazione oculare, G. Ital. Oftalmol. **2:**169-184, 1949.
2. Lapière, S.: La pemphigoïde (W. Lever) peut-elle être considérée comme une entité morbide séparée de la dermatite polymorphe de Dühring-Brocq? Dermatol. Congr. Budapest 1965.
3. Lever, W. F.: Differentialdiagnose zwischen Pemphigus vulgaris, bullösen Pemphigoid und Dermatitis herpetiformis, Med. Klin. **62:**1173-1176, 1967.

Pemphigus foliaceus

1. Amêndola, F.: Ocular manifestation of pemphigus foliaceus, Am. J. Ophthalmol. **32:**35-44, 1949.

ERYTHEMA MULTIFORME

1. Anderes, W.: Über einen Fall von "toxic epidermal necrolysis" (Lyell) mit schweren Augenkomplikationen, Ophthalmologica **145:**291-296, 1963.
2. Brégeat, P., Fougères, R., Hamard, H., and Mondon, H.: À propos d'un syndrome de Lyell, Bull. Soc. Ophtalmol. Fr. **71:**536-541, 1971.
3. Claxton, R. C.: A review of 31 cases of Stevens-Johnson syndrome, Med. J. Aust. **1:**936-966, 1963.
4. Coursin, D. B.: Stevens-Johnson syndrome: Non-specific para-sensitivity reaction, J.A.M.A. **198:**113-116, 1966.
5. Franceschetti, A., Ricci, A., Diallinas, N.: Kératoplastie dans un cas d'épidermolyse nécrosante suraiguë (maladie de Lyell), Bull. Mem. Soc. Fr. Ophtalmol. **78:**339-357, 1965.
6. Greenberg, L. M., Mauriello, D. A., Cinotti, A. A., and Buxton, J. N.: Erythema multiforme exudativum, (Stevens-Johnson syndrome) following sodium diphenylhydantoin therapy, Ann. Ophthalmol. **3:**137-139, 1971.
7. Jensen, S.: A case of Stevens-Johnson's syndrome following antiepileptic medication, Acta Ophthalmol. (Kbh.) **45:**576-581, 1967.
8. Kalkoff, K. W.: Zur Nosologie und Ätiologie des Syndroma muco-cutaneo-oculare acutum Fuchs (syn. Ectodermosis pluriorificialis erosiva; Stevens-Johnson-Syndrom u. a.), Bull. Schweiz. Akad. Med. Wiss. **23:**427-440, 1968.
9. Kawase, S., and Uta, S.: Three cases of ectodermose pluriorificielle, Jap. J. Clin. Ophthalmol. **25:**1981-1985, 1971.
10. Kobzeva, V. I.: Eye involvement in multiforme exudative erythema, Oftalmol. Zh. **23:**119-122, 1968.
11. Lorenz, E.: Wesen und Entstehung des Lyell-Syndroms und ähnlicher Manifestationsformen der akuten toxischen Epidermolyse im Kindesalter, Wien. Klin. Wochenschr. **80:**240-242, 1968.
12. Lyell, A.: A review of toxic epidermal necrolysis in Britain, Br. J. Dermatol. **79:**662-671, 1967.
13. Ostler, B. H., Conant, M. A., and Groundwater, J.: Lyell's disease, the Stevens-Johnson syndrome and exfoliative dermatitis, Trans. Am. Acad. Ophthalmol. Otolaryngol. **74:**1254-1265, 1970.
14. Shapiro, J.: Erythema multiforme with monocular involvement, Am. J. Ophthalmol. **67:**369-371, 1969.

15. Sieber, O. F., Jr., John T., Fulginiti, V. A., and Overholt, E. C.: Stevens-Johnson syndrome associated with *Mycoplasma pneumoniae* infection, J.A.M.A. **200:**79-81, 1967.
16. Ström, J.: Ocular symptoms in febrile mucocutaneous reactions, ectodermosis erosiva pluriorificialis, Stevens-Johnson's syndrome, mucocutaneous syndrome, etc., Acta Ophthalmol. (Kbh.) **44:**411-414, 1966.
17. Van Buskirk, M. E., Lessell, S., and Friedman, E.: Pigmentary epitheliopathy and erythema nodosum, Arch. Ophthalmol. **85:**369-372, 1971.
18. Zuccoli, A.: Allergodermie combustiforme. Contribution clinique, Ophthalmologica **156:**208-217, 1968.

BEHÇET'S DISEASE
1. Aoki, K., and Fujioka, K.: 100 cases of Behçet's disease in Hokkaido, Jap. J. Clin. Ophthalmol. **25:**1751-1754, 1971.
2. Bietti, G. B., and Bruna F.: An ophthalmic report on Behçet's disease. In Monacelli, M., and Nazzaro, P.: Behçet's disease, Basel, 1966, S. Karger, AG.
3. Bietti, G. B., Cerulli, L., and Pivetti, P.: Behçet's syndrome, and immunosuppressive treatment: our personal experience, Symposium on Immunology and Immunopathology of the Eye, Strasbourg, 1974.
4. Bengisu, N.: La maladie de Behçet, Ann. Oculist. **202:**165-176, 1969.
5. Campinchi, R., Rousselie, F., Bernard, J., and Kastler M.: Allergie microbienne dans le syndrome de Behçet, Bull. Soc. Ophthalmol. Fr. **68:**33-37, 1968.
6. Fellner, M. J., and Kantor, I.: Behçet's syndrome: Skin puncture test as guide in therapy, N.Y. State J. Med. **64:**1760-1761, 1964.
7. Futagami, T., Saito, K., Saito, M., Sanefuji, M., and Fujioka, K.: New therapeutic attempts in Behçet's disease, Rinsho Ganka **23:**557-564, 1969.
8. Gills, J. P., Jr., Buckley, C. E., III.: Cyclophosphamide therapy of Behçet's disease, Ann. Ophthalmol. **2:**399-405, 1970.
9. Haim, S.: Contribution of ocular symptoms in the diagnosis of Behçet's study of 23 cases, Arch. Dermatol. **98:**478-480, 1968.
10. Hübner, H.: Zur Therapie des Morbus Gilbert-Behçet, Ber. Dtsch. Ophthalmol. Ges. **70:**430-434, 1970.
11. Kawakita, H., Nishimura, M., Satoh, Y., and Shibata, N.: Neurological aspects of Behçet's disease. A case report and clinico-pathological review of the literature in Japan, J. Neurol. Sci. **5:**417-439, 1967.
12. Kleinhans, K.: Zur Frage der medikamentösen Behandlung des Morbus Behçet, Ber. Dtsch. Ophthalmol. Ges. **70:**425-430, 1970.
13. Mamo, J. B., and Azzam, S. A.: Treatment of Behçet's disease with chlorambucil, Arch. Ophthalmol. **84:**446-450, 1970.
14. Marniya, J.: A sixteen-year survey in Behçet's disease, Rinsho Ganka **22:**105-110, 1968.
15. Monacelli, M., and Nazzaro, P.: Behçet's disease, Basel, 1966, S. Karger, AG.
16. Polychronakos, D. J., and Sarakotsis, G.: Das Adamantiades-Behçet Syndrom, Klin. Monatsbl. Augenheilk. **154:**336-341, 1969.
17. Rossochowitz, W., and Metze, G.: Beitrag zum Adamantiades-Behçet Syndrom, Klin. Monatsbl. Augenheilk. **157:**414-419, 1970.
18. Smith, R. B., Prior, I. A. M., and Sturman, D.: Behçet's disease with retinal vascular lesions, Br. Med. J. **2:**220-221, 1967.
19. Strachan, R. W., and Wigzell, F. W.: Polyarthritis in Behçet's multiple symptom complex, Ann. Rheum. Dis. **22:**26-35, 1963.

Collagenoses
1. Bakerenov, B. T.: Hemorrhage in the retina and conjunctiva of lids in a nodular periarteritis (of a collagenous group), Oftalmol. Zh. **22:**139-140, 1967.
2. Belousova, E. F.: [Symmetrical lesions of the cornea in systemic lupus erythematosus], Vestn. Oftalmol. **79:**71-72, 1966.
3. Belousova, Z. F.: [To the question of ophthalmic symptoms in dermatomyositis], Oftalmol. Zh. **22:**447-449, 1967.
4. Bettman, J. W., Daroff, R. B., and Sanders, M.: Papilledema and asymptomatic intra-

cranial hypertension in a systemic lupus erythematosus. A fluorescein angiographic study of resolving papilledema, Arch. Ophthalmol. **80:**189-193, 1968.

5. Bloch, K. J., and Bunim, J. J.: Sjögren's syndrome and its relation to connective tissues diseases, J. Chronic Dis. **16:**915-927, 1963.
6. Böke, W., and Bäumer, A.: Klinische und histopathologische Augenbefunde beim akuten Lupus erythematodes disseminatus, Klin. Monatsbl. Augenheilk. **146:**175-187, 1965.
7. Bottoni, A.: Il fondo oculare nelle collagenopatie, Aggion. Ter. Oftalmol. **15:**151-204, 1963.
8. Breinin, G. M.: Scleredema adultorum. Ocular manifestations, Arch. Ophthalmol. **50:**155-162, 1953.
9. Capaccini, A., and Del Buono, G.: La dermatomiosite. Contributo clinico, Ann. Ottal. Clin. Ocul. **88:**628-634, 1962.
10. Cogan, D.: Nonsyphilitic interstitial keratitis with vestibuloauditory symptoms, Arch. Ophthalmol. **42:**42, 1949.
11. Cordier, J., Saudax, E., and Mouraux, J. M.: Aspects du fond d'oeil rencontrés au cours de la lupo-érythémato-viscérite maligne et de la périartérite noueuse, Bull. Soc. Ophthalmol. Fr. **60:**518-524, 1960.
12. Cullen, J. F.: Occult temporal arteritis; a common cause of blindness of old age, Br. J. Ophthalmol. **51:**513-525, 1967.
13. Dubois, E. L., and Tuffanelli, P. L.: Clinical manifestations of systemic lupus erythematosus, J.A.M.A. **190:**104-111, 1964.
14. Falk, I., and Zabel, R.: Die Beziehungen klinisch unterschiedlicher Bilder der Sklerodermie zur inneren Medizin, Dermatol. Wochenschr. **152:**593-764, 1966.
15. François, P., Wannebroucq, Ch., and Guilbert-Legrand: Manifestations rétiniennes d'une périartérite noueuse, Bull. Soc. Ophthalmol. Fr. **65:**893-895, 1965.
16. Gärtner, J., Löpping B., and Holzmann, H.: Über Glaskörperveränderungen bei Sklerodermie. Untersuchungen mit Ultraschall, Arch. Klin. Exp. Dermatol. **229:**110-116, 1967.
17. Goldburt, N. N., Likhachev, Yu. P., and Kaminer, L. N.: Concerning temporal arteritis, Arch. Patol. (Mosk.) **30:**20-23, 1968.
18. Halmay, O., Bajan, M., and Felden, E.: Halbseitiges mit Sklerodermie assoziiertes Glaukom, Klin. Monatsbl. Augenheilk. **152:**558-562, 1968.
19. Hammami, H., and Streiff, E. B.: Altérations vasculaires rétiniennes dans un cas de lupus érythémateux disséminé. Evolution après traitement aux immunosuppresseurs, Ophthalmologica **166:**16, 1973.
20. Harayama, T.: A case of scleroderma diffusum with fundus involvement, Rinsho Ganka **20:**857-859, 1966.
21. Harrison, S. M., Frenkel, M., Grossman, B. J., and Matalon, R.: Retinopathy in childhood dermatomyositis, Am. J. Ophthalmol. **76:**786, 1973.
22. Hermans, G., and Mockel-Pohl, S.: Pathologie cornéenne dans le lupus érythémateux disséminé, Bull. Soc. Belge Ophtalmol. **150:**629-644, 1968.
23. Hortz, G.: Augenhintergrundveränderungen bei "Kollagen-krankheiten," Ophthalmologica **133:**354, 1952.
24. Hradský, M., Herout, V., Cernik, F., Sazama, L., Rondiakova, Z., and Kvasnička, J.: Das Gougerot-Houwer-Sjögren-Syndrom und die Polyarteritis nodosa, Z. Gesamte Inn. Med. **23:**25-29, 1968.
25. Klien, B. A.: Die Blutgefässe der Netzhaut und der Aderhaut bei allgemeiner Sklerodermie, Österreichische Ophthalmologische Gesellschaft, 6th Annual Meeting, pp. 31-41, 1961.
26. Kirkham, T. H.: Scleroderma and Sjögren's syndrome, Br. J. Ophthalmol. **53:**131-133, 1969.
27. Lasco, F., and Nicolesco, M.: Les localisations ophtalmologiques des collagénoses, Arch. Ophtalmol. **20:**602-615, 1960.
28. Maione, M.: Su un caso di dermatomiosite con manifestazioni a carico delle palpebre, Ann. Ottalmol. Clin. Ocul. **73:**662, 1947.

29. Manschot, W. A.: The eye in relation to collagen diseases, Trans. Ophthalmol. Soc. U. K. **80:**137-151, 1961.
30. Manschot, W. A.: The eye in collagen diseases, Fortschr. Augenheilk. **11:**1-87, 1961. (Bibl. Ophthalmol. fasc. 58).
31. Manschot, W. A.: Generalized scleroderma with ocular symptoms, Ophthalmologica **149:**131-137, 1965.
32. Marvo, T., and Yamagami, Y.: Fundus appearances of diffuse scleroderma, Rinsho Ganka **56:**30-38, 1962.
33. Meunier, A., and Toussaint, D.: Sclérodermie en "coup de sabre" avec lésion du fond d'oeil, Bull. Soc. Belge Ophtalmol. **118:**369-377, 1958.
34. Moore, G. J., and Sevel, D.: Corneo-scleral ulceration in periarteritis nodosa, Br. J. Ophthalmol. **50:**651-655, 1966.
35. Moro, F.: Sulle manifestazioni oculari delle forme occulte di arterite temporale, Ann. Ottalmol. Clin. Ocul. **89:**631-650, 1963.
36. Pollack, I. P., and Becker, B.: Cytoid bodies of the retina in a patient with scleroderma, Am. J. Ophthalmol. **54:**655-660, 1962.
37. Reeves, J. A.: Keratopathy associated with systemic lupus erythematosus, Arch. Ophthalmol. **74:**159-160, 1961.
38. Sackner, M. A.: Scleroderma. Modern medical monographs, New York, 1966, Grune & Stratton, Inc.
39. Sjögren, H.: Some new investigations concerning the sicca-syndrome, Acta Ophthalmol. (Kbh.) **39:**619-622, 1961.
40. Sjögren, H.: Zur Kenntnis der Keratoconjunctivitis sicca. VII. Das Sicca-Syndrom eine auto-immune Krankheit, Acta Ophthalmol. (Kbh.) **46:**201-206, 1968.
41. Spaeth, G. L.: Corneal staining systemic lupus erythematosus, New Eng. J. Med. **276:**1168-1171, 1967.
42. Stucchi, C. A., and Geiser, J. D.: Manifestations oculaires de la sclérodermie généralisée. (Points communs avec le syndrome de Sjögren), Doc. Ophthalmol. (den Haag) **22:**72-110, 1967.
43. Susac, J. O., García-Mullin, R., and Glaser, J. S.: Ophthalmoplegia in dermatomyositis, Neurology **23:**305, 1973.
44. Svane-Knudsen, P.: Augenveränderungen bei Periarteritis nodosa, Ugeskr. Laeg. **123:**229-232, 1961.
45. Thomas, C., Cordier, J., and Duprez, A.: Manifestations ophthalmoscopiques des dermatomyosites, Bull. Soc. Fr. Dermatol. Syphiligr. **66:**349-350, 1959.
46. Tuovinen, E., and Raudasoja, R.: Poikilodermatomyositis with retinal haemorrhages and secondary glaucoma, Acta Ophthalmol. (Kbh.) **43:**669-672, 1965.
47. Van Wien, S., and Merz, E. H.: Exophthalmus secondary to periarteritis nodosa, Am. J. Ophthalmol. **56:**204-208, 1963.
48. Vilanova, X., Cardenal, C., and Capdevila, J. M.: Chronischer Lupus erythematodes der Conjunctiva, Dermatologica **113:**226-231, 1956.
49. De Vries, S.: Retinopathy in dermatomyositis, Arch. Ophthalmol. **46:**432, 1951.
50. Yoshimoto, H., and Yanagita, Y.: Ocular manifestations of systemic lupus erythematosus, Jap. J. Clin. Ophthalmol. **25:**1841-1846, 1971.

NEVOXANTHOENDOTHELIOMA (JUVENILE XANTHOGRANULOMA)

1. Myška, V., Otradovec, J., Klouček, F., Sobra, J., and Procházka, B.: [Mukokutane Form eines eosinophilen xanthomatosen Granulomes mit schwerer Beteiligung der Hornhäute bei einem Erwachsenen] (In Czech), Cesk. Oftalmol. **20:**360-368, 1964.
2. Sanders, T. E.: Infantile xanthogranuloma of the orbit; a report of three cases, Am. J. Ophthalmol. **61:**1299-1306, 1966.
3. Sanders, T. E.: Intraocular juvenile xanthogranuloma (nevoxanthogranuloma): A survey of 20 cases, Trans. Am. Ophthalmol. Soc. **58:**59-74, 1961.
4. Saraux, H., Brini, A., Dhermy, P., and Brugier, J. C.: Le xantho-granulome juvénile (naevo-xanthoendothéliome), Ann. Oculist. **200:**1036-1065, 1967.
5. Smith, J. L. S., and Ingram, R. M.: Juvenile oculodermal xantho-granuloma, Br. J. Ophthalmol. **52:**696-703, 1968.

6. Zimmerman, L. E.: Ocular lesions of juvenile xanthogranuloma. Nevoxanthoendothelioma, Am. J. Ophthalmol. **60:**1011-1035, 1965.

PORPHYRIA

1. Aguade, J. P., Mascaro, J.-M., Galy-Mascaro, G., and Capdevila, J. M.: Sur quelques manifestations cutanées et oculaires peu connues des porphyries. (Les lymphangiectasies papuleuses centro-faciales de la porphyrie), Ann. Dermatol. Syph. **96:**265-270, 1969.
2. Barth, J., and Barth, C.: Zur Frage der Augenveränderungen bei der Porphyria cutanea tarda, Dermatol. Monatsschr. **158:**122-126, 1972.
3. Calmettes, L., Deodati, F., Bec, P., and Delpech, J.: Manifestations oculaires de la porphyrie chronique, Bull. Mém. Soc. Fr. Ophtalmol. **79:**569-575, 1966.
4. Cullman, B., Denk, R., and Holzmann, H.: Zur Häufung von Farbensinnstörungen bei der Porphyria cutanea tarda (Waldenström), Graefe Arch. Klin. Exp. Ophthalmol. **170:**201-208, 1966.
5. Del Buono, G., and Artifoni, E.: Comportamento dell'apparato oculare in corso di sensibilizzazione fotodinamica. I. Le manifestazioni oculari nella clinica della porfirinopatie, G. Ital. Oftalmol. **15:**283-309, 1962.
6. Toppel, L.: Veränderungen des Augenhintergrundes bei Porphyria cutanea tarda, Munch. Med. Wochenschr. **107:**933-935, 1965.

Hydroa vacciniforme

1. Czukrasz, I., and Schlammadinger, J.: Über mit Hydroa vacciniformis einhergehende Keratitis parenchymatosa, Klin. Monatsbl. Augenheilk. **142:**403-407, 1963.
2. Kochs, A. G., and Libowitzky, H.: Chronisch polymorpher Lichtausschlag mit Frühjahrskatarrh der Bindehäute und Linsenschädigung, Dermatol. Wochenschr. **114:**438-444, 1942.
3. Ullerich, K., Wulf, K., and Wiskemann, A.: Augenaffektionen infolge Lichtsensibilisierung durch eine photodynamisch wirksame Substanz, Klin. Monatsbl. Augenheilk. **131:**30-46, 1957.

SEBACEOUS NEVUS

1. Baquis, G.: Sulla possibilità di localizzazione del nevo sebaceo precanceroso di Jadassohn agli annessi oculari, Ann. Ottalmol. Clin. Ocul. **95:**35-48, 1969.
2. Lantis, S., Leyden, J., Thew, M., and Heaton, C.: Naevus sebaceus of Jadassohn, Arch. Dermatol. **98:**117-123, 1968.

PIGMENTED TUMORS (MELANOMAS)

1. Alezzandrini, A., Cremona, E., and Thierer, B.: Precancerous melanosis of lids and conjunctiva, Arch. Oftalmol. Buenos Aires **37:**105-110, 1962.
2. Bessière, E., Léger, M., Verin, P., and Le Rebeller, M. J.: Mélanome malin conjonctival associé à une cystomatose sudoripare (hidrocystomatose à contenu graisseux), Bull. Mém. Soc. Fr. Ophtalmol. **78:**484-496, 1965.
3. Böck, J., and Feyrter, F.: Über die Beziehungen zwischen dem Naevus der Haut, dem Naevus der Augenbindehaut und dem Melanom der Aderhaut. I. Der Naevus der Haut, insbesondere der Lidhaut, Graefes Arch. Klin. Exp. Ophthalmol. **178:**51-66, 1969.
4. Clune, J. P.: Primary malignant melanoma of the cornea. A review and case report, Am. J. Ophthalmol. **55:**147-150, 1963.
5. Collier, M.: Le naevus "partagé" des paupières, Bull. Soc. Ophtalmol. Fr. **64:**1028-1031, 1964.
6. Covell, L. L., and Markiewitz, H. H.: The choroid as site of prime manifestation of systemic involvement in skin melanoma. Report of a case, Am. J. Ophthalmol. **51:**1296-1303, 1961.
7. Daicker, B.: Cancerous melanosis, Arch. Ophthalmol. **75:**404-406, 1966.
8. Dhermy, M. P., and Dugelay-Magnaud, J.: Mélanome juvénile de la paupière, Bull. Soc. Ophtalmol. Fr. **64:**503-512, 1964.
9. Ehlers, N.: A case of divided nevus, Arch. Ophthalmol. **73:**664-666, 1965.
10. Feyrter, F.: and Böck, J.: Über die Beziehungen zwischen dem Naevus der Haut, dem Naevus der Augenbindehaut und dem Melanom der Aderhaut. II. Der Naevus der Augenbindehaut und der Carunkel, Graefes Arch. Klin. Exp. Ophthalmol. **178:**67-71, 1969.

11. Font, R. L., Naumann, G., and Zimmermann, L. E.: Primary malignant melanoma of the skin metastatic to the eye and orbit. Report of ten cases and review of the literature, Am. J. Ophthalmol. **63:**738-754, 1967.
12. Greither, A.: Nävus und malignes Melanom, Internistische Praxis **3:**303-312, 1963.
13. Hogan, M. J.: Tumores pigmentados externos del ojo, Ann. Soc. Mex. Oftalmol. **31:** 155-159, 1958.
14. Jay, B.: Naevi and melanomata of the conjunctiva, Br. J. Ophthalmol. **49:**169-204, 1965.
15. Manschot, W. A.: Congenital ocular melanosis, conjunctival naevus, conjunctival melanosis, conjunctival melanoma, Ophthalmologica **152:**495-505, 1966.
16. Reese, A. B.: Precancerous and cancerous melanosis, Am. J. Ophthalmol. **61:**1272-1277, 1966.
17. Vancea, P., and Vancea, P. P.: Epithélioma intraépithélial pigmenté développé dans un "junctional naevus" de la conjonctive bulbaire, Arch. Ophtalmol. (Paris) **23:**35-45, 1963.
18. Wollensak, J., and Meythaler, H.: Histologie der Lidtumoren mit besonderer Berücksichtigung von juvenilem Melanom (Spitz) und Hidradenoma papilliferum, Klin. Monatsbl. Augenheilk. **150:**388-397, 1967.

Hereditary dermatoses with eye findings

PSEUDOXANTHOMA ELASTICUM
1. Caravati, C. M., Jr., Richardson, D. R., and Bradley, J. E.: Blue sclerae associated with pseudoxanthoma elasticum, Arch. Dermatol. (Chicago) **96:**699-700, 1967.
2. Erbakan, S.: Groenblad-Strandberg syndrome. Report of two cases in which macular degeneration occurred before angioid streaks, Am. J. Ophthalmol. **51:**704-706, 1961.
3. Franceschetti, A.: Importance génétique des altérations atypiques du fond de l'oeil dans le syndrome de Groenblad-Strandberg (pseudoxanthome élastique et stries angioïdes). 13. Congr. Int. Dermatol. 1967, 553-557, 1968.
4. Gills, J. P., Jr., and Paton, D.: Mottled fundus oculi in pseudoxanthoma elasticum. A report of two siblings, Arch. Ophthalmol. (Chicago) **73:**792-795, 1965.
5. Magdalena-Castinera, J.: Estrías angioides y luxación de cristalinos, Arch. Soc. Oftalmol. Hisp.-Amer. **21:**63-73, 1961.
6. Majláth, E., Fülöp, E., Masszi, J., and Pajor R.: Die Bedeutung des Pseudoxanthoma elasticum für die Augenheilkunde, Klin. Monatsbl. Augenheilk. **159:**632-638, 1971.
7. Matsui, M.: ["Peau d'orange" fundus in a case of pseudoxanthoma elasticum] (In Japanese), Jap. J. Clin. Ophthalmol. **24:**951-952, 1970.
8. Mazalton, A., and Messimy, R.: Maladie de Paget et syndrome de Groenblad-Strandberg, Sem. Hop. Paris **37:**3591-3596, 1961.
9. Paton, D.: The relation of angioid streaks to systemic disease, Springfield, Ill., 1972, Charles C Thomas, Publisher.
10. Shimizu, K.: [Mottled fundus in association with pseudoxanthoma elasticum] (In Japanese), Jap. J. Ophthalmol. **5:**1-12, 1962.

INCONTINENTIA PIGMENTI
1. Brégeat, P., Duperrot, B., Juge, P., Mascaro-Galy, and Hamard, H.: Incontinentia pigmenti et atrophie optique unilatérale, Bull. Mem. Soc. Fr. Ophtalmol. **77:**185-196, 1964.
2. Crislain, J.-R., Mussini, J., De Berranger, P., Le Bodic, M. F., and Dubigeon, P.: Incontinentia pigmenti. (À propos d'une nouvelle observation), Pédiatrie **23:**67-79, 1968.
3. Graciansky, P., Timsit, E., Heuet De Barochet, Y., and Larregue, M.: Incontinenta pigmenti; lésions initiales, Ann. Dermatol. Syph. **94:**410-411, 1967.
4. Gross, H.: Frühstadium des Syndroms der Incontinentia pigmenti (Bloch-Sulzberger), Paediatrische Praxis **6:**631-634, 1967.
5. Lieb, W. A., and Guerry, D.: Fundus changes in incontinentia pigmenti, Am. J. Ophthalmol. **45:**265, 1958.
6. McCrary, J. A., III, and Smith, L. J.: Conjunctival and retinal incontinentia pigmenti, Arch. Ophthalmol. (Chicago) **79:**417-422, 1968.

7. Wilk, A.: [Bloch-Sulzberger syndrome (incontinentia pigmenti)] (In Polish), Klin. Oczna **42:**793-795, 1972.
8. Wollensak, J.: Charakteristiche Augenbefunde beim Syndroma Bloch-Sulzberger (Incontinentia pigmenti), Klin. Monatsbl. Augenheilk. **134:**692-706, 1959.
9. Zweifach, P. H.: Incontinentia pigmenti: Its association with retinal dysplasia, Am. J. Ophthalmol. **62:**716-722, 1966.

XERODERMA PIGMENTOSUM

1. Delogu, A., and Fusco, G.: Su di un caso di xeroderma pigmentoso con lesioni oculari, Ann. Ottalmol. Clin. Ocul. **93:**31-38, 1967.
2. Gulati, G. C., and Ahluwalia, B. K.: Ocular involvement in xeroderma pigmentosum, J. All-India Ophthalmol. Soc. **15:**233-235, 1967.
3. Haim, S., and Zonis, S.: Squamous cell carcinoma of the conjunctiva in xeroderma pigmentosum, Israel J. Med. Sci. **1:**431-434, 1965.
4. Lynch, H. T., Anderson, D. E., Smith, J. L., Jr., Howell, J. B., Krush, A. J.: Xeroderma pigmentosum, malignant melanoma, and congenital ichthyosis; a family study, Arch. Dermatol. (Chicago) **96:**625-635, 1967.
5. Oláh, Z.: [Malignant tumour of the cornea and xeroderma pigmentosum] (In Czech), Cesk. Oftalmol. **24:**119-122, 1968.
6. Perron, R., et al.: Un cas de xeroderma pigmentosum avec manifestations oculaires, Bull. Soc. Ophtalmol. Fr. **68:**520-522, 1968.

ANHIDROTIC ECTODERMAL DYSPLASIA

1. Jung, E. G., and Vogel, M.: Anhidrotische Ektodermaldysplasie mit Hornhautdystrophie, Schweiz. Med. Wochenschr. **96:**1477-1483, 1966.

ICHTHYOSES

1. Artifoni, E., and Campana, G.: Distrofia corneale primitiva in soggetto affetto da ittiosi, congenita, Ann. Ottalmol. Clin. Ocul. **92:**1274-1282, 1966.
2. Böck, J., and Niebauer, G.: Über zwei Kranke mit Ichthyosis vulgaris und Netzhautgefässerkrankung, Wien. Klin. Wochenschr. **76:**758-760, 1964.
3. Franceschetti, A., Amann, F., Bamatter, F., and Brocher, J. E. W.: Dégénérescence tapéto-rétinienne dans un cas de syndrome de Sjögren-Larsson (hyperkératose ichthyosiforme congénitale, diplégie spastique, retard mental) avec dysplasies osseuses et ectodermiques associées à une "incontinentia pigmenti histologica," Confin. Neurol. **23:**334-342, 1963.
4. Jay, B., Blach, R. K., and Wells, R. S.: Ocular manifestations of ichthyosis, Br. J. Ophthalmol. **52:**217-226, 1968.
5. Klein, D., and Franceschetti, A.: Missbildung und Krankheiten des Auges. In Becker, P. E.: Humangenetik, vol. IV, Stuttgart, 1964, Georg Thieme Verlag.
6. Koleszar, G., and Papp, G.: Gemeinsames Vorkommen von Ichthyosis congenita, Ektropium, Esotropie und Ektrodaktylie, Klin. Monatsbl. Augenheilk. **152:**575-577, 1968.
7. Korting, G. W., and Ruther, H.: Ichthyosis vulgaris und akrofaciale Dysostose, Arch. Dermatol. Syph. (Berlin) **197:**91-104, 1953/54.
8. Padron, O., Vargas, J., and García Ocampo, N.: Ictiosis generalizada con manifestaciones corneales progresivas, Rev. Oftal. Venezuela **26:**45-48, 1970.
9. Reich, H.: Sjögren-Larsson-Syndrom, Med. Klin. **67:**909-912, 1972.
10. Rose, H. M.: Lid changes in non-bullous ichthyosiform erythrodermia, Br. J. Ophthalmol. **55:**750-752, 1971.
11. Schindle, R. D., Houston, C. R., and Leone, C. R.: Cicatricial ectropion associated with lamellar ichthyosis, Arch. Ophthalmol. **89:**62, 1973.

EPIDERMOLYSIS BULLOSA

1. Baidan, N., Daniluc, T., and Chiriac, N.: [Corneo-conjunctival lesions in dystrophic bullous epidermolysis] (In Rumanian), Oftalmologia (Bucaresti) **14:**251-260, 1970.
2. Cordella, M., and Peralta, S.: Lagoftalmo cicatriziale in un caso di epidermolisi bullosa distrofica poliplastica, Minerva Oftalmol. **8:**155-157, 1966.
3. Hill, J. C., and Rodrigue, D.: Cicatricial ectropion in epidermolysis bullosa and in congenital ichthyosis; its plastic repair, Can. J. Ophthalmol. **6:**89-97, 1971.

4. Miron, M. S., Marinov, I., and Pascu, M.: Epidermolyse bulleuse et décollement bilatéral de la rétine, Arch. Ophtalmol. (Paris) **21:**778-782, 1961.

Infections

PYOGENICS
1. Mann, R. A., and Rosborough, D.: Pyoderma gangrenosum. A case report, Br. J. Surg. **55:**718-720, 1968.

Leprosy
1. Choyce, D. P.: Diagnosis and management of ocular leprosy, Br. J. Ophthalmol. **53:** 217-223, 1969.
2. Garus, Y. J.: Fundus changes in leprosy, Vestn. Oftalmol. **80:**66-69, 1967.
3. Garus, Y. J.: The early diagnosis of leprotic iritis, Oftalmol. Zh. **23:**201-205, 1968.
4. Gupta, S.: Ocular involvement in leprosy, Proc. All-India Ophthalmol. Soc. **23:**189-194, 1968.
5. Santonastaso, A.: Alterazioni oculari nella lebbra, Ann. Ottalmol. **60:**21-37, 107-124, 276-300, 796-835, 1932.

Tuberculosis
1. De Voe, A. G., and Locatcher-Khorazo, D.: The external manifestations of ocular tuberculosis, Trans. Am. Ophthalmol. Soc. **62:**203-212, 1964.
2. Doden, W.: Über die Tuberkulöse des Auges und Adnexe, Wien. Klin. Wochenschr. **79:**569-574, 1967.
3. Scuderi, G., and Cardia, L.: Nodular tuberculosis of the skin of the lids and of the regional lymph nodes, Rev. Brasil. Oftalmol. **23:**183-191, 1964.

VIRUSES
1. Bietti, G. B., Cerulli, L., and Moschini, G. B.: Die Viruskeratitiden, Ber. Dtsch. Ophthalmol. Ges. **71:**141-171, 1971.
2. Cavara, V., and Bietti, G. B.: Manifestazioni oculari da virus e da rickettsie, Relazione al 39. Congresso della Società Oftalmologica d'Italia, Torino, 1952, Bologna, 1952, Casa Editrice Licinio Cappelli.

Herpes zoster of the first branch of the trigeminus
1. Acres, T. E.: Herpes zoster ophthalmicus with controlateral hemiplegia, Arch. Ophthalmol. **71:**371-376, 1964.
2. Bietti, G. B., Cerulli, L., and Moschini, G. B.: Die Viruskeratitiden, Ber. Dtsch. Ophthalmol. Ges. **71:**141-171, 1971.
3. Blodi, F. C.: Ophthalmic zoster in malignant diseases, Am. J. Ophthalmol. **65:**686-688, 1968.
4. Bouzas, A.: L'Atteinte des voies lacrymales dans le zona ophtalmique, Bull. Mém. Soc. Fr. Ophtalmol. **77:**171-184, 1964.
5. Chinaglia, V., and Belci, C.: Herpes zoster e ipertensione oculare, Ann. Ottalmol. Clin. Ocul. **90:**273-284, 1964.
6. Falcinelli, G.: Paralisi muscolari ed esoftalmo nell'erpes zoster, Boll. Oculist. **41:**938-947, 1962.
7. Goldsmith, M. O.: Herpes zoster ophthalmicus with sixth nerve palsy, Can. J. Ophthalmol. **3:**279-283, 1968.
8. Guyard, M., Perdriel, G., and Ceruti, F.: A propos de cas atypiques de zona ophtalmique, Bull. Soc. Ophtal. Fr. **68:**287-290, 1968.
9. Hudson, C. D., and Vickers, R. A.: Clinicopathologic observations in prodromal herpes zoster of the fifth cranial nerve: report of a case, Oral. Surg. **31:**494-501, 1971.
10. Juel-Jensen, B. E.: Results of the treatment of zoster with idoxuridine in dimethylsulphoxide, Ann. N. Y. Acad. Sci. **173:**74-82, 1970.
11. Kielar, R. A., Cunningham, G. C., and Gerson, K. L.: Occurrence of herpes zoster ophthalmicus in a child with absent immunoglobulin A and deficiency of delayed hypersensitivity, Am. J. Ophthalmol. **72:**555-557, 1971.
12. Passeri, S., Vinciguerra, E., and Mammarella E.: Neurite ottica retrobulbare acuta in corso di herpes zoster oticus con paralisi del facciale e disturbi cocleo-vestibolari, Ann. Ottalmol. Clin. Ocul. **94:**1573-1581, 1968.

13. Romani, E.: Emianopsia omonima a quadrante post-zosteriana, Boll. Oculist. **49:**177-183, 1970.

14. Sod, N. N.: Herpes zoster ophthalmicus and varicella, Orient. Arch. Ophthalmol. **7:**40-41, 1969.

Herpes simplex

1. Bietti, G. B., Cerulli, L., and Moschini, G. B.: Die Viruskeratitiden, Ber. Dtsch. Ophthalmol. Ges. **71:**141-171, 1971.

2. Cavara, V., and Bietti, G. B.: Manifestazioni oculari da virus e da rickettsie, Relazione al 39. Congresso della Società Oftalmologica d'Italia, Torino, 1952, Bologna, 1952, Casa Editrice Licinio Cappelli.

3. Kaufman, H. E.: The natural history and diagnosis of herpes corneae. In Michaelson, I. C., and Berman E. R.: Causes and prevention of blindness, Jerusalem seminar, New York, 1972, Academic Press Inc., p. 192.

4. Nauheim, J. S.: Herpes simplex der Lider und ihrer Umgebung, Trans. Am. Acad. Ophthalmol. Otolaryngol. **75:**1236-1241, 1971.

Vaccinia

1. Capolongo, G.: Contributo allo studio delle manifestazioni oculari nel vaiolo, Riv. Oftalmol. **1:**578, 1946.

2. Coskey, H. J., Bryan, H. G.: Vaccinia of the ocular region, J. Pediatr. Ophthalmol. **5:**157-159, 1968.

3. Ruben, F. L., and Lane, J. M.: Ocular vaccinia. An epidemiologic analysis of 348 cases, Arch. Ophthalmol. **84:**45-48, 1970.

MOLLUSCUM CONTAGIOSUM

1. Bietti, G. B., Cerulli, L., and Moschini, G. B.: Die Viruskeratitiden, Ber. Dtsch. Ophthalmol. Ges. **71:**141-171, 1971.

2. Cavara, V., and Bietti, G. B.: Manifestazioni oculari da virus e da rickettsie, Relazione al 39. Congresso della Società Oftalmologica d'Italia, Torino, 1952, Bologna, 1952, Casa Editrice Licinio Cappelli.

3. Haellmigk, C.: Keratokonjunktivitis bei Molluscum contagiosum der Lider, Klin. Monatsbl. Augenheilk. **148:**87-91, 1966.

4. Marisi, F.: Sulle alterazioni della cornea da mollusco contagioso e da verruca volgare del bordo palpebrale, Boll. Oculist. **24:**337, 1945.

5. Nover, A.: Recidivierende Keratitis durch Molluscum contagiosum des Unterlides, Klin. Monatsbl. Augenheilk. **117:**302-304, 1950.

6. Sysi, R.: Molluscum contagiosum corneae, Acta Ophthalmol. (Kbh.) **19:**25-27, 1941.

VERRUCA VULGARIS

1. Noojin, R. O.: Multiple ophthalmic verrucae, Arch. Dermatol. Syph. **97:**176-177, 1968.

2. Vito, P.: Sulla congiuntivite da verruca del bordo libero delle palpebre, Boll. Oculist. **15:**627-634, 1936.

RICKETTSIOSIS

1. Cavara, V., and Bietti, G. B.: Manifestazioni oculari da virus e da rickettsie, Relazione al 39. Congresso della Società Oftalmologica d'Italia, Torino, 1952, Bologna, 1952, Casa Editrice Licinio Cappelli.

CHLAMYDIOSIS

1. Alfano, J. E., and Perez, A. T.: Cat-scratch disease, Am. J. Ophthalmol. **55:**99-103, 1963.

2. Bietti, G. B., Cerulli, L., and Moschini, G. B.: Die Viruskeratitiden, Ber. Dtsch. Ophthalmol. Ges. **71:**144-171, 1971.

3. Cassady, J. V., and Culbertson, C. S.: Cat-scratch disease and Parinaud's oculoglandular syndrome, Arch. Ophthalmol. **50:**68-74, 1953.

4. Cavara, V., and Bietti, G. B.: Manifestazioni oculari da virus e da rickettsie, Relazione al 39. Congresso della Società Oftalmologica d'Italia, Torino, 1952, Bologna, 1952, Casa Editrice Licinio Cappelli.

5. Farber, G. A., Forshner, J. G., and O'Quinn, S. E.: Reiter's syndrome. Treatment with methotrexate, J.A.M.A. **200:**171-173, 1967.

6. Freedman, A., and al-Hussaini, M. K., Dunlop, E. M. C., et al.: Infection by TRIC agent and other members of the *Bedsonia* group; with a note on Reiter's disease. II.

Ophthalmia neonatorum due to TRIC agent, Trans. Ophthalmol. Soc. U. K. **86:**313-320, 1966.

7. Jones, B. R., al-Hussaini, M. K., Dunlop, E. M. C., et al.: Infection by TRIC agent and other members of the *Bedsonia* group: With a note on Reiter's disease. I. Ocular disease in the adult, Trans. Ophthalmol. Soc. U. K. **86:**291-312, 1966.
8. McEwen, C.: Reiter's disease: Its nature and relationship to other diseases, Trans. Stud. Coll. Physicians Phila. **34:**39-46, 1966.
9. Noer, H. R.: An "experimental" epidemic of Reiter's syndrome, J.A.M.A. **198:**693-698, 1966.
10. Ostler, B. H., et al.: Reiter's syndrome, Am. J. Ophthalmol. **71:**986-991, 1971.
11. Sabella, G.: La sindrome di Reiter. Contributo casistico e critico, G. Clin. Med. **48:**366-393, 1967.
12. Schachter, J., and Barnes, M. G., et al.: Isolation of bedsoniae from joints of patients with Reiter's syndrome, Proc. Soc. Exp. Biol. Med. **122:**283-285, 1966.
13. Vasquez Barriere, A.: El ojo en la enfermedad de Nicolas-Favre, Arch. Oftalmol. Buenos Aires **16:**653, 1941.
14. Volpi, U., and Focosi, F.: Reiter's disease. Clinical and histopathological studies, Ann. Ottalmol. Clin. Ocul. **94:**120-132, 1968.

SYPHILIS

1. MacFaul, P. A., and Catterall, R. D.: Acute choroido-retinitis in secondary syphilis; presence of spiral organisms in acqueous humor, Br. J. Vener. Dis. **47:**159-161, 1971.
2. Rice, N. S. C., et al.: Study of late ocular syphilis. Demonstration of treponemes in acqueous humor and cerebro-spinal fluid. II. Ocular findings: Trans. Opthalmol. Soc. U. K. **88:**251-256, 1968.
3. Ryan, S. J., Hardy, P. H., Hardy, J. M., and Oppenheimer, E. H.: Persistence of virulent treponema pallidum despite penicillin therapy in congenital syphilis, Am. J. Ophthalmol. **73:**258-261, 1972.
4. Wilkinson, A. E.: Study of late ocular syphilis. Demonstration of treponemes in acqueous humor and cerebro-spinal fluid. I. Methods of demonstration of treponemes, Trans. Ophthalmol. Soc. U. K. **88:**251-256, 1968.

MYCOSES

1. Calmettes, L., Deodati, F., and Bazex, A.: Dermatose mycosique et uvéite, Bull. Soc. Belge Ophtalmol. **124:**878-881, 1960.
2. Cavara, V.: Le micosi oculari, Siena, 1928, Libreria Editrice Senese.
3. Cramer, H. J., Liendloff, H., and Koch, A.: Singuläres Candida-Granulom der Haut mit Hornhaut-Candidose durch eine seltene Hefeart, Dtsch. Gesundheitsw. **23:**1554-1558, 1968.
4. François, J., and Elewaut-Rijsselaere, M.: Mycoses oculaires, Bull. Soc. Belge Ophtalmol. **148:**361-380, 1968.
5. McGrand, J. C.: Symposium on direct fungal infection of the eye. Keratomycosis due to *Aspergillus fumigatus* cured by Nystatin, Trans. Ophthalmol. Soc. U. K. **89:**799-802, 1969.
6. McLean, J. M.: Oculomycosis. (The XIX Jackson Memorial Lecture), Am. J. Ophthalmol. **56:**537-549, 1963.
7. Olson, C. L.: Fungal contamination of conjunctiva and lid margin, Arch. Ophthalmol. **81:**351-355, 1969.
8. Persaud, V., and Holroyd, J. B. M.: Mycetoma of the palpebral conjunctiva caused by *Allescheria boydii (Monosporium apiospermum)*, Br. J. Ophthalmol. **52:**857-859, 1968.
9. Viallefont, H., and Costeau, J.: A propos des localisations oculaires de la candidose, J. Med. Montpellier **3:**45-46, 1968.
10. Vozza, R., and Bagolini, B.: Su di un caso di grave ulcerazione bilaterale delle palpebre da *Candida albicans,* Boll. Oculist. **43:**433-439, 1964.

ZOONOSES

1. Korting, G. W.: Phthiriasis palpebrarum—und ihre ersten historischen Erwähnungen, Hautarzt **18:**73-74, 1967.
2. Stargardt, K.: Phthiriasis der Lider und Follikularkatarrh, Z. Augenheilk. **38:**288, 1918.

3. Beasley, F. J.: Phthiriasis palpebrarum, report of a case, J. Fla. Med. Assoc. **51:**533-534, 1961.

Syndromes with skin and eye findings

NEUROFIBROMATOSIS

1. Agoston, I.: Beidseitige symmetrische sektorenförmige Pigmentveränderung der Netzhaut bei der Recklinghausenschen Neurofibromatosis, Acta Ophthalmol. (Kbh.) **46:**41-48, 1968.
2. Arai, Y.: Two cases of von Recklinghausen's disease associated with ocular symptoms, Jap. J. Clin. Ophthalmol. **21:**1165-1171, 1967.
3. Arseni, C., Maretsis, M., and Maretsis, M. S.: Unilateral pulsating exophthalmos in von Recklinghausen's disease, Ophthalmologica **153:**409-418, 1967.
4. Babel, J., and Younessian, S.: Buphthalmie ohne Hypertension. Ein Fall von familiärer Neurofibromatose, Ber. Dtsch. Ophthalmol. Ges. **69:**221-224, 1968.
5. Bengisu, U., Tahsinoglu, M., and Toker, G.: La neurofibromatose associée au choristome cartilagineux de l'épisclère, Ann. Oculist. **206:**401, 1973.
6. Bracher, R.: Buphthalmus und Neurofibromatose Recklinghausen, Graefes Arch. Ophthalmol. **173:**351-368, 1967.
7. Brini, A., Sibilly, A., and Fontaine, R.: Glaucome congénital et maladie de von Recklinghausen uvéale. Anévrysme cirsoïde et neurofibromatose cutanée de la région temporale homolatérale, Bull. Soc. Ophtalmol. Fr. **65:**665-671, 1965.
8. Cernea, P., and Dobrescu, C.: Mélanome malin uvéal, manifestations de la maladie de Recklinghausen, Ophthalmologica **166:**161, 1973.
9. Ehlers, H.: Die Augensymptome bei der Recklinghausenschen Neurofibromatose, Ophthalmologica **151:**284-308, 1966.
10. El-Shewy, T. M., and Koura, F. M. A.: Chiasmal syndrome as a manifestation of intracranial neurofibromatosis, Bull. Ophthalmol. Soc. Egypt **64:**555, 1971.
11. Frenkel, M.: Retinal angiomatosis in a patient with neurofibromatosis, Am. J. Ophthalmol. **63:**804-808, 1967.
12. Grant, W. M., and Walton, D. S.: Distinctive gonioscopic findings in glaucoma due to neurofibromatosis, Arch. Ophthalmol. (Chicago) **79:**127-134, 1968.
13. Jefferson, M.: Pulsating exophthalmos in von Recklinghausen's disease, Trans. Ophthalmol. Soc. U. K. **85:**527-536, 1966.
14. Mortada, A.: Orbital neurilemmoma with café-au-lait pigmentation of the skin, Br. J. Ophthalmol. **52:**262, 1968.
15. Pestre, A.: Syndrome de Recklinghausen et buphtalmie glaucomateuse chez un nouveauné, Bull. Soc. Ophtalmol. Fr. **71:**1034-1038, 1971.
16. Roveda, K. M., and Courtis, J. M.: "Verrugosidades" del iris en la enfermedad de Recklinghausen, Arch. Soc. Oftal. Hisp.-Amer. **29:**409-412, 1969.
17. Saran, N., and Winter, F. C.: Bilateral gliomas of the optic discs associated with neurofibromatosis, Am. J. Ophthalmol. **64:**607-612, 1967.
18. Sokolova, O. N., and Cherepanov, A. N.: [Ocular symptoms of Recklinghausen's central neurofibromatosis] (In Russian), Oftalmol. Zh. **20:**261-265, 1965.

MULTIPLE MUCOSAL NEUROMAS

1. Perry, H. O., Kiely, J. M., and Moertel, C. G.: Cutaneous clues to visceral cancer, Minn. Med. **51:**1719-1726, Dec. 1968.

SCLEROSIS TUBEROSA

1. Andreani, D.: Su di un caso di malattia di Bourneville con compromissione del corpo ciliare, Boll. Oculist. **39:**319-327, 1960.
2. Anglani, D., and Piccione, P.: La malattia di Bourneville. Quadri anatomico-clinici e radiologici, Arch. De Vecchi Anat. Patol. **48:**845-862, 1967.
3. Atkinson, A., Sanders, M. D., and Wong, V.: Vitreous haemorrhage in tuberous sclerosis, Br. J. Ophthalmol. **57:**773, 1973.
4. Chepaldi, A., and Villano, V.: Su di un caso di malattia di Bourneville. Ann. Ottalmol. Clin. Ocul. **90:**230-244, 1964.
5. Dyer, A. M., Hill, R., Rowan, R. M., and Taylor, W. O. G.: Case of tuberous sclerosis

and haemorragic retinopathy (with fundus photographs), Br. J. Med. **67**(II):398-399, 1967.

6. Garron, L. K., and Spencer, W. H.: Retinal glioneuroma associated with tuberous sclerosis, Trans. Am. Acad. Ophthalmol. Otolaryngol. **68**:1018-1021, 1964.

7. Ravault, M. P., Lequin, and Durant, M. L.: Phakomatose de Bourneville à manifestations oculaires, Bull. Soc. Ophtalmol. Fr. **66**:760-763, 1966.

8. Remenár, L., and Pál, M.: [Über die Augenhintergrundsymptome der Sclerosis tuberosa] (In Hungarian), Szemészet **184**:216-220, 1967.

9. Rettinger, E., and Wessing, A.: Seltene Hautveränderungen bei Morbus Bourneville, Ber. Dtsch. Ophthalmol. Ges. **68**:228-234, 1967.

10. Rollin, J. P., Laugier, P., and Royer, J.: La sclérose tubéreuse de Bourneville et ses manifestations oculaires, Clinique Ophtalmol. **5**:31-67, 1966.

VASCULAR PHAKOMATOSES

Meningo-oculofacial angiomatosis

1. Arlt, K.: Das Sturge-Weber-Krabbe-Syndrom. Operationsindikation und Operationstechnik, Chirurgische Praxis **12**:171-177, 1968.

2. Arseni, C., and Carp, N.: La maladie de Sturge-Weber. Observations anatomocliniques et histopathologiques, Ann. Anat. Pathol. **12**:411-422, 1967.

3. Berkow, J. W.: Retinitis pigmentosa associated with Sturge-Weber syndrome, Arch. Ophthalmol. (Chicago) **75**:72-76, 1966.

4. Bölcs, S., and Bajnok G.: Über die meningo-oculo-faciale Angiomatose. Klin. Monatsbl. Augenheilk. **150**:702-706, 1967.

5. François, J.: Angiomatose oculo-cutanée de Lawford. (Angiome facial et Glaucome tardif), Ophthalmologica **122**:215-227, 1951.

6. Grasso Cannizzo, E.: Considerazioni sull'insorgenza del glaucoma nella sindrome di Sturge-Weber, Studi Sassaresi **20**:1-23, 1942.

7. Kalina, R.: Facial angiomatosis with angioid streaks; association of angioid streaks with a component of the Sturge-Weber syndrome, Arch. Ophthalmol. (Chicago) **84**:528-531, 1970.

8. Rizzo, P.: Considerazioni su di un caso di sindrome di Lawford (naevus flammeus del viso e glaucoma cronico senza ingrandimento del globo oculare), Ann. Ottalmol. Clin. Ocul. **81**:607-620, 1955.

9. Sbordone, M., and Apponi Battini, G.: Sindrome di Sturge-Weber; contributo alla terapia chirurgica, Arch. Ottalmol. Clin. Ocul. **68**:453-461, 1964.

10. Strazzi, A.: La sindrome di Surge-Weber. Considerazioni su 14 casi, Riv. Otoneurooftalmol. **35**:621-640, 1960.

11. Wirth, A.: Glaucoma associato a naevus flammeus bilaterale: Osservazioni patogenetiche e terapeutiche, Boll. Oculist. **36**:619-624, 1957.

Von Hippel-Lindau disease, or angiomatosis of the retina and cerebellum

1. Arseni, C., Maretsis, M., and Vasilesco, A.: La maladie de von Hippel–Lindau; à propos d'un cas, Rev. Otoneuroophtalmol. **39**:174-182, 1967.

2. Cordier, J., Saraux, E., Watrin, E., and Raspiller, A.: Angiomatose rétino-cérébelleuse (maladie de von Hippel–Lindau): à propos d'une observation, Bull. Soc. Ophtalmol. Fr. **67**:951-958, 1967.

3. Coriglione, G., and Schiallaci, C.: Malattia di von Hippel–Lindau; contributo clinico, Minerva Oftalmol. **9**:62-66, 1967.

4. Goldberg, M. F., and Duke, J. R.: Von Hippel-Lindau disease; histopathologic findings in a treated and an untreated eye, Am. J. Ophthalmol. **66**:693-705, 1968.

5. Macrae, H. M., and Newbigin, B.: Von Hippel-Lindau disease: A family history, Can. J. Ophthalmol. **3**:28-34, 1968.

6. Paufique, L., Ravault, M. P., and Durand, L.: Maladie de von Hippel à localisation papillaire, Bull. Soc. Ophtalmol. Fr. **66**:755-757, 1966.

7. Sedan, R., and Farnarier, G.: Angiomatose rétino-cérébelleuse de von Hippel-Lindau, Bull. Soc. Ophtalmol. Fr. **67**:612-613, 1967.

8. Wessing, A.: Lichtkoagulation bei Angiomatosis retinae (v. Hippel-Lindausche Erkrankung), Ophthalmologica **151**:874-877, 1966.

Telangiectatic ataxia, or Louis-Bar syndrome
1. Arthuis, M.: L'Ataxie-télangiectasie, Médecine Infantile **75**:213-230, 1968.
2. François, J., and Neetens, A.: Syndrome "ataxie-télangiectasies" de Louis-Bar, Bull. Soc. Ophtalmol. Fr. **4**:288-292, 1961.
3. Giménez-Roldán, S., Negrete, O. A., and Pérez Sotelo, M.: La motilidad ocular en el sindrome de Louis Bar (ataxia teleangiectasia); estudio sobre 4 casos, Rev. Esp. Otoneurooftalmol. Neurocir. **26**:30-38, 1967.
4. Grützner, P.: Augensymptome bei Ataxia teleangiectatica, Klin. Monatsl. Augenheilk. **135**:712-717, 1959.
5. Harley, R. D., Baird, H. W., and Craven, E. M.: Ataxia telangiectasia. Report of seven cases, Arch. Ophthalmol. (Chicago) **77**:582-592, 1967.
6. Hermans, E. H., Grossfeld, J. C. M., and Spaas, J. A. J.: The fifth phacomatosis, Dermatologica **130**:446-476, 1965.
7. Kojima, K., Takayanagi, Y., Watanabe, I., and Niimi, K.: Ataxia-telangiectasia (Louis-Bar syndrome), Acta Soc. Ophthalmol. Jap. **72**:625-637, 1968.
8. Nemeth, E.: Louis-Bar-artiges Syndrom im Erwachsenenalter, Klin. Monatsbl. Augenheilk. **153**:655-660, 1968.
9. Quick, A. J.: Teleangiectasia: Its relationship to the Minot-von Willebrand syndrome, Am. J. Med. Sci. **254**:585-601, 1967.

Klippel-Trénaunay-Weber syndrome
1. Bietti, G. B.: Angiomatöse dermatooculäre Syndrome, Ber. Dtsch. Ophthalmol. Ges. **68**:529-530, 1967. (Discussion to Meyer-Schwickerath and von Barsevich)
2. François, J., and Neetens, A.: Angiomatose de la face, de la conjonctive et de la rétine, Bull. Soc. Belge Ophtalmol. **125**:1028-1936, 1960.
3. Gautier-Smith, P. C., Danders, M. D., and Sanderson, K. V.: Atteintes oculaires et nerveuses dans l'angiome serpigineux. (Ocular and nervous system involvement in angioma serpiginosum), Ann. Ocul. (Paris) **206**:356, 1973.
4. Heidrich, R., and Siegek, E.: Klippel-Trénaunay-Parkes-Syndrom mit Dystrophia musculorum progressiva (Erb) und bilateralem Gesichtsnävus, Med. Bild. **10**:146-147, 1967.
5. Ortiz García, and Piñuero Carrión: Angioma capilar de la orbita, Arch. Soc. Oftalmol. Hisp.-Amer. **29**:601-605, 1969.
6. Reuter, G.: Über das Syndrom des Klippel-Trénaunay-Parkes-Weber. Bericht über zwei klinikeigene Fälle, Z. Kinderchir. **5**:251-258, 1967.
7. Ruiz-Barranco, F.: Angiomatosis encéfalo-orbitaria, Arch. Soc. Oftalmol. Hisp.-Amer. **25**:158-167, 1965.
8. Valenzano, L., and Testa, V.: Sindrome di Klippel-Trénaunay-Parkes-Weber associata con la sindrome di Sturge-Weber-Krabbe, Boll. Ist. Dermatol. S. Gallicano **4**:47-58, 1967.
9. Weber, G., and Roth, W. G.: Generalisierte essentielle Teleangiektasien an Haut und Conjunctiven, Z. Haut Geschlechtskr. **42**:655-658, 1967.

Rendu-Osler-Weber syndrome
1. Wolper, J., and Laibson, P. R.: Hereditary hemorrhagic telangiectasis (Rendu-Osler-Weber disease) with filamentary keratitis, Arch. Ophthalmol. **81**:272-277, 1969.

Bonnet-Dechaume-Blanc syndrome
1. Bonnet, P. J., Dechaume, J., and Blanc, E.: L'Anévrysme cirsoïde de la rétine. (Anévrysme racémeux). Ses rélations avec l'anévrysme cirsoïde de la face et avec l'anévrysme cirsoïde du cerveau, J. Med. Lyon **18**:165-178, 1937.
2. Saraux, H., Le Besnerais, Y., Graveleau, Janet, L. G., and Chatellier, P.: Les formes atypiques du syndrome de Bonnet, Dechaume et Blanc, Bull. Mém. Soc. Fr. Ophtalmol. **80**:326-333, 1967.
3. Unger, H. H.: Zum Wyburn-Mason-Syndrome (angiomatose cirsoïde meningo-retino-faciale de Bonnet), Ber. Dtsch. Ophthalmol. Ges. **67**:418-420, 1965.

Weskamp-Cotlier-Gass nevo-oculocutaneous syndrome
1. Frasca, G., and Belmonte, M.: Angiomatosi neuro-cutanea e cheratocono; una nuova entità sindromica? Riv. Otoneurooftalmol. **41**:119-130, 1966.
2. Gass, J. D. M.: Cavernous hemangioma of the retina. A neuro-oculo-cutaneous syndrome, Am. J. Ophthalmol. **71**:799-814, 1971.

3. Mildner, I.: Kavernöse Hämangiome der Retina als Symptom einer Phakomatose, Ber. Dtsch. Ophthalmol. Ges. **71:**610, 1971.

BASAL CELL NEVUS SYNDROME

1. Herzberg, J. J., and Wiskemann, A.: Die fünfte Phakomatose. Basal-zellnaevus mit familiärer Belastung und Medulloblastom, Dermatologica **126:**106-123, 1963.
2. Laugier, P., Oppermann, A., and Pageaut, G.: Syndrome naevique a prédominance basocellulaire (5ᵉ phacomatose)? Ann. Dermatol. Syph. **93:**361-372, 1966.
3. Rater, C. J., Selke, A. C., and Van Epps, E. F.: Basel cell nevus syndrome, Am. J. Roentgenol. **103:**589-594, 1968.

WISKOTT-ALDRICH SYNDROME

1. Korting, G. W.: Lentiginosis profusa perigenito-axillaris, Z. Haut. Geschlechtskr. **42:**19-22, 1967.
2. Michalowski, R.: Naevus sébacé de Jadassohn—un état précancéreux, Dermatologica **124:**326-340, 1962.
3. Mills, S. D., and Winkelmann, R. K.: Eczema, thrombocytopenic purpura and recurring infections, A.M.A. Arch. Dermatol. **79:**446-472, 1959.
4. Podos, S. M., Einaugler, R. B., Albert, D. M., and Blaese, R. M.: Ophthalmic manifestations of the Wiskott-Aldrich syndrome, Arch. Ophthalmol. **82:**322-329, 1969.

ALOPECIA

1. Langhof, H., and Lemke, L.: Ophthalmologische Befunde bei Alopecia areata, Dermatol. Wochenschr. **146:**585-590, 1962.
2. Lemke, L.: Ophthalmologische Befunde bei der Alopecia areata, Klin. Monatsbl. Augenheilk. **144:**306, 1964.
3. Ludvig, J.: Tapetoretinale Degeneration mit totaler Alopezie bei Geschwistern, Österreichische Ophthalmologische Gesellschaft, 8 Jahreshauptversammlung 24 (bis):63-70, 1963.
4. Salamon, T., and Stojakovic, M.: Über einen Fall con Alopecia areata maligna bei einer Patientin mit Retinitis pigmentosa (tapetoretinale Degeneration) und anderen multiplen kongenitalen Anomalien, Z. Haut Geschlechtskr. **43:**267-272, 1968.

VOGT-KOYANAGI-HARADA SYNDROME

1. Bhatnagar, B. S., and Nahar, S.: Vogt-Koyanagi syndrome with optic neuritis, J. All-India Ophthalmol. Soc. **14:**128-130, 1966.
2. Cavara, V., and Bietti, G. B.: Manifestazioni oculari da virus e da rickettsie. Relazione al 39 Congresso della Società Oftalmologica d'Italia, Torino, 1952, Bologna, 1952, Casa Editrice Licinio Cappelli.
3. Diallo, J., Privat, Y., and Faye, I.: Syndrome de Vogt-Koyanagi-Harada chez une jeune femme noire; considérations nosologiques et étiopathogénetiques, Bull. Soc. Fr. Dermatol. Syphiligr. **75:**308-311, 1968.
4. Girard, P. T., Tommasi, M., Bonamour, G., and Garde, A.: Encéphalite nécrosante uvéite postérieure de Harada, aphtose scrotale, Rev. Neurol. **108:**13-22, 1963.
5. Haddad, N., M'Rad, R., Moins, J. H., and Stora, J.: Syndrome d'uvéo-névraxite Vogt-Koyanagi. (A propos d'un cas), Rev. Assoc. Med. Langue Fr. **3:**142-147, 1967.
6. Ikui, H., Furuyoshi, Y., Nakamizo, K., Sunigo, M., Onishi, T., and Ono, H.: Histopathological studies on cutaneous lesions in sympathetic ophthalmia and Vogt-Koyanagi-Harada Syndrome, Acta Soc. Ophthalmol. Jap. **65:**1057-1059, 1961.
7. Jacobson, J. H., Popkin, A., and Hirose, T.: The electroretinogram in Harada's disease, Am. J. Ophthalmol. **64:**1152-1154, 1967.
8. Kahan, A., Sztanojevits, A., Szabados, F., Vass, Z., and Szabo, M.: Pigmentautoaggression in der Pathogenese des Vogt-Koyanagi-Harada-Syndroms, Graefes Arch. Ophthalmol. **167:**246-264, 1964.
9. Manor, R. S.: Particular aspects of the Vogt-Koyanagi-Harada syndrome. Ophthalmologica **165:**425, 1972.
10. Seals, R. L., and Rise, E. N.: Vogt-Koyanagi-Harada syndrome, Arch. Otolaryngol. (Chicago) **86:**419-423, 1967.
11. Wilson, P.: Sympathetic ophthalmitis simulating Harada's disease, Br. J. Ophthalmol. **46:**626-628, 1962.

12. Yoshioka, H.: Early fundus changes in Harada's syndrome, Jap. J. Clin. Ophthalmol. **21:**135-141, 1967.

Focal dermal hypoplasia

1. Goltz, R. W., Peterson, W. C., and Goltz, R. W.: Focal dermal hypoplasia syndrome, Acta Derm. Venereol. **43:**421-440, 1963.
2. Gorlin, R. J., Meskin, L. H., Peterson, W. C., and Goltz, R. W.: Focal dermal hypoplasia syndrome, Acta Derm. Venereol. **43:**421-440, 1963.

Dyskeratosis congenita

1. Collier, M.: Les signes oculaires associés à l'aplasie cutanée circonscrite, Bull. Soc. Ophtalmol. Fr. **61:**191-195, 1961.
2. Reich, H.: Augenbeteiligung bei Dyskeratosis congenita (Zinsser-Cole-Engman-Syndrom), Klin. Monatsbl. Augenheilk. **161:**288, 1972.

Marfan's syndrome

1. Loveman, A. B., Gordon, A. M., Fliegelman, M. T.: Marfan's syndrome. Some cutaneous aspects, Arch. Dermatol. (Chicago) **87:**428-435, 1963.
2. Ramsey, M. S., Fine, B. S., and Shields, J. A.: The Marfan syndrome. A histopathology study of ocular findings, Am. J. Ophthalmol. **76:**102-116, 1973.
3. Wachtel, J. G.: The ocular pathology of Marfan's syndrome. Including a clinico-pathological correlation and an explanation of ectopia lentis, Arch. Ophthalmol. (Chicago) **76:**512-522, 1966.
4. Wollensak, J.: Syndroma Marfan und Homocystinurie, Ber. Dtsch. Ophthalmol. Ges. **68:** 404-407, 1967.

Bonnevie-Ullrich-Turner syndrome

1. Noonan, J. A.: Hypertelorism with Turner phenotype. A new syndrome with associated congenital heart disease, Am. J. Dis. Child. **116:**373-380, 1968.
2. Ullrich, O., and Fremerey-Dohna, H.: Dyskephalie mit Cataracta congenita und Hypotrichose als typischer Merkmalskomplex, Ophthalmologica **125:**73-90, 1953.
3. Zunin, C., and Mariotti, L.: Le anomalie oculari nello status Bonnevie-Ullrich, Ann. Ottalmol. Clin. Ocul. **79:**359-376, 1953.

Dyskeratosis palmoplantaris

1. Bardelli, A. M.: Distrofia corneale erpetiforme e cheratosi palmoplantare. Sindrome di Richner-Hanhart, Minerva Oftalmol. **8:**133-138, 1966.
2. Grayson, M.: Corneal manifestations of keratosis and palmaris, Am. J. Ophthalmol. **59:** 483-486, 1965.
3. Franceschetti, A., and Thier, C. J.: Über Hornhautdystrophien bei Genodermatosen unter besonderer Berücksichtigung der Palmoplantarkeratosen. (Klinische, genetische und histologische Studien), Graefes Arch. Ophthalmol. **162:**610-670, 1961.
4. Ventura, G., Biasini, G., and Petrozzi, M.: Cheratoma palmoplantare dissipatum associato a lesioni corneali in due fratelli, Boll. Oculist. **44:**497-510, 1965.
5. Westmore, R., and Billson, F. A.: Pseudoherpetic keratitis. Corneal changes in circumscribed palmoplantar keratoderma, Br. J. Ophthalmol. **57:**654, 1973.

Cockayne's syndrome

1. Brodrick, J. D., and Dark, A. J.: Corneal dystrophy in Cockayne's syndrome, Br. J. Ophthalmol. **57:**391-399, 1973.
2. Cockayne, E. A.: Dwarfism with retinal atrophy and deafness, Arch. Dis. Child. **11:**1, 1936.
3. Felgenhauer, W. R., and Ammann, F.: Syndrome de Cockayne fruste associé à la neurofibromatose de Recklinghausen, J. Genet. Hum. **16:**6-24, 1967.

Waardenburg-Klein syndrome

1. Bernabei, L., Pierangeli, C. E., Di Brino, M., and Baldisseri, L.: Sulla sindrome di Waardenburg, Otorinolaringol. Ital. **36:**333-347, 1968.
2. Cant, J. S., and Martin, A. J.: Waardenburg's syndrome. Report of a family, Br. J. Ophthalmol. **51:**755-759, 1967.
3. Fauci, A., and Jemma, S.: Sindrome di Waardenburg e Klein. Studio su di un ceppo familiare, Arch. Ottalmol. Clin. Ocul. **67:**345-358, 1963.

4. Hoffmann, D. H., and Schulze, U.: Zur Abgrenzung und genetischen Deutung des Van-der-Hoeve-Waardenburg-Syndroms, Klin. Monatsbl. Augenheilk. **151:**766, 1967.

5. Marx, P., and Bertrand, J.: Un cas de syndrome de Waardenburg, Bull. Soc. Ophtalmol. Fr. **68:**444-447, 1968.

6. Matsuyama, S., Miyagi, I., Tamura, H., Ohnuma, T., and Sugawara, H.: [A case of interoculo-irido-dermato-auditive syndrome (Waardenburg)] (In Japanese), Jap. J. Clin. Ophthalmol. **21:**643-647, 1967.

7. Rysenaer, L.: Le syndrome de Waardenburg, Acta Otorhinolaryngol. Belg. **21:**167-178, 1967.

DERMOCHONDROCORNEAL DYSTROPHY

1. Ardouin, M., Urvoy, M., and Bezier, J.: Dyscéphalie avec "tête d'oiseau," cataracte bilatérale et kératite en bandelette, Bull. Soc. Ophtalmol. Fr. **62:**438-442, 1962.

2. François, J.: Dystrophie dermo-chondro-cornéenne familiale, Ann. Ocul. (Paris) **182:** 409, 1949.

3. Paufique, L., Didierlaurent, A., Cotton, J. B., and Maugery, J.: Trois nouveaux cas de syndrome de François (dyscéphalie avec tête d'oiseau), Bull. Soc. Ophtalmol. Fr. **67:** 315-316, 1967.

4. Remky, H., and Engelbrecht, G.: Dystrophia dermo-chondro-cornealis (François), Klin. Monatsbl. Augenheilk. **151:**319-331, 1967.

CROUZON'S DISEASE

1. Bietti, G. B.: Forme rare ed atipiche di disostosi craniche e cranio-facciali con compli-canze oculari: acrocranio-aracnodattilia; disostosi cranio-facciali a carattere familiare ereditario (tipo Crouzon, tipo emifacio-craniosico ecc.) con sindattilia, Boll. Oculist. **24:** 83-136, 1945.

2. Crouzon, O.: Dysostose cranio-faciale héréditaire, Bull. Soc. Med. Hop. (Paris) **33:**545, 1912.

3. Gorlin, R. J., Chaudhry, A. P., and Moss, M. L.: Craniofacial dysostosis, patent ductus arteriosus, hypertrichosis, hypoplasia of labia majora, dental and eye anomalies—a new syndrome? J. Pediatr. **56:**778-785, 1960.

4. Iannone, D.: Disostosi cranio-faciale di Crouzon complicata, Riv. Patol. Clin. Sper. **22:** 45-57, 1967.

HALLERMANN-STREIFF-FRANÇOIS SYNDROME

1. Hallermann, W.: Vogelsicht und Cataracta, Klin. Monatsbl. Augenheilk. **113:**115, 1948.

2. Iuglio, N.: Su di un caso di sindrome di Hallermann e Streiff, nuova sindrome di Fran-çois, Ann. Ottalmol. Clin. Ocul. **93:**655-660, 1967.

3. Streiff, E. B.: Dysmorphie mandibulo-faciale (tête d'oiseau) et altérations oculaires, Ophthalmologica **120:**79, 1950.

4. Torres Marty, L., and Dolcet, L.: Sindrome de François-Hallermann-Streiff, Arch. Soc. Oftalmol. Hisp.-Amer. **24:**474-478, 1964.

TREACHER-COLLINS SYNDROME

1. Brehm, G.: Alopecie, Dysgammaglobulinaemie und mandibulo-faciale Dysostosis (Fran-ceschetti-Zwahlen), Aesthet. Med. (Berlin) **15:**226-229, 1966.

2. Franceschetti, A., Klein, D., Brocher, J. E. W., and Ammann, F.: Eine ausgeprägte Form der Dysmorphia cervico-oculofacialis (Wildervanck-Franceschetti-Klein), Acta Fac. Med. Univ. Brunen. **25:**53-61, 1965.

3. Morra, M.: Disostosi cranio-facciale e sublussazione del cristallino, Arch. Ottalmol. Clin. Ocul. **69:**15-21, 1967.

4. Saraux, H., and Besnainou, L.: Les syndromes maxillo-oculaires, Ann. Ocul. (Paris) **198:** 953-971, 1965.

5. Sartoris, A., and Busca, G. P.: La sindrome di Franceschetti-Zwahlen, Minerva Otorino-laringol. **16:**85-105, 1966.

6. Sugar, H. S., and Berman, M.: Relationship between the mandibulo-facial dysostosis syn-drome of Franceschetti and the oculo-auriculovertebral dysplasia syndrome of Goldenhar, Am. J. Ophthalmol. **66:**510-514, 1968.

PROGERIA

1. Arnould, G., Cordier, J., Tridon, P., Laxenaire, M., and Thiriet, M.: La progeria de l'adulte: syndrome de Werner, Rev. Otoneuroophtalmol. **38**:257-264, 1966.
2. Curth, H. O.: Progeria with erythema on hands and feet, parietal alopecia, congenital coloboma and osteoporosis, Arch. Dermatol. **60**:439-441, 1949.
3. Nemec, J., Jakubicek, R., and Malinsky, J.: Augenkomplikationen bei Progerie, Klin. Monatsbl. Augenheilk. **144**:308, 1964.
4. Wieser, D.: Zur Differentialdiagnose und ocularen Symptomatologie der Cutis marmorata teleangiectatica congenita und der Progerie, Ophthalmologica **143**:300-304, 1962.

EHLERS-DANLOS SYNDROME

1. Adriaenssens, A.: Le syndrome de Groenblad-Strandberg et la maladie d'Ehlers-Danlos, Ann. Ocul. (Paris) **198**:656-670, 1965.
2. Cordella, M., and Vinciguerra, E.: Le manifestazioni oculari nella sindrome di Ehlers-Danlos, Minerva Oftalmol. **8**:103-107, 1966.
3. Durham, D. G.: Cutis hyperelastica (Ehlers-Danlos syndrome) with blue scleras, microcornea, and glaucoma, Arch. Ophthalmol. **49**:220-221, 1953.
4. Goodman, R. M., Wooley, C. F., Frazier, R. L., and Covault, L.: Ehlers-Danlos syndrome occurring together with the Marfan syndrome. Report of a case with other family members affected, New Eng. J. Med. **273**:514-519, 1965.
5. Green, W. R., Friedman-Kien, A., and Banfield, W. G.: Angioid streaks in Ehlers-Danlos syndrome, Arch. Ophthalmol. **76**:197-204, 1966.
6. Hirthe, D., and Lindenhayn, K.: Ein Beitrag zum Ehlers-Danlos-Syndrome, Paediatr. Grenzgeb. **6**:213-223, 1967.
7. Modugno, G. C.: Sindrome di Ascher associata ad ipogenitalismo ed alterata eliminazione dei 17-chetosteroidi urinari, Boll. Oculist. **46**:400-405, 1967.
8. Pemberton, J. W., Freeman, H., and Schepens, C. L.: Familial retinal detachment and the Ehlers-Danlos syndrome, Arch. Ophthalmol. **76**:817-824, 1966.
9. Rahn, E. K., Falls, H. F., Knaggs, J. G., and Proux, D. J.: Leber's congenital amaurosis with an Ehlers-Danlos–like syndrome. Study on an American family, Arch. Ophthalmol. **79**:135-141, 1968.
10. Rozman, C., Jurado-Grau, J., and Elizalde, C.: Sindrome de Ehlers-Danlos con linfedema. Presentación familiar, Med. Clin. (Barcelona) **49**:237-242, 1967.
11. Scullica, L., and Masci, E.: Contributo alla conoscenza dell'associazione del cheratocono con alterazioni cutanee. (Sindrome di Ehlers-Danlos; neurodermite), Boll. Oculist. **41**:350-360, 1962.

MUCOPOLYSACCHARIDOSES

1. Breinin, G. M.: Scleredema adultorum. Ocular manifestations, Arch. Ophthalmol. **50**:155-162, 1953.
2. Danes, S. B., and Bearn, A.: Hurler's syndrome: A genetical study of clones in cell culture with particular reference to the Lyon hypothesis, J. Exp. Med. **126**:509-522, 1967.
3. Desvignes, P., Pouliquen, Y., Legras, M., and Guyot, J. D.: Aspect clinique, examen histologique et structural d'une cornée dystrophique de la maladie de Hurler, Bull. Mém. Soc. Fr. Ophtalmol. **80**:43-48, 1967.
4. Konstas, P., Ikonomou, A., Minas, B., and Tsitros, A.: Atypisches Hurler-Syndrom (Scheie's syndrom), Arch. Soc. Grèce Nord. **16**:111-118, 1967.
5. Sagnet, H., Morineaud, J. P., Revil, H., Thomas, J., and Marfert, Y.: A propos d'une observation de maladie de Hurler chez un enfant vietnamien. Commentaires sur les mucopolysaccharidoses, Ann. Pediatr. (Paris) **44**:136-140, 1968.
6. Steinbach, H. L., Preger, L., Williams, H. E., and Cohen, P.: The Hurler syndrome without abnormal mucopolysacchariduria, Radiology **90**:472-478, 1968.
7. Van Hoof, F., and Hers, H. G.: Mucopolysaccharidosis by absence of α-fucosidase, Lancet **1**:1198, 1968.
8. Watrin, J., Michon, P., and Michon, C.: Un cas de sclérœdème de Buschke, Bull. Soc. Fr. Dermatol. Syphiligr. **60**:349-352, 1953.

Syndermatotic cataracts

1. Alfano, J. E.: Ocular aspects of the maternal rubella syndrome. Trans. Am. Acad. Ophthalmol. Otolaryngol. **70:**235-266, 1966.
2. Algan, B.: "Atopic cataracte" et prurigo de Besnier. A propos d'une observation, Bull. Soc. Belge Ophtalmol. **124:**887-890, 1960.
3. Andogsky, N.: Cataracta dermatogenes. Beitrag zur Aetiologie der Linsentrübung, Klin. Monatsbl. Augenheilk. **52:**824-831, 1914.
4. Arrechea, A., Benzecry, E., and Zigaler, J. S.: Sindrome de Werner-Klinefelter, Arch. Oftalmol. Buenos Aires **41:**97-108, 1966.
5. Bellafiore, V., Giuffré, L., and Scialfa, A.: La sindrome di Rothmund. (Studio istologico cutaneo-lenticolare e citogenetico), Ann. Ottalmol. Clin. Ocul. **92:**394-407, 1966.
6. Bernard, P., Bernard, P., Lacourt, J., and De Rollat, G.: A propos d'un cas de cataracte dermatosique atopique, Ann. Ocul. (Paris) **199:**1068-1078, 1966.
7. Bertoni, G., and Lostia, A.: Sulla sindrome di Werner. Contributo clinico e istologico, Ann. Ottalmol. Clin. Ocul. **93:**1130-1144, 1967.
8. Blodi, F.: Cataracta syndermatotica bei Prurigo aestivalis, Acta Ophthalmologica **26:**379-384, 1948.
9. Brihaye, M., Dumoulin, P., Content, J., Dachy, A., and Nameche, J.: Etude virologique d'une embryopathie oculaire rubeoleuse, Bull. Soc. Belge Ophtalmol. **144:**878-899, 1966.
10. Cardarelli, J.: Congenital rubella syndrome: Clinical and virological studies, Can. J. Ophthalmol. **3:**213-217, 1968.
11. Castrow, F. F., II, and Beukelaer, M.: Congenital rubella syndrome; unusual cutaneous manifestations, Arch. Dermatol. **98:**260-262, 1968.
12. Collier, M.: Les modifications du cristallin chez les porteurs de psoriasis, Bull. Soc. Ophtalmol. Fr. **62:**59-65, 1962.
13. Cowan, A., and Klauder, J. V.: Frequency of occurrence of cataract in atopic dermatitis, Arch. Ophthalmol. **43:**759-768, 1950.
14. Daniel, R. K.: Alergía y cataratas (estudios adicionales), Semana Med. **107:**185-187, 1955.
15. De Bernardini, S. E.: Contributo allo studio delle cataratte sindermatotiche. Un caso tipico di sindrome di Werner, G. Ital. Oftalmol. **7:**3-10, 1954.
16. Degos, R., and Tchao, J. S.: Syndrome de Rothmund (dermite atrophique réticulée associée à une cataracte bilatérale précoce), Bull. Soc. Fr. Dermatol. Syphiligr. **56:**266-268, 1949.
17. Doak, P. B., and Eyre, K. E. D.: Werner's syndrome, N. Z. Med. J. **59:**574-577, 1960.
18. Franceschetti, A., and Carones, A. V.: Su di un caso di cheratocono familiare con neurodermite disseminata, cataratta, associato a dei sintomi di una displasia ectodermica. Con uno studio statistico sulla correlazione fra cheratocono e nevrodermite disseminata. G. Ital. Oftal. **13:**143-160, 1960.
19. Franceschetti, A., and Maeder, G.: Cataracte et affections cutanées du type poïkiloderme (syndrome de Rothmund) et du type sclérodermie (syndrome de Werner), Ophthalmologica **117:**196-198, 1949.
19a. Franceschetti, T. A.: Étude ophtalmologique génétique et biochimique de la maladie de Fabry, Chronica Dermatologica (Roma) **3-4:**369-591, 1973 (thesis no. 3346 of Geneva and Zurich).
20. François, J.: Syndromes with congenital cataract, Trans. Am. Acad. Ophthalmol. Otolaryngol. **64:**433-471, 1960.
21. García-Perez, A., et al.: La cataracta de la dermitis atopica, Rev. Clin. Esp. **115:**51-54, 1969.
22.. Gingrich, R. E., Jr., and Fusaro, R. M.: The lens and the skin. I. Common antigens of the skin and crystalline lens, J. Invest. Dermatol. **43:**235-236, 1964.
23. Gloria, E.: Cataratte sindermatotiche e xeroderma pigmentoso, Ann. Ottalmol. Clin. Ocul. **92:**436-450, 1966.
24. Gorgone, G., and Coriglione, G.: Anetodermia di Jadassohn con complicanze oculari. (Contributo clinico), Atti L. Congr. Soc. Oftalmol. Ital. Firenze **24:**373-380, 1967.

25. Heijer, A., and Reed, W. B.: Sjögren-Larsson syndrome. Congenital ichthyosis, spastic paralysis and oligophrenia, Arch. Dermatol. (Chicago) **92**:545-552, 1965.

26. Hermann, P.: La cataracte de l'embryopathie rubéoleuse, Sem. Med. Prof. Med. Soc. **38**:622-623, 1962.

27. Herz, M., and Łańcucki, J.: [Cataract in the course of prurigo. Report of six cases] (In Polish), Pol. Tyg. Lek. **18**:857-861, 1963.

28. Höpping, W.: Hautatrophie und Cataract, S.-B. Verein Rhein-Westfal. Augenaerzte (Klin. Monatsbl. Augenheilkd.) **146**:291, 1965.

29. Howell, J. B., Anderson, D. E., and McClendon, J. L.: The basal cell nevus syndrome, J.A.M.A. **190**:274-277, 1964.

30. Hughes, D. W. O'G., and Parkinson, R., et al.: The expanded congenital rubella syndrome. Report of two cases with neonatal purpura and review of the recent literature, Med. J. Aust. **1**:420-425, 1967.

31. Ingram, R. M.: Retinal detachment associated with atopic dermatitis and cataract, Br. J. Ophthalmol. **49**:96-97, 1965.

32. Janke, G.: Cataracta syndermatotica und Ichthyosis congenita, Klin. Monatsbl. Augenheilk. **117**:286, 1950.

33. Jütte, A., and Lemke, L.: Amotio-Katarakt-Keratoconus als okularer Symptomkomplex bei endogenem Ekzem, Klin. Monatsbl. Augenheilk. **147**:12-25, 1965.

34. Klemens, F.: Dermatose, Katarakt und Ablatio retinae, Klin. Monatsbl. Augenheilk. **140**:657-663, 1962.

35. Kózmińska, A., and Filipowicz-Banachowa, A.: [Atopic dermatitis, cataract and retinal detachment. A rare oculo-cutaneous syndrome] (In Polish), Przegl. Dermatol. **52**:589-592, 1965.

36. Krasnov, B. I., and Kamenetsky, I. C.: [Of the Werner's syndrome] (In Russian), Oftalmol. Zh. **22**:142-143, 1967.

37. Von Kugelberg, I.: Juvenile Katarakt bei Dermatosen. Cataracta syndermatotica, Klin. Monatsbl. Augenheilk. **92**:484-508, 1934.

38. Lebas, P.: Les syndromes oculo-cutanés, Bull. Soc. Belge Ophthalmol. **124**:1-837, 1960.

39. Leite, M., Vaz, F., and Vaz, B.: [Sindermatotic cataract] (In Portuguese), Rev. Brasil. Oftalmol. **31**:83-86, 1972.

40. Lyevre, J. J., and Levy, J. F.: A propos de la cataracte syndermatotique, Arch. Ophtalmol. (Paris) **26**:545-556, 1966.

41. Maeder, G.: Le syndrome de Rothmund et le syndrome de Werner, Ann. Ocul. (Paris) **182**:809-854, 1949.

42. Manna, F., and Jankowski, W.: [Biomicroscopic examination of the lens in psoriasis] (In Polish), Klin. Oczna **36**:371-374, 1966.

43. Marena, F.: Considerazioni cliniche su alcuni casi di cataratta atopica. Ann. Ottalmol. Clin. Ocul. **88**:513-522, 1962.

44. Menser, M. A., Dods, L., and Harley, J. D.: A twenty-five-year follow-up of congenital rubella, Lancet **67**(II):1347-1350, 1967.

45. Meyer, A.: [Alopecia and cataract] (In German), Ther. Umsch. **19**:497-502, 1962.

46. Monnet, P., Paufique, L., Salle, B., Rosenberg, D., Pasquier, N., and Picaud, S.: Syndrome familial associant cataracte, érythème télangiectasique des joues, nanisme sans retard osseux, amyotrophie des extrémités et implantation proximale du pouce, Bull. Soc. Ophtalmol. Fr. **68**:677-678, 1968.

47. Müller, S. A., and Brunsting, L. A.: Cataracts associated with dermatologic disorders, Arch. Dermatol. **88**:330-339, 1963.

48. Müller, S. A., and Winkelmann, R. K.: Cataracts in alopecia areata. Report of five cases, Arch. Dermatol. **88**:202-206, 1963.

49. Nordmann, J., and Gerhard, J.-P.: Cataracte "atopique" et troubles endocriniens, Bull. Soc. Ophtalmol. Fr. **66**:1233-1238, 1966.

50. Ostfeld, I., Mitrea, N., and Achim, D.: [Xeroderma pigmentosum and cataract] (In Rumanian), Oftalmologia (Bucuresti) **12**:153-156, 1968.

51. Paufique, L., Ravault, M.-P., Moulin, G., and Bonnet-Géhin: Cataracte et ichthyose congénitale, Bull. Soc. Ophtalmol. Fr. **63**:240-241, 1963.

52. Petersen, H. P.: Teleangiectasias and cataract, Acta Ophthalmol. (Kbh.) **32:**565-571, 1954.
53. Pinkerton, O. D.: Cataract associated with congenital ichthyosis, Arch. Ophthalmol. **60:**393-396, 1958.
54. Reid, R. R., Murphy, A. M., Gillespie, A. M., et al.: Isolation of rubella virus from congenital cataracts removed at operation, Med. J. Aust. **1:**540-542, 1966.
55. Ring, C. C.: Atopic dermatitis with cataracts. A report of three cases, one with keratoconus, Trans. Ophthalmol. Soc. N. Z. **10:**41-47, 1958.
56. Rook, A., Davis, R., and Stevanovic, D.: Poikiloderma congenitale. Rothmund-Thomson syndrome, Acta Derm. Venereol. (Stockh.) **39:**392-420, 1959.
57. Roy, F. H., Fuste, F., et al.: The congenital rubella syndrome with virus recovery. Ocular pathology and literature review, Am. J. Ophthalmol. **62:**222-232, 1966.
58. Roy, F. H., Hiatt, R. L., Korones, S. B., and Roane, J.: Ocular manifestations of congenital rubella syndrome; recovery of virus from affected infants, Arch. Ophthalmol. (Chicago) **75:**601-607, 1966.
59. Rubenstein, R. A., and Eggleston, T. F.: Congenital cataracts associated with congenital ichthyosiform erythroderma, J. Pediatr. Ophthalmol. **2:**53-56, 1965.
60. Schultheisz, E., and Schultheisz, F.: Zwei Fälle von Werner-Syndrom, Wien. Klin. Wochenschr. **68:**855-857, 1956.
61. Scialdone, D., and Artifoni, E.: Un insolito quadro di dermopatia pigmentaria associato a retinite pigmentosa, cataratta e sordità congenite, oligofrenia ed atassia cerebellare, G. Ital. Oftalmol. **17:**49-60, 1964.
62. Selzer, G.: Rubella in pregnancy. Virus isolation and inclusion bodies, South Afr. J. Obstet. Gynaecol. **2:**5-9, 1964.
63. Shukla, B., Srivastava, S. P., and Jain, S. C.: Unilateral vitiligo iridis, Br. J. Ophthalmol. **50:**436-437, 1966.
64. Silver, H. K.: Rothmund-Thomson syndrome: an oculo-cutaneous disorder, Am. J. Dis. Child. **111:**182-190, 1966.
65. Singh, G., and Mathur, J. S.: Atopic erythroderma with bilateral cataract, unilateral keratoconus and undescended testes, Br. J. Ophthalmol. **52:**61-63, 1968.
66. Sprafke, H.: Cataracta juvenilis syndermatotica, Dermatol. Wochenschr. **152:**928-932, 1966.
67. Summerly, R., et al.: Alopecia areata and cataract, Arch. Dermatol. **93:**411-412, 1965.
68. Szewczykowa-Bocheńska, N., and Łańcucki, J.: [Cataracta dermatogenes, Andogsky's syndrome] (In Polish), Klin. Oczna **36:**375-378, 1966.
69. Suzi, V. P., Lal, H., et al.: Werner's syndrome, J. Indian Med. Assoc. **47:**34-36, 1966.
70. Tamura, H., and Uemura, Y.: A case report of the comedo-cataract syndrome, Acta Soc. Ophthalmol. Jap. **73:**738-744, 1969.
71. Thiel, H. J., Manzke, H., and Gunschera, H.: Katarakt bei Chondrodystrophia calcificans connata (Conradi-Hunermann-Syndrom), Klin. Monatsbl. Augenheilk. **154:**536-545, 1969.
72. Trénel, M., and Prieur, M.: Alopécie congénitale familiale héréditaire avec cataracte précoce, Rev. Neurol. **2:**561, 1930.
73. Vlad, P., Mirodon, E., and Mitrea, N.: [A case of dermatogenic cataract] (In Rumanian), Oftalmologia (Bucuresti) **9:**335-338, 1965.
74. Wahl, J. W., and Ellis, P. P.: Rothmund-Thomson syndrome, Am. J. Ophthalmol. **60:**722-726, 1965.
75. Weill, G., and Nordmann, J.: La cataracte et ses rapports avec la pathologie générale, Ann. Ocul. (Paris) **163:**401-421, 1926.
76. Whyte, H. J.: Unilateral comedo naevus and cataract, Arch. Dermatol. **97:**533-535, 1968.
77. Zaun, H.: Zur Kenntnis des Werner-Syndroms, Med. Welt **62:**2725-2727, 1962.
78. Zimmermann, L. E.: Histopathologic basis for ocular manifestations of congenital rubella syndrome, Am. J. Ophthalmol. **65:**837-862, 1968.
79. Zoldan, T.: Su di un caso di cataratta in associazione a lichen follicolare cheratosico atrofizzante, Boll. Oculist. **41:**613-616, 1962.
80. Zucker-Franklin, D., Rifkin, H., and Jacobson, H. G.: Werner's syndrome. An analysis of ten cases, Geriatrics **23**(8):123-135, 1968.

Ocular involvement in dermatologic disease

CHAIRMAN: **Frederick C. Blodi***

Dr. Blodi: While you bring the written questions forward to the podium, I would like to ask Professor Ramalho from Portugal to say a few words about Behçet's disease.

Dr. Ramalho: Many systemic diseases and syndromes affect simultaneously the eyes, skin, and mucous membranes as we have seen in different papers in this symposium. Behçet's disease is well known for its multiple manifestations affecting various organs and tissues of the body, besides the skin, the mucous membranes, the eyes, the central nervous system, and the joints. Reports of involvement of other sites have been published.

Although it is claimed to be of probable viral origin, its etiology is still not known. Our studies with electron microscopy using various staining techniques in the specimens of skin lesions failed to show any suggestions of virus particles.

The clinical evolution of the disease is variable and presents multiple forms. It can be self-limiting, or on the contrary it can progress with periods of remission during months and years, involving seriously and fatally the central nervous system.

It usually affects young males, between 24 and 35 years of age. It is a rare disease, although more commonly seen in Mediterranean countries and in Japan where about 30% of all uveitis are thought to be Behçet's disease. Since it presents usually with variable and different symptoms with rather slow progression, sometimes with long periods of remission, it can be difficult to diagnose in the beginning, especially when all the typical aspects are not present.

Usually the dermotologic component is seen first and consists of aphthous ulcers in the mucosa of the mouth and genital area (tongue, lips, vagina, and scrotum) and erythema nodosum (Figs. 1 and 2, *A*). Although classically it is said to cause anterior uveitis with relapsing hypopion (iridocyclitis) in the eyes, we, like other investigators, have often seen retinal vasculitis (migrating phlebitis, Fig. 2, *B* and *C*), optic neuritis (Fig. 4, *C*), central serous chorioretinitis (Fig. 3, *A* and *B*), juxtapapillary chorioretinitis (Fig. 3, *C*), episcleritis (Fig. 4, *A*), central retinal vein thrombosis (phlebitis), and ocular

*Department of Ophthalmology, University of Iowa College of Medicine, Iowa City, Iowa.

muscle involvement (palsies with diplopia and ptosis). We have also noticed, as an early sign in the ocular fundus, vitreous haze with dilatation of retinal venules (Figs. 4, *B* and *C*). On fluorescein angiography in late stages of transit, leakage of the dye at the disk area and geographic pigment epithelium disturbances in the retina were seen (Fig. 5). Enlargement of blindspots and central scotomas were also found in our studies. Secondary glaucoma after central vein thrombosis was seen in one of our patients as an initial symptom. Later he developed typical skin and mucous membrane involvement and hypopion uveitis. At last his central nervous system was affected by showing signs and involvement of vital brain centers. He died about 3 years after starting his first complaints, with convulsions and coma.

Neurologic symptoms involving brain and meninges are normally seen only in the later stages and can prove fatal when progressively causing damage to the vital centers. In our studies we have found meningeal signs with intracranial hypertension; focal signs as diplopia and ptosis (III, IV, and VI), hemiparesis, quadriparesis, involvement of respiration, deglutition, and speech centers; other focal palsies; convulsions; and coma. Behavior changes and mental abnormalities with hypereuphoria, which was conflicting with the general state of health, were also recorded in two of our cases.

General symptoms and signs such as fever, malaise, myalgia, and arthritis affecting different joints were also present. Biopsies taken from synovial tissue during exacerbation periods showed nonspecific inflammatory changes in our specimens. Electron microscopy studies carried on the specimens of the skin lesions in our patients, using the standard procedures showed thickening of the

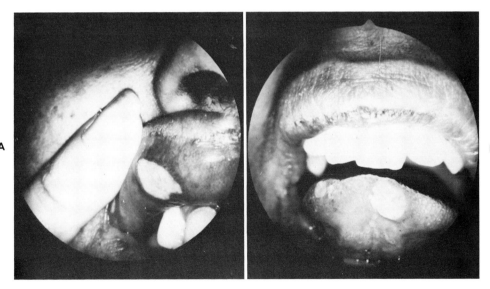

A   B

Fig. 1. A, Aphthous ulcer of upper lip, during period of exacerbation on 35-year-old woman with Behçet's disease. **B,** Two ulcers on tip of tongue of same patient as in **A,** during the acute phase with high fever, hyperleukocytosis, and high sedimentation rate in premenstrual period. Note filiform papillae at tip of tongue.

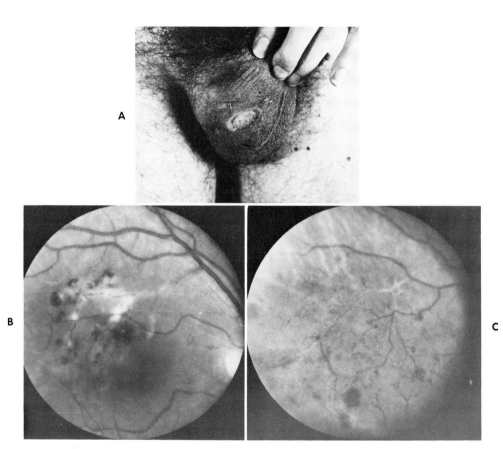

Fig. 2. A, Large scrotal ulcer in 24-year-old male patient with Behçet's disease. He also had aphthous ulceration in his mouth. **B,** Right fundus photograph of same patient as in **A,** showing phlebitis of macular branch of superior temporal venule. **C,** Same fundus 6 months later showing further involvement of venules, now more temporally (phlebitis migrans).

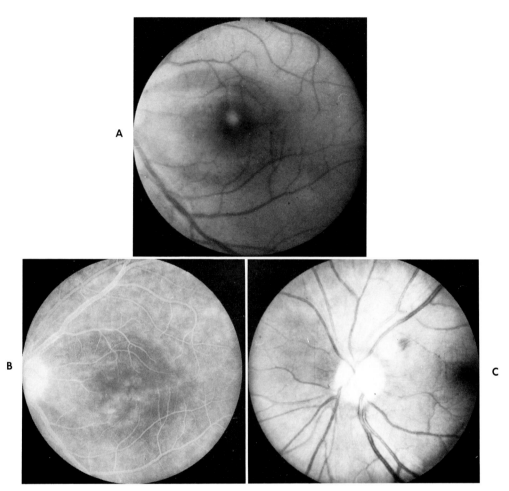

Fig. 3. A, Left fundus of young man of 27 years of age, showing macular edema with great reduction of vision (4/20) and central scotoma. **B,** Fluorescein angiography of same retina as in **A,** 76 seconds after injection of sodium fluorescein, showing leaking spots at macular area (central serous retinopathy). Note also increased fluorescence of disk and staining of venular walls (superior temporal). **C,** Right fundus of same patient 7 months later, showing juxtapapillary chorioretinitis.

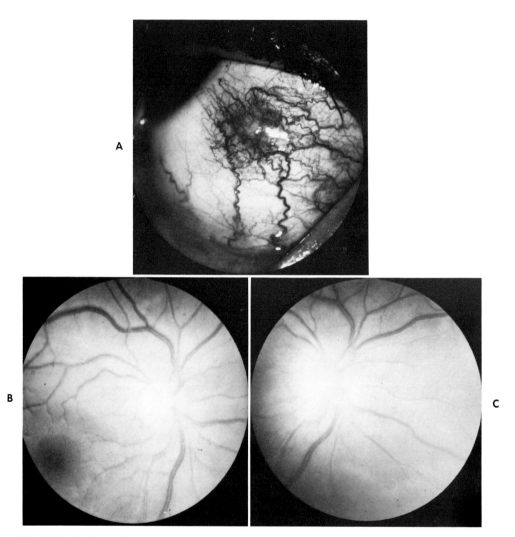

Fig. 4. A, Left eye showing nodule of episcleritis during one of the periods of exacerbation. **B,** Right fundus showing venous dilatation of same patient. Vision was 20/20 in both eyes. **C,** Two months later showing optic neuritis (papilledema) and vitreous haze.

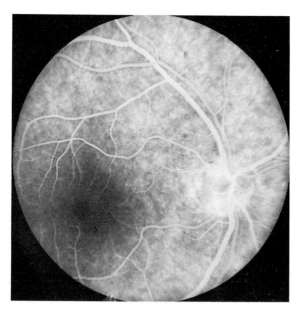

Fig. 5. Right fundus fluorescein photography (late stage, 73 seconds), showing slight dye leakage at disk area and geographic mottled appearance in the whole retina (pigment epithelium disturbance).

vascular wall mainly because of the multilamination of the basal membrane and swelling of endothelial cells. There was also a separation of the cellular elements with infiltration of leukocytes in the wall of the blood vessels. At the beginning, involvement of the skin and the mucous membranes is usual. Its progression can be slow, taking sometimes months or even years before it affects the eyes, when the diagnosis is easy. Arthritis and fever can be the starting complaints in some instances. High white blood cell count and high sedimentation rate were often observed during the exacerbation periods. The nonspecific pustule formation in the skin within 24 to 48 hours at the sight of sterile needle puncture is almost pathognomonic. All our patients had a positive skin test. At least two main components of the syndrome must be present in order to have the diagnosis made. Dermatologic symptoms were always present (in all the cases) on our patients and similarly ocular involvement. In one instance the only ocular involvement was the recurrent ocular palsies (extrinsic ocular muscles) with diplopia.

The treatment of the disease has been difficult and nonrewarding in the long run. Steroids and other anti-inflammatory drugs usually give relief during the acute phases, but do not seem to arrest the progression and the natural course of the disease in most instances. Chloroquine type of anti-inflammatory agents and immunosuppressive drugs have been tried without great success. We have lately been trying, with success, long-acting ACTH (depot),* gamma globulins, vasodilators, and plasma expanders during the acute stages of vital center involvement in the central nervous system.

*In acute intracranial hypertension, heavy doses of intravenous dexamethasone with hypertonic mannitol have been used.

During the last few years we have been interested in Behcet's disease and have already reported some of our results on clinical findings, microcirculation and fluorographic aspects in the retina, vascular permeability, and ultrastructural changes. All our reported patients were young males as usual, except one 35-year-old woman who started with dermatologic symptoms (ulcers in the mouth, tongue, lips, and vagina). Later she was admitted to the hospital with high fever of unknown etiology. This patient's exacerbations coincided with her menstrual periods. All her mucocutaneous and other symptoms and signs showed regression soon after the menstrual periods. This type of periodicity, although reported by some authors, is neither sufficiently stressed nor properly studied. This patient also showed small red spots in the nail bed of her fingers, during the acute phases. Preliminary studies carried on this patient suggested vascular permeability changes in the retina and in the brain (rupture of blood-retina and blood-brain barriers). Fluorescein angiography in her retina showed dye leakage in the disk area and vascular wall staining. Plasma and cerebrospinal fluid protein and immunoglobulin studies (electroimmunodiffusion [Schuller]) suggested an increase of permeability of cerebral blood vessels during the periods of exacerbation. Total proteins are raised in cerebrospinal fluid, especially during the periods of exacerbation. Absolute values of total albumins, alpha$_2$ and gamma globulins are also increased in the cerebrospinal fluid during acute phases of the disease. Urinary excretion of pregnanediol and plasma progesterone levels were found to be on the lower side in the second half of the menstrual cycle. No changes of estrogens, gonadotropins, pregnanediol, and plasma progesterone were noticed in the first half of the cycle. These changes should be further investigated in order to understand better the relationship between the hormonal activity and the exacerbation of symptoms. It is well known that certain synthetic progesterone-like substances have a strong anti-inflammatory activity. On the other hand Behçet's disease is rarely seen in females. It affects usually young males.

Although the etiology of this disease is not yet known, it is a well accepted fact that the multiple manifestations in the eyes, skin, mucous membranes, nervous system, joints, and various other organs are associated with pronounced vascular changes. Initially these changes are functional (permeability to fluorescein in the retina) without any visible lesions, and only later there is an organic and visible vasculitis (phlebitis usually) with edema multilamination of basal membrane infiltration of vascular wall with leukocytes and occlusion of the lumen. This systemic vascular involvement (diffuse vasculitis) with oculomucocutaneous and visceral manifestations look similar to that seen in the collagen type of disease.

Dr. Blodi: Dr. Zahoruk has two questions.

Dr. Zahoruk: Either one of the panelists on dermatology and perhaps Dr. Halasa might give me some help here. I recently saw a child about 2 weeks old with a capillary hemangioma of the face. Now my question in regard to this patient is, Are we to call it a Sturge-Weber disease just on the basis of this hemangioma alone or do we have to have the neurologic signs? At the moment there are no EEG changes and there are no ocular lesions. My question basically with regards to this case is, When do you call it a Sturge-Weber syndrome?

Dr. Perry: I believe that one must appreciate that the Sturge-Weber syndrome is that of a nevus flammeus with, at times, involvement of the cerebral substance. I believe one must think in terms of a syndrome here rather than of specific diagnostic criteria. The patient may be involved minimally or more extensively. In this particular patient, who is only 2 weeks of age, I would not be so certain. Because there are no cerebral involvements at this time, it does not mean that they will not occur in the future, and one must wait a period of time. You should be aware, however, that the mental deterioration seems to bear little relationship to the degree of cerebral calcification that can occur. I believe that under these circumstances this patient with the unilateral nevus flammeus is the prototype of a Sturge-Weber syndrome. The lesion may not develop all of the manifestations, but I think this patient must be followed for a period of time to know just what is going to develop. I am inclined to say, even at this stage, that this is a Sturge-Weber syndrome until proved otherwise. I would not just dismiss this case as a simple nevus flammeus of the skin.

Dr. Zahoruk: The next case is the 5-year-old daughter of one of our medical students. The mother said her daughter could have some serious systemic disease because she was always rubbing her eyes and there were ecchymotic areas under both lower lids. When I looked at the upper lid, I could see red spots between the cilia. Is this pediculosis? Apparently these are the excreta. The excreta are red because the lice suck blood. My question in regard to this patient is, How do you treat the ocular manifestations of pediculosis?

Dr. Blodi: The second question obviously should be answered by somebody who comes from an area where they have the most experience with pediculosis.

Dr. Knox: I did not know that I came to Iowa to learn that. That the dermatologist from the Mayo Clinic has seen so much of this was rather surprising in view of the article in *Time* magazine about clean Minnesota! Somehow in the back of my mind we hear about using pilocarpine ointment on the eyelids for pediculosis. This was something taught to me during my residency. But since I left the army, I have not had occasion to see a case.

Dr. Blodi: Dr. Perry, does Crohn's disease occur with psoriasis?

Dr. Perry: I do not recall Crohn's disease being particularly associated with psoriasis, but psoriasis is such a common disease that I would not be surprised if it did occur. Ordinarily the cutaneous signs of Crohn's are peculiar ulcerations around the anal area. They consist of peripapillary, vegetating lesions in the anogenital area, a folliculitis, but not commonly psoriasis that I am aware of. The British have reported on the association of cutaneous periarteritis with Crohn's disease so that one must be aware of this finding.

Dr. Blodi: Professor Bietti, one question, we can ask you. One aspect of this subject is not too well known in the Western hemisphere that you pointed out on your tables, and that aspect is the association of atopic dermatitis with two eye conditions: one is vernal catarrh and the other one is keratoconus. Now are these associations causally connected, and how come you see them so often and we don't?

Dr. Bietti: I am happy you have put this question to me because this association of vernal catarrh with keratoconus (leaving aside atopic dermatitis) was first described by Gonzalez, a Mexican ophthalmologist, in 1904. He considered that keratoconus was a secondary occurrence. There was a weakening of the cornea, and therefore there was a secondary ectasia. So, we did research in central and southern Italy where vernal catarrh is rather frequent. We made a statistical analysis of the occurrence of the two together—keratoconus and vernal catarrh—and we found that there was a reliable, significant association, not an occasional one. Recently somebody in South America said that they found the same as we did, a statistical reliability of this association. But they went back to the idea of Gonzalez. I disagree completely with their interpretation, and the fact that in atopic dermatitis you may have both keratoconus or vernal catarrh shows that there is a common cause for the two or that there is a common disposition. We had a family of two brothers, one was affected by keratoconus and the other one by vernal catarrh without keratoconus. Therefore, the two manifestations are parallel manifestations of a single predisposition. The keratoconus is not a secondary manifestation of vernal catarrh. By the way, we see many, many cases of slight vernal catarrh that have no corneal involvement and later develop a keratoconus. This is an additional fact to be remembered.

19

Systemic disease and the eye: implications for research and clinical diagnosis

Frank W. Newell

The assignment today is a little anomalous. I find this so because I had not seen the papers of earlier speakers and did not know what they were going to say until I had the pleasure of listening. Presumably, though, anything that I do not understand should be classed as an implication for more research. Anything that appears applicable to the diagnosis and management of a patient should be designated as an implication for clinical practice.

Professor Bean's opening remarks reflect his unique position in American medicine as a historian, a sensitive observer of the passing scene, and chief editor of the *Archives of Internal Medicine*. Surely as a worthy literary successor to William Osler, it is appropriate that he be designated the Osler Professor.

I thought that ophthalmic history was too briefly encapsulated in passing from Bacon to Donders to deaf-mutes to eye, ear, nose, and throat practice. In the university in which the department of ophthalmology is headed by Professor Frederick Blodi, a graduate of the University of Vienna, it is worth noting that the first chair of ophthalmology was established in Vienna in 1733. However, ophthalmology, and indeed most older specialties, developed in the United States in a manner quite different from that in Europe. With our historic emphasis upon the equality of man, it was considered inappropriate in the early United States that any physician designate himself as more able to treat a particular disease than his fellow physician. Thus it was considered unethical to designate oneself a specialist long after specialism was established in Europe.

Although eye hospitals were established in the United States in the 1820's, shortly after the hospitals stimulated by the spread of trachoma acquired in Napoleon's Egyptian campaign necessitated similar hospitals in Europe, ophthalmology did not emerge as a definite specialty until shortly after the Civil War. Despite this, the first national ophthalmic society was established in the

These studies were supported in part by Grants EY-00523 and RR-51 from National Institutes of Health, U. S. Public Health Service.

423

United States in 1864. Many of the founding and early members of the American Ophthalmological Society were surgeons who did not restrict themselves to ophthalmology. Several years ago, when he was guest of honor of the American Academy of Ophthalmology and Otolaryngology, Vail[5] pointed out that the combination of eye and ear, nose, and throat as a specialty emerged at the end of the nineteenth century, mainly as a midwestern phenomenon.

I share with Professor Bean the sense of disservice that sometimes occurs between ophthalmology and medicine and between specialties and medicine. Some of this ophthalmic disservice may arise because many ophthalmologists provide the services of a primary physician and see many patients who do not have a family physician. Additionally, because of the predilection of certain disorders to cause predominantly ocular symptoms, many ophthalmologists have become skilled in esoteric areas: toxoplasmosis, ectopic calcification, and uncommon metabolic diseases. Thus, sometimes when we seek the skills of our friends in medicine for help in the management of these abnormalities, we find that we do not share common concepts concerning their management.

I believe that many ophthalmologists fail their patients when they observe signs of vascular hypertension or the signs of localized arteriosclerosis. Management is sometimes difficult, inasmuch as the patient is often seeking correction of an ocular defect, has no systemic symptoms, and is unwilling to undergo the laboratory and diagnostic studies required to clarify the abnormality. Sometimes, too, the ocular changes are so subtle that the internist discounts the ophthalmologist's finding, and an exceptional opportunity to correct a disease in its first stages is missed.

The many formal reports from the University of Iowa indicate that a successful collaboration in the investigation of disease by the departments of medicine and ophthalmology is possible and that a most beneficial association may be arranged.

As I attempt to encapsulate the messages of 18 speakers discussing 10 topics, I recall particularly Garrod's 1906 statement "to treasure the exceptional" and Pope's earlier statement, "The proper study of man is man." I am impressed that the speakers during the past 3 days emphasized strongly the similarity between hereditary and acquired disease so that their distinction becomes less and less possible. Thus conditions that we often regard as acquired are modified greatly by the genetic background of the individual, and environmental and physical factors may play a major role in the manifestations of hereditary diseases. This viewpoint I believe was particularly emphasized in the consideration of rheumatic diseases and the discussion of obvious hereditary diseases by Dr. Fredrickson and Dr. Podos.

Dr. Fredrickson indicated the unusual value of fibroblast cultures in the diagnosis of a number of metabolic diseases. Each of us who has facilities for this work feels fortunate in that once the fibroblasts are available, it is possible to return to studies years later and do tests that were not available when the cells were initially acquired. This provides some patients with an unusual immortality inasmuch as the individual may die, but his fibroblast cultures remain available. Thus, although there may have been but one or two instances of the abnormality described, the researcher is able to continue his studies concerning the enzymatic defect even though the patient cannot be seen. (Workers in these fields are extremely interested in children with rare metabolic disorders and will go to exceptional lengths to assist the clinician in studies.)

The outline Dr. Fredrickson provided dividing hereditary diseases into those involving connective tissue, elastic tissue, and collagen tissue disorders emphasizes the difficulties associated in studying these disorders. Thus, one finds that connective tissue abnormalities merge into abnormalities of the lysosomal hydrolases and then into other biochemical disorders.

Both Dr. Podos and Dr. Fredrickson emphasized the importance of studying every child with congenital cataracts for galactose transferase (galactose-1-phosphate uridyl transferase) deficiency. The cataract caused by deficiency of galactose transferase is much less severe than that caused by a deficiency of galactose kinase. The kinase cataract tends to resemble concentric rings and does not have the snowflake appearance of transferase deficiency.*

The amino acid abnormalities for the most part involve the metabolism of phenylalanine. Because of the role of this amino acid in melanin synthesis, children with these disorders often have very little skin pigmentation and tend to be blond with rosy cheeks.

The ocular involvement in ochronosis should present little diagnostic difficulty, although the ophthalmologist must consider symmetric nevi, scleral nerve loops, or premature senile scleral plaque. One problem arises in that the typical black appearance of alkaptonuric urine does not occur until the urine sample oxidizes, a reaction that takes several hours to occur.

Pronounced albinism presents the ophthalmologist with no particular problem when he observes the individual with nystagmus, bilateral reduced vision, and a conspicuous choroidal circulation. I think, though, that ophthalmologists sometimes fail to appreciate that less severe albinism might be responsible for minor degrees of bilateral reduction in vision. All of us should be aware that the nystagmus is less severe for near than for far sight, and although distance vision may be greatly reduced, vision for near is often good enough to permit schooling with normally sighted children. Studies on tyrosinase of hair follicles provide us with information as to which individual is going to develop pigmentation later in life. This increase in pigmentation may be associated with an improvement in vision and decreased nystagmus.

Information concerning mucopolysaccharidosis has increased enormously in recent years. Although gargoylism was described many years ago, it was only in 1954 that the involvement of the mucopolysaccharides was recognized. Sometime after that, the abnormal excretion of mucopolysaccharides in the urine was found to provide us with a sensitive screening test. The diagnosis of Hurler and the Hunter types of mucopolysaccharidosis was always fairly simple, but since those early reports at least seven different types of mucopolysaccharidosis have been described. Additional types based upon results when tissue cultures of different individuals are mixed seem to be emerging. In gargoylism, the opacification of

---

*Assays for galactose kinase activities may be obtained from Dr. Ernest Beutler, City of Hope Medical Center, 1500 East Duarte Road, Duarte, California 91010. Full instructions are contained in Am. J. Ophthalmol. **77:**291, 1974.

the cornea seems to be more noticeable centrally than peripherally, yet on histologic studies, the main storage is in the peripheral cornea. The deposits in the corneal endothelium, the iris, and the ciliary body have not been emphasized. The defects in the ganglion cell layer of the retina were described many years ago, but, additionally, there appears to be a disorder of the retinal pigment epithelium deserving further study.

The clinical changes in these children are becoming increasingly well recognized at autopsy and an accumulation of gangliosides and mucopolysaccharides is found responsible for the papilledema sometimes seen. Although the ganglioside was earlier believed to be an incidental finding occurring in degenerated nervous tissue, it now seems to be related to lysosomal hydrolase deficiencies as occurs in Tay-Sachs disease.

The concentration of gangliosides in the brains of individuals dying with mucopolysaccharidosis links these disorders to those characterized by cherry-red spots at the fovea. A large number of studies have become available since O'Brien[3] indicated a deficiency of hexosaminidase in Tay-Sachs disease in 1970. Since then, we have seen the whole pattern of enzyme defects described with deficiencies of hexosamidase A and B, a deficiency of hexosamidase A only, and a deficiency of hexosamidase B solely. A Tay-Sachs disease league has been formed, and testing is available so that two heterozygotes for this gene do not marry and run the one in four risk of having a homozygote infant. Inasmuch as the prevalence of this gene is probably 1 in 30 in those of East European Jewish background, the testing should be encouraged.

Ophthalmologists must be alerted to the importance of treating Wilson's disease at the first sign of a Kayser-Fleischer ring, even though hepatic and neurologic complications have not yet occurred. This disorder may have its onset with predominantly ocular hepatic or central nervous system disorders. It is often possible to prevent deterioration and progression by the use of penicillamine. It is thus not fair to ignore the ocular sign when we observe it even though other changes have not yet occurred.

The vortex pattern that develops in the carriers of Fabry's disease is of unusual interest. Earlier this was diagnosed as Fleischer's corneal dystrophy. Additionally, the pattern of deposition of chloroquine in the cornea gives rise to nearly the same appearance, except that it disappears when chloroquine is discontinued. Recognition of this disorder is of importance to the offspring, inasmuch as early renal transplant appears to be beneficial.

Fredrickson's description of lipid disorders emphasized the association of hereditary and secondary types. We in ophthalmology are in a particularly key position to insist on studies of cholesterol and of triglycerides and to obtain lipoprotein electrophoresis in patients with xanthelasma, lipemia retinalis, or corneal arcus occurring in youthful patients.

Ophthalmologists tend to think most commonly of lipemia retinalis as occurring in diabetic acidosis, but it also occurs in type IV hyperlipidemia, a group of individuals who are exquisitely sensitive to an increase in blood triglycerides.

Earlier in this meeting, a participant asked if it were not expensive and unrewarding to measure cholesterol and triglycerides in patients with xanthelasma, corneal arcus, and other ophthalmic indications of disturbed lipid metabolism.

The tests may be costly, though not extremely so, but they are unusually rewarding. Costs are reduced if one limits lipoprotein electrophoresis to those patients who have elevated levels of cholesterol or triglycerides, or whose plasma sample becomes turbid with standing. Dietary control of the secondary hyperlipidemias is well worthwhile and may minimize subsequent cardiovascular and cerebral vascular disease.

Dr. Bole's classification of rheumatoid disease appears unusually useful and was complemented beautifully by Dr. Kearn's clinical presentation. Dr. Bole provided us with the diagnostic categories of the American Rheumatism Association, which closely parallels any classification a group of ophthalmologists would develop for etiologic factors in uveitis. Dr. Kearns emphasized the absence of systemic disease in episcleritis and contrasted it with the some 70% of patients with scleritis associated with rheumatoid arthritis. This observation should be coupled with Dr. Bole's statement that seronegative rheumatoid arthritis is seldom associated with systemic signs, whereas seropositive arthritis is often associated with complications.

The unusual value of penicillamine in the management of scleromalacia perforans should be emphasized. The surgical treatment of scleromalacia perforans is complicated by conjunctival necrosis. Thus, as long as the sclera is covered with conjunctiva, the disease, though serious, is not disastrous. Once the conjunctiva erodes, the scleral defect rapidly progresses. A scleral graft in such eyes is foredoomed to failure because of the absence of conjunctiva. Successful surgery must be carried out therefore relatively early in the disease but only when one is certain that it will not be medically arrested.

I sense that internists and ophthalmologists do not discuss the same entity in considering Sjögren's disease. The internist knows it to be a most serious generalized abnormality with an unusual number of systemic changes involving almost every organ and sometimes progressing to fatal lymphomas. The ophthalmologist often tends to equate Sjögren's syndrome with elderly patients with a mild keratoconjunctivitis sicca. These patients do not have autoantibodies and are not troubled with a dry mouth, and if they have rheumatoid arthritis, it is extremely mild. They do not develop the systemic complications of Sjögren's disease and may well have nothing more severe than senile atrophy of lacrimal function. Filamentary keratitis occurring in some eyes after cataract extractions should be mentioned inasmuch as it may be mistaken for that occurring in keratoconjunctivitis sicca. The superiority of bengal rose or a mixture of bengal rose and fluorescein in the diagnosis of conjunctival and corneal exfoliation in keratoconjunctivitis should be emphasized.

Dr. Kearns described the wide variation of clinical signs observed in acute necrotizing arteritis and the importance of obtaining sedimentation rates in our patients who have obscure disorders, particularly those involving headache and reduced vision. It is easy to be misled inasmuch as these patients typically do not complain of severe sympoms, and we may believe that they are not seriously ill. In two recent patients, a necrotizing giant cell arteritis was not diagnosed because they were in the immediate postoperative period of cataract extraction and their diminution of vision led to inappropriate studies for macular edema and complications of the cataract surgery.

Reiter's disease provides an area in which there will be much useful study in the next several years. It presents a curious combination of infection combined with an altered immune response and suggests an unusual disease mechanism. The possibility of a *Chlamydia* infection seems remote inasmuch as, if this were the causative organism, it would have been discovered by now or basophilic inclusion bodies would have been found. Mycoplasma disorders are currently tempting. In one patient, Reiter's disease appeared to be venereal, and since then we have studied both marital partners in those patients with recurrent Reiter's disease.

The description of patients with systemic lupus erythematosus or dermatomyositis indicated the occurrence of cotton-wool patches in youthful patients who do not have vascular hypertension. The remarkable number of these cotton-wool deposits seen in these disorders is impressive, and there are no other abnormalities that cause so many. It is tempting to speculate why the youthful retina is more vulnerable to such patches than is the older retina.

Dr. McLaren and Dr. Halasa presented a most scholarly discussion of vitamin A deficiency and the triad of night blindness, xerophthalmia, and keratomalacia. The hospitality and meals have been so generous at this meeting that it is easy to forget that 5 or 10 cents per person could provide enough vitamin A to prevent the deficiency. In the Middle East, of course, the vitamin A deficiency is associated with a low protein intake and may be combined with kwashiorkor. In the United States, vitamin A deficiency is associated mainly with poor absorption of the vitamin from the gastrointestinal tract and occurs with systemic disorders. Public health education is poor in many countries in which vitamin A deficiency is a problem. Infants go blind surrounded by green vegetables that contain enough vegetable carotene to prevent the disease. They drink milk from which the cream has been skimmed, which removes vitamin A. Breast feeding, too, is unpopular. Combined with this is the deficiency of β-lactase in black individuals, which causes them to dislike milk as a staple of diet. It is evident that on the world scene, not only public health education is required, but also some type of vitamin A that can be administered with ease, absorbed by children who have poor nutrition, and preferably stored in the body for a long period without toxicity.

The discussion of pernicious anemia and its relationship to tobacco amblyopia emphasized the difference of opinion concerning the role of cyanates in metabolism in Great Britain and this country. We rarely make a diagnosis of tobacco amblyopia in the United States and additionally see little pernicious anemia. The current status of the disagreement has been neatly summarized by Potts[4] in a review that is followed by an able defense of the role of cyanide.

Last evening Dr. McLaren impressed me with the importance he placed upon the role of obesity control in nutrition. He emphasized a low-cholesterol diet, exercise, not smoking, and slimness to prevent coronary artery disease. Stamler in Chicago has emphasized this, and I believe that many feel that overnutrition is a far more serious problem in the United States than vitamin deficiency. This is emphasized by the current Cecil and Loeb *Textbook of Medicine,* in which atherosclerosis is indexed under obesity and not under atherosclerosis.

Professor Solomon emphasized the triad of thyroid hyperplasia, infiltrative ophthalmopathy, and infiltrative dermatopathy. The classification of ocular signs of hyperthyroidism was published in both major United States ophthalmic journals but has not been adopted widely by ophthalmologists. Some find the classification an oversimplification. Thus a vision decrease may reflect an optic neuropathy, or an exposure keratitis, or may be an abnormality unrelated to thyroid disease. Each ophthalmologist must be interested in the relationship of Graves' disease to autoimmune disorders. I was impressed that we had come the full circle in considering thyroid signs as being related to an imbalance in the pituitary hormone and the thyroid hormone. The compressibility of the orbit provides a useful prognostic sign in thyroid disease. Many of the ocular signs of hyperthyroidism may spontaneously disappear if the proptosis is compressible, whereas, if it is not compressible, spontaneous improvement is unlikely.

The large number of individuals pleased with Ogura's technique is most impressive. The good results seem to occur because of the usual course we observe in a blowout fracture of the orbit: the orbital contents settle into the maxilla, the eye recedes, and the upper lid droops. Thus the changes we dread so much in blowout fractures are quite desirable in the management of proptosis.

Dr. David Knox's recommendation to use a suction cup to move the eye to differentiate between paralysis of an ocular muscle and contracture of its direct antagonist is excellent.

Professor Dardenne designed an exquisite experiment to study a topic that was carefully reviewed previously. His demonstration of a difference in amino acid content in exophthalmos-producing substance and in the thyroid-stimulating hormone appears important. Certainly his standardization of study by use of small fish of uniform size, the use of plasma mixed with dye to make certain that the substance is retained after injection, and the use of the profile projector to study proptosis are all necessary quantifications in a difficult area. I look forward with considerable interest to further studies.

Patients who develop some of the ocular signs of thyroid disease in the absence of either hyperthyroidism or a history of previous thyroid abnormality present a particular problem. I believe that recent development of sensitive measurements of the two principal thyroid hormones, thyroxin (T_4) and triiodothyronine (T_3), provides us with diagnostic information previously available only indirectly. Bioassay of the *long-acting thyroid stimulator* (LATS) may be valuable in patients who do not have thyrotoxicosis but have other manifestations of Graves' syndrome, such as ophthalmopathy or pretibial myxedema. Werner's triiodothyronine suppression test may be of unusual value.

Some of the most severe instances of thyroid ophthalmopathy occur in patients who have not had hyperthyroidism but have been treated with uracil salts. These cases are reminiscent of those seen nearly 50 years ago that involved thyroidectomy in the absence of hyperthyroidism and developed malignant exophthalmos. We should keep in mind the value of von Graefe's lid lag in the diagnosis of thyroid abnormalities. Additionally, I do not recall observing spontaneous contracture of the vertically acting ocular muscles in any disorder other than thyroid ophthalmopathy.

Dr. Ditzel provided us with much brilliant original material. He has an intriguing explanation that diabetic retinopathy arises from the increased affinity of hemoglobin for oxygen so that it is not released to tissues and thus retinal anoxia occurs. His demonstration of the balance existing between organic phosphates and 2-diphosphoglycerate erythrocytes provides an inexpensive prophylactic treatment.

Possibly the calcium would additionally assist in combating osteoporosis and it might well be used empirically. (AFTERTHOUGHT: Overdosage of calcium phosphate or administration of excess phosphate in the presence of renal disease may lead to ectopic calcification. The use of calcium phosphate must be carefully supervised, and it is by no means a completely innocuous medication.)

Dr. Henkind delivered a classic description of the variety of changes in diabetes. I concur in his views concerning the value of fluorescein angiography in the diagnosis of diabetic retinopathy. Further, I believe that photocoagulation is indicated in every patient with neovascularization. His emphasis on the use of specular reflection to detect Descemet's membranal wrinkling in diabetics is interesting, and once again I will employ it carefully. His emphasis on increased incidence of ectropion uveas is also worthy of systematic study.

The association of capillary nonperfusion with retinal edema residues is significant as is macular edema causing loss of vision in diabetics. The occurrence of cotton-wool deposits in diabetes mellitus in the absence of hypertension has been emphasized only recently.

The hypothesis that fluid vitreous in myopia of more than 5 diopters prevents proliferative retinopathy because there is no vitreous support for neovascularization is challenging. It suggests measures to assure a fluid vitreous in patients with diabetic retinopathy. Ischemic optic neuropathy in diabetics does not seem to be a major problem. Indeed, there seems to be an adequate blood supply to the optic nerve in many small blood vessel disorders.

The lectures of Professors Kirkendall and Cogan complemented each other. Present-day ophthalmologists classify the fundus appearance of vascular hypertension much less frequently than was done a generation ago. Possibly this arises because of the difficulty in distinguishing the localized changes of involutionary sclerosis in the aged from the generalized changes of arteriolosclerosis and the associated vascular hypertension. There is seldom a problem in diagnosing vascular hypertension when attenuated arterioles occur with cotton-wool patches, hemorrhage, and sometimes papilledema. However, in less severe involvement the changes are more subtle. Thus, Michaelson[1] found that ophthalmologists interpreting fundus photographs of patients with hypertension had an extremely large number of errors, even by the same examiner when grading a picture the second time.

Arteriolosclerosis is the anatomic reflection of a prolonged significant increase in blood pressure that results in thickening of the walls and narrowing of the lumen of arterioles in response to the vascular hypertension. The vascular involvement is generalized; thus all arterioles throughout the body are affected to a similar degree.

Two types of changes may occur in arteriosclerosis: (1) Replacement fibrosis may develop when patients who have a slowly progressive, moderately severe hypertension associated chiefly with elevation of the systolic blood pressure in the range of 170 to 200 mm. Hg, with a diastolic pressure usually less than 100 mm. Hg. There is increased collagen and elastic tissue in all layers of the blood vessel wall. (2) Hyperplastic thickening in fibrinoid necrosis occurs as an acute severe reaction to sudden pronounced elevation of the blood pressure in which the systolic blood pressure exceeds 200 mm. Hg and the diastolic blood pressure exceeds 120 mm. Hg. Hyperplastic thickening and fibrinoid necrosis occur only in vessels containing muscle fibers. Vessels that are the site of previous involutionary sclerosis or replacement fibrosis are not involved in fibrinoid necrosis. These changes protect the arterioles from the effects of severe vascular hypertension and explain the infrequency with which hyperplastic thickening and fibrinoid necrosis are seen in elderly patients with pronounced elevated blood pressures.

It is important to recognize that the Keith-Wagener-Barker[2] classification relates solely to the grouping of retinal changes associated with hypertension. It loses its prognostic and diagnostic value when applied to involutionary sclerosis or arteriosclerosis. Inasmuch as hypertension causes generalized diffuse arteriolar changes, one should not use the classification to systematize focal changes or those secondary to retinal inflammation with venous stasis. Both eyes should have a similar degree of change; involvement of one eye only suggests impaired internal carotid artery circulation on the side of the normal eye or sometimes monocular glaucoma.

I sense a curious division of labor here. Professor Kirkendall urges that ophthalmologists direct more attention to the subtle vascular changes occurring in early vascular hypertension. Conversely, I believe that ophthalmologists might derive more information by measurement of the blood pressure on the occasion of an ocular examination.

David Cogan presented an unusually diverse collection of examples of occlusive disease of the retina. I thought that his patients could be classed fairly well as showing necrotizing arteritis, calcific lipid, platelet, fibrous, myxomatous, and bacterial emboli. Most important is to recognize the emboli of atrial myxoma inasmuch as this lesion is amenable to surgery.

The most important point concerning central vein closure is close observation of the second eye and treatment if necessary. Moreover, we need much more information concerning decompression of the optic nerve by opening of its meningeal sheaths.

The discussion of Dr. Brain and Dr. Luxenburg presented a comprehensive consideration of the various defects of the blood and its contents. Abnormalities arising from erythrocytes, leukocytes, and platelets in terms of shape, size, number, oxygen affinity, electrical charge, solubility, and life-span provided a useful method for considering the major hemoglobinopathies and anemias. I look forward to seeing Dr. Luxenburg's classification enjoy widespread usage and was impressed with his emphasis on the appearance of dilated tortuous vessels in the ocular fundus and their occurrence in abnormalities of the plasma proteins, leukemias, polycythemia, hemoglobinopathies, and diabetes mellitus. I believe that his recommendations concerning the H factor in the treatment of hemophilia are of unusual importance to every ophthalmologist who does cataract surgery or other surgery in patients with hemophilia.

Dr. Knox has been unusually helpful to each of us in emphasizing the importance of Crohn's disease and Whipple's disease to the ophthalmologist. We are all familiar with the possibility of uveitis occurring in the course of Crohn's disease and, inasmuch as this appears to be an autoimmune disorder, are not particularly surprised that it occurs. There is much more to learn concerning the unusual vitreous observed in Whipple's disease, and this may be a key to understanding this abnormality.

Professor Perry presented an excellent classification of the dermatologic diseases with ocular findings. He indicated the important role the ophthalmologist has in preventing dermatitis venenata. We probably all regret that the dictates of time prevented a greater discussion of the hemangiomas about the eye inasmuch as these are difficult to manage.

Professor Bietti presented a most comprehensive study of ocular diseases and once again demonstrated his encyclopedic knowledge of these conditions.

The presentation of the past 3 days indicates the wide spectrum of disease that may affect the eye. This meeting has indicated the possibilities of unusually useful collaboration between the ophthalmologist, internist, dermatologist, hematologist, rheumatologist, and other specialists. We will all leave this meeting better physicians than before, and I join you in thanking our hosts for making it possible.

REFERENCES

1. Ballantyne, A. J., and Michaelson, I. C.: Textbook of the fundus of the eye, ed. 2, Baltimore, 1970, The Williams & Wilkins Co.
2. Keith, N. M., Wagener, H. P., and Barker, N. W.: Some different types of essential hypertension: their course and prognosis, Am. J. Med. Sci. **197:**332, 1939.
3. O'Brien, J. S., Okada, S., Chen, A., and Fillerup, D.: Tay-Sachs disease. Detection of heterozygotes and homozygotes by serum hexosaminidase assay, New Eng. J. Med. **283:**15, 1970.
4. Potts, A. M.: Tobacco amblyopia, Survey Ophthalmol. **17:**313, 1973.
5. Vail, D. T.: The rise and fall of EENT, Trans. Am. Acad. Ophthalmol. Otolaryngol. **74:**11, 1970.

Index

A

Abetalipoproteinemia, 15, 16, 37-39, 137
Acantholysis, 301, 303, 342
N-Acetyl-α-D-glucosaminidase deficiency, 28, 47
Acid hydrolase deficiency, 18
Acne rosacea, 298-299, 354-356
Acrodermatitis enteropathica, 16
Acrosclerosis, 95
Addison's disease, 6, 156
Adrenal cortex, 156
Adrenal medulla, 156
Albinism, 11, 14, 50-52, 425
Alcohol amblyopia, 132, 147, 152, 153-154
Aldose reductase, 72
Aliments, 124
Alkaptonuria, 6, 14, 52
Allelism, 19
Allergic dermatitis, 294-296
Allergic granulomatous angiitis, 99
Allergy, food, 287-288
Alopecia, 341, 382
Amaurosis fugax, 115, 224, 225, 246
Amaurotic idiocy, 23, 39, 44
Amblyopia, 132-133
    alcohol, 132, 147, 152, 153-154
    nutritional, 136, 147, 153-154
    tobacco, 147, 148, 152, 153-154, 428
Amebiasis, 279, 289
American Ophthalmological Society, 424
Amino acid metabolism disorders, 12, 49-61, 425
    eye signs, 13, 14, 49-50, 61
Aminoaciduria, 14
    primary, 52-56
    secondary, 56-61
Amniocentesis, 20, 73-74
Amyloidosis, in rheumatoid arthritis, 83
Anemia, 243, 258-259
    pernicious, 132, 133, 148, 428
    spherocytic hemolytic, 244

Anetodermia erythematosa, 390
Angiitis
    allergic granulomatous, 99
    hypersensitivity, 100
Angiohemophilia, 259
Angioid streak, 366
    in Ehlers-Danlos syndrome, 386
    in pseudoxanthoma elasticum, 5, 311, 365
    in sickle-cell disease, 273
Angiokeratoma corporis diffusum, 23, 390
Angiomatosis
    meningo-oculofacial, 378
    of retina and cerebellum, 379
Angiopathy, congenital dysplastic, 6
Anhidrotic ectodermal dysplasia, 314-315, 367-368
Ankylosing spondylitis, 86-87
    clinical findings, 86
    laboratory findings, 86-87
    ocular involvement, 109-110
    treatment, 87
Anterior pituitary tumor, 156
Anterior segment
    in vitamin A deficiency, 137-140
    in vitamin B–complex deficiency, 146
Antibodies; see specific classes
Anticoagulation therapy, 246
    in retinal vein occlusion, 236-237, 238
Anticollagenase, 151
Antideoxyribonucleic acid antibodies, in lupus erythematosus (systemic), 90, 93
Antimalarial therapy
    in lupus erythematosus (systemic), 93
    ophthalmologic evaluation and, 83
    in psoriatic arthritis, 88
    in rheumatoid arthritis, 83
Antimetabolites, in psoriatic arthritis, 88
Antinuclear antibodies
    in juvenile rheumatoid arthritis, 86
    in lupus erythematosus (systemic), 90, 93
    in progressive systemic sclerosis, 96

433

Psoriatic arthritis, 87-88
  clinical findings, 87-88
  laboratory findings, 88
  ocular involvement, 110
  treatment, 88
"Pulseless disease," 101
Pyogenics, 370
Pyridoxine, 71

R

Radiography
  in ankylosing spondylitis, 87
  in juvenile rheumatoid arthritis, 86
  in progressive systemic sclerosis, 96
  in psoriatic arthritis, 88
  in rheumatoid arthritis, 83
Radiotherapy
  in Graves' disease, 165-166
  of orbit, 177
Raynaud's phenomena, 82, 97
Recklinghausen's disease, von; *see* Neurofi-
    bromatosis
Red blood cells; *see* Erythrocytes
Refractive error
  in diabetes mellitus, 199
  malnutrition and, 146, 152-153
Refsum's disease, 13, 35-36, 369
Reiter's syndrome, 88-90, 289, 331-332, 372-
    373, 427-428
  clinical findings, 89
  laboratory findings, 89-90
  ocular involvement, 110
  treatment, 90
Renal biopsy, in lupus erythematosus (sys-
    temic), 93
Renal transplantation, in Fabry's disease, 20,
    42
Rendu-Osler-Weber syndrome, 335-336, 379
Research, 423-432
Reticuloendothelial disease, 242-249, 260-261
  ocular manifestations, 250-265, 266-273
Reticulum cell sarcoma, 254, 266-267, 270-
    272
Retina; *see also* Macula; Optic disk; Optic
    nerve
  in abetalipoproteinemia, 15
  in albinism, 50-51, 52
  in anemia, 243, 258-259
  in Bassen-Kornzweig syndrome, 37-39
  in Behçet's disease, 414, 420
  in coagulation disorders, 259
  in Crohn's disease, 275-276, 288
  in cystinosis, 14, 57
  in dermatomyositis, 114
  in Fabry's disease, 23, 42
  in Farber's disease, 25, 40

Retina—cont'd
  in gargoylism, 426
  in GM₁ gangliosidosis, 45
  in GM₂ gangliosidosis, 23
  in hereditary hemorrhagic telangiectasia, 7
  in hereditary metabolic disorders, 10, 11,
    60-61
  in Hodgkin's disease, 254
  in homocystinuria, 53-54
  in Hooft's syndrome, 39
  in Hunter's syndrome, 28, 47
  in Hurler's syndrome, 46
  in hyperlipoproteinemia, 36-37
  in hypertension, 221-222, 430, 431
  in hyperviscosity syndrome, 250, 251
  in hypophosphatasia, 56
  in ichthyosis, 317
  in immunoglobin disorders, 245
  intestinal parasites and, 279
  in leukemia, 244, 245, 254, 268
  in lipidoses, 11
  in lupus erythematosus (systemic), 110-
    112, 120
  in Marfan's syndrome, 384
  in Maroteaux-Lamy syndrome, 47-48
  in Menkes' disease, 61
  in neurofibromatosis, 376
  in Niemann-Pick disease, 40
  platelet emboli and, 267
  in polycythemia, 243-244, 256
  in pseudoxanthoma elasticum, 311, 365-366
  in Refsum's disease, 13, 35
  in Rendu-Osler-Weber syndrome, 336
  in Sanfilippo syndrome, 47
  in Scheie's syndrome, 47
  in scleroderma, 113, 114
  in sclerosis tuberosa, 377-378
  in sickle-cell disease, 14, 244, 257-258, 267
  in Tay-Sachs disease, 44
  in temporal (cranial) arteritis, 115-116
  in thrombocytopenia, 246
  in tuberous sclerosis, 327
  in vitamin A deficiency, 136, 137, 141,
    143-144, 145-146
  in Vogt-Koyanagi-Harada syndrome, 382
  in von Hippel–Lindau disease, 379
  in Waardenburg syndrome, 52
  in Whipple's disease, 286
Retinal, 141-144
Retinal arterioles, in hypertension, 213-214
Retinal artery; *see* Central retinal artery
Retinal capillaries, 231
Retinal capillary obstruction, 231-233
Retinal exudates
  in diabetic retinopathy, 201-202
  in hypertension, 214-216